CLINICAL TRIALS OF DRUGS AND BIOPHARMACEUTICALS

CLINICAL TRIALS OF DRUGS AND BIOPHARMACEUTICALS

Chi-Jen Lee
Lucia H. Lee
Christopher L. Wu
Benjamin R. Lee
Mei-Ling Chen

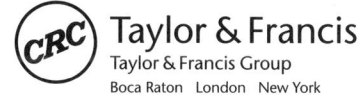

Taylor & Francis
Taylor & Francis Group
Boca Raton London New York

A CRC title, part of the Taylor & Francis imprint, a member of the
Taylor & Francis Group, the academic division of T&F Informa plc.

FIRST INDIAN REPRINT, 2011

Published in 2006 by
CRC Press
Taylor & Francis Group
6000 Broken Sound Parkway NW, Suite 300
Boca Raton, FL 33487-2742

Printed and bound in India by Replika Press Pvt. Ltd.

International Standard Book Number-10: 0-8493-2185-9 (Hardcover)
International Standard Book Number-13: 978-0-8493-2185-6 (Hardcover)
Library of Congress Card Number 2005043902

Library of Congress Cataloging-in-Publication Data

Clinical trials of drugs and biopharmaceuticals / edited by Chi-Jen Lee ... [et al.].
    p. ; cm.
    Rev. ed. of: Handbook of phase I/II clinical drug trials. 1997.
  Includes bibliographical references and index.
  ISBN 0-8493-2185-9 (alk. paper)
  1. Drugs--Testing. 2. Clinical trials. I. Lee, Chi-Jen. II. Handbook of phase I/II clinical drug trials.
  [DNLM: 1. Drug Evaluation--methods. 2. Clinical Trials, Phase I--methods. 3. Clinical Trials, Phase II--methods. 4. Clinical Trials, Phase III--methods. 5. Clinical Trials, Phase IV--methods. QV 771 C6419 2005]

RM301.27.E37 2005
615'.704'0287--dc22   2005043902

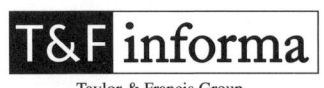

Preface

This book is a revised edition of the *Handbook of Phase I/II Clinical Drug Trials*, which was published in 1996. A number of the former authors have moved on to other interests and have transferred their tasks to a new generation of authors. Our challenge as editors is to introduce fresh ideas and alternative perspectives for a rapidly evolving field. Much of the previous content has been consolidated and reorganized into a practical format for use by pharmaceutical and biopharmaceutical companies, university scientists, ministries of health, and health authorities. Several chapters have been revised and new chapters added to highlight critical chemical and biological considerations for drug development and all phases of clinical trials (I through IV). The new edition also provides information pertaining to early preclinical evaluations, which have become an important transitional step before proceeding with initiation of human trials. Likewise, assessments of pharmacological activities for many drugs in clinical trials are discussed.

With advances in modern pharmaceutical sciences, the processes of discovery and development of new therapeutic drugs have changed dramatically, and, in turn, resulted in an extraordinary improvement in potential prophylactic and therapeutic interventions. Cooperative efforts among academic institutes, government agencies, and the pharmaceutical industry have helped to facilitate these advances. The predicted benefits for disease treatment and prevention will result from a better understanding of disease pathogenesis and expanded knowledge of immune mechanisms, the molecular structures of drugs and biologics, and biotechnology. At present, many new classes of vaccines are being developed to prevent infection and to treat cancers and chronic diseases.

Drug therapy is becoming more complicated due not only to the sheer number of new drugs available but also to the broad armamentarium of therapeutic options available for individual complex diseases. Complex drug regimens increase the potential for drug interactions to occur; thus, it is even more critical for biomedical scientists to understand the mechanisms of pharmacokinetic and pharmacodynamic activity and processes of drug evaluation within the context of preventing clinically undesirable adverse reactions.

Finally, *Clinical Trials of Drugs and Biopharmaceuticals* provides an overview of the current procedures and major issues involved in the clinical aspects of drug and biopharmaceutical development. This textbook provides both a conceptual approach and specific information about each phase of clinical development prior to licensure. It also describes the design of postmarketing studies. This new edition examines how recent advances in pharmaceutical sciences and increased demand for safer and more effective drugs have changed the processes in which drugs are developed and approved.

Acknowledgments

The authors thank colleagues and friends, including Dr. Joan C. May and Dr. Richard Walker, Center for Biologics Evaluation and Research, U.S. Food and Drug Administration; Dr. Dong-Sheng Chen, formerly of the Center for Drug Evaluation and Research, U.S. Food and Drug Administration; and Dr. Yi-Jiun Huang and Dr. Hui-Po Wang, Bureau of Pharmaceutical Affairs, Department of Health, Taiwan, for their review of the manuscripts, comments, and constructive suggestions. The content of this book is the authors' own and does not represent the position and opinion of the institutes they serve.

The Editors

Chi-Jen Lee, Sc.D., is Supervisory Research Chemist, Center for Biologics Evaluation and Research, U.S. Food and Drug Administration, Bethesda, Maryland. He has served as chief of the Polysaccharide and Conjugate Vaccine Quality Control section since 1974. Dr. Lee graduated in 1957 from National Taiwan University, College of Medicine, School of Pharmacy, with a B.S. in Pharmacy. He obtained his Sc.D. in Biochemistry in 1966 from the Johns Hopkins University, Bloomberg School of Public Health, Department of Biochemistry. He served as an Assistant Professor at the Rockefeller University in New York from 1968 to 1973. He was a Visiting Professor at the National Cheng Kung University, College of Medicine, Taiwan, in 1984. He was given the Honorary Professor Award in 2000 by Inner Mongolia Medical College, China; the Congress Award at the Fifth International Congress on Natural Medicine, Shengyang, China, in 2004; and the Distinguished Service Award, National Taiwan University, School of Pharmacy Alumni Association–North America in 2003. He has received several FDA Awards of Merit and FDA Commendable Service Awards. Dr. Lee is the author of *Development and Evaluation of Drugs: From Laboratory Through Licensure to Market* (1993, CRC Press; second edition, 2003) and *Managing Biotechnology in Drug Development* (1996, CRC Press); coauthor of *Polysaccharides in Medicine and Biotechnology* (1996, Marcel Dekker); and editor of *Professional Frontiers in 21st Century* (2002, Chinese–American Professionals Association). He has published more than 150 research papers and abstracts. He has served as a thesis director for doctoral candidates in the Department of Microbiology, The George Washington University Medical Center, Washington D.C., and as President of the Chinese–American Professionals Association of Greater Washington.

Lucia H. Lee, M.D., is currently a medical officer at the Center for Biologics Evaluation and Research, U.S. Food and Drug Administration, Bethesda, Maryland. Dr. Lee received her medical degree at the University of Rochester School of Medicine. She completed her pediatric training at The Johns Hopkins Hospital and then returned to Rochester, New York, for her pediatric infectious diseases fellowship. There, she worked to clone and characterize the cDNA encoding a kexin-like protease in mouse *Pneumocystis carinii* that was also found to be cross-reactive with human *P. carinii*. Dr. Lee's research has been recognized by awards from the Pediatric Infectious Diseases Society and Eli Lilly and Company. Dr. Lee has extensive training and experience in clinical trial design. Prior to coming to the FDA, Dr. Lee served in several capacities as a coinvestigator and research coordinator for studies conducted in collaboration with the NICHD Pediatric AIDS Clinical Trials Unit and Vaccine Trial Evaluation Unit at the University of Rochester. At the FDA, she is involved in the design of vaccine clinical trials conducted in the United States, Europe, Africa, South America, and Australia. She serves on committees on both a national and international level. Dr. Lee is also a fellow of the American Academy of Pediatrics and a member of the Pediatric Infectious Disease Society.

Christopher L. Wu, M.D., is Associate Professor, Department of Anesthesiology/CCM, Division of Pain Medicine, Division of Obstetric Anesthesia, The Johns Hopkins University, Baltimore, Maryland. Dr. Wu received his M.D. degree from Albany Medical College in New York in 1989. He then completed his residency training at The University of Rochester Medical Center and served as Assistant Professor in the Department of Anesthesiology at Rochester Medical Center from 1994 to 1999 and at The Johns Hopkins University from 1999 to 2001. He is certified by the American Board of Anesthesiology. He has received many honors and awards from the University of Rochester, Department of Anesthesiology, and was named Teacher of the Year twice by The Johns Hopkins University, Department of Anesthesiology and Critical Care Medicine. He is a member of editorial boards of *Anesthesiology, Faculty of 1000 Medicine, Regional Anesthesia, Pain Medicine*, and other medical journals. Dr. Wu has served as a reviewer for several journals, including

American Journal of Anesthesiology, *Anesthesia & Analgesia*, *Anesthesiology*, and more than 10 other medical journals. He is also a member of the American Society of Anesthesiology Committee on Regional Anesthesia, American Society of Regional Anesthesia, New York State Society of Anesthesiologists, and three other professional societies. Dr. Wu has published numerous original peer-reviewed research papers, reviews, and abstracts in the areas of anesthesiology and critical care medicine, more than 8 articles in book chapters, and 16 editorials and letters in medical journals. He has presented over 45 invited lectures at international and national meetings, universities, and medical societies. He has been invited to serve as session chair for medical professional meetings in regional anesthesis, evidence-based medicine, and developments in pain management, among others.

Benjamin R. Lee, M.D., is Director, Laparoscopy Section in the Department of Urology at Long Island Jewish Medical Center, New Hyde Park, New York, and Associate Professor of Urology, Albert Einstein College of Medicine. After graduating *magna cum laude* from the College of Arts and Sciences, Cornell University, in 1990, Dr. Lee received his M.D. degree from The Johns Hopkins School of Medicine in 1994. He then completed his residency training at the Brady Urological Institute at Johns Hopkins in 2000 under Dr. Patrick C. Walsh. Dr. Lee is the author or coauthor of more than 70 scientific papers, 100 abstracts, and 15 videos. His research has been recognized by many awards and honors from the American Urological Association, the Endourological Society, *Urology Journal*, and other organizations. He is currently section editor of the "Techniques in Endourology and Video CD-ROM" section of the *Journal of Endourology* and has been elected to the New York Academy of Medicine. He is certified under the American Board of Urology. Dr. Lee serves as a reviewer for several journals, including *Urology*, *Journal of Urology*, and *Journal of Endourology*. He served as Visiting Professor, Department of Urology, at University of Patras, Greece, in 2002, and at Singapore General Hospital, Singapore, in 2004. He has presented over 100 invited lectures at international and national meetings, universities, and research institutes. Dr. Lee is an academic urologist whose practice is dedicated to the treatment of urologic disease in a minimally invasive fashion. He has extensive experience with minimally invasive approaches to treat renal masses, prostate cancer, kidney disease, stricture disease, kidney stones, and benign prostate hyperplasia. At Long Island Jewish Medical Center, his practice focuses on urologic laparoscopy techniques, the physiology of laparoscopy, and other minimally invasive techniques.

Mei-Ling Chen, Ph.D., is Associate Director, Office of Pharmaceutical Science, Center for Drug Evaluation and Research, U.S. Food and Drug Administration, Bethesda, Maryland. Dr. Chen received her B.S. in Pharmacy from the National Taiwan University and Ph.D. in Pharmacokinetics and Biopharmaceutics from the University of Illinois at Chicago. Following her postdoctoral training, she joined the FDA in 1984 and became a Regulatory Expert in 1990. She was subsequently promoted to Chief of Pharmacokinetics Evaluation Branch, Division of Biopharmaceutics, and then Director, Division of Pharmaceutical Evaluation II, Office of Clinical Pharmacology and Biopharmaceutics. In 2000, Dr. Chen advanced to her current position, providing guidance in scientific direction and regulatory policy in the Office of Pharmaceutical Science. During her tenure in the FDA, Dr. Chen has served as the Topic Lead of the Biopharmaceutics Coordinating Committee in CDER, and cochaired the Complex Drug Substances Coordinating Committee in the FDA. She has also been appointed as chairperson or cochairperson of several working groups on important scientific issues in the agency. She has been instrumental in the development of many guidance and policy documents for pharmaceutical industry and FDA reviewers on bioavailability and bioequivalence. Dr. Chen has received numerous merit awards for the FDA. She is on the U.S. Pharmacopoeia Expert Committee of Bioavailability and Nutrient Absorption, as well as on the Expert Panel for Active Complexes. As a regulatory and scientific expert, Dr. Chen has been frequently requested as a speaker or moderator at national and international meetings. Dr. Chen has published numerous review articles, research papers, and abstracts in the area of clinical pharmacology and biopharmaceutics. She is the author of several book chapters and currently on the editorial board of *Clinical Pharmacokinetics*. She has been invited as a referee for several prestigious journals, including *Clinical Pharmacology and Therapeutics, Clinical Pharmacokinetics, European Journal of Pharmaceutical Sciences, Journal of Pharmaceutical Sciences, Pharmaceutical Research, Journal of Pharmacokinetics and Pharmacodynamics,* and *Pharmacogenetics.* Dr. Chen has been Fellow of the American Association of Pharmaceutical Scientist since 2001.

Contributors

Yasir Al-Rawi, M.B.Ch.B.
PAION Deutschland GmbH
Aachen, Germany

Renzo Canetta, M.D.
Vice President
Clinical Oncology Research
Bristol-Myers-Squibb
Wallingford, Connecticut

Mei-Ling Chen, Ph.D.
Associate Director
Office of Pharmaceutical Science
Center for Drug Evaluation and Research
U.S. Food and Drug Administration
Bethesda, Maryland

Peter I. Folb, M.D., FRCP, FRS (SAF)
Chief Specialist Scientist
Medical Research Council of South Africa
Cape Town, South Africa

Muzlifah A. Haniffa, M.B.Ch.B., MRCP
Specialist Registrar in Dermatology
Royal Victoria Infirmary
Newcastle upon Tyne, United Kingdom

Mark Hovde, M.B.A.
Vice President, Business Development
Fast Track
Kennett Square, Pennsylvania

Robert W. Hurley, M.D., Ph.D.
Resident in Anesthesiology
The Johns Hopkins University
Baltimore, Maryland

Christiane Langer, M.D.
Associate Director
Clinical Oncology Research
Bristol-Myers-Squibb
Wallingford, Connecticut

Clifford M. Lawrence, M.D., FRCP
Consultant Dermatologist
Royal Victoria Infirmary
Newcastle upon Tyne, United Kingdom

Benjamin R. Lee, M.D.
Director, Laparoscopy Section
Department of Urology
Long Island Jewish Medical Center
New Hyde Park, New York
and
Associate Professor of Urology
Albert Einstein College of Medicine
Bronx, New York

Chi-Jen Lee, Sc.D.
Supervisory Research Chemist
Center for Biologics Evaluation and Research
U.S. Food and Drug Administration
Bethesda, Maryland

Lucia H. Lee, M.D.
Medical Officer
Center for Biologics Evaluation and Research
U.S. Food and Drug Administration
Bethesda, Maryland

Suzy N. Leech, M.B.Ch.B., MRCP
Post CCST Clinical Fellow
Royal Victoria Infirmary
Newcastle upon Tyne, United Kingdom

Robert E. Martell, M.D., Ph.D.
Vice President, Chief Medical Officer
MethylGene, Inc.
Montreal, Quebec, Canada

Joseph Mattana, M.D.
Department of Medicine
Long Island Jewish Medical Center
New Hyde Park, New York
and
Albert Einstein College of Medicine
Bronx, New York

Graham R. McClelland, Ph.D.
Global Head, Clinical Pharmacology
  Operations
Roche Products, Ltd.
Welwyn Garden City
Hertfordshire, United Kingdom

Valeria Molnar, M.Sc.Pharm.
Director, Clinical Pharmacology Consulting
Torquay, United Kingdom

Georges Moroz, M.D.
Clinical Science Leader
Hoffmann–La Roche, Inc.
Nutley, New Jersey

Nancy C. Pauly, M.D.
Head, Cardiovascular and Thrombosis Unit,
  Investigational Drugs, Global
  Pharmacovigilance and Epidemiology
Sanofi-Aventis
Bridgewater, New Jersey

Paul E. Rolan, M.D., FRACP, FFPM
Professor of Clinical Pharmacology
Department of Clinical and Experimental
  Pharmacology
Medical School
University of Adelaide
Adelaide, Australia

Edmond Roland, M.D., FAHA
Cardiology Department
G. Pompidou European Hospital
Paris, France

Hitesh H. Shah, M.D.
Department of Medicine
Long Island Jewish Medical Center
New Hyde Park, New York
and
Albert Einstein College of Medicine
Bronx, New York

Pravin C. Singhal, M.D.
Department of Medicine
Long Island Jewish Medical Center
New Hyde Park, New York
and
Albert Einstein College of Medicine
Bronx, New York

Mariola Soehgren, M.D.
PAION AG
Aachen, Germany

Wolfgang Soehgen, M.D.
PAION AG
Aachen, Germany

Joseph W. Stauffer, M.D.
Vice President of Medical Affairs
Alpharma Incorporated
Fort Lee, New Jersey

Shri C. Valvani, Ph.D.
Pharmaceutical Consultant
Former Director, Pharmaceutics and Drug
  Delivery Systems Research
Pharmacia & Upjohn Company
Kalamazoo, Michigan

Anton B. Alexandroff Vrach, Ph.D., MRCP
Specialist Registrar in Dermatology
Royal Victoria Infirmary
Newcastle upon Tyne, United Kingdom

**W. Stephen Waring, B.Med.Sci., MRCP,
  Ph.D.**
Consultant Physician and Honorary Senior
  Lecturer
Scottish Poisons Information Bureau
Royal Infirmary of Edinburgh
Edinburgh, Scotland

**David J. Webb, M.D., D.Sc., FRCP, FRSE,
  F.Med.Sci.**
Professor of Therapeutics and Clinical
  Pharmacology and Consultant Physician
Clinical Research Centre
University of Edinburgh
Western General Hospital
Edinburgh, Scotland

Christopher L. Wu, M.D.
Associate Professor
Department of Anesthesiology/CCM
Division of Pain Medicine, Division of
  Obstetric Anesthesia
The Johns Hopkins University
Baltimore, Maryland

Contents

PART I

Preparation for Clinical Trials

A clinical trial is a research study in human volunteers to determine whether experimental treatments are safe and effective under controlled conditions and whether they should be approved for wider use in the general population. Potential treatments must be studied first in laboratory animals to examine potential toxicity before they can be tried in humans. Treatments having acceptable safety profiles and promising pharmacological activity are then moved into clinical trials.

Clinical trials are the most critical steps in the process of drug development and evaluation. Among hundreds and thousands of isolated or synthesized chemicals, many compounds that look interesting in preclinical studies do not make it to clinical trials. They may lack specific pharmacological activity, are highly toxic, are difficult to produce on a large scale, or are of limited usefulness due to the high cost of development. Chemicals and biologics that do show promise in preclinical studies face extensive, strict, and thorough clinical trials in healthy volunteers and in high-risk populations. Usually only 1 of every 20 compounds tested in clinical trials will be found sufficiently safe and effective to receive FDA approval for marketing.

Regulatory agencies make great efforts to protect the participants of clinical trials. Some risk, however, may be unavoidable because of the uncertainty factor in new medical products. Participating in a clinical trial has both benefits and risks. For example, eligible participants are able to:

- Play an active role in their own health care.
- Gain access to new treatments before they are widely available.
- Receive medical care at adequate healthcare facilities during the trial.
- Help others by contributing to medical knowledge.

Risks of participating include the following:

- The treatment may have unpleasant or serious side effects.
- The treatment may not be effective for the participant.
- The treatment may require extensive time and attention, including trips to the study site, hospital stays, and health examination.

In a 2000 Harris poll of cancer clinical trial participants, 76% of the respondents mentioned the reason they participated was that the trial offered the best quality of care for their disease. Other important reasons include helping other people and receiving more and better attention for their own specific diseases. Some treatments being studied can have unpleasant or even serious side effects; often these are temporary and disappear when the treatment is discontinued. Some side effects may appear during treatment or may not show up until later. All known risks should be explained to participants before the trial begins.

The informed consent provides an opportunity for the investigator and participant to exchange information and ask questions. Patients invited to enter a trial are not obliged to join but can consent to participate if they consider the potential risks and benefits acceptable. Participants also have the right to leave a trial at any time. At the same time, people need to realize that under certain risk circumstances their participation may be discontinued without their consent.

The various types of clinical trials include:

- Treatment trials, which test new treatments, new combinations of drugs, or new approaches to therapies
- Prevention trials, which search for more effective ways to prevent disease in new patient or prevent a disease from returning
- Diagnostic trials, which find better tests for diagnosing a particular disease
- Screening trials, which examine the best way to detect certain diseases
- Quality of life trials, which explore ways to improve comfort and the quality of life for patients with a chronic disease

Most use of investigational new drugs takes place in controlled clinical trials to assess the safety and efficacy of new drugs. Sometimes patients do not qualify for these conditions because of other health problems, age, or other factors. For patients who may benefit from the drug use but do not qualify for the trials, the experimental drugs may be provided by *expanded access* use of the drug. For example, a treatment investigational new drug (IND) provides for access to the new drug by patients with life-threatening or serious diseases for which no good alternative treatment exists. Another purpose for a treatment IND is to look for additional information about the drug, especially its safety. Some investigational drugs are available from pharmaceutical manufacturers through expanded access programs, which are generally managed by the manufacturers, with the investigational treatment being administered by investigators or physicians in practice.

In the past, most clinical trials for new drugs had been performed in Caucasian men. Groups such as women, African–Americans, Hispanics, and Asians often were not adequately represented. It is important to evaluate new drugs and biologics in a wide variety of people because they can work differently in people of different ages, races, ethnicity, and gender. Trial guidelines are developed to indicate inclusion or exclusion criteria — medical or social factors used to determine whether a person may or may not be allowed to enter a clinical trial. These criteria help to identify appropriate participants and exclude those who may be at risk or unsuitable.

Information on clinical trials can be obtained from the Food and Drug Administration (FDA) Office of Special Health Issues (301-827-4460). The ClinicalTrials.gov website also gives patients, family members, healthcare professionals, and members of the public access to information about a wide range of diseases and conditions. The site contains information on about 8200 clinical trials sponsored by the National Institutes of Health (NIH), other federal agencies, and the pharmaceutical industry in over 99,000 locations worldwide. It provides information about the purpose of a trial, eligible participants, locations, and phone numbers for more details.

CHAPTER 1

Drug Discovery and Preclinical Research

Chi-Jen Lee, Lucia H. Lee, Christopher L. Wu, and Benjamin R. Lee

CONTENTS

1.1   INTRODUCTION

The potential to prevent and treat disease has improved extraordinarily due to the discovery and development of new drugs and biopharmaceuticals. The pathogenesis of many disorders has become better understood as our knowledge of immune mechanisms, molecular structures of drugs and biologics, and biotechnology has expanded. Many new antibiotics to treat infections and therapeutics to treat cancers and chronic diseases have been developed over the past decades. Biotechnology provides effective methods for identifying new molecules for the pharmaceutical industry and facilitates the process of drug development. Preclinical research allows evaluation of the pharmacokinetics, pharmacodynamics, dose–response profiles, and toxicological potential of a drug. Preclinical studies also determine the optimal formulation and dose for phase I clinical trials, analyze physicochemical characteristics of the testing compound, and provide the rationale for the proposed therapeutic indication. The information gained from animal safety tests is used to predict and characterize potential adverse effects in humans. The new drug candidates also undergo analysis for physicochemical characterization, including identity, strength, purity, and stability.

A drug is a chemical agent used for treatment of disease. More broadly, a drug is defined as any chemical agent or biological product that affects life processes. Many drugs, including taxol, reserpine, and other alkaloids, are of plant origin. Drugs may also be isolated from animal or mineral sources or from microorganisms. Many hormones, such as insulin, growth hormone, and corticosteroids, for example, are obtained from animal tissues, and various antibiotics (e.g., penicillin, streptomycin, and tetracycline) are derived from living organisms, including bacteria, fungi, and actinomyces. The active ingredients from natural products are isolated and purified by chemical methods.

1.2 DRUG DISCOVERY TO CONQUER DISEASES

At the beginning of the 20th century, a metabolic approach was applied to the formulation of new drugs. Because various cells of the body and of certain microorganisms could be selectively stained by certain dyes, it was suggested that drugs of the dye type might attach to specific active groups in cells of the human body and in microorganisms. Such a drug would then act as a "magic bullet," attacking the target cells specifically and killing only the microorganisms while leaving the human body unaffected. In this way, Salvarsan™ was developed by Paul Ehrlich for the treatment of syphilis. This approach required a knowledge of the biochemical processes involved in the metabolism of the body. Attempts to cure diseases were then made by using drugs to alter the body's metabolism.

Drug development made a great leap forward with the discovery of antibiotics. The golden age of antimicrobial therapy began in the 1940s, and it produced large quantities of antibiotics leading to clinical trials and subsequent treatment of infectious diseases. Antibiotics have almost entirely replaced sulfonamides in the treatment of bacterial infection. Because bacteria mutate easily, however, drug-resistant strains of bacteria develop quickly. As a result, investigators are forced to develop new antibiotics to stay ahead of the steady emergence of drug-resistant strains.

Furthermore, many modern drug are synthesized by the techniques of organic chemistry.[1,2] As the biochemical and molecular basis of drug actions became better understood, many new drugs were developed by systematic molecular modification facilitated by the quantitative structure–activity relationship (QSAR), resulting in the improvement of the pharmacokinetic (PK) properties (absorption, distribution, metabolism, and elimination) or pharmacodynamic (PD) properties (mechanism of drug action, cell binding sites) of drugs. Today, molecular modeling and computer science are assuming an increasingly important role in improving our understanding of the basis of drug receptor interactions and in assisting development of new therapeutic agents. Thus, in the next several years, progress in the development of a sound theoretical basis will make molecular design a realistic aid for drug discovery for biomedical investigators and the pharmaceutical industry.

Since the 1980s, many proteins that coordinate vital functions of human life and health have been synthesized. Biotechnology produces diverse new products for the pharmaceutical industry and enhances the treatment of disease. The advances brought by biotechnology involve the areas of recombinant DNA (rDNA) technology, genetic engineering, molecular biology, and immunology. For example, the first recombinant human insulin was manufactured by producing the alpha and beta chains separately in *Escherichia coli* and subsequently combining them. The thrombolytic agent, tissue plasminogen activator (tPA), has been produced by a similar method. Biotechnology and related products have had a major impact on many aspects of our lives and will continue to do so in the future; examples include the developments of a hepatitis B virus vaccine and protein biopharmaceuticals that coordinate chemical messages. Many biological products, including vaccines, anticoagulants, colony-stimulating factors, interferons, interleukins, and monoclonal antibodies, have been produced using the biotechnology techniques that allow the isolation, identification, and production of very small amounts of proteins present in the body. Furthermore, the genes that control protein biosynthesis can be analyzed and their DNA structures sequenced. The isolated gene DNA can be inserted into a bacterial plasmid and cloned into *E. coli* or yeast. This method permits the isolation of specific proteins and their mass production by rapidly growing microorganisms.

In the early period of biotechnology development, newly formed companies were usually managed by scientific investigators. Their lack of management and licensing experience frequently led them to transfer technology to the pharmaceutical industry in exchange for research funding and a 4 to 10% royalty fee on product sales.[3] With growing experience, the larger and better-funded biotechnology companies have progressed to joint cooperative research and product development. Agreements on strategic alliances have been reached between U.S. and foreign companies.

The traditional pharmaceutical approach for drug development entails the screening of a large number of trial compounds, leading to progressively narrower selection regimes. Drugs are either chemically synthesized or isolated from natural products. The success of a new drug, after going through all these steps, is based largely on empirical experience or the luck of trial and error. Such an approach, however, is extremely inefficient and expensive. The rational approach to biotechnology drug development utilizes precise knowledge of the key molecular reactions to define the structure–activity relationship or receptor–ligand interaction and then to intervene precisely at these reactions. It is the access to these experimental models that enables the rational drug design programs to be effective as well as efficient.

1.3 DRUG DEVELOPMENT IN THE BIOTECHNOLOGY ERA

Biotechnology research identifies new molecules for the pharmaceutical industry, enables development of lifesaving medical treatment regimens, and improves the specificity of diagnostic reagents. Continued application of technologic innovations in the biomedical and pharmaceutical fields offers exciting prospects in drug development. The outcome of this new approach will certainly play a major role in shaping the future of pharmaceutical sciences. Molecular biology concepts applied to established disciplines of medicinal chemistry and pharmaceutical sciences allow the introduction of numerous new biopharmaceuticals into the international market. The products represent innovative and unique molecules developed as biological response modifiers, colony-stimulating factors, enzymes, hormones, monoclonal antibodies, and vaccines. Over the past several years, more than 1300 biotechnology companies in the United States have been involved in basic research and product development, and more than 250 molecules have been evaluated in human clinical trials.[4]

Biotechnology has been applied in many areas. During the 1980s, the use of transgenic techniques in cell and tissue cultures helped investigators to understand the action mechanism of proteins essential for eliciting specific biochemical responses; for example, erythropoietin, which stimulates bone marrow to produce red blood cells, is produced by kidney cells and secreted into the blood. Genome mapping and proteomic sequencing applied to small molecules provide an effective screening method to identify promising drug candidates. Combinatorial chemistry, a powerful tool developed in the 1990s, utilizes a mix-and-match process in which a simple subunit is joined to one or more other subunits in every possible combination.[5] Combinatorial chemistry, which generates compounds through rapid simultaneous, parallel, or automated synthesis, is replacing complicated chemical synthesis, a process in which investigators make one compound at a time. Combinatorial chemistry is expected to increase the speed of drug discovery and the pace of drug development.

Completion of the Human Genome Project has contributed a comprehensive resource for identification and localization of gene sequence databases and the prospect of continued genome-sequencing research. Extrapolation from detailed genetic maps of 23 human chromosomes that indicate the location and identity of individual genes offers limitless possibilities to detect, treat, and prevent inherited diseases. Characterization of known diseases and as yet unknown diseases by genetic components provides opportunities for early medical intervention. In addition, gene therapy involves the integration of specific genes into the genome of body disorders. The Human Genome Project will affect every branch of molecular biology and drug development. Having the complete DNA sequencing of humans and animals will provide answers to many important questions regarding the treatment of a wide range of diseases and medical disorders by gaining an understanding of the proteins encoded by the genes. To understand the basic functions of life, it is important to elucidate all the proteins produced within a human body and to grasp how the genes that encode the proteins are expressed, how genes vary within our species and other animal species, and how DNA sequences affect the biologic characteristics of proteins. Genomics will enhance our knowledge of mechanisms involved in preventive, diagnostic, and therapeutic medicine. Investigators will uncover the molecular bases of diseases, will be able to prevent many diseases, and will design individual therapies to treat medical disorders. When the DNA sequence of the human genome is known, scientists will be able to identify common genetic variations and determine how particular variations correlate with risks for certain diseases; they will also be able to examine the interactions between genes and environmental influences such as diet, infection, and pollution.

Improvements in biomedical science techniques have had a significant impact on drug development. A greater understanding of the relationships among protein structure, function, and mechanisms of action is now being realized. Polymerase chain reaction (PCR), transgenic animals, peptide chemistry, recombinant DNA technology, catalytic antibodies, and biosensors are tools that have expanded our capacity to produce purified drug and biological products.[6] These bioengineered drugs can be prepared by direct chemical synthesis and, therefore, can be prepared with greater accuracy at lower cost. Low-molecular-mass drugs capable of highly specific target interaction can mimic important biological functions and offer possible diagnostic and therapeutic application. Small molecules designed to bind to particular hormone receptors are an attractive option to conventional cancer therapeutic agents. Also promising is the role of receptor inhibitors in the prevention of pathological processes leading to malignant tumor development. Recent years have witnessed an increasing interest in developing biologically derived agents as commercially produced pharmaceuticals. Most of such drugs are comprised of proteins and glycoproteins. The number of these biologic products with potential therapeutic application continues to grow.

In the near future, novel drugs will become available that are derived from a detailed molecular understanding of chronic diseases such as diabetes and hypertension. The drugs will target molecules specifically and more accurately, thus reducing adverse reactions. Drugs for the treatment of cancer and cardiovascular diseases will routinely be matched to a patient's likely response, as predicted by molecular fingerprinting; for example, a physician will know which genes are responsible and what medicines will work best for a particular patient with high cholesterol. When people become ill, therapists will be able to examine individual genes to provide precise and specific treatment. The average life span will reach 90 to 95 years, and our understanding of the human aging process will expand the maximum length of human life.[7,8]

1.4 DRUG EVALUATION IN PRECLINICAL RESEARCH

Preclinical research,[9] the initial process of drug development, is intended to provide a preliminary evaluation of the pharmacokinetics, pharmacodynamics, dose–response profiles, and toxicological potential of a drug. In addition to providing basic information about the pharmacology and safety of a drug candidate, preclinical studies also determine the optimal formulation and dose for phase I clinical trials, analyze physicochemical characteristics of the testing compound, and provide the rationale for the proposed therapeutic indication. Approval to initiate human clinical trials is based on the results from preclinical pharmacological and animal toxicity studies. In many instances, agreements on criteria for proposed pharmacological outcomes and the methodology of toxicity testing are reached on a case-by-case basis. Regulatory agencies provide guidelines for preclinical studies. The major tests performed on a drug candidate during preclinical trials involve:

- PK and PD studies
- Bioequivalence and bioavailability
- Acute and chronic toxicity
- Mutagenicity or carcinogenicity
- Immunotoxicity and other tests

Study designs and methods for these tests have been described in detail.[10,11] Various issues frequently arise during the planning of preclinical studies regarding the preliminary formulation of test material, selection of animal species and number, duration of toxicity studies, frequency and routes of drug administration, proposed human clinical dose in relation to animal studies, and validation of a modified test system. Usually, many discussions throughout the drug evaluation process are conducted between manufacturer representatives and regulatory scientists in order to reach an agreement on conditions for testing and product approval.

Most drugs on the market today were developed by trial and error or by mass screening of natural products and synthetic compounds. These traditional approaches to drug discovery have now been modified by a more direct strategy of structure-based drug design. The important starting point is the molecular target or cell receptor in the body for a specific drug. The specific drug is designed to fit the target and alter its biological activity. Enzyme inhibitors have been developed using this structure-based drug design method — for example, the potent enzyme inhibitor of purine nucleotide phosphorylase which has been tested in animals for the treatment of arthritis. A closely related compound is in clinical trials as a therapy for psoriasis and for one form of cancer. Designed enzyme blockers are useful cancer therapeutic agents, as thymidilate synthase catalyzes nucleotide synthesis in cancer cells, a process that is essential for DNA replication and proliferation. An inhibitor prepared by Merck is being studied for treatment of glaucoma by interfering with the enzyme carbonic anhydrase. Merck is also developing another drug to treat emphysema which inhibits human neutrophil elastase, an enzyme involved in damaging lung tissue, rheumatoid arthritis, and acute respiratory distress syndrome.[11]

The information from animal safety tests can be used as an initial guide for comparing clinical benefits and risks for human trials. Likewise, animal toxicity studies are used to predict and characterize potential adverse effects in humans. These guidelines are intended to provide general methods of toxicological studies to appropriately evaluate drug safety and applications for drug approval; however, unified methods and routine studies cannot be expected to reveal all adverse reactions of a specific drug, and it is often necessary to perform additional tests or modify the procedures of the basic guidelines. Good laboratory practice (GLP) regulations were established to ensure the quality and integrity of bioresearch and animal test data submitted to the regulatory agency.[12,13]

A pharmacokinetic study is conducted to establish the parameters for drug actions and to examine how the drug affects biological function. The processes that relate to the fate of a drug in the body involve absorption, distribution, metabolism, and excretion. The pharmacokinetic study helps to identify any toxic effect and estimates the most appropriate method of drug administration and optimum effective dosage for administration. Pharmacodynamic studies examine more specifically how a drug exerts its pharmacological effects. This type of study looks at how a drug interacts with cells or organs, drug effects and adverse reactions, and characteristics or dose–response curves. Information on the pharmacokinetics and pharmacodynamics of a drug in laboratory animals and humans is important for selecting dose levels and dose regimens. It is also important for the design of toxicology studies as well as in evaluating safety and extrapolating toxicological data to humans.

In the search for new drug candidates, the compounds that pass through the screening tests are scaled up to mass production. The active raw materials, synthetic intermediates, drug compound, and final formulated product are analyzed for physicochemical characterization, including identity, strength, quality, purity, and stability. The information from these studies is used to identify potential safety problems in the product, to meet the requirements of regulatory agencies, and to serve as a basis for establishing quality controls and specifications for the product.[14]

REFERENCES

1. Burgen, A.S.V., The road to rational drug design, in *Innovative Approaches in Drug Research*, Harms, A.F., Ed., Elsevier, San Diego, CA, 1986, pp. 1–7.
2. Sarel, S., Mechoulam, R., and Agrana, I., Eds., *Trends in Medicinal Chemistry, Proceedings of the XIth International Symposium on Medicinal Chemistry*, Blackwell Scientific, Oxford, 1992, pp. 55–61.

3. Gordon, S.L., Overview of the commercial prospects for biotechnology products in health care, in *Genetically Engineered Human Therapeutic Drugs,* Copsey, D.N. and Delnatte, S.Y.J., Eds., Macmillan, New York, 1988, pp. 137–142.

4. PRMA, *Biotechnology Medicines in Development,* Pharmaceutical Research and Manufacturers of America, Washington, D.C., 1996.

5. Lee, Jr., K.B. and Burrill, G.S., *Biotech '96, The Industry Annual Report*, Ernst and Young, New York, 1995.

6. Sindelar, R.D., Additional biotechnology-related technique, in *Pharmaceutical Biotechnology*, Crommelin, D.A. and Sindelar, R.D., Eds., Harwood Academic, Amsterdam, 1997, pp. 123–166.

7. Collins, F.S. and Jegalian, K.G., Deciphering the code of life, *Sci. Am.*, 281(6), 86–91, 1999.

8. Collins, F.S., Genome Project, *N. Engl. J. Med.*, 341, 28–37, 1999.

9. Lee, C.J., Lee, L.H., and Lu, C.H., *Development and Evaluation of Drugs: From Laboratory through Licensure to Market*, 2nd ed., CRC Press, Boca Raton, FL, 2003, pp. 31–116.

10. Walsh, G., The drug development process, in *Biopharmaceuticals: Biochemistry and Biotechnology*, John Wiley & Sons, New York, 1998, pp. 37–74.

11. Bugg, C.E., Carson, W.M., and Montgomery, J.A., Drugs by design, *Sci. Am.*, 269(6), 92–98, 1993.

12. Code of Federal Regulations, Nonclinical Laboratory Studies: Good Laboratory Practice (GLP) Regulations, Title 21, Part 58, Food and Drug Administration, Rockville, MD, 1991, pp. 233–246.

13. Lee, C.J., Ishimura, K., Nakajima, T. et al., New drug development and good laboratory practice (GLP) in the United States [Japanese], *Lab. Animal Sci. Technol.*, 2, 95–105, 1990.

14. Schirmer, R.E., *Modern Methods of Pharmaceutical Analysis*, 2nd ed., CRC Press, Boca Raton, FL, 1991.

CHAPTER 2

The Pharmaceutical Background

Shri C. Valvani

CONTENTS

2.1 INTRODUCTION

The primary goal of research-based pharmaceutical organizations around the globe is to discover, develop, and procure regulatory approvals for marketing new drugs for the treatment or prevention of diseases in humans and animals. This chapter deals primarily with pharmaceutical considerations for the development of new chemical or molecular entities for human therapeutic applications. A comprehensive discussion of all pharmaceutical considerations in the design and development of every type of dosage forms or drug delivery systems for all available routes of administration is beyond the scope of this chapter; rather, it focuses on pharmaceutical considerations for dosage forms generally developed for preclinical safety and pharmacology assessment and early testing in humans. However, the information presented and the concepts covered in this chapter are applicable to the development of pharmaceutical drugs, biopharmaceutical products, and medical devices during most stages of the drug development process.

Over the last several years, the amount of scientific data required for preclinical and clinical testing and registration of new products has increased significantly. Global consolidation of the pharmaceutical industry with strategic mergers and acquisitions and competitive market forces continue to exert pressures for accelerating drug development. A delay of even a single day in obtaining regulatory approvals for marketing a new drug can translate into significant loss in sales of a product with major market potential. It is generally recognized that the requirements for registration of new pharmaceutical products from many countries have differed not only in content but also in how the scientific data are compiled and formatted for regulatory reviews. This has culminated in the desire to harmonize registration requirements across most parts of the world. The International Conference on Harmonisation (ICH) of Technical Requirements for Registration of Pharmaceuticals for Human Use has achieved an excellent track record in establishing guidelines that help reduce or eliminate redundant technical requirements for testing and registration of products. While ICH does not cover the entire world, it is focused toward development of unified standards for new drug review and registrations for the three largest consumers of pharmaceutical products and consequently sales of drug products: the United States, the European Community, and Japan. The ICH is cosponsored by regulatory agencies, compendial groups, and major industrial organizations from these three regions. Major topics related to pharmaceutical development that address quality, safety, and efficacy of new products in different stages of harmonization include stability testing, impurities in drug substances and products, validation, light stability, and stability of biotechnology products. In addition, several ICH guidelines cover various aspects of conducting and managing clinical trials of new pharmaceutical and biopharmaceutical products.

2.2 BACKGROUND

The discovery phase of new chemical or molecular entities often involves chemical synthesis or an identification of a lead from a high throughput screen, such as those driven by combinatorial chemistry efforts or isolation from natural sources. With the advent of genetic and protein engineering, a new generation of drugs, protein or polypeptide molecules, has continued to emerge not only for therapeutic application but also for diagnostic treatments. During the past several years, many new drugs derived from biotechnology sources, such as cytokines, erythropoietins, plasminogen activators, blood-plasma factors, hormones, growth factors, insulin, monoclonal antibodies, and rDNA vaccines, have appeared in global markets, and numerous products are in the late stages of development. Because most protein drugs and large peptides cannot be synthesized, they are produced via genetic engineering or recombinant DNA techniques, fermentation or cell culture, isolation, and purification steps. A decision to develop new drugs often depends on the results of early screening, which involves testing new drug molecules in one or more biologically relevant animal models or *in vitro* and *ex vivo* techniques to determine the pharmacological response that reflects potential therapeutic benefits or unmet medical needs.

When the new drug has been shown to possess the desirable therapeutic or pharmacological promise during initial screening in appropriate animal models, it must undergo evaluation of purity, potency, stability, and other pharmaceutical properties leading to development of early dosage forms or delivery systems for extensive evaluation of preclinical safety and pharmacological testing before early testing in humans for safety and tolerance can begin. The requirements for initiating clinical trials of new drugs vary considerably depending on the regulations within each country. Initial testing of new drugs in humans requires a comprehensive dossier of information for the regulatory review and approval process. Specific guidelines for the format, content, and submission of regulatory documents for pharmaceutical development and other sections must be rigorously followed before studies in humans can be undertaken. The use of sound scientific principles, adherence to regulatory guidelines, and application of rational science-based approaches are critical to successful testing and development of new drugs in humans and for veterinary applications.

When the decision is made to develop a new compound, usually the first step is to prepare a sufficient quantity of active pharmaceutical ingredient or drug substance so the multidisciplinary approach to early investigation and development can begin. The synthesis or manufacture of bulk drug substances at this early stage is often carried out on a small laboratory scale, from several tens of grams to a few kilograms, depending on the expected dosage and toxicology testing protocol needs. The quantities of drug substance required for animal safety testing is highly dependent on the therapeutic indication (e.g., acute or chronic use). Chronic use requires larger quantities of drugs and more extensive repeat-dose testing in animals to establish the safety of the drug.

For preclinical safety assessment, usually in two different animal species (e.g., rodents and nonrodents), new drugs must be formulated in an appropriate dosage form that will deliver the drug in a way that maximizes the availability of the drug for thorough evaluation of drug-related toxicity or adverse effects. Drug formulation development for toxicological evaluation must be optimized to deliver the drug to the animal species in question and also to minimize any non-drug-related issues. Often a placebo or control must also be developed to sort out any toxicological or methodology findings related to formulation or vehicle. The design and development of early formulations for preclinical testing and for early testing in humans require an interplay of physicochemical, biological, and dosage form considerations.

For new drugs, preclinical or nonclinical studies are expected to provide multifaceted toxicity data that should help establish the dose–activity relationship, the dose–toxicity relationship, the relationship of route of administration and dose frequency response to activity and toxicity, and the potential risk for clinical toxicity. The determination of no-observed-adverse-effect levels (NOAELs) or toxic levels in animals should involve not just maximizing the dosage administered but also achieving the highest systemic or local level of drug exposure with the lowest dosage administered. Therefore, the toxicology-formulation development phase may require the design and development of several drug formulations of varying compositions where the availability of the drug may be affected (e.g., vehicles, additives, pH, physical properties). The goal during the preclinical development phase is to identify a formulation that will achieve the highest drug exposure with the lowest dosage and yet is tolerated by the animal species involved for the duration of toxicity studies. An important aspect is to minimize any non-drug-related events and outcomes. Sometimes exposures high enough to produce a true toxic level may not be achievable because of the limitations imposed by the physicochemical properties of the drug; for example, any solution or suspension has a limit volume that can be administered safely to a given animal species for a given route of administration. Administration of volumes or amounts exceeding those limits can lead to non-drug-related observations. The pharmaceutical scientist must strive to achieve a balance between maximum tolerated dose of the drug in a given volume of vehicle and maximum tolerated volume of the vehicle.

2.3 PREFORMULATION CONSIDERATIONS

The development process usually begins with the preformulation characterization of a drug substance. Preformulation evaluation is the study of critical physicochemical or mechanical properties that could affect the biological performance of the drug, processing, design, and development of an efficacious dosage form. Critical physicochemical properties of a drug molecule include its solubility, lipophilicity, physical and chemical stability, diffusivity, particle size, ionization constants (pKa), and crystal form. Table 2.1 lists these and other parameters that may be evaluated during the preformulation investigation stage. Most of these are molecular properties of the drug and provide a sort of fingerprint of the drug molecule. A thorough understanding of these characteristics and their impact on safety and pharmacology is important for successful formulation design and development.

Most of the above properties are governed by the chemical or molecular structure of the drug substance. Some of the preformulation parameters are derived properties, which are affected by processing; for example, the *in vitro* or *in vivo* rate of dissolution, specific surface area, or flow properties of the drug may be affected by particle size reduction via micronization, milling, or manipulation of crystallization techniques. The development of formulations for toxicology testing, early human evaluation, or marketing may not require extensive in-depth evaluation of all of these parameters. It largely depends on the therapeutic application, type of drug, dosage form, or route of administration. For example, for solid oral dosage forms, the stability of the drug in the solid state with regard to various environmental factors (e.g., temperature, humidity, light) and processing-related factors must be investigated in greater detail, while the design of solution formulations

Table 2.1   Preformulation Characterization of Drug Substances or Active Pharmaceutical Ingredients

Chemical structure and molecular weight	*Nonaqueous solubility:*
	  Pure solvents
	  Mixed cosolvents
	  Effect of pH
		Mechanical properties:
		  Viscoelastic properties
		  Compressibility
		  Flowability

Organoleptic properties: Color, odor, taste		

Chemical purity and identity:
  Level and identification of
    impurities
  Spectral properties (infrared,
    ultraviolet)
	In vitro dissolution or drug release rate:
	  Bulk drug and pure drug compact
	  Effect of particle size, surface area
		Solution stability:
		  pH rate profile
		  Degradation rate and
		    mechanism
		  Effect of temperature

	Partition coefficient or lipophilicity:
	  Octanol/water systems
	  Alkane/water systems
		Photolytic degradation
		Oxidation/hydrolysis
		Presence of metals

Physical properties:
  Particle size, shape, and
    frequency distribution
  Bulk density
  Microscopic characterization
  Surface area
  Surface activity
  Effect of milling/micronization
	Ionization constants (pKa):
	  Aqueous and nonaqueous systems
		Nonaqueous solution
		  stability
		Ionic strength
		Effect of additives

	Biopharmaceutics properties:
	  In vitro absorption/transport
	    properties
	  Permeability in humans	

Aqueous solubility:
  pH solubility profile
  Effect of temperature
  Effect of solubilizing agents
  Effect of buffers, ionic strength
	Crystalline properties:
	  Melting point
	  Polymorphism (effect on
	    bioavailability)
	  Thermal analysis (e.g., differential
	    scanning calorimetry, thermal
	    gravimetric analysis)
	  Isomerism
		Solid-state stability:
		  Effect of temperature
		  Effect of humidity
		  Effect of light
		  Effect of oxygen/nitrogen
		  Effect of additives

(parenteral or oral), degradation mechanisms, and kinetics of solution stability may require an in-depth critical evaluation as compared to its solid-state behavior.

Specialized delivery systems, such as aerosol delivery systems for inhalation or for intranasal delivery and those intended for delivery to the lungs for local or systemic effects, are often used with nebulizers or other devices. This type of delivery system requires consideration of such critical factors as metering and a pump mechanism for production of spraying patterns, which are dependent on orifice, nozzle, or jets used in the device. Inhalation drug products are one of the most complex pharmaceutical products, thus they present the formidable challenge for pharmaceutical scientists. An inhalation product represents a combination of drug product formulation and a complex container closure system, which are much more closely tied with each other in this case as opposed to those for conventional dosage forms. Because of these complexities, unique regulatory requirements exist for the development of inhalation drug products, whether they are pressurized metered dose inhalations systems or dry powder inhalation systems. Some of the important parameters requiring a thorough evaluation include particle size and shape, distribution and surface characterization, dose content uniformity, amount delivered per actuation, number of doses delivered, spray pattern and plume geometry of valves and actuators used, and leakage rate.[1,2]

For proteins and polypeptide macromolecular drugs, biological activity is often dictated by molecular conformation and, thus, is largely governed by noncovalent forces; therefore, conformational stability, including denaturation and aggregation, and an assessment of biological activity must be addressed during formulation development of proteinaceous or biological drugs. For larger macromolecules, unlike small molecules, much more extensive analytical testing is required to establish the stability behavior and biological performance of large molecules. This is because no single test can provide a comprehensive picture of the integrity, potency, and activity of the molecule. For example, when large molecules are subjected to thermal stability, it is not uncommon to detect little or no change in strength or potency when observed using high-performance chromatographic procedures; yet, they might show a significant drop in biological activity as measured by activity-based assays. For targeted or site-specific drug delivery systems (e.g., monoclonal antibodies), consideration of biochemical and transcellular events at the cellular level is important.

Preformulation investigation usually commences with complete analytical characterization of the drug substance with regard to its chemical purity, including the level and nature of impurities. For proteins, peptides, and other biologicals, evaluation of trace contaminants (e.g., viral, nucleic acid, endotoxin, antigen, foreign protein, microbial contamination) may be carried out as part of the initial characterization in addition to other specific tests for purity and identity. For conventional organic drug molecules, early chemical synthesis often is directed toward maximizing the chemical purity of the drug while minimizing the impurities and residual organic volatile solvents.

The isolation and identification of impurities that may be present in the drug substance beyond a certain threshold level are required by most regulatory agencies worldwide. In this regard, under ICH guidelines on impurities in new drug substances, applications for marketing new drugs would have to demonstrate that all impurities above a certain level (e.g., 0.1%) have been identified.[3] Specific guidelines on testing and qualification of process and drug-related organic impurities, inorganic impurities, and residual solvents are discussed in the guidelines.[4] The ICH guidelines emphasize the importance of specification limits for purity and potency of the drug substance. A scientific rationale for impurities specification based on safety considerations must be provided. The guidelines clearly state that the limits for impurities should be set no higher than the level that can be justified by the safety data and no lower than the level that can be achieved by the manufacturing process and analytical capability. In general, it is better to test the drug substance batch with the highest level of impurities for toxicology studies so a higher level of safety profile for impurities can be established.

Early evaluation of chemical purity and impurities characterization is critical to ensure that drugs with no additional or higher level of impurities, as compared with what has been used for toxicology assessment in animals, will be used in the formulations for early human testing. Generally, the process involves determination of impurities, quantitation of impurities, and isolation and identification of impurities above a threshold level. For new drug molecules with one or more assymetric (chiral) centers, where two or more enantiomers are possible, characterization of stereoisomeric composition as well as preclinical evaluation of enantiomers are required.[5] Drug-specific, stability-indicating assay methodology that will resolve process-related impurities, as well as degradation products, must be developed and validated for bulk drug substances and for formulations for animal and human testing. In addition to analytical characterization, determination of important physicochemical properties, such as melting point or boiling point, ionization constants for electrolyte drugs, partition coefficients, isoelectric point for protein drugs, spectroscopic properties (e.g., ultraviolet, infrared), and polymorphic characterization, is critical to establishing the identity and purity of the drug molecule.

From a physical standpoint, the goal of the pharmaceutical scientist is to design and develop a dosage form for marketing that is stable at labeled storage (at least for a period required for successful marketing — usually two years), is elegant, contains the precise amount of drug, will deliver the drug in the most available form, and can be consistently manufactured on a large production scale in an economic manner to meet market needs after regulatory approvals. Because formulations and processes intended for large-scale marketing may be different from those used for early testing in humans, a link between the pivotal clinical batches and commercial process must be established. This is accomplished by demonstration of their bioequivalence between clinical formulations and marketable products.

2.4 DOSAGE FORM CONSIDERATIONS

A review of pharmaceutical dosage forms available in global markets would indicate that tablets and capsules are by far the most widely used dosage forms, primarily because of advances in the technology of manufacture, flexibility in dosing, stability, elegance, and ease of ingestion, among other factors. Another advantage of tablet and capsule dosage forms is that the duration of action

Table 2.2   Dosage Form or Drug Delivery System Considerations

Tablets:	Emulsions	Liposomes
Compressed	Microemulsions	Transdermal patches
Layered	Gels/creams/ointments	Biodegradable polymer systems
Sugar coated	Oral solutions	Bioerodible polymer systems
Film coated	Parenteral solutions	Microspheres
Enteric coated	Ophthalmic solutions	Nanoparticles
Chewable	Aerosols	Surgical foams
Delayed release	Pressurized metered dose	Edible foams
Extended release	inhalation systems	Softgels/hydrogels
Sublingual	Dry powder inhalation systems	Micellar solutions
Buccal	Nasal sprays	Monoclonal antibodies
Effervescent	Suspensions	Implants/pumps
Hard filled capsules	Lyophilized powders	Microsponges
Soft gelatin capsules	Ready-to-use injections	Vaccines
Suppositories		

can be modulated by controlling the delivery of active drug molecule. Extended release, controlled release, or sustained release solid-dosage products of already approved drugs are being developed to improve consumer or patient compliance or to improve therapeutic profiles. A list of the major pharmaceutical dosage forms and drug delivery systems in use today is provided in Table 2.2. A detailed listing of various types of tablet dosage forms appears within the table. Similar listings can be constructed for each of the other types of dosage forms; however, for brevity, other dosage forms are listed in their simplest form.

Because the goal of toxicology and pharmacology testing is to define the toxicity, activity, and safety relationships, administration of very high concentrations or doses of formulations for pre-clinical safety testing in animals is usually required during early stages. This leads to the development of solution or suspension formulations of the drug for toxicological testing. For early metabolic or bioavailability studies in animals or humans, a parenteral solution, for intravenous administration, is often required in order to assess drug disposition and clinical pharmacology. Other dosage forms, such as tablets, capsules, liquids, semisolids, and other delivery systems, may also be used for animal toxicology testing and for early human studies. One of the key requirements for these formulations is that they must present the drug in the most bioavailable form in order to achieve the highest *in vivo* exposure (usually denoted by maximum concentration and area under the curve), and they must be stable for the duration of investigational studies. Isotonicity, osmomolality, and physiological pH are important considerations for parenteral formulations for toxicology testing. Parenteral formulations must not cause excessive hemolysis upon injection, neither should they cause precipitation in the blood when injected. Suspension formulations must possess good homogeneity to deliver uniform dosing and should demonstrate acceptable physical stability, especially minimal settling tendency with good resuspendability. The U.S. regulations require that the formulations for toxicology testing must be manufactured in accordance with good laboratory practices (GLPs). Similar regulatory requirements are generally recommended in other parts of the world for the conduct of toxicology studies and clinical studies.

2.5 BIOLOGICAL CONSIDERATIONS

The ultimate goal in the drug design and development process is to improve or optimize the biological performance of drugs to maximize the therapeutic ratio. Biological performance can be regarded as the most efficient delivery of drug substance to the site at which it is needed the most and at such a rate of delivery that it elicits the most beneficial therapeutic response while minimizing undesirable side effects. It is generally recognized that physical chemical properties of the drug and pharmaceutical considerations with regard to route of administration play a critical role in

Table 2.3   Biological Considerations for Oral Drug Delivery

Membrane transport mechanism:	*Stomach emptying and*	*Bile acid secretions*
Active transport	*gastrointestinal motility:*	*Intestinal flora*
Passive diffusion	Fasting	
Facilitated diffusion	Nonfasting	*Malabsorption due to disease*
Gastrointestinal pH:	Hydrodynamics	*state*
Stomach	Type of food	*Pharmacological drug effects*
Duodenum	*Enzymes of the gastrointestinal tract:*	
Jejunum	Lumenal	
Ileum	Surface bounds	
Colon	Intercellular	
Surface and bulk pH	Specificity and distribution	

governing the overall biological performance of drugs. Some of the important parameters influencing biological performance are the absorption and transport processes across biological barriers. The nature of these biological barriers and the enzymatic, metabolic, or biochemical events associated with these barriers largely depends on the route of administration. For example, endothelial barriers are important for target-specific delivery to liver, lungs, or the reticular endothelial system; cellular barriers, for targeting to tumor and other specific cells; and epithelial barriers, for oral, topical, or transdermal delivery. Because a majority of the drugs are administered by the oral route, we will critically examine the factors influencing the gastrointestinal process for drug absorption and transport. This requires consideration of biological and physicochemical factors.

Some of the important biological factors that govern gastrointestinal absorption are shown in Table 2.3. The absorption process depends on the complex interplay of most of these factors. Drug absorption, whether through the gastrointestinal tract, nasal cavity, buccal mucosa, transdermal route, or other barriers, requires that the drug be transported in a molecular form across the barrier membrane. Biological membranes are composed of small amphipathic molecules, phospholipids, and cholesterol, the association of which creates lipoidal bilayers in an aqueous environment. Embedded in the matrix of lipid molecules are proteins, which are generally hydrophobic in nature. It is generally recognized that most lipid-soluble drugs can pass by passive diffusion through the lipid membrane from regions of high concentration to regions of low concentration. A smaller majority of drugs can pass through active transport, often by carrier-mediated transport or through specific transporters.

Similarly, the pH of the intestinal contents in various segments, the presence of biliary salts, enzymes, the type and nature of food, presence or absence of food, the intestinal flora, and the disease state will all influence the drug absorption process. It is commonly accepted that the presence of enzymes (e.g., proteolytic enzymes and other specific enzymes) may inhibit or limit the absorption of the large peptide or protein drugs. In addition, the extent of absorption in the gastrointestinal tract for drugs is largely influenced by the gastric emptying time as well as the transit time through the small intestine.[6–9] In this regard, gamma scintigraphy and other techniques have been extensively used to evaluate food effects and other variables such as stress, exercise, or density.[10,11] Interactions with other concomitantly administered drugs, protein binding, and disease state can also significantly affect the absorption process. A thorough consideration of these factors in the design of formulations for animal and human studies is required by the pharmaceutical scientist.

Most solid dosage forms for oral administration (tablets, capsules, and powders) must first undergo disintegration followed by dissolution of drug particles and transport of drug molecules into the gut. Oral suspensions require dissolution and molecular transport for absorption to occur. Extended- or modified-release oral dosage forms may release the drug by surface erosion, biodegradation, osmotic pressure, or other mechanisms. Diffusion of the active drug molecules across the gut mucosa into the systemic circulation occurs either by active transport or by passive diffusion process. The drug may undergo a variety of enzymatic or metabolic conversions, transport and

Table 2.4 Physicochemical Considerations for Drug Delivery

Drug molecular properties:	Solubility:	Molecular interactions:
Lipophilicity	Crystal form	Drug–drug complexation
Molecular weight/size	Coprecipitates	Drug–drug interactions
pKa of the weak acid/base	Particles size	Drug–mucoid polysaccharides
Chemical stability	Dissolution	Drug–heavy metal ions
Enzymatic stability	Micellar solubilization	Protein binding
	Cosolvent solubilization	Adsorption
	Polymer complexation	
	In vitro precipitation	
	Hemolysis	

deposition into several organs, possible biotransformation, and finally excretion by one or more specific routes. Depending on the permeability and solubility of the drug molecule, a small fraction or most of the drug may eventually reach the receptor site where the desired therapeutic response is achieved.

2.6 PHYSICOCHEMICAL CONSIDERATIONS

Table 2.4 shows some of the physicochemical properties involved in drug absorption and transport processes. Lipophilicity of the drug or the membrane–water partition coefficient and solubility are two of the most important properties of the drug molecule that have a profound influence on these processes. The parameters listed in Table 2.4 are extremely important in formulation design and development for preclinical testing or for evaluation in humans. For example, drugs must be formulated in the solution form for parenteral administration via the intravenous route. Similarly, the sterile solution or sterile suspension forms of drugs may be used for other routes of administration. Solubility of the drug in a particular aqueous system or a mixed organic cosolvent system will determine the limitation within which the drug may be formulated. Often, during the preclinical investigation phase, high concentrations or doses of drugs must be administered to animals to determine the toxicological response. This creates a challenge for the pharmaceutical scientist, who must develop a formulation that not only will be in the solution form but also must remain so without precipitation at the site of injection and in the body tissues and fluids. Furthermore, the drug or the formulation intended for the intravenous route should not cause significant hemolysis, local irritation, or incompatibility with blood components. In vitro and in vivo techniques for studying the precipitation potential upon injection and the hemolysis potential have been reported and must be considered in drug development.[12–17]

The drug must be available in the solution form regardless of whatever form it is administered. The dissolution of solid dosage forms is a prerequisite, before absorption across biological barriers can occur. Even when solutions with limited aqueous solubility are given via the oral route, they may precipitate in the stomach or intestinal region, because of either pH changes or solubility limitations, and then they must redissolve before absorption can occur. Drugs with low solubility may dissolve slowly in the gastrointestinal tract. The rate of in vivo dissolution may be the rate-determining step in the absorption process. Development of a method for determining the in vitro dissolution rate for solid dosage forms is of vital importance in the characterization of bioavailability because the rate of in vivo dissolution determines the rate and extent to which the substance is absorbed. Establishment of an in vitro dissolution and in vivo bioavailability correlation has increasingly become an industry practice to ensure bioequivalence. Drugs with poor or low aqueous solubility often present the greatest challenge for pharmaceutical scientists and frequently may be associated with bioavailability problems. For example, digitoxin, griseofulvin, some steroids, indomethacin, chlorpropamide, and other drugs with low solubility are considered to have large variation in biological availability. These types of drugs present significant challenges to demonstrating bioequivalence to link early formulations with those developed for commercial use.

Because of limitations in aqueous solubility, various solubilization techniques may be investigated to increase the apparent solubility to achieve the desired formulation goal. Solubilization techniques, including the use of surface-active agents (e.g., polysorbates, sorbitan esters, quaternary ammonium compounds, and sodium lauryl sulfates), have been used successfully for formulations of pharmaceutical compounds;[18–21] however, the use of surface-active agents often presents toxicology or hypersensitivity problems and cannot be used for certain routes of administration.

Cosolvents, such as polyethylene glycols, propylene glycol, glycerin, alcohol, and other solvents, are often employed to improve the solubility behavior of drugs with low solubility or poor stability in aqueous solutions. The solubility of a drug increases exponentially as a function of cosolvent concentration. In general, most nonpolar drugs with lower aqueous solubility demonstrate a greater solubilizing capacity by most cosolvents. Several drugs, such as digoxin, phenytoin sodium, diazepam, and chlordiazepoxide, are formulated in a variety of cosolvent systems.[22–27] Of course, some of these and other cosolvents have toxicological implications, primarily muscle damage or tissue damage and constraints on the route of administration.[28–31] Such drugs must be injected slowly to avoid precipitation or pain upon injection.[32–34]

For drugs with weak ionizable groups, an improvement in solubility for drug formulation can be accomplished by controlling the pH within reasonable limits, depending on the ionization constant (pKa) of the drug molecule. Alternatively, an improvement in solubility can be accomplished by formation of a salt by chemical modification, complexation with cyclodextrins, coprecipitate formation, and a variety of other techniques.[35–37]

While low aqueous solubility may be a problem or limitation for conventional drug delivery, it is often an asset or a desirable parameter for the development of most controlled-release or sustained-release delivery systems.[38] It is not uncommon to employ prodrug modifications or other chemical modifications to achieve a reduction in the solubility or to improve the solution stability of a drug molecule.[39–42] The taste of organic drug molecules has a good correlation with its aqueous solubility. For example, increasing the chain length of clindamycin esters, thus reducing the aqueous solubility, dramatically improves the taste.[43] An inhibition or reduction in bitterness of drug molecules can be accomplished by cationic or anionic salt formation.[44]

For poorly absorbed drugs that do not undergo significant degradation or first-pass metabolism, membrane permeability and the dose-to-solubility ratio are the key parameters controlling oral drug absorption. The membrane permeability for drugs absorbed by passive diffusion depends on the membrane–water or oil–water partition coefficient (a measure of lipophilicity). While aqueous solubility is one of the most important limiting factors in governing the flux across biological membranes, it is the combination of solubility and partition coefficient that influences the absorption and transport processes. It can be shown that biological activity may be dependent on concentration or dose and partition coefficient, concentration alone, solubility alone, or the product of solubility and partition coefficient.

Because of the interdependence of solubility and the partition coefficient, no single value for either parameter can be assigned for optimum performance. For example, an aqueous solubility of several micrograms/milliliter for a very potent drug requiring a therapeutic dose of only a few milligrams may suffice, but inadequate bioavailability may result for a drug with similar solubility that requires a larger therapeutic dose of several hundreds of milligrams. Similarly, a highly lipophilic drug may have low bioavailability because of its poor solubility and dissolution characteristics, while a drug that is too polar will probably exhibit poor transport properties.

The above concepts have been studied extensively and have resulted in a series of scientific publications and culminated in a biopharmaceutics classification system (BCS). The BCS provides a scientific rationale and framework for classifying an orally administered drug based on its aqueous solubility and its intestinal permeability. This, in combination with the *in vitro* dissolution characteristics of the drug product, allows identification of three critical factors: solubility, permeability, and dissolution rate, all of which control the rate and extent of absorption of immediate release solid dosage form.[45] The biopharmaceutics classification system has been the subject of extensive research with much discussion on its applications and limitations.[46–48]

A consideration of the BCS has led the Food and Drug Administration to issue guidance on classifying the drug substances for immediate-release, solid, oral dosage forms into four distinct classes.[49] The four classes represent drugs that demonstrate: (1) high permeability and high solubility, (2) high permeability and low solubility, (3) low permeability and high solubility, and (4) low permeability and low solubility. The guidance defines drugs as being highly soluble when the highest dose is soluble in 250 mL or a lower volume of water over a pH range of 1 to 7.5. The drugs are considered highly permeable when the extent of absorption in humans is determined to be at least 90% of an administered dose, based on mass balance or as compared to an intravenous reference dose. The guidance provides information for the waiver of bioequivalence studies when the drugs possess high solubility and high permeability, with rapid dissolution, a wide therapeutic window, and the use of previously accepted excipients.

Most drugs and drug products undergo chemical and physical decomposition and degradation continually as a function of storage. When the active pharmaceutical ingredient in drug formulations loses its potency by chemical degradation, the chemical potency should not fall below acceptable registered specification (usually 90% of the labeled potency). The physical appearance, as well as other performance characteristics such as dissolution, hardness, taste, and odor, for solid oral dosage forms also must be within acceptable limits; otherwise, the products are considered subpotent and may no longer produce the desired pharmacological response. Thus, the chemical and physical stability of the drug substance in solid and solution states under a variety of environmental conditions (e.g., light, humidity, temperature, pH, buffers, oxidation, solvents, physical stress) provides the limitations and opportunities for successful design and development of dosage forms. Similarly, investigating the stability of formulations under most of these conditions, including testing under accelerated conditions, is critical to successful development for early clinical evaluation as well as for marketing. Thanks to the harmonization efforts, the finalized ICH guidelines for conducting physical and chemical stability for both drug substances and products including biotechnology and biological products have been issued.[50–51] These guidelines allow uniform testing of drug substances and drug products for registration in Europe, Japan, the United States, and Canada. Stability testing under more stringent conditions is required for marketing in tropical countries because of extreme climate conditions.[52] Process development, optimization of formulations, and validation are other important activities that must be carried out in the later stages for large-scale manufacturing required for continued clinical evaluation or for marketing after regulatory approval.

2.7 SUMMARY

The drug discovery and development process involves complex interplay of physicochemical, biological, dosage form, and route of administration considerations. These factors have significant impact on the biological performance of drugs by modulating transport across biological barriers as well as affecting other biochemical events. A combination of these factors may be regarded as critical for successful formulation design and pharmaceutical development. A thorough understanding and consideration of these factors by pharmaceutical scientists, medicinal chemists, pharmacologists, biologists, clinicians, toxicologists, and others involved in the drug discovery, design, and development process can significantly improve the rational selection or design of drug molecules for early evaluation in animals and humans.

REFERENCES

1. FDA, *Guidance for Industry: Nasal Spray and Inhalation Solution, Suspension, and Spray Drug Products — Chemistry, Manufacturing, and Controls Documentation*, draft guidance, Center for Drug Evaluation and Research, U.S. Food and Drug Administration, Washington, D.C., 1999.

2. FDA, *Guidance for Industry: Metered Dose Inhaler (MDI) and Dry Powder Inhaler (DPI) Drug Products — Chemistry, Manufacturing, and Controls Documentation*, draft guidance, Center for Drug Evaluation and Research, U.S. Food and Drug Administration, Washington, D.C., 1998.

3. International Conference on Harmonisation, Guidance for industry: Q3A impurities in new drug substances, *Fed. Reg.*, 68(28), 6924–6925, 2003.

4. International Conference on Harmonisation, Guidance for industry: Q3C impurities — residual solvents, *Fed. Reg.*, 62(247), 67377, 1997.

5. FDA, *Policy Statement for the Development of New Stereoisomeric Drugs*, Center for Drug Evaluation and Research, U.S. Food and Drug Administration, Washington, D.C., 1992.

6. Davis, S.S., Hardy, G., and Fara, J.W., Transit of pharmaceutical dosage forms through the small intestine, *Gut*, 27, 886, 1986.

7. Chloe, S.Y. et al., Novel method to assess gastric emptying in humans: the pellet gastric emptying test, *Eur. J. Pharm. Sci.*, 14, 347, 2001.

8. Coupe, A.J., Davis, S.S., and Wilding, I.R., Variation in gastrointestinal transit of pharmaceutical dosage forms in healthy subjects, *Pharm. Res.*, 8, 360, 1991.

9. Kaus, L.C., Gilespie, W.R., Hussain, A.S., and Amidon, G.L., The effect of *in vivo* dissolution, gastric emptying rate, and intestinal transit time on the peak concentration and area under the curve of drugs with different gastrointestinal permeabilities, *Pharm. Res.*, 16, 272, 1999.

10. Christensen, F.N., Davis, S.S., Hardy, J.G., Taylor, M.J., Whalley, D.R., and Wilson, C.G., The use of gamma scintigraphy to follow the gastrointestinal transit of pharmaceutical formulations, *J. Pharm. Pharmacol.*, 37, 91, 1985.

11. Wilding, I.R., Coupe, A.J., and Davis, S.S., The role of gamma-scintigraphy in oral drug delivery, *Adv. Drug. Deliv. Rev.*, 46, 103, 2001.

12. Reed, K.W. and Yalkowsky, S.H., Lysis of human red blood cells in the presence of various cosolvents. III. The relationship between hemolytic potential and structure, *J. Parenter. Sci. Technol.*, 41, 37, 1987.

13. Obeng, E.K. and Cadwallader, D.E., *In vitro* dynamic method for evaluating the hemolytic potential of intravenous solution, *J. Parenter. Sci. Technol.*, 43, 167, 1989.

14. Cox J.W., Sage, G.P., Wynalda, M.A., Ulrich, R.G., Larson, P.G., and Su, C.C., Plasma compatibility of injectables: comparison of intravenous U74006F, a 21-aminosteroid antioxidant, with Dilantin brand of phenytoin, *J. Pharm. Sci.*, 80, 371, 1991.

15. Davio, S.R., McShane, M.M., Kakuk, T.J., Zaya, R.M., and Cole, S.L., Precipitation of renin inhibitor ditekerin upon i.v. infusion: *in vitro* studies and their relationship to *in vivo* precipitation in the cynomolgus monkey, *Pharm. Res.*, 8, 80, 1991.

16. Krzyaniak, J.F., Raymond, D.M., and Yalkowsky, S.H., Lysis of human red blood cells. I. Effect of contact time on water induced hemolysis, *J. Pharm. Sci. Technol.*, 50, 223, 1996.

17. Krzyaniak, J.F., Raymond, D.M., and Yalkowsky, S.H., Lysis of human red blood cells. II. Effect of contact time on cosolvent induced hemolysis, *Int. J. Pharm.*, 152, 193, 1997.

18. Li, P. and Zhao, L., Cosolubilization of non-polar drugs in polysorbate 80 solutions, *Int. J. Pharm.*, 249, 211, 2002.

19. Alkhamis, K.A., Allaboun, H., and Al-Momani, W.Y., Study of the solubilization of gliclazide by aqueous micellar solutions, *J. Pharm. Sci.*, 92, 839, 2003.

20. Li, P. and Zhao, L., Solubilization of flurbiprofen in pH-surfactant solutions, *J. Pharm. Sci.*, 92, 951, 2003.

21. Fahelelbom, K.M., Timoney, R.F., and Corrigan, O.I., Micellar solubilization of clofazimine analogues in aqueous solutions of ionic and nonionic surfactants, *Pharm. Res.*, 10, 631, 1993.

22. Jouyban-Gharamaleki, A. et al., Comparison of various cosolvency models for calculating solute solubility in water-cosolvent mixtures, *Int. J. Pharm.*, 15, 177, 1999.

23. Millard, J., Alvarez-Nunez, F., and Yalkowsky, S., Solubilization by cosolvents: establishing useful constants for the log-linear model, *Int. J. Pharm.*, 245, 153, 2002.

24. Jouyban, A. et al., A cosolvency model to predict solubility of drugs at several temperatures from a limited number of solubility measurements, *Chem. Pharm. Bull. (Tokyo)*, 50, 594, 2002.
25. Li, P., Zhao, L., and Yalkowsky, S.H., Combined effect of cosolvent and cyclodextrin on solubilization of nonpolar drugs, *J. Pharm. Sci.*, 88, 1107, 1999.
26. Stephens, D., Li, L.C., Pec, E., and Robinson, D., A statistical experimental approach to cosolvent formulation of a water-insoluble drug, *Drug Dev. Ind. Pharm.*, 25, 961, 1999.
27. Tongaree, S., Flanagan, D.R., and Poust, R.I., The effects of pH and mixed solvent systems on the solubility of oxytetracycline, *Pharm. Dev. Technol.*, 4, 571, 1999.
28. Brazeau, G.A. and Fung, H.L., Physicochemical properties of binary organic cosolvent–water mixtures and their relationships to muscle damage following intramuscular injection, *J. Parenter. Sci. Technol.*, 43, 144, 1989.
29. Brazeau, G.A. and Fung, H.L., Use of an *in vitro* model for the assessment of muscle damage from intramuscular injections: *in vitro–in vivo* correlation and predictability with mixed cosolvent systems, *Pharm. Res.*, 6, 766, 1989.
30. Brazeau, G.A. and Fung, H.L., Effect of organic solvent-induced skeletal muscle damage on the bioavailability of intramuscular [14C] diazepam, *J. Pharm. Sci.*, 79, 773, 1990.
31. Montaguti, P., Melloni, E., and Cavaletti, E., Acute intravenous toxicity of dimethyl sulfoxide, poly-ethylene glycol 400, dimethyl formamide, absolute ethanol, and benzyl alcohol in inbred mouse strains, *Arzneim.-Forsch/Drug Res.*, 44, 566, 1994.
32. Brazeau, G.A., Cooper, B., Svetic, K.A., Smith, C.L., and Gupta, P., Current perspectives on pain upon injection of drugs, *J. Pharm. Sci.*, 87, 667, 1998.
33. Yalkowsky, S.H., Valvani, S.C., and Johnson B.W., *In vitro* method for detecting precipitation of parenteral formulations after injection, *J. Pharm. Sci.*, 72, 1014–1017, 1983.
34. Alvarez-Nunez, F.A. and Yalkowsky, S.H., Buffer capacity and precipitation control of pH solubilized phenytoin formulations, *Int. J. Pharm.*, 185, 45, 1999.
35. Manolikar, M.K. and Sawant, M.R., Study of solubility of isoproturon by its complexation with beta-cyclodextrin, *Chemosphere*, 51, 811, 2003.
36. Sjostrom, B., Kronberg, B., and Carlfors, J., A method for the preparation of submicron particles of sparingly water-soluble drugs by precipitation in oil-in-water emulsions. I. Influence of emulsification and surfactant concentration, *J. Pharm. Sci.*, 82, 579, 1993.
37. He, Y., Li, P., and Yalkowsky S.H., Solubilization of fluasterone in cosolvent/cyclodextrin combinations, *Int. J. Pharm.*, 264, 25, 2003.
38. Shah, K.P. and Chafetz, L., Use of sparingly soluble salts to prepare oral sustained release suspensions, *Int. J. Pharm.*, 109, 271–281, 1994.
39. Beaumont, K., Webster, R., Gardner, I., and Dack, K., Design of ester prodrugs to enhance oral absorption of poorly permeable compounds: challenges to the discovery scientist, *Curr. Drug. Metab.*, 4, 461, 2003.
40. Juntunen, J. et al., Anandamide prodrugs. 1. Water-soluble phosphate esters of arachidonylethanolamide and R-methanandamide, *Eur. J. Pharm. Sci.*, 19, 37, 2003.
41. Hayashi, Y. et al., A novel approach of water-soluble paclitaxel prodrug with no auxiliary and no byproduct: design and synthesis of isotaxel, *J. Med. Chem.*, 46, 3782, 2003.
42. Hecker, S.J. et al., Prodrugs of cephalosporin RWJ-333441 (MC-04,546) with improved aqueous solubility, *Antimicrob. Agents Chemother.*, 47, 2043, 2003.
43. Sinkula, A.A., Morozowich, W., and Rowe E.L., Chemical modification of clindamycin: synthesis and evaluation of selected esters, *J. Pharm. Sci.*, 62, 1106, 1973.
44. Keast, R.S.J. and Breslin, P.A.S., Modifying the bitterness of selected oral pharmaceuticals with cation and anion series of salts, *Pharm. Res.*, 19, 1019, 2002.
45. Yu, L. et al., Biopharmaceutics classification system: the scientific basis for biowaiver extensions, *Pharm. Res.*, 19, 921, 2002.
46. Rinaki, E., Valsami, G., and Macheras, P., Quantitative biopharmaceutics classification system: the central role of dose/solubility ratio, *Pharm. Res.*, 20, 1917, 2003.
47. Yazdanian, M., Briggs, K., Jnakovsky, C., and Hawi, A., The "high solubility" definition of the current FDA guidance on biopharmaceutic classification system may be too strict for acidic drugs, *Pharm. Res.*, 21, 293, 2004.

48. Martinez, M. et al., Applying the biopharmaceutics classification system to veterinary pharmaceutical products. Part 2. Physiological considerations, *Adv. Drug Deliv. Rev.*, 54, 825, 2002.
49. FDA, *Guidance for Industry: Waiver of In Vivo Bioavailability and Bioequivalence Studies for Immediate Release Solid Oral Dosage Forms Based on a Biopharmaceutics Classification System*, Center for Drug Evaluation and Research, U.S. Food and Drug Administration, Washington, D.C., 2000.
50. International Conference on Harmonisation, Guidance for industry: Q1A(R2) stability testing of new drug substances and products, *Fed. Reg.*, 68(225), 65717–65718, 2003.
51. International conference on Harmonisation, Final guideline on stability testing of biotechnology/biological products: availability, *Fed. Reg.*, 61(133), 36466, 1996.
52. International Conference on Harmonisation, Guidance for industry: Q1F stability data package for registration applications in climatic zones III and IV, *Fed. Reg.*, 68(225), 65717–65718, 2003.

CHAPTER **3**

The Pharmacological Background for Drug Evaluation

Lucia H. Lee, Christopher L. Wu, Benjamin R. Lee, and Chi-Jen Lee

CONTENTS

3.1 INTRODUCTION

Drug discovery, in most cases, relates to an efficient, insightful interpretation of biochemical knowledge and logical application to pharmacological activities. Traditionally, the drug discovery process has relied on screening a large number of chemical and biological specimens to identify potential candidates. Many years ago, crude substances were initially extracted from plants. Plant derivatives were modified to become the active compounds found in aspirin, reserpine, and taxol. Large quantities of the plant material were collected and purified to yield the active component, known as a "lead compound." Chemists then attempted to modify the lead compound to make it more pharmacologically active, reduce potential toxicity, or change its hydrophobicity so it could easily pass through cell membranes — all properties that rendered the compound more effective as a pharmaceutical agent. Purification of crude substances was gradually replaced by large-scale systemic screening of natural and synthetic compounds. Today, more thorough and efficient knowledge-based strategies are utilized to identify new compounds. Structure-based drug design using computer modeling is also used to simulate chemical modifications. In this way, modification of an existing leading drug or designing a new drug is achieved without physically manipulating every possible compound.

Preclinical research, the initial process of drug development, is intended to provide a preliminary assessment of the pharmacological activities, dose–response profiles, and toxicological potential of a drug. In addition to providing basic information about the pharmacology and safety of the test drug, preclinical studies determine the optimal formulation and dose for phase I clinical trials, identify potential toxic adverse effects, and provide the rationale for the proposed therapeutic indication.

Approval to initiate human clinical trials is based largely on the results from preclinical pharmacological and toxicological studies. In many situations, agreements on criteria for proposed pharmacological outcomes and methods of toxicity testing are approached on a case-by-case basis. Regulatory authorities provide guidelines to outline general considerations for preclinical pharmacological studies. Studies on acute toxicity, subchronic and chronic toxicity, reproductive and developmental toxicity, mutagenicity, teratogenicity, and carcinogenicity should be well designed and performed. The major tests performed on a drug candidate during preclinical stage include:

- Pharmacodynamic studies
- Pharmacokinetic studies
- Bioequivalence and bioavailability
- Acute toxicity
- Chronic toxicity
- Reproductive toxicity and teratogenicity
- Mutagenicity or carcinogenicity
- Immunotoxicity
- Local toxicity and other tests

Both the regulatory agency and the manufacturer must be satisfied that the testing conditions are common, acceptable procedures that achieve accurate and consistent experimental results.

Pharmacology is the study of the activities of drugs and how they interact with the body. Pharmacodynamics (PD) examines more specifically how the drug exerts its pharmacological effects. The study emphasizes how a drug interacts with cells or organs, drug effects and adverse reactions, and the characteristics of dose–response curves. The information on the pharmacokinetics and pharmacodynamics of a drug in laboratory animals and humans is important for the design of toxicology studies as well as in evaluating safety and extrapolating toxicological data to humans. A pharmacokinetic (PK) study is conducted to establish the parameters for drug actions. The processes that relate to the fate of a drug in the body involve absorption (A), distribution (D), metabolism (M), and excretion (E). This study helps to identify any toxic effect and estimates the most appropriate method of drug administration and the optimum effective dosage for administration.[1,2] Generally, ADME studies are conducted on two species, usually rats and dogs, at various dosage levels and in both male and female animals. Most of the time, ADME studies are not performed for biopharmaceuticals.

Proteins are catabolized by proteolytic enzymes into amino acid fragments and reutilized in the synthesis of endogenous proteins. Their end-products of metabolism are not considered to be a safety issue. This is in contrast to chemical drugs, which can form potentially toxic metabolites. After glomerular filtration, protein drugs are actively reabsorbed by the proximal tubules through endocytosis and then hydrolyzed within the cell to peptide fragments and amino acids and returned to the blood circulation; consequently, only small amounts of intact protein are detected in the urine.

The binding of drugs to plasma proteins can influence both their distribution and elimination and, consequently, their pharmacological activity. For chemical drugs and small peptides, it is generally considered that only the free molecules can pass through membranes; therefore, the distribution and elimination clearance of total drugs are usually less than those of free drugs. The drug activity is more closely related to the free drug concentration than to the total plasma concentration. For large protein drugs such as tissue plasminogen activator (tPA), growth hormone, and interferon, however, plasma binding proteins may act as facilitators of cellular uptake processes for protein drugs to interact with receptors. As a result, the amount of bound product directly influences its pharmacodynamics.

Prediction of the rate and extent of oral absorption of drugs in humans is important in drug development. In some cases, the rat model is a suitable model for predicting the extent of oral absorption in humans. Drug stability and gastrointestinal (GI) absorption may differ depending on whether a drug is formulated as a solution, suspension, or other rapid-release dosage form. Absorption also depends on the dosage given. The nonlinear extent between the human and the rat can be extrapolated by normalizing doses according to body surface area and body weight. In contrast, several drugs have shown much better absorption in dogs than in humans, and marked differences in the nonlinear absorption profiles of the two species have been found for some drugs. Some drugs have also had much longer T_{max} values and more prolonged absorption in humans than in dogs. Oral absorption data obtained from experimental dogs, therefore, should be confirmed in another animal species.[3,4]

The toxicological and ADME studies that are required for submission of an investigational new drug (IND) are defined in general terms by the Department of Health in the United Kingdom, by the European Drug Regulatory Authorities, and by the U.S. Food and Drug Administration (FDA). These regulatory agencies also require the review of suitable PK and PD information about a new chemical entity (NCE). In contrast, the Japanese Ministry of Health, Labour, and Welfare lists an intensive series of pharmacological tests that must be conducted and reported before receiving permission to conduct clinical trials for NCEs. The required format of the pharmacology reports for the different regulatory authorities is similar, and they provide guidance for the style and format for reporting the appropriate data.

Each regulatory authority requires presentation of the pharmacological properties of the NCE in two separate sections: (1) the primary pharmacology, which examines the pharmacological actions related to the proposed therapeutic use, and (2) the second pharmacology, which describes other relevant activities of the drug, sometimes referred to as the safety pharmacology evaluation. The primary safety tests are conducted as part of the toxicological submission package and may follow the good laboratory practice (GLP) procedures. Another section on drug interactions is also required by the regulatory agencies.

3.2 EVALUATION OF PHARMACOLOGICAL ACTIVITIES FOR PROPOSED THERAPEUTIC USE

The primary pharmacological activities of the NCE should be demonstrated using scientifically acceptable experimental methods, and it should be shown that these activities can be determined in clinical trials. The regulatory agencies require a review of data that establish the mechanism of the principal pharmacological action. The type and extent of these studies depend on the particular NCE and are evaluated on a case-by-case basis. Appropriate validation of the experimental models and technical procedures used is also required. The laboratory must use procedures that are generally accepted by the scientific community as appropriate and reliable and must present information that demonstrates the validity of the techniques and data. The guidelines recommend that, if feasible, the evaluation of the NCE should be performed in parallel with a standard drug for the same therapy. The data should be expressed and presented in quantitative terms. The regulatory reviewers will examine dose-related effects and the time-course of the activity; thus, the PK and PD profiles of the NCE must be studied within the same series of experiments in the same animals.

The primary safety evaluation of the NCE will be reported in the toxicology section of an investigational new drug (IND) application; however, a general pharmacological profile of the NCE is also required, with special attention paid to any effect additional to the primary pharmacological action. The objective of secondary pharmacological studies is to establish the effects on the major biological system using a variety of experimental models. Japanese scientists suggest that the secondary pharmacological tests be conducted to explore whether the NCE has other potential clinical applications — for example, possible effects of the NCE on the cardiovascular and respiratory systems and on the overall behavior of laboratory animals. The purpose of performing secondary pharmacological studies is to explore whether the primary activity is specific or selective. When a primary therapeutic dose also causes significant secondary effects, then more extensive study is necessary to address the selectivity of the drug candidate.

The particular series of experiments for the secondary pharmacological evaluation depends on the research approach of the manufacturer. An institute that relies on random screening for drug discovery often includes a large number of routine screens and tests that may not be related to the proposed therapeutic use, such as determination of the antiinflammatory activities of a new antihypertensive agent. In contrast, a company that has a focused drug discovery program conducts only selected experiments for specific needs. Appropriate scientific judgment is therefore required to decide on the nature and profile of these pharmacological studies.

The guidelines published by the U.S., U.K., and European regulatory agencies suggest that studies on the secondary pharmacological activities of NCEs should include these evaluations:

- *United States:*
  Neuropharmacology
  Cardiovascular or respiratory
  Gastrointestinal
  Genitourinary
  Endocrine
  Antiinflammatory
  Immunoactive
  Chemotherapeutic
  Enzyme effects and other

- *United Kingdom and Europe:*
  Central nervous system
  Autonomic system
  Cardiovascular system
  Gastrointestinal system
  Other systems, where relevant

Additional studies may be conducted in response to particular observations from the primary studies. For example, an unexpected vascular response elicited during a cardiovascular study *in vivo* may be followed up with an assessment of the effects of the NCE on isolated preparations of heart or other organs *in vitro* for establishing its mechanism of action.

Regulatory agencies also require reporting of relevant pharmacological studies on the interaction of NCEs with other drugs that patients may receive. Furthermore, interaction studies are required with regard to anticipated components of the drug delivery systems for NCEs. The European Expert Report must include a critical evaluation of the experimental studies and interpretation of the pharmacological data, with additional discussion on their relationship to the ADME and toxicological results. The Expert Report is thus a medium for justifying and explaining the preclinical development of the product. Much of the key experimental data are included as appendices.

3.3 PHARMACOKINETIC ASSESSMENTS

In vitro studies are necessary to examine the biochemical processes and provide extensive insight into the metabolism and disposition of drugs and their mechanism of action. Furthermore, *in vivo* studies are critical for pharmacokinetic assessments for drug activity and disposition. *In vivo* studies are more complicated in that:

- The administered drug must pass through tissue barriers to reach its site of action.
- Many drugs are bound to blood components in the vascular system from which they may be slowly released.
- The drug may be metabolized to active, inactive, or reactive metabolites in various tissues.
- The drug is distributed to tissues where it exerts a pharmacological effect but will also be distributed to other tissues from which it may be slowly released.
- The drug and its metabolites are eliminated from the body by excretion.

The intensity and duration of action of drugs are greatly affected by the rates of drug absorption, distribution to tissues, and elimination by metabolism or excretion.[5] For drugs that produce their effects indirectly by depletion of pharmacologically active endogenous substances, the intensity and duration of drug response depend on the rate of biosynthesis of the endogenous substance.

3.3.1 Absorption

A drug must enter the body to exert its pharmacological activity. Absorption refers to the entry of a drug into the blood mucous membranes, respiratory tract, skin, or sites of injection. Drugs administered by intravenous injection are considered 100% available. Intramuscular and subcutaneous injections are considered highly available. Drugs administered by the oral route must first pass through the GI tract and then enter the portal circulation before reaching the systemic circulation; thus, these drugs are less available. The larger the fraction of drug absorbed from the GI tract, the more bioavailable the product will become.

Some drugs vary greatly in their absorption, depending on the physiological conditions. Other factors might also affect drug absorption, such as pH, certain disease states, drug interactions, and aging. Many drugs cannot be given orally because they are destroyed by the strong acids of the stomach. Proteins, such as insulin and hormones, are given only by injection. Other drugs alter the pH either by blocking the acid production of the cell (e.g., proton pump inhibitors) or by acting as buffers, thus reducing the effect of the acid produced.

Absorption and pharmacokinetic studies should be conducted early in the drug evaluation, during pharmacology and toxicology studies, to determine the relationship between systemic drug levels and pharmacological and toxicological effects. Such studies provide insight into the rate and extent of absorption and allow quantitative assessment of the extent and duration of systemic exposure to the drug.

The pharmacological activity and toxicity of drugs should be considered when evaluating the potential of a lead compound as a drug. For orally administered drugs, the form of the drug having the greatest potential for absorption should be selected. Dogs, pigs, and rhesus monkeys all have simple stomachs that can readily accommodate a human-scale dosage formulation. The dog represents the most convenient animal species for conducting biopharmaceutical studies, as unit dosage formulations can be administered and serial blood specimens can be collected.[6]

The most direct way of assessing drug absorption *in vivo* is to compare blood and urinary levels of the parent drug following administration by the intended route and by the intravenous route. If absorption is low, then blood levels of intact drug will differ after extravascular and intravenous administration. The ratio between the areas under the concentration–time curves by the intended route and the intravenous injection indicates the systemic bioavailability and provides a quantitative measure of the extent to which the drug reaches the circulatory system. In addition, the systemic bioavailability of drugs with nonlinear kinetics should be determined at equivalent drug doses by the intended route of administration and by intravenous injection.

An important factor involved in determining body drug concentration is how much of it is bound to plasma protein. The amount of free drug concentration is directly related to the activity of the drug. Thus, the drugs that bind readily to protein may require higher doses to elicit a therapeutic response. Most acidic drugs are bound to serum albumin, whereas many basic drugs bind to alpha-acid glycoprotein. Changes in the number or amount of these binding sites can alter the concentration at the receptor sites.

The patient's nutritional status and age substantially affect the quantity and quality of the plasma proteins present. In elderly and malnourished patients, the plasma albumin may have less affinity for the drug, fewer binding sites available, or smaller volume of distribution. Because of these possible variations, healthy human volunteers, rather than a diseased population, are used in phase I clinical trials. Furthermore, the absorbed materials from the GI tract must pass through the portal circulation before gaining access to the blood circulation. This process exposes the drugs to liver enzymes and to potential metabolism. Some drugs, such as oral nitrates, are removed to a great extent by the hepatic first-pass metabolism; thus, larger doses should be given orally to achieve therapeutic concentrations in the blood. Intestinal flora also cause changes in drug metabolism in the GI tract.

3.3.2 Distribution

Distribution refers to the movement of drug between the water, lipid, and protein constituents or other tissues in the body. Drug distribution is a function of the molecular properties of the product and interaction with the biochemical reactions that drive tissue perfusion. The volume of distribution indicates the ratio of drug concentration in the body to the amount found in plasma. Drug transfer between body compartments is proportional to the amount of drug in the plasma. Drug binding to plasma protein and the quantity of water in the body compartment can significantly affect the volume of distribution. The distribution of a drug and its metabolites and the factors that affect this distribution are important in pharmacokinetic assessment, as the intensity of a pharmacological response and potential toxic effects are related to the concentration of the active component at the site of action. The physical chemical properties of drugs have a major impact on their distribution. When a drug is absorbed, it should reach its target site in sufficient concentration to produce a therapeutic effect. Drug effectiveness is directly proportional to the amount of drug that is distributed to the target site and recognized by the receptor. Pharmacokinetic studies examine how much of the drug disperses throughout the body.

The distribution of drugs depends highly on the lipophilicity of the drugs and the extent to which they are ionized at physiological pH (7.4). Lipophilic drugs are readily transported by passive diffusion across cell membranes and have a high affinity for adipose tissue and lipid components of cells; thus, these drugs are extensively distributed. Weak acids tend to be distributed less extensively than weak bases. Polar compounds do not enter the brain readily because of the endothelial lining that separates the brain from the circulation. Highly polar and ionized drugs are restricted to the vascular system and tend to have low volumes of distribution.

The plasma-protein binding characteristics of drugs should be evaluated to examine the binding capacity of plasma proteins and the affinity of drugs to these proteins. The protein binding must be evaluated over the range of drug concentrations used in pharmacology and safety studies.[7,8] It is useful to conduct competitive protein-binding studies to assess the effects of other drugs on the protein binding of the new drug candidate. A useful method for evaluation of tissue distribution is whole-body autoradiography.[9] In this method, animals are frozen in an organic solvent at predetermined times after administration of radiolabeled drug and embedded in carboxymethylcellulose ice prior to being sectioned in a microtome. Sections of the animal are then examined by x-ray to determine the distribution of radioactivity in the animal.

Disease, age, and genetic defects are the most common factors that affect the sensitivity of the drug receptor — that is, the minimal concentration of a drug that elicits a pharmacological activity. In sensitive patients, less drug is necessary to stimulate the receptor to induce a therapeutic effect. This phenomenon might be caused by genetic modifications, disease states, or other drug interactions.

3.3.3 Metabolism

Metabolism is involved with the chemical process of biotransformation as a mechanism of detox-ification or activation. Drug metabolism is a complex process involving hepatic and other enzymatic system. The duration and intensity of action of lipophilic drugs depend highly on their rate of metabolism. The liver is the main metabolic site. The kidneys, lungs, and other organs are also involved in metabolism.[10] Many drugs form active metabolites; thus, the pharmacological activity induced by the drug is also elicited by its metabolites. Under such situations, the activity of the administered drug is prolonged. Usually, the radioactive-labeled drugs are used to measure the metabolic pathway and formed products.

Liver function is one of the most important factors in metabolism. Several conditions drastically decrease the activity of liver enzymes and prolong the drug effect. Liver function is affected by various factors including disease, age, drug abuse, malnutrition, and smoking. Many biochemical pathways are involved in inactivating drugs and foreign harmful materials. As a result, metabolites are more easily excreted from the body. Certain adverse reactions may result from accumulation of the drug or its metabolites in the liver and other tissues.

The initial phase of metabolism consists of chemical reactions involving oxidation, reduction, and hydrolysis introducing or changing the functional groups (e.g., $-COOH$, $-OH$, $-NH_2$, $-SH_2$), followed by a second phase of synthetic reactions involving conjugations of the drug or its metabolites with endogenous compounds such as glycine or other amino acids, glucuronic acid, and sulfate ions. The resulting conjugates are usually less active than the parent molecules. This process makes the drugs more polar and water soluble, enabling rapid excretion by the kidneys. Differences in metabolism among species may cause difficulty in extrapolating animal pharmacol-ogy and toxicity data to humans.[11] The physical chemical characteristics of drugs are important in evaluating metabolism studies. In general, drugs with low lipid solubility at physiological pH (e.g., several antibiotics and quaternary ammonium drugs) are not metabolized but are eliminated by excretion.[12] In contrast, lipophilic drugs are extensively metabolized and are species dependent with regard to the rate, extent, and pathway of metabolism. It is important to characterize the metabolism and examine factors that may affect the metabolism of these drugs.

Orally administered drugs are absorbed from the small intestine directly through the portal system to the liver. Some drugs may be metabolized in a single passage through the liver or GI tract. This process is referred to as *first-pass metabolism*. In most cases, the bioavailability of orally absorbed drugs is lower than that of drugs given intravenously due to metabolism. Various prodrugs are prepared in order to bypass the breakdown of stomach acid or the first-pass effect. These products are biologically active compounds with their structure modified so they maintain the inactive form and then transform into the active form through metabolism.

3.3.4 Excretion

Excretion is the removal of the drug and its metabolites from the body. Drugs are eliminated from the body primarily through the kidney and liver; however, many other organs may also be involved in the removal process. An assessment of the rate and routes of excretion of a drug and its metabolites is essential during a preclinical drug evaluation. Drugs can be filtered out in the kidney, secreted into the urine, or reabsorbed back into the blood. Renal clearance is the result of filtration through the glomeruli, secretion into the tubules, and reabsorption from the tubules. The rate of renal elimination depends on the renal blood flow, protein-binding capacity, and the physical chemical properties of the drug molecules. After filtration into the renal tubules, lipid-soluble drugs are often reabsorbed back into the bloodstream, depending on their ionization constants.

Kidney dysfunction can result in decreased drug elimination and consequent toxicity. Due to reduced states of cardiac output, aging, and disease, the glomerular filtration rate (GFR) and tubular secretions are reduced, resulting in higher serum drug concentrations. Renal clearance can be accurately measured by collecting 24-hour urine samples to determine the creatine content. In clinical laboratory testing, creatinine clearance is partially determined by measurement of the serum creatinine level. Creatinine clearance is a more sensitive indicator of kidney function than using only the serum creatinine level. The half-life of a drug is the amount of time required to remove 50% of the drug from the body and is commonly used to express the elimination rate of a new drug.[13]

Although fewer drugs are excreted in the bile than in urine, the hepatobiliary system ranks next in importance to the kidney as an excretory organ. Drugs that are distributed to the bile are secreted into the small intestine and then reabsorbed. Biliary excretion often involves drugs and conjugates of metabolites with large molecules. Drugs excreted in urine and bile are usually unbound; as a result, free drug concentrations in the urinary and biliary tract are several times higher than in blood. Excretion of drugs through the saliva is used as a noninvasive monitoring of drug concentrations in the body. The physicochemical properties of drugs and physiological conditions play important roles in determining the extent of drug elimination through extrarenal routes.

REFERENCES

1. Wasan, K.M., Peteherych, K.D., Najafi, S. et al., Assessing the plasma pharmacokinetics, tissue distribution, excretion and effects on cholesterol pharmacokinetics of a novel hydrophilic compound, FM-VP4, following administration to rats, *J. Pharm. Pharm. Sci.*, 4(3), 207–216, 2001.

2. Johnson, K., Shah, A., Tsai, S.J. et al., Metabolism, pharmacokinetics, and excretion of a highly selective *N*-methyl-D-aspartate receptor antagonist, Traxoprodil, in human cytochrome P450 2D6 extensive and poor metabolizers, *Drug Metab. Dispos.*, 31, 76–87, 2003.

3. Chiou, W.L., Ma., C., Chung, S.M. et al., Similarity in the linear and non-linear oral absorption of drugs between human and rat, *Int. J. Clin. Pharm. Ther.*, 38, 532–539, 2000.

4. Chiou, W.L., Jeong, H.Y., Chung, S.M., and Wu, T.C., Evaluation of using dog as an animal model to study the fraction of oral close absorbed of 43 drugs in humans, *Pharm. Res.*, 17, 135–140, 2000.

5. Ariens, E.J., Receptor theory and structure–action relationships, *Adv. Drug Res.*, 3, 235–285, 1966.

6. Adams, W.J., Animal models and their role in bioequivalence studies, in *Generics and Bioequivalence*, Jackson, A.J., Ed., CRC Press, Boca Raton, FL, 1994, pp. 137–177.

7. Chignell, C.F., in *Drug Fate and Metabolism*, Vol. 1, Garrett, E.R. and Hirtz, J.L., Eds., Marcel Dekker, New York, 1978, pp. 187–228.

8. Davidson, C., in *Fundamentals of Drug Metabolism and Drug Disposition*, LaDu, B.N., Mandel, H.G., and Way, E.L., Eds., Williams & Wilkins, Baltimore, MD, 1971, pp. 63–75.

9. Waddell, W.J. and Marlowe, C., Autoradiography, in *Drug Fate and Metabolism*, Vol. 1, Garrett, E.R. and Hirtz, J.L., Eds., Marcel Dekker, New York, 1977, pp. 1–25.

10. Selen, A., Factors influencing bioavailability and bioequivalence, in *Pharmaceutical Bioequivalence*, Welling, P.G., Tse, F.L.S., and Dighe, S.V., Eds., Marcel Dekker, New York, 1991, pp. 117–148.

11. Williams, R.T., in *Fundamentals of Drug Metabolism and Drug Disposition*, LaDu, B.N., Mandel, H.G., and Way, E.L., Eds., Williams & Wilkins, Baltimore, MD, 1971, pp. 187–205.

12. Renwick, A.G., in *Biological Basis of Detoxification*, Caldwell, J. and Jakoby, W.B., Eds., Academic Press, San Diego, CA, pp. 151–179, 1983.

13. Hussein, G. and Bleidt, B., Pharmacokinetics: interactions of new drugs and the human body, in *Clinical Research in Pharmaceutical Development*, Bleidt, B. and Montagne, M., Eds., Marcel Dekker, New York, 1997, pp. 109–124.

CHAPTER 4

Animal Tests as Predictors of Human Response

Peter I. Folb

CONTENTS

4.1 INTRODUCTION

The purpose of this chapter is to place in context, and to set out in broad scope, the place of preclinical animal testing of new chemical entities in the scientific development of medicines. Two interlinked themes emerge. First, early animal testing provides a special and indispensable opportunity for developing proof of concept of novel drugs, on the basis of which efficacy, safety, and quality can subsequently be established in appropriate human studies. Second, and in qualification of the first, it has been increasingly recognized that there are strict limits to the extent to which animal data can be extrapolated to human experience — limits that are determined by the pharmacokinetics, pharmacodynamics, and genetic, immunological, and metabolic responses that may be special and even unique to individual species. The International Conference on Harmonisation (ICH) of Technical Requirements for Registration of Pharmaceuticals for Human Use has set out guidelines for the use of healthy animals and animal models of disease in predicting drug action and safety in humans. An important, and useful, aspect of the ICH approach has been to stress the need for pragmatism in planning animal studies in new drug development. Equally important have been the efforts of animal ethicists and the general public in insisting on careful, strict, and limited use of animals in drug testing.

Many serious toxic reactions caused by new chemical entities may reliably be detected by routine toxicological testing. Experience has shown that predictable dose- and time-dependent reactions are likely to be revealed in animal experiments. It is the detail of these that forms the basis of the experimental toxicology applied to new drug development. Unpredictable idiosyncratic adverse effects, not related to time of administration or dose, are considerably more difficult to identify in preclinical drug evaluation. The focus of what follows is on the former; the latter remains a challenge to drug development science, as does the comprehensive preclinical testing of biopharmaceuticals (including vaccines) in animals, with particular reference to prediction of safety. Tests routinely employed in the past that are wasteful and that have (or should have) been superseded by more thoughtful alternatives (the LD_{50} and Draize tests are examples) should become obsolete and are dealt with in this chapter accordingly.

4.2 LIMITS TO EXTRAPOLATING ANIMAL DATA IN PREDICTING THE HUMAN RESPONSE

The limits to extrapolating animal toxicology data to prediction of the human response, with special reference to safety, include the following:[2,68]

- Pharmacokinetic differences between the test animals and humans
- Idiosyncratic adverse events in humans, the mechanisms of which are not understood and are not demonstrable in animals by ordinary toxicological and pharmacological investigation

- Underlying pathological condition — drugs may exacerbate underlying diseases in humans that do not exist in animals; relationships that exist between the drug and its metabolites, on the one hand, and underlying disease, on the other, cannot adequately be investigated or predicted from studies conducted in healthy animals
- Species differences in anatomy and physiological functions and in tolerance and enzyme induction
- Adverse drug events that can only be communicated verbally and are not normally recognized in animals

4.3 ACUTE TOXICITY TESTING

Acute exposure of experimental animals to a toxic agent may express itself directly in one or more tissues or systemically after absorption from a local site.

4.3.1 Direct Toxic Effects on Tissues

The skin, eyes, gastrointestinal mucosa, vagina, and respiratory tract are the most susceptible to topical toxic effects of drugs. When a substance is known to be locally irritant or corrosive it is not necessary for animal tests to be conducted to confirm what is already established. On the other hand, local irritation may be influenced by the conditions of exposure, such as local pH. Topical toxicity testing is required to determine this. The ICH has set out general guidelines for nonclinical local tolerance testing.[5] Testing should distinguish mechanical aspects of administration or purely physicochemical actions of the compound from toxicological or pharmacodynamic ones. This refers particularly to skin testing for dermatological products and ocular testing for ophthalmological medicines. Acute toxicity testing should be by a route of administration that allows for adequate systemic exposure, except when systemic absorption will be low or when the product is absorbed systemically and its systemic toxicity has been previously investigated. Usually only one animal species must be tested. Frequency and duration of administration are determined according to the anticipated use of the drug. Duration of exposure normally does not exceed 4 weeks. Evaluation of reversibility should be included. Controls are the vehicle or excipients, and positive controls should be used where possible. The same actual concentrations should be used in animal tests as are proposed for use in humans. The overriding concern governing acute toxicity testing in animals is to minimize painful and traumatic exposure and to terminate experiments when severe adverse reactions are noted.

4.3.1.1 Skin

To evaluate the degree of skin irritation that may be exerted by a potentially toxic substance it is necessary to examine the effect in human subjects. Due to enormous variability in the response of the skin of different animal species to toxic chemicals, there is little value in skin irritancy testing that requires extrapolation of findings from one species to another. When dermal tolerance testing in animals is considered justified, a single-dose dermal tolerance test is normally conducted in the rabbit on both shaved intact skin and shaved abraded skin. The exposed skin is examined for erythema, edema, desquamation, scab formation, and other lesions, with changes being noted at 24, 48, and 72 hours. It may be necessary to follow up for up to 8 days. Repeated-dose dermal tolerance testing is usually conducted in rabbits, on both intact and abraded shaved skin, for periods of up to 4 weeks.[5]

4.3.1.2 Eyes

Any chemical with irritant or corrosive properties when applied to the skin is also likely to be an irritant to the cornea and conjunctiva, and in these cases it is not necessary to carry out ocular irritancy tests. The most widely used test for prediction of ophthalmological irritancy is still the Draize test in rabbits,[14] although the test is now widely regarded as having become obsolete because it is unduly injurious to the experimental animals concerned. When local ocular toxicity and tolerance testing is required for products due to be used by topical application to the eye or close to the eye, such as the face or hair (including medicated shampoos), single administration is usually applied in the rabbit. The test should include examination for anesthetizing properties. When repeat ocular dosing is indicated, testing should be by daily administration in the rabbit for not more than 4 weeks. In single-dose testing, evaluation of the eyes, lids, conjunctivae, nictitating membrane, cornea, and iris in one eye is necessary, with the other eye serving as a control. Repeated-dose ocular toxicity testing should take into account the results of the acute, single-dose outcome.*

4.3.1.3 Mucosal Surfaces

Irritancy testing of mucosal surfaces is necessary when substances are intended for application to surfaces such as the vagina, where local factors such as pH have to be considered. Little difference exists between species and between individuals in mucosal responses to toxic injury.

4.3.2 Lethal Dose 50 (LD$_{50}$) Test**

The LD$_{50}$ test[47,51,71] is aimed at determining the dose of a toxic substance that kills 50% of the animals that receive it. The LD$_{50}$ test has formed a standard part of the early assessment of a new medicine, on the grounds that it allows precise study of the nature of the acute toxicity of a compound; however, the concept of killing animals in this way has proved objectionable to many, necessitating a critical review of the justification for the test.

4.3.2.1 Value of the LD$_{50}$ Test

The value of the LD$_{50}$ test in acute toxicity testing is twofold.[47] First, it makes it possible to determine the therapeutic margin — the margin between effective and toxic doses. Compounds can be compared, allowing for those with the widest margin of safety to be selected for further development. When significant species variation is found, this is regarded as having implications for human use. Second, the test makes it possible for lethal effects to be compared with blood levels of the active principle and with the findings obtained in repeated-dose studies (toxicokinetic evaluation).

---

* Kaufman[35] has pointed out the problems with the Draize test and the argument for an alternative approach from the perspective of an ophthalmologist. Besides the general doubt that the test has application in clinical medicine, Kaufman points out in some detail the fundamental anatomical differences between the rabbit and human eyelid, tearing mechanism, and cornea. These include: (1) the rabbit epithelial surface layer is tenfold more permeable to hydrophilic solutes than the human eye; (2) Bowman's layer (the next layer) is six times thicker in humans; (3) the rabbit's threshold of pain in the eye is much higher than that of humans, so irritating substances are not washed away as readily; (4) rabbits have a less efficient tearing system than humans; (5) unlike humans, rabbits have a nictitating (winking) membrane (a third eyelid), which has an unclear effect on elimination of foreign materials; (6) humans develop corneal epithelial vacuoles in response to some toxic substances, while rabbits do not; (7) the rabbit mean corneal thickness is 0.37 mm, while that of humans is 0.51 mm; (8) rabbits are more susceptible to damage from alkaline materials because the pH of their aqueous humor is 8.2 compared with 7.1 to 7.3 in humans; and (9) the cornea represents 25% of the rabbit eye surface area and only 7% of the surface area in humans. For these reasons, Kaufman suggests, correlation between the Draize test and actual human experience is weak. Moreover, it is argued, the severity of the rabbit eye response predicts poorly the degree of human ocular injury. The Draize rabbit eye irritation test has never been validated against a reported human database. The position of the United Kingdom on the Draize test has been explained in the House of Commons.[28] The government of the United Kingdom has placed a ban on testing cosmetic products and ingredients by the Draize test. Testing of noncosmetic products, such as medical eye drops, in this manner is still allowed. Such animal testing only takes place after *in vitro* screening tests have been used to identify, classify, and eliminate materials with obvious irritant potential. The Draize test is not carried out on strongly acid or alkaline substances, on substances demonstrated to have severe adverse skin effects in dermal tests, or on substances that have potential corrosive effects or severe irritancy in the alternative tests currently available. The Draize test is not permitted in some states in Australia.

** The LD$_{50}$ test identifies the single lethal dose of a substance that kills half the animals in a test group. It is becoming obsolete but has traditionally been used to: (1) classify substances or products for regulatory purposes, (2) provide information for treatment of acute intoxications, (3) standardize biological products, (4) set dose levels for subsequent toxicity studies, (5) provide comparative information on the dose–response curve, and (6) provide data for evaluation and validation of alternative test methods (see NIH Recommendations at www.iacuc.cwru.edu/policy/nihpolicies).

4.3.2.2 Limits to Extrapolation

The objections that have been raised to the LD_{50} test and the caveats to extrapolation of data derived from it should be carefully considered.[71] Even when conducted with care, the results of the LD_{50} test must be regarded as an isolated finding and considered in conjunction with other findings from acute toxicity testing. Zbinden and Flury-Roversi[71] have suggested the following guidelines for the LD_{50} test, and these are now widely accepted.

- LD_{50} data should always be considered in conjunction with other relevant information, not in isolation.
- Conducting the LD_{50} test on large animals should be discontinued; a test on a limited number of small animals, including detailed recording of symptoms and pathology, should be done instead.
- No LD_{50} test should be conducted with pharmacologically inert substances (a maximum dose of 5 g/kg for oral administration and 2 g/kg for parenteral administration should be sufficient if death or acute symptoms are not produced).
- The test should not be conducted in newborn animals.

In summary, the LD_{50} test represents a comparatively small part of the information that can be gained from acute toxicity studies. If the LD_{50} test is carefully performed, with appropriate concern for the humane issues that should be associated with it, it can provide useful information on the biological and toxicological properties of a new chemical entity; however, alternative tests are proving to be equally useful.

Instead of the LD_{50} test, two alternative animal tests have significantly improved the prospects of animal welfare: the acute toxic class method and the limit test procedure. The acute toxic class method is a stepwise procedure that uses three animals of a single sex per step. Depending on mortality or the moribund status of the animals, on average two to four steps may be necessary to allow judgment on the acute toxicity of the test substance. This procedure is reproducible, uses few animals, and is able to rank substances in a manner similar to other acute toxicity testing methods. The acute toxic class method is based on biometric evaluations with fixed doses sufficiently separated to enable a substance to be ranked for classification purposes and hazard assessment. The absence or presence of compound-related mortality of the animals dosed at one step will determine the next step: (1) no further testing, (2) dosing of three additional animals with the same dose, or (3) dosing of three additional animals at the next higher or lower dose level. The method has been validated *in vivo* against LD_{50} data obtained from the literature (see the Organisation for Economic Cooperation and Development's *Guidelines for Testing Chemicals*, adopted December 17, 2001; www.oecd.og).

The limit test is primarily used in situations where prior information indicates that the test material is likely to be nontoxic, with toxicity only above regulatory limit doses. Information about the toxicity of the test material can be gained from similar previously tested compounds or similar tested mixtures or products, taking into account the identity and percentage of compounds known to be of toxicological significance. A limit test at one dose level of 2000 mg/kg body weight may be carried out with six animals (three animals per step). Exceptionally, a limit test at one dose level of 5000 mg/kg may be carried out with three animals. If test-substance-related mortality is produced, further testing at the next lower dose level may be necessary. A chemical may be regarded as having an equivalent LD_{50} of 4000 mg/kg or higher when no mortality occurs at 2000 mg/kg. A chemical with such low toxicity does not require further testing for lethal effects. This method obviates the need for a full LD_{50} test.[67] In the guidelines of the U.S. Environmental Protection Agency,[72] 2000 mg/kg is an acceptable limit test for the dermal route, and 5000 mg/kg for the oral route. This simple test permits important information such as signs of intoxication, identification of target organs, and reversibility of toxicity to be obtained from careful observation in a small number of animals.

4.3.3   Fixed-Dose Oral Toxicity Testing

In an international study involving 33 laboratories in 11 countries, the acute oral toxicity in rats of 20 substances was evaluated using a fixed-dose procedure.[59] The results were compared with those obtained for test materials using the standard LD_{50} test. The study showed that fixed-dose testing makes possible the following: (1) consistent results that are not seriously affected by interlaboratory variation; (2) adequate information for risk assessment of acute toxicity, including its nature, time to onset, duration, and outcome, for the substances concerned; (3) use of fewer animals than the current internationally agreed-upon procedures; (4) less pain and distress to the animals than the LD_{50} test, as well as less compound-related mortality; and (5) ranking according to standard classification systems and to acute oral toxicity, such ranking being consistent with that achieved by standard LD_{50} testing.

4.3.4   Testing for Systemic Toxicity

Systemic effects resulting from short-term exposure to chemicals may develop either rapidly or after delayed onset, and the result may be transient, prolonged, or irreversible. The systemic toxicity of any substance is likely to be determined by the combined effects of the exposure, route of administration, and physical presentation of the product. For an animal model to provide meaningful results it should be comparable physiologically with humans, and toxicokinetic (pharmacokinetic) similarities should be observed between the new chemical entity in the test animal and in humans.

4.4 LONG-TERM (CHRONIC) TOXICITY TESTING

The principles underpinning long-term toxicity testing in animals are well established.[1,9,20,24,34,43,50,65,66] For many years, the value of such testing has been seriously questioned, and it has been hoped that a more complete understanding of the relevant pharmacology and of the physiological changes caused by acute exposure to a new drug might provide sufficient information to anticipate adverse long-term effects. It was thought that in this way animal testing might be replaced or at least considerably reduced. That has not been achieved, and there remains for the time being much to be done in seeking an alternative. Dayan[9] pointed out that with repeated-dose testing most structural lesions that are likely to be produced should be identifiable, and that knowledge can also be gained of functional disturbances, although the latter are unlikely to be quantifiable. Long-term animal studies only partly reveal functional disorders, and the influence on toxicity of drugs of factors such as aging, disease, and diet remains uncertain.

4.4.1   Mechanisms of Drug Injury from Long-Term Exposure

In planning and evaluating long-term toxicity studies in animals, several possible mechanisms of drug injury are considered:[43]

- Accumulation of the parent drug or its metabolites in the tissues, with consequent toxic injury
- Repeated or low-grade continuous injury to DNA or to the hereditable DNA expression during cell differentiation
- Disturbance of the adaptive synthesis of cell receptors
- Damage to repair responses, rendering such an animal sensitive to an additional toxic insult

4.4.2   Dose Considerations

The normal practice is to employ a minimum of three treatment groups, divided according to dose, and one control group. An additional group may be added if it is necessary to examine a toxic effect in relation to a particular dose. The lowest dose is conventionally set at the equivalent of five times the projected therapeutic dose to establish a nontoxic dose level. The mid-dose usually represents the geometric mean between the low and high doses, but pharmacokinetic considerations have to be considered when selecting this. The high-dose level is calculated so as to identify toxic effects but not to a degree that might jeopardize successful completion of the study.

4.4.3 Frequency of Administration

In general, adequate exposure of the experimental animal to a drug is achieved by once-daily dosing, 7 days a week, but more frequent administration may be necessary for drugs with a very short half-life or brief duration of action.

4.4.4 Route of Administration

The route of administration in animal studies of an investigational new drug should ideally be the same as that proposed for clinical use.[34] This can be problematic if a high dose is required that cannot be tolerated when given by a particular route. If use of an alternative route is unavoidable, comparative pharmacokinetic data will be required.

4.4.5 Duration of Study*

In rodents, the number of incidental (spontaneous) lesions begins to rise from 15 to 18 months of age onward.[9] This reduces the discriminatory power of any study by reason of the lesions themselves and the impairment that they might cause to the usual response of the animals. In the dog and primate (and other nonrodent species), on the other hand, an 18-month-old animal might not yet have reached the pubertal stage of development.

4.5 PHARMACOKINETICS AND TOXICOKINETICS**

4.5.1 General Principles

Pharmacokinetic results from single-dose kinetic studies may help in the choice of formulation and in prediction of the rate and duration of exposure during a dosing interval. This may assist in the selection of appropriate dose levels for use in later studies. The treatment regimen and species should be selected whenever possible with regard to pharmacodynamic and pharmacokinetic principles. This may not be achievable for the very first studies, at a time when neither animal nor human pharmacokinetic data are available. Toxicokinetics should be incorporated appropriately into the design of the studies.

4.5.2 Specific Aspects of Toxicokinetics Testing

Toxicokinetics is the generation of pharmacokinetic data to assess systemic exposure, either as an integral component in the conduct of nonclinical toxicity studies or as specially designed supportive studies. The data may be used in interpretation of toxicology findings and their relevance to clinical

---

* Glockin[24] has explained the FDA requirement for 12-month, long-term animal toxicity studies (both rodent and nonrodent studies). The study should be extended beyond 12 months when warranted by a specific concern or by an unusual condition of use. Lumley and Walker[42] and Worden[65] have suggested that a 6-month study should be sufficient to establish the toxicity profile of new drugs, and that no-effect levels can also be predicted within that period. This is only true if reliance is not placed solely on histopathological changes.

** This section is based on the Guidelines for Industry developed within the Expert Working Group (Safety) of the ICH which can be found at http://www.nihs.go.jp/dig/ich/safety (CDER FTP of the FDA: CDVS2.CDER.FDA.GOV).

safety. Toxicokinetic data focus on the kinetics of a new therapeutic agent under the conditions of toxicity studies. Toxicokinetic data enhance the value of the toxicological data in terms of both understanding the toxicity tests and comparing results with clinical data. The emphasis is on interpretation of toxicity tests and not on characterizing the pharmacokinetic parameters of the substance studied. No rigid detailed procedures for conducting toxicokinetic studies are recommended. In addition to the principal objective of describing the systemic exposure achieved and its relationship to dose and the time course, the study relates drug exposure in toxicity studies to toxicity findings, thus contributing to assessment of the relevance of the findings to clinical safety. It further supports the choice of species and treatment regimen in nonclinical toxicity studies and provides information which, in conjunction with toxicity studies, contributes to the design of subsequent studies. These objectives may be achieved by the derivation of one or more of the following measurements made at appropriate time points: plasma (or whole blood or serum) AUC, C_{max}, and $C_{(time)}$, which are the most commonly used in assessing exposure. Toxicity studies that usefully support toxicokinetic information are single- and repeated-dose toxicity studies and reproductive, genotoxicity, and carcinogenicity studies. Toxicokinetic information may also be of value in assessing the implications of a proposed change in the clinical route of administration. Toxicokinetic monitoring may also serve to alert to nonlinear, dose-related changes in exposure that may have occurred. Toxicokinetic information allows for better interspecies comparisons than simple dose/body weight (or surface area) comparisons.

4.5.3 Repeated-Dose Tissue Distribution Studies*

Tissue distribution studies provide information on the distribution and accumulation of the test compound and metabolites, especially in relation to their potential sites of action. Repeated-dose tissue distribution studies are considered when:

- Single-dose distribution studies suggest that the half-life of the test compound (or metabolites) in organs or tissues significantly exceeds the apparent half-life of the elimination phase in plasma or is also more than twice the dosing interval in the toxicity studies.
- Steady-state levels of a compound or metabolite in the circulation, determined in repeated-dose pharmacokinetic or toxicokinetic studies, are markedly higher than those predicted from single-dose kinetic studies.
- Histopathological changes are observed that would not be predicted from short-term toxicity studies or from single-dose tissue distribution and pharmacological studies. Those organs or tissues that were sites of the lesions should be the focus of such studies.
- The pharmaceutical is being developed for site-specific targeted delivery, so repeated-dose tissue distribution studies may be appropriate.

---

* The following principles underpin the setting of dose levels: (1) At a low dose, preferably a no-toxic-effect dose level, the exposure in any toxicity study should ideally equal or just exceed the maximum expected dose (or known to be attained) in patients. (2) Exposure at intermediate dose levels should normally represent an appropriate multiple or fraction of the exposure at lower (or higher) dose levels, depending on the objectives of the toxicity study. (3) The high dose levels in toxicity studies are normally determined by toxicological considerations. (Careful attention should be paid to interpretation of toxicological findings when the dose levels result in nonlinear kinetics; nevertheless, toxicokinetics can be very helpful in assessing the relationship between dose and exposure in this situation.) (4) The toxicokinetic strategy to be adopted for alternative routes of administration should be based on the pharmacokinetic properties of the substance administered by the intended route. The toxicokinetic profile helps to determine whether changing the clinical route will significantly reduce the safety margin. (5) A primary objective is to describe the systemic exposure to the administered compound in the species examined. In some circumstances measurement of metabolite concentrations in plasma or other body fluids is especially important in the conduct of toxicokinetics — for example, when the administered compound acts as a prodrug and the delivered metabolite is acknowledged to be the primary active entity; when the compound is metabolized to one or more pharmacologically or toxicologically active metabolites that could make a significant contribution to tissue or organ responses; or when the administered compound is extensively metabolized and the measurement of plasma or tissue concentrations of a major metabolite is the only practical means of estimating the drug exposure following administration.

Table 4.1 Duration of Studies Required in Repeated-Dose Toxicity Testing To Support Phase I and II Trials in the European Union and Phase I, II, and III Trials in the United States and Japan

Duration of Clinical Trials	Minimum Duration of Repeated-Dose Toxicity Studies	
	Rodents	Nonrodents
Single dose	2 weeks[a]	2 weeks
Up to 2 weeks	2 weeks[a]	2 weeks
Up to 1 month	1 month	1 month
Up to 3 months	3 months	3 months
Up to 6 months	6 months	6 months
>6 months	6 months	Chronic

[a] In the United States, as an alternative to 2-week studies, single-dose toxicity studies with extended examinations can support single-dose human trials.

Source: CPMP, *Non-Clinical Safety Studies for the Conduct of Human Clinical Trials for Pharmaceuticals*, CPMP/ICH/286/95 (modification), Committee for Proprietary Medicinal Products, European Agency for the Evaluation of Medicinal Products, London, 2000.

Table 4.2 Duration of Repeated-Dose Toxicity Studies To Support Phase III Trials in the European Union and Marketing in All Regions

Duration of Clinical Trials	Minimum Duration of Repeated-Dose Toxicity Studies	
	Rodents	Nonrodents
Up to 2 weeks	1 month	1 month
Up to 1 month	3 months	3 months
Up to 3 months	6 months	3 months
>3 months	6 months	Chronic

Source: CPMP, *Non-Clinical Safety Studies for the Conduct of Human Clinical Trials for Pharmaceuticals*, CPMP/ICH/286/95 (modification), Committee for Proprietary Medicinal Products, European Agency for the Evaluation of Medicinal Products, London, 2000.

4.4.5 Duration of Studies

The durations of studies required in repeated-dose toxicity testing to support phase I and II trials in the European Union (EU) and phase I, II, and III trials in the United States and Japan are set out in Table 4.1. The durations of repeated-dose toxicity studies to support phase III trials in the EU and marketing in all regions are set out in Table 4.2.

4.6 CARCINOGENICITY TESTING

Several considerations guide preclinical testing for carcinogenicity of a new chemical entity, including:[73]

- Tumors develop spontaneously, in animals and humans, with varying frequency, and allowance must be made for this in the interpretation of results.
- Many different types of tumors affect different organs and tissues; the pattern of pathological response to any particular carcinogen may differ from animal to animal and from humans to animals.

- Technical factors, such as dosage, frequency of administration, and duration of action of the test substance, and the actual interpretation of results may have different relevance in humans and test animals.
- Carcinogenic action in humans frequently involves ill-defined mixtures of substances and ancillary factors distinct from carcinogenesis caused by single, pure compounds.

Suspicion is attached to a particular substance when epidemiological data point to an association, when structural resemblances to known carcinogens are observed, when the drug has hormone-like or tissue-growth promoting effects, when the drug has mutagenic or antimitotic activity, or when other suggestive toxicity data exist.

Testing for the carcinogenic potential of a new chemical entity should be guided by consideration of a number of issues that include the intended patient population, clinical dosage regimen, dose–response effects, selectivity in animals and in humans, and the outcome of repeated-dose toxicology studies. If the latter indicate immunosuppressant properties, hormonal activity, or other activity considered to be a risk factor for humans, this information should be considered in the design of further studies of carcinogenic potential.[6]* The choice of animal tested is based on considerations of pharmacology, repeated-dose toxicology, metabolism, toxicokinetics, and route of administration. In the absence of clear evidence favoring one species, it is recommended that the rat be selected. If the results of a carcinogenicity study and of genotoxicity tests and other data indicate that a substance clearly poses a carcinogenic hazard to humans, a second carcinogenicity study would not usually be helpful.[6]

The majority of human carcinogens have also been shown to be carcinogenic in animals, and virtually all, when tested appropriately, induce cancer in several animal species.[23,27,30,36,49,63] It is not unusual for 80 to 100% of test animals to be affected within a latent period of 12 to 18 months. Human carcinogens that are genotoxic (most are) also reliably display activity in standard short-term *in vitro* mutagenicity tests.

Conversely, a chemical that is (1) consistently genotoxic in a number (not just one) of short-term *in vitro* tests, (2) active in several *in vivo* bioassay systems (giving a high yield of tumors with a latent period of less than 18 months), and (3) active over a range of dose levels is a probable human cancer risk. On the other hand, when an unknown test chemical is active only in a single bioassay system or in a small number of *in vitro* systems, its classification as a genotoxin and potential carcinogen requires careful analysis of the positive and negative data. It may be that in the intact mammalian system (that is, in the whole animal) biochemical defense systems adequately protect against reactive radicals, giving a negative test result despite evidence of genotoxicity that may be found with *in vitro* testing.[63]

The ICH has proposed that conducting one long-term carcinogenicity study (rather than two long-term studies), using a "weight of evidence" approach whereby the use of scientific judgment is used in evaluation of the totality of the data, along with other appropriate experimental investigations should enhance the assessment of carcinogenic risk to humans while reducing the extent and number of animals used for the purpose.[6]

For biotechnology-derived pharmaceuticals, standard carcinogenicity bioassays are generally not required;[7] however, in certain product-specific cases concerns about carcinogenic potential (such

---

* In general, the following are regarded as indicative of carcinogenic potential, justifying further animal testing: suggestive cellular changes such as apoptosis, cell proliferation, liver foci of cellular alteration, or changes in intercellular communication; biochemical effects such as actions on plasma hormone levels, growth factors, binding to proteins such as alpha-2u globulin, and tissue enzyme activity; suggestive effects on the P-450 enzymes that mediate biotransformation of drugs; and metabolism of the pharmaceutical in the animal model that might affect the carcinogenic risk for humans. The latter effects are more likely to be found in testing rats than mice. In some special circumstances, however, the mouse would be preferred to the rat as the more appropriate species for human carcinogenicity risk assessment. The overall "weight of evidence" would take into account the scientific status of the test systems, tumor incidence and latency, pharmacokinetics of the drug in the rodent models compared with humans, and data from ancillary or mechanistic studies.[53]

as growth factors, immunosuppressive agents, etc.) would justify special testing to evaluate risk. The *in vitro* potential to support or induce proliferation of transformed cells and clonal expansion, possibly leading to neoplasia, justifies further studies in relevant animal models. When other studies do not make possible an adequate assessment of carcinogenic potential, testing in a single rodent species might be considered. A rationale should be provided for the selection of doses.[7]

4.6.1 *In Vivo* Carcinogenicity Testing

The most practical investigations for predicting chemical carcinogenesis in humans are those in which mitotic lesions are induced in the livers of rats, skin tumors in mice, mammary tumors in female rats, and pulmonary tumors in certain sensitive strains of mice. The majority of such tumors are induced in less than a year. The test compound is compared with a known positive control, at several dose levels, so as to provide an estimate of the dose–response relationship. Agents thought to act as promoters are administered together with a genotoxic carcinogen appropriate for the relevant target organ. The test substance is administered in four or five dose levels. Comparison with the appropriate positive control provides an indication of the relative potency of the test substance. Some authorities[23,36] have pointed out how important it is in the evaluation of the data to conduct a comprehensive pathological and toxicological assessment of individual animals in carcinogenicity testing, including comparison with controls and evaluation of case histories. The response in intact experimental animals reflects at best a potential for human risk, but not an order of risk.[56]

4.6.2 Database for Carcinogenicity Risk Assessment

A global database is required for the carcinogenicity risk assessment of new chemical entities that includes the following: (1) structure–activity relationships of the chemical and its similarity to known carcinogens, (2) known results of short-term genotoxicity tests, and (3) outcome of *in vivo* studies in which evidence is sought in mice, rats, or hamsters of a statistically significant incidence of cancer. (Whole-animal studies would be selected on the basis of comprehensive assessment of the probable mechanisms of action, whether genotoxic or promoting, of the chemical under consideration.) Carcinogenesis is often organ specific, as a result of the formation of locally produced reactive metabolites. It is highly improbable that any human carcinogen would yield negative results for all three components of such a screening procedure.

4.6.3 Special Considerations in Extrapolating Carcinogenicity Data

Purchase[49] found in a study of the carcinogenicity potential of 250 compounds that both the specificity (prediction of carcinogenicity) and the sensitivity (prediction of noncarcinogenicity) in rat and mouse studies are approximately 85%. Of the chemicals studied, 64% consistently produced cancer at the same site. The chemical and the host are each involved in the expression of a carcinogen. Potency may vary between hosts, depending on tumor type, nutritional status, environmental conditions, and other variables. This explains any differences between laboratories and between test systems. It is generally accepted that chemicals should be tested under constraints that minimize the number of false-negative results. The maximum dose chosen is usually larger than the dose that is likely to be given to humans. Results from animal studies are extrapolated to humans on the (erroneous) assumption that the most sensitive outcome from the most sensitive species is appropriate to humans and that a simple quantitative correlation can be made. Animal data are neither quantitatively nor qualitatively reliable for such extrapolation, and the dose–response relationship cannot be assumed to be linear at low levels of exposure.

4.7 IMMUNOTOXICOLOGY EVALUATION*

Routine assessment should be made of any adverse effects on immune function of investigational new drugs. This includes immunosuppression (effects on the immune system that result in decreased immune function), immunogenicity (immune reactions elicited by the drug or its metabolites), hypersensitivity (immunological sensitization due to the drug or its metabolites), autoimmunity (immune reactions to self-antigens), and adverse immunostimulation (activation of immune system effector mechanisms). Any results suggestive of adverse immune effects observed in nonclinical toxicology studies should be further evaluated. When signs consistent with immune suppression are observed in clinical trials, such as drug-related increases in the incidence of infections, conducting appropriate nonclinical studies to determine drug effect on immune function might be useful in understanding the clinical data. The CDER recommends that a weight-of-evidence approach should be followed in which all adverse effects observed in nonclinical toxicology studies are considered in determining whether follow-up immune studies should be conducted. The latter include treatment parameters (dose, duration, route of administration), degree of change in immunological measurements, numbers of studies, different species in which adverse effects are observed, and number of concurrent immune-related adverse effects.

In standard nonclinical toxicology studies, indicators of immunosuppression include evidence of:

- Myelosuppression, such as pancytopenia, leucopenia, lymphopenia, or other blood dyscrasias
- Alterations in immune system organ weights and histology (for example, hypocellularity of immune system tissues such as the thymus, spleen, lymph nodes, or bone marrow)
- Decreased globulin levels
- Increased incidence of infections or increased incidence of tumors

Where possible in repeated-dose toxicology studies, organ weights and histological examination should be conducted on the spleen, thymus, lymph nodes, and bone marrow. The lymphoid tissue that drains or contacts the site of drug administration (and therefore is exposed to the highest concentration of the drug) should be specifically examined. When effects suggestive of immune suppression are observed, such as depletion or hyperplasia in lymph nodes or splenic white pulp or changes in cortical (T-cell) or medullary (B-cell) areas, these should be noted.** Other indicators of immune suppression in nonclinical toxicology include treatment-related infections and lymphoproliferative tumors. Infections caused by weakly pathogenic organisms may be an indicator of immune suppression.

With regard to their immunogenicity, drugs can be grouped into two major classes: (1) polypeptides or proteins with molecular weights greater than 10,000, and (2) low-molecular-weight compounds (less than 1000). The former are usually immunogenic if administered to a mammalian species in which the molecule does not naturally occur. Immune responses to smaller peptides or proteins in the 5000 to 10,000 range may also be immunogenic. Immunogenicity is unpredictable for compounds in the 1000 to 5000 range. Low-molecular-weight compounds are immunogenic

---

* This section is based on, and partly reproduced from, the U.S. Food and Drug Administration Center for Drug Evaluation and Research (CDER) document *Immunotoxicology Evaluation of Investigational New Drugs*, dated October 2002.

** Useful information for determining the effects of drugs on immune function has been obtained from assays of natural killer (NK) cell function, *in vitro* blastogenesis, cytotoxic T-cell function, cytokine and chemokine production, delayed-type hypersensitivity response, and host resistance to experimental infections or implanted tumors. Assays for drug effects on various cytokines and chemokines have been used to help understand the mechanism of immunosuppression as well as to identify potential biomarkers useful in clinical trials. Drug-induced suppression of the cutaneous delayed hypersensitivity response to contact allergens such as oxalazolone has been shown to be a sensitive and useful method. Assays might be performed for drug effects on bone marrow progenitor cells, macrophage or neutrophil function, or complement activation. The dose, duration, and route of administration used in functional assays should be consistent, where possible, with the nonclinical toxicology study in which an adverse immune effect was observed. In humans, a decrease of more than 40% in total lymphocytes or 75% in granulocyte counts is regarded as clinically significant.

only if covalently bound to proteins to form hapten–protein complexes (such as sulfonamides or penicillin). Two major concerns in human medicine associated with drug immunogenicity are (1) drug allergenicity, and (2) the ability of antidrug immune responses to alter the biological activities of the drug (pharmacokinetics, pharmacodynamics, or toxicities).

Predictive testing of drug hypersensitivity reactions depends on the type of reaction: type I (immediate), type II (antibody-mediated cytotoxic reactions), type III (immunoglobulin G [IgG]-mediated immune complex reactions), or type IV (T-lymphocyte-mediated–delayed-type hypersensitivity response). A panel of suggested tests has now been identified by CDER and others. Type I reactions should be distinguished from pseudoallergic (anaphylactiod) reactions resulting from activation of inflammatory or anaphylactic mechanisms independent of antigen-specific immune responses. The latter may result from non-immune-mediated histamine release or complement activation, and the reaction is likely to be dose related. There are no known standard methods for determining the potential of experimental drugs to produce autoimmune reactions. If a drug is expected to be used in pregnant women and has been shown to induce immune suppression in adults, incorporation into reproductive toxicology studies should be considered. The effect of maternal drug exposure on lymphoid system organ weights, histology, and hematology in the F1 generation offspring should be included in the terminal examination. If chronic toxicology studies or rodent bioassays indicate carcinogenic potential, determination of a potential role for drug-induced immunosuppression is helpful. Tumor host resistance models may be useful for evaluating the potential role of immunosuppression in carcinogenicity findings.

In the future, it is anticipated that new methods (genomics, proteomics, transgenic animals) will become available for determining useful endpoints for drug safety assessment, especially those tests concerning hypersensitivity, autoimmunity, and photoallergy.

4.8 REPRODUCTIVE AND DEVELOPMENTAL TOXICITY TESTING

The major manifestations of developmental toxicity are (1) death of the developing organism, (2) structural abnormality, (3) altered growth, and (4) functional deficiency. The scope of tests includes determining the effects of the test drug on reproductive competence of adult animals, developmental toxicity (any adverse effect prior to attainment of adult life), embryotoxicity, fetal toxicity, and embryo–fetal toxicity. The testing strategy for reproductive and developmental toxicity should be determined by the following:[29]

- Anticipated drug use, especially in relation to reproduction
- Form of the substance and routes of administration intended for humans
- Any existing data on toxicity, pharmacodynamics, kinetics, and similarity to other compounds in structure or activity

Data on likely human exposure, comparative pharmacokinetics in test animals and in humans, and an understanding of the mechanisms of reproductive toxicity will enable extrapolation of the results to humans. A combination of studies is necessary that allows exposure of mature adults and all stages of development from conception to sexual maturity. To allow detection of immediate and latent effects of exposure, observations should be continued through one complete life-cycle, from conception in one generation through conception in the following generation. Studies should take into account preexisting knowledge of class-related effects on reproduction. Rats are the preferred rodent species because of the large amount of background knowledge already available. The rabbit has been used as a second mammalian species and is required in embryotoxicity studies only.*

---

* If it can be shown, by kinetic, pharmacological, and toxicological studies, that the species is a relevant model for humans, a single species may be sufficient. *In vitro* systems, while reducing the numbers required in experimentation, lack the complexity of the developmental processes and the dynamic interchange between the maternal and the developing organism.[29]

The results of human and animal exposure to teratogens and other reproductive toxins depend precisely on the extent, duration, and time of exposure and on the chemical entity concerned. Any of the following may be found: impaired ability of the female to conceive, abortion, dysmorphogenesis, premature birth, low birth weight, perinatal mortality and morbidity, cancer, and dysfunctional growth and development after birth.[37–39,44,46,64] Hundreds of chemical agents are injurious to the experimental animal. They include poisons, therapeutic agents, and industrial and agricultural chemicals. However, proof of dysmorphogenesis and other teratogenic and reproductive toxic effects on the human fetus as a result of maternal exposure during pregnancy has been shown for only a very small number of chemicals: thalidomide, androgens, virilizing progestagens, cytotoxic drugs, antithyroid drugs, and certain anticonvulsants. For a number of reasons, reproductive toxicity data derived from animal experiments have inherent limitations in their application to humans. These include the following:

- Species differences exist between test animals and humans in drug distribution and action and in tissue and organ responses.
- Differences in the method of dosing and route and duration of administration: Excessive doses might invalidate the test by killing the animals, and doses that are too low might give a misleading impression of safety. Humans tend to be 2 to 50 times more sensitive than animals on a dose-per-weight basis.
- A variety of teratogens may produce the same malformation, and, conversely, a variety of malformations may be produced by the same teratogen; moreover, an established teratogen is not necessarily deleterious with every exposure. In such circumstances, attribution of causation can be difficult.
- No clear relationship exists between a particular chemical or pharmacological class and specific effects on the embryo. For example, one sulfonylurea may cause a high percentage of malformations in animals, while another has little or no effect.

Precision in preclinical reproductive toxicity testing is all the more important given the difficulties inherent in applying epidemiological methods in human teratology. The effects of "low-grade" human teratogens may not be discernible from the normal background incidence of major congenital malformations (2 to 3%). Accurate information regarding time of exposure of the pregnant mother to the suspected teratogen may be lacking. Any association may be further complicated by agents that enhance the expression of the primary offender, such as food additives, cigarette smoking, and alcohol.

The principles and methods underpinning the detection of reproductive toxicity of medicinal products have been set out in ICH guidelines,[29] which serve as a *vade mecum* for those planning reproductive toxicology studies on new chemical entities and for reviewers of reproductive toxicity data. What follows is a précis of the content of the ICH guideline, with emphasis on the underlying scientific and logical principles, based on study designs currently in use for testing of medicinal products.

Most studies are likely to be combined so as to show effects on:

- Fertility and early embryonic development
- Pre- and postnatal development, including maternal function
- Embryo–fetal development

Toxicity to male fertility is assessed for effects on spermatogenesis, histopathology, and weight of reproductive organs, as well as, in some cases, hormone assays and genotoxicity data, following premating repeated-dose administration for 4 weeks.[31] Increasing evidence from both animal and human studies indicate male-mediated developmental effects. The proposed mechanisms for detecting such effects include transmission of chemicals from the father to the conceptus by the seminal fluid, indirect contamination of the mother and the conceptus by substances carried from the workplace into the home environment through personal contact, and paternal preconception exposure that results in transmissible genetic changes.[32]

Increased attention is now being given to screening new vaccines for developmental toxicity in animals before use in humans, on the grounds that the developing conceptus may theoretically be exposed to the induced antibodies or sensitized T-cells. Evaluation includes postnatal examination to detect all possible manifestations of developmental toxicity through effects on the immune system. Species selection for the preclinical studies is based on immunogenicity to the vaccine and the relative timing and rate of transfer of maternal antibodies to the offspring.[61]* Assessment should include: (1) detection of antibody production in the pregnant animal; (2) antibody transfer from the pregnant female to the fetus through antibody measurements in the newborn; and (3) the presence, persistence, and effects of the antibody response in the newborn.

4.9 NEUROTOXICITY TESTING

Neurotoxicity evaluation[12,55] is an important part of toxicology, in recognition that the nervous system is a critical target for hazardous substances. Testing has been made possible by advances in the neurosciences, but limitations remain in techniques and methods of evaluation. Effects of the test substance on the central nervous system are normally assessed by evaluation of motor activity, behavioral changes, coordination, sensory/motor reflex responses, and body temperature.[33] Behavioral change is likely to be the earliest detectable expression of toxic injury to the nervous system, as adverse biochemical or pathological effects exceed the homeostatic capacity of the central nervous system.[12] It may be difficult, or impossible, to detect intellectual impairment (a common expression of neurotoxicity in humans) by animal tests, particularly as distinctions are relative rather than absolute. Age is another complicating issue in assessing toxic insult to the central nervous system. The immature and developing brain is especially susceptible to toxic injury at the time of active cellular proliferation, myelination, and synaptogenesis. The aging central nervous system is also vulnerable.

Where relevant, effects of the test substance on the autonomic nervous system should also be assessed. This includes drug or metabolite binding to receptors relevant for the autonomic nervous system, functional responses to agonists or antagonists *in vivo* and *in vitro*, direct stimulation of autonomic nerves, and measurement of cardiovascular responses, baroreflex responses, and heart rate variability.[33]

4.10 CATEGORIZING THE TOXICOLOGICAL RESPONSE

The outcome of a toxicological study in animals may fall into one of four categories:[30]

1. Sufficient evidence exists of an association between the toxic agent and the purported outcome. This is based on findings in multiple species or strains or in multiple experiments, preferably with different routes of administration or different doses, or both, or the incidence of the finding is unusual in degree, site, type, or age of onset. Additional data on dose–response effects, short-term studies, and chemical structure may be available.
2. Limited evidence — The data suggest a causative effect but are insufficient because: (a) a single species or strain was examined or the results were derived from a single experiment; (b) the experiments were conducted with inadequate dose levels, too brief duration of exposure, inadequate period of follow-up, or poor animal survival and too few animals or the reporting was inadequate; or (c) the lesions produced often occur spontaneously.

---

* The FDA has pointed out that virtually no scientific literature on animal reproductive toxicity testing for vaccine products exists. Their document *Considerations for Reproductive Toxicity Studies for Preventive Vaccines for Infectious Diseases Indications* sets out a framework for such testing.[17] Broadly, the FDA (Center for Biologics Evaluation and Research) is recommending the ICH S5A guidance document *Detection of Toxicity to Reproduction for Medicinal Products* as a point of reference to assist the design of reproductive toxicity studies to assess the potential teratogenic effect of biological products in general.

3. Inadequate evidence — Because of major qualitative or quantitative limitations the studies cannot be interpreted as showing either the presence or absence of an effect or, within the limits of the test, the chemical has not been shown conclusively to produce the lesions concerned.
4. No data are available.

The first two categories provide an indication only of the strength of the experimental evidence, and not of the extent of the activity of the chemical entity under review or the mechanism of its toxic effect.

4.11 PRECLINICAL PHARMACOLOGICAL AND TOXICOLOGICAL TESTING OF VACCINES*

Verdier[60] has pointed out that the safety evaluation of vaccines is complex, as they act through a multistage mechanism in which the vaccine may serve as a prodrug, or antibodies or activated lymphocytes may be the actual effectors; therefore, several potential toxicities have to be considered: direct toxicity of the test article; toxicity linked to the pharmacodynamic activity of the vaccine; activation of preexisting disorders; toxicity of contaminants and impurities; and other adverse reactions due to interaction between the various components. Repeated-dose studies are pivotal. The animal model and treatment schedule selection and the parameters investigated are critical for the relevance of the safety assessment. Tests for detecting hypersensitivity or autoimmune reactions exist but they require further validation. Any adjuvant or active component added to the vaccine formulation necessitates special assessment using studies routinely performed for new drugs.

Vaccines for human use may contain:

- Organisms that have been inactivated by chemical or physical means and maintain immunogenic properties
- Living organisms that are naturally avirulent or that have been treated to attenuate their virulence while retaining immunogenic properties
- Antigens extracted from organisms, secreted by them, or produced by recombinant DNA technology

Antigens may be used in their native state or detoxified by chemical or physical means and may be aggregated, polymerized, or conjugated to a carrier to increase their immunogenicity.[74]

Suitable animal models are not always available, and responses in such models may not be predictive of human responses. Selection of animal species should be made on a case-by-case basis. For new vaccine products, preclinical safety tests should be part of the testing program, even though full testing may not be necessary to the extent required for non-vaccine medicinal products. For combined vaccines containing known antigens, preclinical toxicity testing may not be necessary. The route of administration should be as close as possible to the proposed clinical route. If for practical reasons this is not possible, then another route of administration may be acceptable, but that should be justified. Studies to address specific safety concerns such as neurovirulence often require other routes of administration.

Single-dose toxicity data from at least one animal species should be performed with a dose providing an adequate safety margin in relation to the human dose. If toxic effects are seen in the study, the dose–response relationship should be further characterized. A study on repeated-dose toxicity in one animal species is normally required for vaccines that require multiple doses. The selection of an appropriate animal species should be decided on a case-by-case basis.

---

* This section draws on the note for guidance on preclinical pharmacological and toxicological testing of vaccines issued by the European Agency for the Evaluation of Medicinal Products (EMEA) in 1997 (CPMP/SWP/465/95) and on the work of Verdier.[60]

The route and dosing regimen in the experimental animal should reflect intended clinical use. Where appropriate, consideration should be given to immunological aspects of toxicity, such as production of complexes with host immunoglobulins (antibody-dependent enhancement of disease) or release of immunofunctional molecules (cytokines) affecting functions of the immune system.

Only when a vaccine is intended for use in women of child-bearing age or during pregnancy do reproductive toxicity studies become necessary. The guidelines for such testing of vaccines have been set out by Verdier and colleagues.[61] As most vaccines will be administered intramuscularly, subcutaneously, or intracutaneously, local tolerance should be evaluated.

4.12 IMPROVING THE RELEVANCE AND HUMANE CONDUCT OF TOXICOLOGY TESTING

A number of recommendations have been made for improving the relevance of toxicology testing in animals.[16,40,42,68–70] These include:

- Establishment of databanks for the collection of results would provide a valuable resource for design and analysis of future experiments.[41]
- The methodology in experimental toxicology must advance to the extent that subjective effects in humans, such as hallucinations, dizziness, difficulty in concentrating, and disturbance in memory, might be assessed in animals by behavioral testing.[68]
- Improved comparative evaluation of anatomical structure, physiological function, and pathology in test animals and in humans, including patients with the diseases for which the medicine is intended, would improve extrapolation and reduce the difficulties inherent in species differences in metabolism, distribution, and elimination.

Any prospective researcher should be required to submit a rationale and detailed protocol for using animals for careful and independent ethics review. The proposal would include a complete list of drugs to be used and an inventory of surgical procedures. Each proposal is carefully reviewed. No animal studies may proceed without the approval of the scientific panel and ethics committee. Strict adherence to the protocol of investigation throughout the study would be required. Although such measures do not provide certain protection against abuse of animals in research, they do decrease the risk, and they provide for sanctions if transgressions occur.

In any animal study, the choice of test should depend on the nature and stage of the research. The decision is likely to be guided by three considerations: (1) the likelihood that the study will answer the scientific question being asked; (2) the social attitudes, legal codes, and ethical standards that are affected by the study; and (3) economic considerations. The use of research animals is expensive, research in non-animal models less so; the latter are simpler to control and provide fewer ethical hurdles. Before commencing animal studies, the investigator needs to pose a specific question and describe the expected answer, needs to be familiar with the relevant scientific literature, and needs to be able to show that the available models can answer the scientific question being posed. If several models might provide a reasonable prospect of useful information, the researcher needs to decide which is likely to be best. Protocols of study should include animal care and management guidelines. It is imperative that all such animal work be underpinned by humane treatment. This places the researcher under an obligation to prevent undue pain and suffering, but it does not address the issue of animal rights. It denies the view of those animal rights advocates who maintain that animal and human rights in experimentation should be equal, and it admits that certain things done to animals may not be done to humans. The injunction of "humane treatment" of animals in this context establishes a double standard for animals and humans.[4]

Pakes[48] has pointed out that good science and good conscience go hand in hand in the sound care of experimental animals. Animals' feelings, such as pain and distress, affect the subjects' physiological responses. The researcher needs to be on the lookout for disturbances of sleeping, drinking, feeding, locomotion, grooming, exploration, learning, mating, and reproduction. Physiological signs include pupil dilation, increased blood pressure and heart rate, increased respiration, and an arousal response on electroencephalography (EEG). Signs of acute pain, guarding, moving away, biting, self-mutilation, restlessness, salivation, impaired ambulation, changes in respiration, and assuming abnormal positions may give the researcher some insight into the feelings of a test animal. Animals experiencing chronic pain may become quiet and withdrawn, lose appetite and weight, change their urinary and bowel activity, and develop abnormal grooming behavior. Chronic pain is more difficult to recognize than acute pain.

Laboratory veterinarians play an important role in detecting and minimizing the pain and distress that animals may experience. They are needed in the planning and supervision of studies and for maintaining watch on the treatment of the animals. There are numerous ways in which pain may be avoided or minimized, including reducing the level of surrounding noxious stimuli, avoiding stressful and other situations that lower the threshold of pain tolerance, and improving methods and procedures aimed at raising pain tolerance. Gentle handling and special attention such as petting and talking to the test animal may reduce stress levels. If an animal has to be restrained, the restraining devices should be the correct size and as comfortable as possible. The animal should be conditioned to the environment prior to the start of the experiment. Records should be kept of the entire procedure.

Recent studies have shown that handling or maternal contact stimulates growth and decreases blood levels of beta-endorphins in rat pups which in turn reduce variances of data and increase the level of significance of observed changes. Certain species, however, do not react positively to handling; for example, young hamsters may react adversely. Thus, handling can significantly influence physiological responses such as release of prolactin, corticosterone, thyroxine, and other hormones. Heart function and hematological values may also be affected. Stress causes an elevation in circulating catecholamines, which in turn mobilize fats from adipose tissues, with a resultant rise in free fatty acids in the blood.[52]

Environmental factors that affect the outcome of an animal experiment can be physical (temperature, light, noise), chemical (food, water, detergents, pesticides, gases), biological (disease), or social (isolation, grouping, handling, and maternal influences). Another consideration is choice of the most appropriate animal. Species, strain, and gender are important. Other necessary considerations are specific disease profiles such as tumor type (which may vary between animal species), strain, gender, and age. Traditional methods of assessment and measurement must be critically reexamined; for example, death need not necessarily be the endpoint of a study. Specific signs of disease or illness, such as impaired ambulation, muscle atrophy, rapid weight loss, paralysis, and central nervous system disturbances, may be sufficient. The route of administration of a test substance can affect the pain and stress of the animal. As far as possible, routes of administration should closely mimic the anticipated human exposure and be balanced against the discomfort and pain that the animal might experience.

4.12.1 The Three R's

It has been suggested that the modern approach to toxicological testing should be based on three R's — reduction, refinement, and replacement — to optimize the balance between the needs of society and the welfare of animals:[13,21,48,52,54,57]

- *Reduction* — The number of animals should be reduced to the absolute minimum that will achieve the necessary result by placing greater focus on the objectives of the study, achieving better experimental design, and minimizing the need for repeat studies. Reassessing lethal tests such as the LD_{50} test, using prescreening, using *in vitro* tests where possible, and promoting greater sharing and dissemination of test data worldwide would contribute to a reduction in animal testing. Reusing animals or using them for multiple tests (for example, ocular and dermal), might be considered.

- *Refinement* — Adjustments to study designs and techniques have led to a reduction in the number of animals used, and in many cases they have made testing more humane, without reducing scientific validity and in some cases improving it. Examples include the fixed-dose scheme, limit tests, and modifications to ocular irritation tests (the low-volume test, a tiered approach, and use of sequential tests).
- *Replacement* — A number of alternative tests have been studied, and significant progress has been made in developing *in vitro* replacement models. These include eye, muscle, and skin irritation; phototoxicity; photosensitization; and target organ toxicity testing.

4.13 *IN VITRO* TOXICITY TESTING AND COMPUTER-BASED SYSTEMS

It has been predicted that *in vitro* toxicity tests will play an increasingly important role in chemical safety evaluation. They are commonly used as screens to provide data for product development priorities, and they are being incorporated into drug regulatory testing. They will maximize the opportunities for identifying highly toxic materials at an early stage in the process of evaluation, and they reduce the excessive need for *in vivo* testing.[19] An evaluation process that is provided entirely by *in vitro* testing requires a far deeper knowledge base than is currently available. *In vitro* toxicity and toxicokinetic studies, combined with physiologically based toxicokinetic modeling and quantitative structure–activity testing, will form the basis for such an approach. Computer-based structure–activity relationships combined with cell culture testing systems provide valuable toxicological data for hazard and risk assessments, and *in vitro* systems allow for more rapid identification of toxic compounds.[11] They can also be utilized to study the mechanisms of toxicity at cellular and subcellular levels. The data derived from these studies can be used to improve the predictability of standard animal models for chemical and drug toxicity. It is not realistic to expect that *in vitro* methods will entirely replace testing in the whole animal. Numerous interrelationships exist among structure, function, and behavior in toxicology that require the intact animal for study. Examples include measurement of the neurobehavioral effects of toxic substances, strain and species differences with regard to the metabolic fate of test compounds, the role of the intestinal flora, enterohepatic circulation in influencing metabolic pathways of test compounds, and differential distribution within an organ and biotransformation due to variations in organ architecture and cell polarity.

4.14 SEQUENTIAL STUDIES AND A DECISION TREE

Gad et al.[22] reported their experience over 4 years, during which they conducted 124 acute systemic toxicity studies (64 oral, 39 dermal, and 21 by inhalation), throughout which they altered study and program designs with the purpose of maximizing information and minimizing animal usage. By employing dose-selection strategies, probes, and lethality limits, with staggered sequential dosing, and by conducting studies in batteries, animal usage was reduced by 48% below the average number regarded as necessary for an LD_{50} study. The authors suggested that the combined use of a neurobehavioral screen, adjunct studies, and flexible study design results in significant improvement in the information obtained from such studies. The use of a decision tree approach for selecting tissues for histopathology was proposed by the same workers.[22] Specific indicators such as organ weights for selecting organs for microscopic examination were evaluated. The result has been to increase the flexibility of the standard approach to the design and conduct of acute systemic toxicity studies and in general to subject standard procedures to more critical consideration.

Table 4.3   Comparative Weights of Organs in the Mouse, Rat, Rabbit, Rhesus Monkey, Dog, and Human

	Weight (g)						
	Adrenal	Brain	Lung	Liver	Kidney	Heart	Spleen
Mouse (0.02 kg)	0.36	1.75	0.32	0.08	0.1	0.004	0.12
Rat (0.25 kg)	1.8	10.0	2.0	1.0	0.75	0.05	1.5
Rabbit (2.5 kg)	14	77	13	5	1	0.5	18
Rhesus monkey (5 kg)	90	150	25	18.5	8	1.2	33
Dog (10 kg)	80	320	50	80	25	1	100
Human (70 kg)	1400	1800	310	330	180	14	1000

Source: Davies, B. and Morris, T., *Pharmacol. Res.*, 10, 1093, 1993. With permission.

Table 4.4   Volumes of Various Body Fluids and Organs in the Mouse, Rat, Rabbit, Monkey, Dog, and Human

	Volume (mL)					
	Mouse	Rat	Rabbit	Monkey	Dog	Human
Brain	—	1.2	—	—	72	1450
Liver	1.3	19.6	100	135	480	1690
Kidneys	0.34	3.7	15	30	60	280
Heart	0.1	1.2	6	17	120	310
Spleen	0.1	1.3	1	—	36	192
Lungs	0.1	2.1	17	—	120	1170
Gut	1.5	11.3	120	230	480	1650
Muscle	10	245	1350	2500	5530	35,000
Adipose tissue	—	10	120	—	—	10,000
Skin	2.9	40	110	500	—	7800
Blood	17	13.5	165	367	900	5200
Total body water	14.5	167	1790	3465	6036	42,000
Intracellular fluid	—	92.8	1165	2425	3276	23,800
Extracellular fluid	—	74.2	625	1040	2760	18,200
Plasma volume	1	7.8	110	224	515	3000

Note: The weights for the various species are the same as those given in Table 4.3.

Source: Davies, B. and Morris, T., *Pharmacol. Res.*, 10, 1093, 1993. With permission.

4.15 AGING STUDIES

In recent years, increasing attention has been paid to models and systems for research into aging to replace studies that may not be done in humans for ethical, legal, or technical reasons but which are nevertheless indispensable for progress in biomedical research into aging.[26] It is clear that the diverse processes of senescence have the common outcome of accelerating mortality rates in different animal species. The use of a broad range of animal models allows for generalization of findings and facilitates an understanding of primary aging processes. A variety of animal models exists that have advantages or special features that might contribute to research on aging. The appropriate choice of a model will require a number of conditions, the most important of which should allow for manipulation of the genetic system, characterization of physiological data, and easy and affordable husbandry.

4.16 PHYSIOLOGICAL MEASUREMENTS

Physiological parameters for different laboratory animal species are diverse and difficult to quantify. The work of Davies and Morris,[8] which is reproduced here with permission in a series of tables (Table 4.3 through Table 4.7), is helpful in assisting researchers to make practical physiological and biochemical decisions when testing animals.

Table 4.5 Flow of Blood through the Major Organs and Other Fluids in the Mouse, Rat, Rabbit, Monkey, Dog, and Human

	Blood Flow (mL/min)					
	Mouse	Rat	Rabbit	Monkey	Dog	Human
Brain	—	1.3	—	72	45	700
Liver	1.8	13.8	177	218	309	1450
Kidneys	1.3	9.2	80	138	216	1240
Heart	0.28	3.9	16	60	54	240
Spleen	0.09	0.6	9	21	25	77
Gut	1.5	7.5	111	125	216	1100
Muscle	0.91	7.5	155	90	250	750
Adipose tissue	—	0.4	32	20	35	260
Skin	0.41	5.8	—	54	100	300
Hepatic artery	0.35	2	37	51	79	300
Portal vein	1.45	9.8	140	167	230	1150
Cardiac output	8	74	530	1086	1200	5600
Urine flow[a]	1	50	150	375	300	1400
Bile flow[a]	2	22.5	300	125	120	350
GFR	0.28	1.3	7.8	10.4	61.3	125

[a] Measurements of urine flow and bile flow are given in mL/day.

Note: The weights for the various species are the same as those given in Table 4.3. GFR, glomerular filtration rate (mL/min).

Source: Davies, B. and Morris, T., *Pharmacol. Res.*, 10, 1093, 1993. With permission.

Table 4.6 Transit Time, pH, and Enzyme Activity of the Gastrointestinal Tract of the Mouse, Rat, Rabbit, Monkey, Dog, and Human

	Transit Time (min)					
	Mouse	Rat	Rabbit	Monkey	Dog	Human
Stomach	—	—	—	—	96	78
Small intestine	—	88	—	—	110	238
Whole gut	—	—	—	—	770	2350
Stomach (anterior)	4.5	5	1.9	4.8	5.5	—
Stomach (posterior)	3.1	3.8	1.9	2.8	3.4	5
Small intestine (beginning)	—	6.5	6	5.6	6.2	5.4
Small intestine (end)	—	7.1	8	6	7.5	7.5
Cecum	—	6.8	6.6	5	6.4	6
Colon	—	6.6	7.2	5.1	6.5	7.5
Feces	—	6.9	7.2	5.5	6.2	—

	Beta-Glucuronidation Activity (nmol substrate/hr/g of contents)					
	Mouse	Rat	Rabbit	Monkey	Dog	Human
Proximal small intestine	1200	304	2.4	—	—	0.02
Distal small intestine	5015	1341	45.4	—	—	0.9

Note: The weights for the various species are the same as those given in Table 4.3.

Source: Davies, B. and Morris, T., *Pharmacol. Res.*, 10, 1093, 1993. With permission.

4.17 CONCLUSION

Much of the wasteful, meaningless, and thus profligate use of experimental animals in the scientific development of new medicines should be curtailed. The widespread recognition of this idea today is gratifying. Much remains to be done, however. This chapter set out to confirm the essential role of animal testing in the process of new drug development, while adding voice to the need expressed by animal ethicists, the public, and indeed the scientific community to reduce to a minimum the

Table 4.7   Miscellaneous Physiological Parameters of the Mouse, Rat, Rabbit, Monkey, Dog, and Human

	Mouse	Rat	Rabbit	Monkey	Dog	Human
Surface area (m²)	0.008	0.023	0.17	0.32	0.51	1.85
Mean lifespan (yr)	2.7	4.7	8.0	22	20	93
Total plasma protein (g/100 mL)	6.2	6.7	5.7	8.8	9.0	7.4
Plasma albumin (g/100 mL)	3.27	3.16	3.87	4.93	2.63	4.18
Plasma alpha-1-AGP (g/100 mL)	1.25	1.81	0.13	0.24	0.37	0.18
Hematocrit (%)	45	46	36	41	42	44
Total ventilation (L/min)	0.025	0.12	0.8	1.67	1.5	7.98
Respiratory rate (per min)	163	85	51	38	23	12
Heart rate (per min)	624	362	213	192	96	65
Oxygen consumption (mL/hr/g body weight)	1.59	0.84	0.48	0.43	0.34	0.2

Note: The weights for the various species are the same as those given in Table 4.3.

Source: Davies, B. and Morris, T., *Pharmacol. Res.*, 10, 1093, 1993. With permission.

use of animals and optimize their participation in the process. Tests that are unduly harmful to animals and are wasteful or unnecessary should be dispensed with. The LD_{50} and Draize tests have become obsolete. Tests of reproductive toxicity, carcinogenicity, etc. are of considerable value, and no alternatives to their use are available. More than anything else, the chapter aims to demonstrate the importance of a rational and flexible approach to the use of animals in the scientific development of new medicines. The question of how best to conduct those tests that are essential — and how to discontinue the inessential — lies at the heart of what has been stated here. The scientific community, pharmaceutical industry, and not least the drug regulators have a collective and crucial role to play in ensuring that this happens.

REFERENCES

1. Aldridge, W.N., Chronic toxicity as an acute phenomenon: introduction to symposium, *Proc. Eur. Soc. Toxicol.*, 17, 5–6, 1976.
2. Balazs, T., Development of tissue resistance to toxic effects of chemicals, *Toxicology*, 2, 247–55, 1974.
3. Brown, V.K., Animal models of responses resulting from short-term exposures, in *The Future of Predictive Safety Evaluation*, Vol. 2, Worden, A., Parke, D., and Marks, J., Eds., MTP Press, Lancaster, U.K., 1987, pp. 47–55.
4. Cohen, C., The case for the use of animals in biochemical research, *N. Engl. J. Med.*, 315, 865, 1986.
5. CPMP, *Note for Guidance on Non-Clinical Local Tolerance Testing of Medicinal Products*, CPMP/SWP/2145/00, Committee for Proprietary Medicinal Products, European Agency for the Evaluation of Medicinal Products, London, 2001.
6. CPMP, *Note for Guidance on Carcinogenicity: Testing for Carcinogenicity of Pharmaceuticals*, CPMP/ICH/299/95, Committee for Proprietary Medicinal Products, European Agency for the Evaluation of Medicinal Products, London, 1997.
7. CPMP, *Note for Guidance on Preclinical Safety Evaluation of Biotechnology-Derived Pharmaceuticals*, CPMP/ICH/302/95, Committee for Proprietary Medicinal Products, European Agency for the Evaluation of Medicinal Products, London, 1997.
8. Davies, B. and Morris, T., Physiological parameters in laboratory animals and humans, *Pharmacol. Res.*, 10, 1093, 1993.
9. Dayan, A.D., The scientific basis for long-term animal studies: what can and cannot be detected, in *Long-Term Animal Studies: Their Predictive Value for Man*, Walker, S.R. and Dayan, A.D., Eds., MTP Press, Lancaster, U.K., 1986, pp. 3–7.
10. Dean, J.H., Luster, M.I., Boorman, G.A., and Lauer, L.D., Procedures available to examine the immunotoxicity of chemicals and drugs, *Pharmacol. Rev.*, 34, 137–148, 1982.

11. DelRaso, N.J., *In vitro* methodologies for enhanced toxicity testing, *Toxicol. Lett.*, 68, 91, 1993.
12. Dewar, A.J., Neurotoxicity, in *The Future of Predictive Safety Evaluation*, Vol. 2. Worden, A., Parke, D., and Marks, J., Eds., MTP Press, Lancaster, U.K., 1987, pp. 107–128.
13. Dorandeu, F. and Lallement, G., Are acute toxicity testing and the three R's rule reconcilable? Example of the lethal dose 50 determination, *Ann. Pharm. Fr.*, 61, 399–411, 2003.
14. Draize, J.H., Woodard, G., and Calvery, H.O., Methods for the study of irritation and toxicity of substances applied topically to the skin and mucous membrane, *J. Pharmacol.*, 82, 377–390, 1944.
15. CPMP, *Non-Clinical Safety Studies for the Conduct of Human Clinical Trials for Pharmaceuticals*, CPMP/ICH/286/95 (modification), Committee for Proprietary Medicinal Products, European Agency for the Evaluation of Medicinal Products, London, 2000.
16. Fletcher, A.P., Drug safety tests and subsequent clinical experience, *J. R. Soc. Med.*, 71, 693–696, 1978.
17. FDA, *Considerations for Reproductive Toxicity Studies for Preventive Vaccines for Infectious Diseases Indications* (draft), U.S. Food and Drug Administration, Washington, D.C., 2000.
18. FDA, *Pharmacogenomics*, U.S. Food and Drug Administration, Washington, D.C. (http://www.fda.gov/cder/pharmtox).
19. Frazier, J.M., *In vitro* models for toxicological research and testing, *Toxicol. Lett.*, 68, 73, 1993.
20. Frederick, G.L., The evidence supporting 18 month animal studies, in *Long-Term Animal Studies: Their Predictive Value for Man*, Walker, S.R. and Dayan, A.D., Eds., MTP Press, Lancaster, U.K., 1986, pp. 65–76.
21. Gad, S.C., Recent developments in replacing, reducing, and refining animal use in toxicologic research and testing, *Fund. Appl. Toxicol.*, 15, 8, 1990.
22. Gad, S.C., Smith, A.C., Cramp, A.L. et al., Innovative designs and practices for acute systemic toxicity studies, *Drug Chem. Toxicol.*, 7, 423, 1984.
23. Gart, J.J., Chu, K.C., and Tarone, R.E., Statistical issues in interpretation of chronic bioassay tests for carcinogenicity, *J. Natl. Cancer Inst.*, 62, 957–974, 1979.
24. Glockin, V.C., Justification for 12 month animal studies, in *Long-Term Animal Studies: Their Predictive Value for Man*, Walker, S.R. and Dayan, A.D., Eds., MTP Press, Lancaster, U.K., 1986, pp. 77–82.
25. Grahame-Smith, D., What is expected from repeated-dose studies by the regulatory authorities, in *Long-Term Animal Studies: Their Predictive Value for Man*, Walker, S.R. and Dayan, A.D., Eds., MTP Press, Lancaster, U.K., 1986, pp. 23–27.
26. Hazzard, D.G., Warner, H.R., and Finch, C.E., National Institute on Aging, NIH: workshop on alternative animal models for research on aging, *Exp. Gerontol.*, 26, 411, 1991.
27. Hoel, D.G., Kaplan, N.L., and Anderson, M.W., Implication of nonlinear kinetics on risk estimation in carcinogenesis, *Science*, 219, 1032–1037, 1983.
28. U.K. House of Commons, Hansard Written Answers for 16 January 2001 (part 21): Draize test.
29. CPMP, *Reproductive Toxicology: Detection of Toxicity to Reproduction for Medicinal Products*, CPMP/ICH/386/95, ICH Topic S5A, Committee for Proprietary Medicinal Products, European Agency for the Evaluation of Medicinal Products, London, 1993.
30. IARC, *Monographs on the Evaluation of the Carcinogenic Risk of Chemicals to Humans*. Suppl. 4. *Chemicals, Industrial Processes and Industries Associated with Cancer in Humans*, Vols. 1–29, IARC Monographs, International Agency for Research on Cancer, Lyon, 1984.
31. ICH, *Detection of Toxicity to Reproduction for Medicinal Products: Addendum on Toxicity to Male Fertility*, ICH-S5B, International Conference on Harmonisation of Technical Requirements for Registration of Pharmaceuticals for Human Use, Geneva, Switzerland, 1996.
32. International Labour Organization, Geneva, Switzerland, 2002 (www.ilo.org).
33. ICH, *Safety Pharmacology Studies for Human Pharmaceuticals*, ICH-S7A, International Conference on Harmonisation of Technical Requirements for Registration of Pharmaceuticals for Human Use, Geneva, Switzerland, 2004.
34. Jackson, M.R., Conventional design of long-term toxicity studies in the pharmaceutical industry, in *Long-Term Animal Studies: Their Predictive Value for Man*, Walker, S.P. and Dayan, A.D., Eds., MTP Press, Lancaster, U.K., 1986, pp. 35–44.
35. Kaufman, S.R., (1989) Perspectives on animal research, *Am. Med. Adv.*, 1, 1–9, 1989 (www.curedisease.com/perspectives).
36. Kodell, R.L., Farmer, J.H., Gaylot, D.W., and Cameron, A.M., Influence of cause of death assignment on time-to-tumor analyses in animal carcinogenesis studies, *J. Natl. Cancer Inst.*, 69, 659–664, 1982.

37. Koeter, H.B.W.M., Relevance of parameters related to fertility and reproduction in toxicity testing, *Am. J. Ind. Med.*, 4, 81–86, 1983.

38. Lansdown, A.B.G., Testing for reproductive toxicity, in *The Future of Predictive Safety Evaluation*, Vol. 2, Worden, A.N., Parke, D.V., and Marks, J., Eds., MTP Press, Lancaster, U.K., 1987, pp. 77–106.

39. Lasagna, L., Regulatory agencies, drugs and the pregnant patient, in *Drug Use in Pregnancy*, Stern, L., Ed., Adis Health Science Press, Sydney, 1984, pp. 12–16.

40. Litchfield, J.T., Evaluation of the safety of new drugs by means of tests in animals, *Clin. Pharmacol. Ther.*, 3, 665–681, 1962.

41. Lumley, C.E. and Walker, S.R., A toxicology databank based on animal safety evaluation studies of pharmaceutical compounds, *Hum. Toxicol.*, 4, 447–460, 1985.

42. Lumley, C.E. and Walker, S.R., What is the value of animal toxicology studies beyond 6 months?, *Br. J. Pharmacol.*, 84(Suppl.), 117P, 1985.

43. McLean, A.E.M., The relationship between animal and human responses, in *Long-Term Animal Studies: Their Predictive Value for Man*, Walker, S.R. and Dayan, A.D., Eds., MTP Press, Lancaster, U.K., 1986, pp. 99–104.

44. Messite, J. and Bond, M.B., Reproductive toxicology and occupational exposure, in *Occupational Medicine: Principles and Practical Applications*, Zenz, C., Ed., Year Book Medical Publishers, Chicago, IL, 1988, pp. 847–903.

45. Miller, K. and Nicklin, S., Immunological aspects, in *The Future of Predictive Safety Evaluation*, Vol. 1, Worden, A., Parke, D., and Marks, J., Eds., MTP Press, Lancaster, U.K., 1987, pp. 181–194.

46. Miller, R.K., Mattison, D.R., Filler, R.S., and Rice, J.M., Reproductive and developmental toxicology, in *Drug Therapy During Pregnancy*, Eskes, T.K.A.B. and Finster, M., Eds., Butterworths, London, 1985, pp. 215–224.

47. Paget, E., The LD_{50} test, *Acta Pharmacol. Toxicol.*, 52(Suppl. 2), 6–19, 1983.

48. Pakes, S.P., Contributions of the laboratory animal veterinarian to refining animal experiments in toxicology, *Fund. Appl. Toxicol.*, 15, 17, 1990.

49. Purchase, I.F.H., Carcinogenic risk assessment: are animals good surrogates for man?, in *Cancer Risks: Strategies for Elimination*, Bannasch, P., Ed., Springer-Verlag, Berlin, 1987, pp. 65–79.

50. Rawlins, M.D., What is expected from repeated-dose studies by clinical pharmacologists, in *Long-Term Animal Studies: Their Predictive Value for Man*, Walker, S.R. and Dayan, A.D., Eds., MTP Press, Lancaster, U.K., 1986, pp. 17–22.

51. Rowan, A., Shortcomings of LD_{50} values and acute toxicity testing in animals, *Acta Pharmacol. Toxicol.*, 52, 52–64, 1983.

52. Rowan, A.N., Refinement of animal research technique and validity of research data, *Fund. Appl. Toxicol.*, 15, 25, 1990.

53. FDA, *S1B Testing for Carcinogenicity of Pharmaceuticals*, U.S. Food and Drug Administration, Washington, D.C., 1997 (www.fda/gov/cber/guidelines.htm).

54. Schechtman, L.M., Implementation of the 3R's (refinement, reduction, and replacement): validation and regulatory acceptance considerations for alternative toxicological test methods, *ILAR J.*, 43(Suppl.), S85–S94, 2002.

55. Silbergeld, E.K., Current status of neurotoxicology: basic and applied, *Trends Neurosci.*, 5, 291–294, 1982.

56. Squire, R.A., Ranking animal carcinogens: a proposed regulatory approach, *Science*, 214, 877–880, 1981.

57. Sterling, S. and Rispin, A., Incorporating the 3R's into regulatory scientific practices, *ILAR J.*, 43(Suppl.), S18–S20, 2002.

58. Thomas, J.A., Ham, T.E., Perkins, P.L., and Raffin, T.A., Animal research at Stanford University, *N. Engl. J. Med.*, 318, 1630, 1988.

59. Van den Heuvel, M.J., Clark, D.G., Fielder, R.J. et al., The international validation of a fixed dose procedure as an alternative to the classical LD_{50} test, *Food Chem. Toxicol.*, 28, 469, 1990.

60. Verdier, F., Non-clinical vaccine safety assessment, *Toxicology*, 174, 37–43, 2002.

61. Verdier, F., Barrow, P.-C., and Burge. J., Reproductive toxicity testing of vaccines, *Toxicology*, 185, 213–219, 2003.

62. Weil, C.S. and Scala, R.A., Study of intra- and interlaboratory variability in the results of rabbit eye and skin irritation tests, *Toxicol. Appl. Pharmacol.*, 19, 276–360, 1971.

63. Weisburger, J.H., Safety evaluation: carcinogenic risks, in *The Future of Predictive Safety Evaluation*, Vol. 2, Worden, A., Parke, D., and Marks, J., Eds., MTP Press, Lancaster, U.K., 1987, pp. 129–152.
64. Wilson, J.G., Experimental studies on congenital malformations, *J. Chron. Dis.*, 10, 111–130, 1959.
65. Worden, A.N., The evidence supporting 6-month animal studies, in *Long-Term Animal Studies: Their Predictive Value for Man*, Walker, S.R. and Dayan, A.D., Eds., MTP Press, Lancaster, U.K., 1986, pp. 83–86.
66. Worden, A.N. and Walker, S.R., Animal models for long term toxic effects, in *The Future of Predictive Safety Evaluation*, Vol. 2, Worden, A., Parke, D., and Marks, J., Eds., MTP Press, Lancaster, U.K., 1987, pp. 57–64.
67. Yamanaka, S., Hashimoto, M., Tobe, M. et al., A simple method for screening assessment of acute toxicity of chemicals, *Arch. Toxicol.*, 64, 262, 1990.
68. Zbinden, G., Predictive value of pre-clinical drug safety evaluation, in *Proceedings of Plenary Lectures Symposia and Therapeutic Sessions of the First World Conference on Clinical Pharmacology and Therapeutics*, Turner, P., Ed., Macmillan Press, London, 1980.
69. Zbinden, G., Risks predicted from animal studies, in *Medicines and Risk/Benefit Decision*, Walker, S.R. and Asscher, A.W., Eds., MTP Press, Lancaster, U.K., 1987, pp. 49–56.
70. Zbinden, G., *Predictive Value of Animal Studies in Toxicology*, Centre for Medicines Research, Carshalton, U.K., 1987.
71. Zbinden, G. and Flury-Roversi, M., Significance of the LD_{50} test for the toxicological evaluation of chemical substances, *Arch. Toxicol.*, 47, 77–99, 1981.
72. USEPA, *Prevention, Pesticides, and Toxic Substances (7101)*, EPA 712-C-96-190, U.S. Environmental Protection Agency, Washington, D.C., 1996 (http://altweb.jhsph.edu/regulations/regulations.htm).
73. Satyavati, G.V., Carcinogenic effects of drugs, *Indian J. Pharmacol.*, 4(2), 57–64, 1972.
74. CPMP, Preclinical Pharmacological and Toxicological Testing of Vaccines, CPMP/SWP/465/9, Committee for Proprietary Medicinal Products, London, 1997 (www.eudra.org/emea.html).

Regulatory Organization and Decision Making

CHAPTER 5

Worldwide Regulatory Agencies

Christopher L. Wu, Benjamin R. Lee, and Mei-Ling Chen

CONTENTS

5.1 INTRODUCTION

The European regulatory system has two routes for the evaluation and approval of medicinal products: (1) The centralized procedure is compulsory for medicinal products derived from biotechnology and other new chemical entities. The European Agency for the Evaluation of Medicinal Products (EMEA) reviews the license application within 210 days, and the European Commission considers the recommendations of EMEA within 90 days to issue a marketing license. (2) The decentralized procedure applies to the majority of conventional medical products.

The U.S. Food and Drug Administration (FDA) includes the Center for Drug Evaluation and Research (CDER) and the Center for Biologics Evaluation and Research (CBER), which evaluate and ensure the safety, efficacy, and purity of drugs and biological products. A recently developed strategic action plan designed to meet new health challenges has five priorities: (1) efficient risk management, (2) improving health through better information, (3) improving patient and consumer safety, (4) protecting the homeland from bioterrorism, and (5) ensuring the safety and security of drugs.

In Japan, the Ministry of Health, Labour, and Welfare (*Kosei-lodo-sho*) regulates drugs and biological products. The Pharmaceutical and Food Safety Bureau evaluates the efficacy, safety, and quality of drugs and biologics based on the Pharmaceutical Affairs Law. A new drug application is reviewed first by the Central Pharmaceutical Affairs Council (CPAC). Based on the advice of the CPAC, the Ministry approves the marketing license. The National Institute of Health Sciences evaluates specifications and testing methods and conducts control tests. A postmarketing surveillance system includes: (1) drug reexamination to monitor the use of new drugs for 4 to 6 years, and (2) drug reexamination to review all prescription drugs every 5 years.

The Department of Health in Taiwan encourages pharmaceutical companies to invest in research and development in drugs and biologics. Good clinical practices (GCPs) were established in 1996 and revised in 2002. Extensive training courses on clinical trials have been given to investigators and healthcare scientists. GCP inspections have been conducted in all clinical trials in Taiwan. A joint institutional review board (IRB) was established in 1997, and the Center for Drug Evaluation (CDE) was established in 1998 to facilitate the effective new drug application (NDA) reviews.

The International Conference on Harmonisation (ICH) of Technical Requirements for Registration of Pharmaceuticals for Human Use brings together the regulatory authorities of Europe, Japan, and the United States and experts from pharmaceutical industries in these three regions in order to eliminate redundant and duplicate technical requirements for drug development. The objective is to expedite the global development and availability of medical products with efficacy, safety, and quality.

5.2 EUROPEAN REGULATORY SYSTEM

The European Union (EU) is composed of 15 member countries: Belgium, Denmark, Germany, Greece, Spain, France, Ireland, Italy, Luxenbourg, Netherlands, Austria, Portugal, Finland, Sweden, and United Kingdom, representing a total population of 371 million, compared to 249 million in the United States and 124 million in Japan, the other two major pharmaceutical groups in the world. The total European pharmaceutical market stands at 41 billion, approximately 33% of world drug sales. In contrast, the United States and Japan account for 31% and 21%, respectively, of world drug sales. Annual expenses for European drug research and development are estimated at about 10 billion. The major regulatory agencies and pharmaceutical groups have managed international drug development and symbolize the importance of harmonization of drug evaluation.

The Pharmaceutical Directive was established in 1965 to create a central coordinating committee in Europe, the Committee on Proprietary Medical Products (CPMP), resulting in establishment of the Multi-State Licensing Procedure, the initiation of a review of older products, and new requirements for the testing and regulation of all medicinal products. In 1995, the regulation of medicines throughout Europe were changed significantly with the foundation of the European Agency for the Evaluation of Medicinal Products (EMEA). The European regulatory system offers two routes for evaluation and approval of medicinal products, and the EMEA plays important role in both procedures. The centralized procedure is compulsory for medicinal products derived from biotechnology and is available at the request of manufacturers for other new chemical entities (NCEs). Applications for a marketing license are forwarded directly to the EMEA. At the conclusion of a scientific review, undertaken within 210 days by the agency, the opinion and recommendation of the review committee are sent to the European Commission for approval and subsequent issuing of a single marketing license, which is applicable to the entire European Union.

The decentralized procedure, based on mutual acceptance or recognition of national authority, applies to the majority of conventional medical products. It provides for the extension of marketing licenses granted by one member state to one or more other member states identified by the applicant. The opinion and recommendation of the review committee are transmitted to the

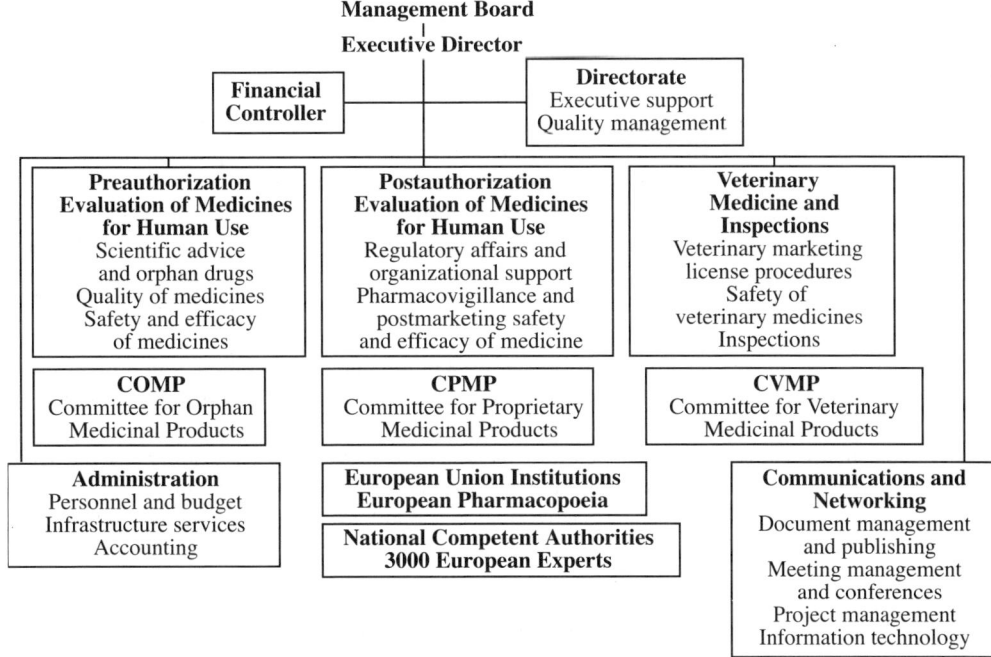

Figure 5.1   Organization of the European Agency for the Evaluation of Medicinal Products (EMEA).

European Commission, which reaches a decision with the assistance of a standing committee composed of representatives of the member states.

The mission of the EMEA is to ensure the protection and promotion of the health of the public and animals by:

- Utilizing the scientific resources of the European Union to provide high-quality evaluations of medical products, to advise on biomedical research and development, and to supply scientific information to health professionals and public
- Developing effective and open procedures to provide access to innovative medicines through a single European marketing license
- Regulating the safety of medicines for humans and animals by means of a pharmacovigilance system and the establishment of safe limits for residues in food-producing animals

The organization of the EMEA is described in Figure 5.1. The EMEA does not directly manage the evaluation of drug applications submitted to support marketing licensure; instead, it forwards drug applications to selected national European Union regulatory agencies for appraisal. The EMEA makes a recommendation to approve or not approve the application based on the report of the national agency. Its overall role is to coordinate and manage the drug regulation system. EMEA has approximately 140 permanent employees and an annual budget of about 20 million.

Under the centralized procedure, drug applications are accepted for such categories as biotechnology products and new chemical entities. This system symbolizes the coordination and cooperation between central management organizations and local national regulatory agencies that facilitate the licensing procedures. Approval of license applications for biotech products must be considered under the centralized procedure, whereas NCEs can be considered under either centralized or decentralized procedures. In the centralized procedure, upon receipt of an application the EMEA staff conducts an initial appraisal with 10 days to verify that sufficient documents have been submitted. At that time, a filing date is assigned. The sponsor also pays an appropriate fee (120,000). The EMEA reviews the submitted documents within 210 days and recommends that the application be accepted or not accepted. This recommendation is then forwarded to the European Commission for its consideration within an additional 90 days; thus, the total evaluation time for a drug application is 300 days. When additional information is required, the 300-day "evaluation clock" stops until the required information is provided. The European Commission has the final authority to issue a marketing license, not the EMEA. The unified marketing authorization is applicable for the entire European Union. It is valid for 5 years and should be renewed thereafter.

The number of new drug applications declined recently from 94 in 2000 to 57 in 2002; however, the number of applications for orphan drugs increased, from 2 in 2000 to 12 in 2002. A sharp increase occurred in the reporting of adverse reactions from both non-European Union countries (11,285 reports in 2000; 27,800 in 2002) and countries in the European Union (14,372 reports in 2000; 14,808 in 2002).

Transparency initiatives regarding the EMEA's operation and collaboration with patient organizations, healthcare professionals, and academic societies were developed in 2002, and the agency's EudraVigilance projects have entered the implementation phase following successful testing by regulatory agencies. The challenges of the future include implementation of a review of the licensing procedures, implications of enlargement, information management for the community system of medicines control, clinical trials, pharmacovigilance support systems, and further extension of transparency for agency operations.

5.3 U.S. FOOD AND DRUG ADMINISTRATION

The U.S. Food and Drug Administration (FDA) is one of the nation's oldest and most respected consumer protection agencies. The FDA is responsible for protecting the public health by ensuring the safety, efficacy, and purity of human and veterinary drugs, biological products, medical devices, and food supplies. It is also responsible for promoting public health by facilitating innovations that make drugs and biologics more effective, safer, and more affordable and by making available to the public accurate scientific information to improve their health.

The FDA is divided into several centers. The Center for Drug Evaluation and Research (CDER; see Figure 5.2) evaluates drug safety and efficacy and is responsible for ensuring accurate product labeling. The Center for Biologics Evaluation and Research (CBER; see Figure 5.3) performs similar duties for biological products intended for human use. Quality assurance of medical products involves establishing specifications and analytical methods regarding identity, strength, quality, purity, bioavailability, and stability. The safety of investigational products is assessed from detailed reviews of the manufacturing process and test procedures, clinical trial results, and control testing of bulk and final lots of products before release to market. Efficacy is examined in one or more controlled clinical trials. Market approval is granted if scientific and clinical data provide sufficient evidence to demonstrate safety and efficacy for the proposed indication. Following licensure, monitoring of product safety and effectiveness continues via postmarketing surveillance of the target population.

A strategic action plan was proposed in 2003 to meet the new public health challenges of making 21st-century knowledge about drugs, biologics, and foods available to the general public. Getting new drugs, biologics, or medical devices into use has grown more difficult, as scientific breakthroughs require more time and higher costs. Because the costs of developing new medical products and using them effectively continue to rise, it has been suggested that an emphasis should be placed on the prevention of obesity, diabetes, and other chronic diseases through better consumer choices and food products. At the same time, we are facing serious threats to the health of the public due to complex, large-scale organized criminal activity. To address these challenges, the FDA has undertaken development of a major strategic action plan that identifies five top priorities for the agency.

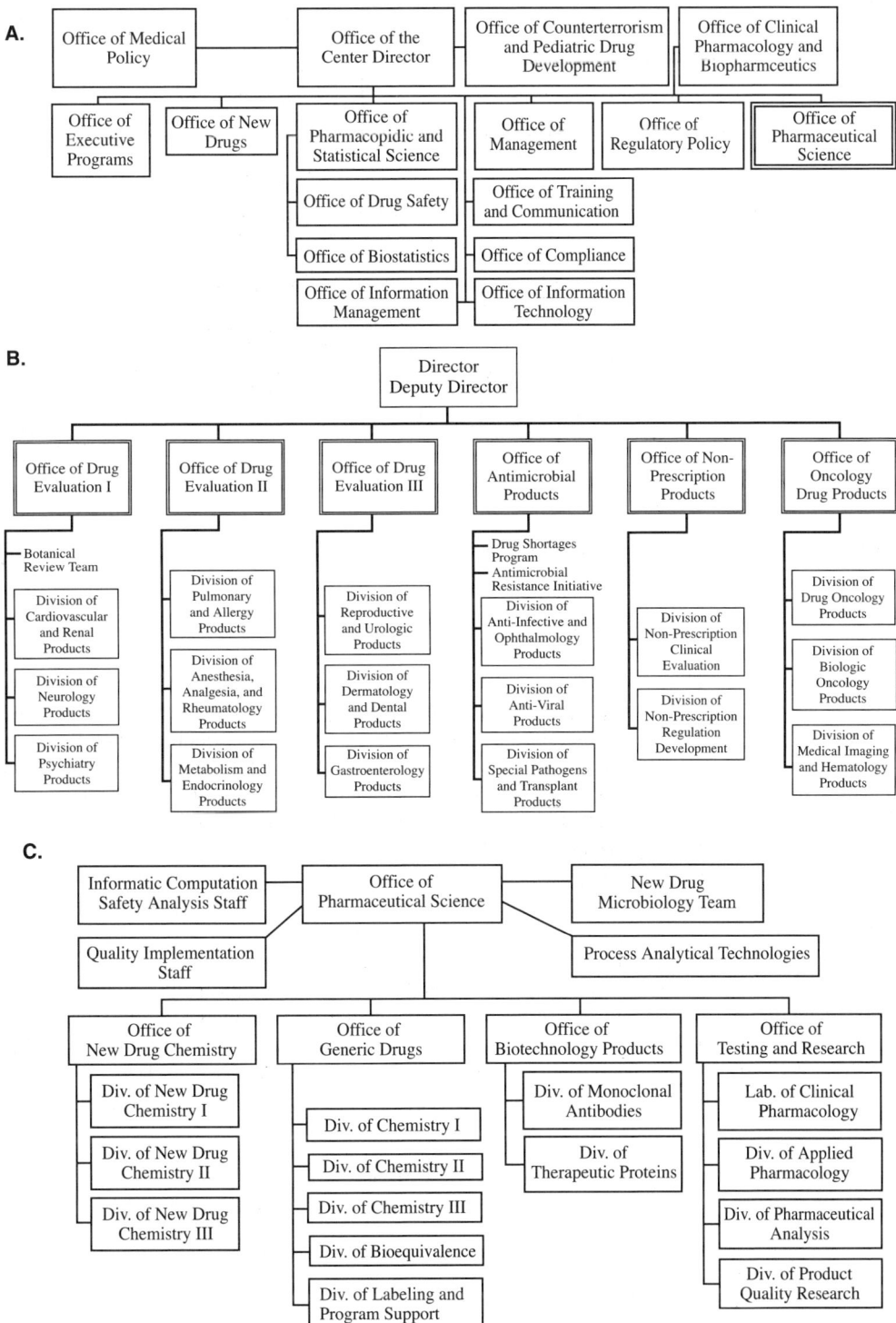

Figure 5.2   (A) Organization chart of the FDA's Center for Drug Evaluation and Research (CDER); (B) Office of New Drugs; (C) Office of Pharmaceutical Science.

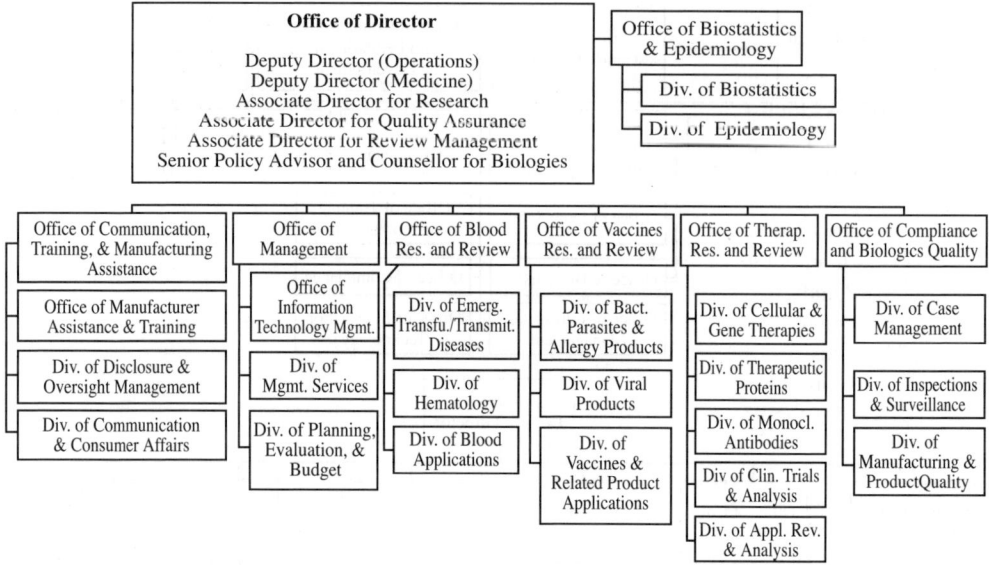

Figure 5.3   The FDA's Center for Biologics Evaluation and Research (CBER).

5.3.1   Efficient Risk Management

The FDA is dealing with new threats in the area of enforcement. Today, organized criminal activity is targeting drugs, infant formula, and other medical products for such illegal operations as selling counterfeit drugs and products contaminated with bacteria, as well as distributing controlled substances through Internet sites. The FDA is also involved in preventing the spread of emerging infections (e.g., recent outbreak of SARS), and threats of bioterrorism require the agency's attention. Recently, the number of new product applications submitted for FDA review has declined significantly. In 2002, the FDA filed 16 priority new drug applications (NDAs), down from a high of 32 in 1997. Standard NDA submissions also decreased — 87 were filed in 2002, down from a high of 101 in 1999. This decrease reflects the importance of facilitating quicker new drug development at lower costs.

The FDA recognizes that efficient risk management is the best way to make the most effective use of agency resources by utilizing the best scientific data, developing quality standards, and applying appropriate decisions for performing regulatory activities. The number of drugs, biologics, and medical devices that the FDA regulates now exceeds 150,000, and almost 3000 investigational new drugs are under development. Also, a growing number of dietary supplements is on the market.

Enforcement by the FDA focuses on the most effective way to promote compliance with regulations:

- By developing and providing clear and consistent guidance
- By encouraging valuable innovation in medical products and food supplies on a strong scientific basis
- By cooperating with other federal and state agencies, academic institutions, and private organizations to perform regulatory responsibilities
- By taking effective actions against criminal activities to maintain public safety

The cost of developing safe and effective new medical products has increased greatly, more than doubling over the past decade; it costs more than $800 million and takes well over 10 years to develop a new drug. According to a recent analysis, of all the new chemical entities that enter clinical testing, only 21.5% will achieve final clinical success and FDA licensure.[1] As a result, the number of new drugs (new molecular entities) approved by the FDA has been declining, falling to 17 in 2002 from a high of 53 in 1996. Over the past decade, however, the number of FDA-regulated imports has increased greatly, growing from 4.2 million in 1997 to 7.8 million in 2002.* The FDA wants to make sure that their standards and guidance encourage the successful development of new drugs and application of imported medical products.

Rising costs of drug development have contributed to rising healthcare costs and hampered timely access to effective treatments; thus, making the process of translating new scientific discoveries into safe and effective treatments more efficient and faster is critical and a high priority for the FDA. Another approach to efficient risk management is the FDA's current standards and guidance to industry. The current good manufacturing practice (CGMP) regulations for drugs and biologics have provided useful and practical information. The FDA's goal for efficient risk management includes the following four objectives and approaches:

- Provide a timely, high-quality, cost-effective process for the review of new product applications.
- Apply the updated scientific knowledge and quality assurance to the FDA's requirements, including CGMP inspections and compliance and enforcement activities.
- Ensure the safety of medical products and the food supply at the least cost to the public.
- Develop strategies and analyses to evaluate options on management and regulatory decision-making.

5.3.2 Improving Health through Better Information

Providing better and clear information to consumers has a great impact on public health. For example, in 2000, the total cost of obesity was estimated to be $117 billion. A lack of physical exercise and inadequate nutrition account for approximately 300,000 deaths each year. Better information allows the general public to make smarter choices that can have a great impact on improving their health. The FDA is undertaking major efforts to help consumers make better-informed decisions; for example, the agency takes steps to ensure that information provided by manufacturers is accurate, and the agency communicates directly with the public to provide information on the risks and benefits of regulated products. Several important strategies have been established to achieve the objective of making the public better informed:

- Develop wider consumer communications (e.g., providing new and better information regarding pediatric labeling to healthcare providers).
- Ensure that manufacturer information for consumers and healthcare providers regarding product risks and benefits is accurate and not misleading. The agency is committed to actively pursuing those who make false and misleading claims. In 2002, the FDA inspected more than 80 dietary supplement firms to correct violations. In 2003, the agency seized dietary supplements from a firm in Florida due to inaccurate claims that the products would treat a variety of medical conditions, including cancer and arthritis.
- Improve and increase FDA-initiated risk–benefit reporting (e.g., educating the public and healthcare providers about antimicrobial resistance).

5.3.3 Improving Patient and Consumer Safety

Adverse events related to medical products, dietary supplements, and foods have had serious consequences on the health of many Americans. Adverse drug reactions alone result in 770,000

---

* The number of line entries is used as an indicator of the relative volume of FDA-regulated imported products. Sources of data include the U.S. Census (1986–1993), U.S. Customs (1994–1996), and FDA OASIS (1997–2002).

injuries and deaths each year. Sometimes problems arise when medical products and dietary supplements are misused because consumers or healthcare providers did not have adequate information about a new treatment. Moreover, unpredictable side effects may occur after licensure of a new product. The FDA has relied on reporting systems to monitor the safety of a new medical product. While these systems are effective in identifying rare and serious adverse events, their reliance on healthcare providers and incomplete reporting means that appropriate detection and response to adverse events may be less timely and effective than is desirable. The FDA is taking steps to achieve direct and secure access to electronic medical record systems. Cooperation with healthcare providers and the Centers for Disease Control and Prevention (CDC) will allow the FDA to access medical records and public health monitoring systems in order to:

- Improve its ability to identify risks associated with medical products.
- Identify adverse events more quickly.
- More accurately analyze risks associated with medical products, dietary supplements, and foods.
- Take effective actions to deal with risks and correct these problems; for example, the FDA will work with the National Library of Medicine to set up DailyMed, a new way to distribute up-to-date and comprehensive medication information in a computerized format for use in healthcare information systems.

5.3.4 Protecting the Homeland from Bioterrorism

September 11, 2001, marked the beginning of a dark autumn. From the moment two hijacked airplanes crashed into the World Trade Center towers, an attack that killed thousands of people, biomedical scientists realized the imminent threat of bioterrorism. The attack showed that these terrorists were sophisticated, organized, and perhaps capable of producing biologic weapons of mass destruction. They were able and willing to destroy large numbers of people. Now, there is widespread concern that naturally occurring pathogens capable of spreading easily through the respiratory tract and food chain could be used as bioterrorist weapons. Such an attack would be particularly dangerous for children, the elderly, and immunocompromised people. The foods most likely to be targets are those that are minimally processed at a central location and are ready to eat, such as milk, fruits, and other fresh foods. In addition to damaging the population's health and safety, bioterrorism against the food supply would also harm the U.S. economy, as bioterrorism incidents could seriously damage public confidence in the effectiveness of the nation's defense of the food supply against infectious diseases.

The FDA has been engaged in developing countermeasures for biological, chemical, and radiological attacks. The agency plays a major role in the nation's defense against bioterrorism, because, for example, terrorists could use FDA-regulated products, such as imported foods, to introduce deadly diseases into the country. In addition, regulated products such as human and animal drugs, vaccines, blood, and blood products would play a central role in countering the terrorist attacks. In 2002, the Public Health Security and Bioterrorism Preparedness and Response Act was passed to provide a total of $2.369 billion for bioterrorism response.

The events of September 11, 2001, and the subsequent anthrax attacks have refocused the FDA's efforts to incorporate enhanced security and safety measures. The agency is expanding its capability to assess and respond to risks associated with terrorist-related health and safety threats to the U.S. homeland. This involves working with industry to develop medical countermeasures using updated science and collaborating with other agencies and organization. For example, the FDA is developing a science-based life-cycle approach to ensuring the safety of medical and food products. In the case of bulk imports, instead of inspecting and sampling a particular shipment at the border, the FDA wants to obtain the complete history of a product, from raw materials through production and transportation to the United States.

The FDA is working to:

- Facilitate the availability of medical measures to counter terrorist attacks on civilian and military populations. Drugs, vaccines, other biological products, and medical devices must be readily available to prevent, diagnose, and treat illnesses resulting from a terrorist attack.
- Enhance the agency's emergency preparedness and response capabilities against terrorist attacks.
- Ensure the security of FDA personnel and sensitive information, as well as the safety of approximately 80% of the nation's food supply.
- Protect the safety and security of drugs, biologics, medical devices, and other FDA-regulated products.

5.3.5   More Effective Regulation through a Strong Workforce

A professional workforce is critically important for the FDA to maintain its effective regulatory activities and the high level of public trust. The agency's regulation depends on solid groups of experienced physicians, immunologists, biochemists, toxicologists, statisticians, and other professionals. Among the staff of the FDA are approximately 1500 with doctorate degrees and more than 400 with medical degrees. Two thirds of the FDA's budget is spent on its workforce. The FDA's accomplishments are primarily a reflection of its professional services. Objectives of the FDA include ensuring a high-quality, diverse, motivated workforce. The FDA provides a working environment in which its scientists have the opportunity for professional training and career development. In addition, the agency is responsive to its employees' diverse workplace needs, such as flexible work schedules for two working parents, care for sick children and elderly parents, and telecommuting. The FDA supports its employees by providing childcare, elder care, and other distinctive needs. To improve the effectiveness of its management, the FDA will modernize its administrative support services and adopt new management practices in order to:

- Improve its information technology capabilities and increase productivity.
- Improve the agency's monitoring of revenues and expenditures.
- Ensure effective communication and working relationships with national and global health organizations.
- Improve its capability to achieve the goals of faster review of new drugs and biologics, more rapid targeting of suspect imports, and quicker identification, analysis, and communication of adverse events.

5.4 REGULATION IN ASIA

The Asian economy has developed rapidly in the past decade. The pharmaceutical industry in Asia is making remarkable changes to expand access to modern science, technology, and healthcare for the people of Asia. With the goal of being recognized as part of a global pharmaceutical industry achieving innovation in novel drugs and biologics, Asian nations are striving to establish their own research-based drug development capability, clinical trials, and regulatory system. Asia hopes to become the third most important pharmaceutical market after the United States and Europe within the next decade.

The low labor costs and high-quality workforce in Asia provide unique opportunities for Asian pharmaceutical companies to actively participate in global drug research and development. Personnel costs in Asia are generally less than one third comparable costs in the United States or Europe. Due to rapid advances in biotechnology, global communication, and information exchange, major pharmaceutical companies are able to increase their global clinical trial activities in Asia. For example, in Taiwan clinical facilities and related contract laboratories have been established for drug development and evaluation.

In many Asian countries, the major drug development programs and international research collaborations are largely sponsored by the governments. Governments in Singapore, Korea, China, Malaysia, and India have actively pursued strategies to attract major global pharmaceutical companies to conduct drug research and clinical trials in their countries. In Asia, diseases such as hepatitis C, severe acute respiratory syndrome (SARS), and liver, brain, and lung cancer are common; therefore, it is convenient and reasonable for foreign drug companies to conduct clinical trials in Asia for these diseases. Asia has played a major role in identifying the etiology of SARS and developing fast diagnostic tools and agents for the effective treatment and prevention of SARS. The disease is highly mutable, and infections are extremely difficult to treat. Without a known therapeutic agent, SARS could become a deadly threat to the United States and other countries. Regions such as Taiwan and China with many SARS-infected patients have attracted foreign research institutes to perform clinical trials for potential anti-SARS agents.

In addition to Japan, several countries, including Taiwan, Singapore, Korea, and China, have aggressively developed biotechnology and pharmaceutical sciences as a major tool for economic growth. Taiwan has many well-educated scientists, a growing number of biomedical research establishments, experience in generic drug manufacturing, access to China's market, and sources of domestic investment capital; however, Taiwan lacks some key technologies and the entrepreneurial management to develop its research-based pharmaceutical companies.

The drug discovery and development process has rapidly moved toward globalization. Asia, with many unique advantages, is becoming one of the major players in the international pharmaceutical community for discovering novel chemical entities and supporting pivotal clinical trials. Japan has played a leading and critical role for drug development in Asia. Although many Asian countries, such as Taiwan, Singapore, Korea, and China, have to strengthen the capability of their research-based pharmaceutical industry, they expect to facilitate solid drug discoveries and clinical trials through significant capital investment and research collaborations with foreign pharmaceutical companies.[3,4]

5.4.1   Clinical Trials and Regulation in Japan

Located in the northeastern part of Asia, Japan has about 2000 pharmaceutical companies, including 80 research-based manufacturers that develop new medical products. Drug production in 2001 was about US$55 billion (6504 billion yen). Japanese people are the greatest consumer of drugs per capita in the world. In Japan, the manufacturing, distribution, and sale of drugs and biological products are regulated by the Ministry of Health, Labour, and Welfare (*Kosei-lodo-sho*).[5] This organization also promotes social welfare, social security, and public health. The Pharmaceutical and Food Safety Bureau, one of ten bureaus under this Ministry, is in charge of issues related to the efficacy, safety, and quality control of drugs, biologics, foods, and cosmetics. It also enforces the Pharmacists Law, the Bleeding and Blood Donor Supply Service Control Law, and the Narcotics and Psychotropics Control Law.

The Pharmaceutical Affairs Law is the supreme law. Its mission is to regulate issues related to drugs, cosmetics, and medical devices to ensure their quality, efficacy, and safety and to promote the development of orphan drugs. According to this law, any sponsor who intends to manufacture or import drugs and other medical products must obtain approval to manufacture (or import) each item and a manufacturer's (importer's) license. Manufacturers or importers of new drugs must apply for reexamination of such drugs 6 years after their initial approval. Manufacturer or importers of other drugs that have already been approved and designated by the minister must apply for reevaluation of the efficacy for such products.

The law also contains provisions involving clinical trials, including requirements of good clinical practices (GCPs) for sponsors of clinical trials, and supports research and development of medical products for rare diseases. Manufacturers or importers must obtain approval for clinical trials from the Minister of Health, Labour, and Welfare or prefectural (local) governor. Before approval is granted, the submitted data and documents, which include the product name, ingredients, composition, administration route, dosage, indications, and adverse reactions, are reviewed and examined in detail. A license to manufacture or import a medical product is granted after sufficient evidence regarding the applicant's capability to manufacture or import the medical product is provided.

Beginning in 1997, the Ministry of Health and Welfare conducted a reform of the new drug application review process. In 2001, the government was reorganized, and the Ministry of Health and Welfare became Ministry of Health, Labour, and Welfare. Objectives of this reform were to strengthen the Ministry's mission and regulations, including review of clinical trial protocols, providing advice on protocols, and verifying compliance of data submitted for NDAs, and to improve the effectiveness of the review process. In 1999, after the reform, the staff in the Ministry increased from 100 to 200. The new system is composed of three sections:

- Ministry of Health and Welfare
- Pharmaceuticals and Medical Devices Evaluation Center, which is a research institute under the National Institute of Health Sciences (also part of the Ministry of Health and Welfare)
- Organization for Pharmaceutical Safety and Research.

5.3.2.1 Current Status of Clinical Trials[5]

Japan introduced its GCPs in October 1989, and they became effective a year later. The first version of the Japanese GCPs differed from those of the United States and Europe; for example, sponsors were allowed to enroll subjects on their oral consent, and the first GCPs did not have a requirement for monitoring of trial sites. In 1997, Japan revised its GCPs for the following reasons:

- Great concern regarding the safety of clinical trials
- Serious adverse reactions that occurred in 1993 in clinical trials for an antiviral agent that caused 15 deaths before being recalled
- Establishment of the ICH good clinical practice guideline

In 1996, the ICH GCP guideline reached step 4 of the ICH process, and incorporating it into the domestic regulations was proposed. As a result, the Ministry of Health and Welfare introduced the ICH GCP in 1997. GCP inspections have been enforced to ensure compliance with regulations. For every NDA, the Ministry inspects two or three randomly selected medical institutions and investigators among dozens of trial sites. GCP inspection is the first and essential step in reaching final approval; thus, meeting GCP requirements is crucial to sponsors. Since inspection was initiated in 1992, 350 medical institutions and investigators and 150 sponsors have been inspected. The majority of them passed the inspection.

The Ministry holds a monthly GCP evaluation committee meeting to examine GCP compliance for every submitted application. The Organization for Pharmaceutical Safety and Research submits inspection reports to this committee. When a clinical trial does not meet requirements, the Ministry has the authority to order the sponsor to delete part or all of the clinical trial data. Among various GCP violations, one of the most common violations is insufficient documentation on the case report form (CRF). The records intentionally or mistakenly omitted from the CRF include:

- Use of prohibited drug prescriptions other than the investigational new drug
- Negative clinical or laboratory test data
- Drug adverse events

Other violations include trials without proper contracts or informed consent by the participants, trials that have not followed the protocol, and occasional falsification or fabrication of data. One cause for these violations is the investigators' lack of quality assurance. In 1998, sponsors enforced the right and responsibility to access and examine source documents at medical institutions to minimize GCP violations.

Since 1998, Japan has experienced two big events in pharmaceutical administration. That year marked a turning point for Japanese GCPs with respect to implementation of the ICH GCP and acceptance of foreign clinical data. When adopting the ICH GCP, the Ministry addressed a number of major issues; (1) requiring proper written informed consent (a change that was resisted by investigators and participants who were previously allowed to rely on oral explanation and consent); (2) a lack of clinical trial coordinators; (3) the need for institutional review boards to add external and nonmedical members; and (4) incentives to encourage subjects to join in clinical trials. Before 1998, the Ministry required domestic data for new drug approval based on the consideration that ethnic factors may affect the clinical data; however, strict application of this requirement would force sponsors to duplicate entire trials, thus delaying the process of drug development. In August 1998, the Ministry set certain conditions for the acceptance of foreign clinical data, and it can request a limited domestic data as a "bridging study."

In 2001 and 2002, Japan revised the Pharmaceutical Affairs Law and established a new evaluation organization. Due to advances in pharmaceutical sciences, it became necessary to revise the act to keep pace with the trend for international harmonization and changes in socioeconomic conditions, scientific progress, and diversification of management. Many new drugs are developed utilizing biotechnology, genomics, nanotechnology, and computer information, and international harmonization will become an even more pressing requirement in the future. The Ministry has carried out these renovations by focusing primarily on safety measures involving medical devices, the accommodation of biologics, and a thorough revision of the approval and licensing system.

5.3.2.2 Drug Approval and Regulation

A manufacturer or drug importer applies to the Ministry of Health, Labour, and Welfare (MHLW) through the prefectural government. The new drug application is reviewed first at the specific division of the Pharmaceutical and Medical Device Evaluation Center (PMDEC) and then forwarded to the specific subcommittee of the Central Pharmaceutical Affairs Council (CPAC) according to the type of drug. PMDEC was established in 1997 to strengthen the government's evaluation capacity for ensuring safety and preventing harmful side effects of pharmaceuticals. Upon acceptance of the application by the MHLW, PMDEC forwards the data to the external medical institution for their reliability survey. Consideration of the data is conducted on a scientific basis by an evaluation team, which prepares a drug evaluation report. The CPAC, an advisory organization to the ministry, is comprised of 15 committees and 75 subcommittees. The council investigates and gives recommendations on important pharmaceutical and health issues. Based on the advice of the CPAC, the Ministry makes a final decision regarding approval of the manufacturer's or importer's drug license application. The processes for drug evaluation and approval are described in Figure 5.4, and the evaluation process of the PMDEC is shown in Figure 5.5.

For drugs containing a new chemical entity, the National Institute of Health Sciences will examine the specifications and testing methods and will also test a few samples. The Institute is responsible for conducting basic research to ensure the quality, efficacy, and safety of a wide range of products that directly and indirectly affect the public's health. Applications for drugs having the same ingredients, efficacy, dosage, and indications as those previously approved are forwarded to the administrative offices for evaluation. Before 1997, the process of drug review from initial submittal of the application to final approval required approximately 18 months for ethical drugs, 10 months for nonprescription drugs, and 6 months for in vitro diagnostic reagents. Since April 2000, the licensing procedure has been reduced to 12 months for new drugs but has not changed for nonprescription drugs and in vitro diagnostic reagents.

5.3.2.3 Postmarketing Surveillance System[6]

The postmarketing surveillance system includes a safety monitoring program for drugs and a policy for promoting the advancement of medicine and pharmacy. The safety monitoring program is carried

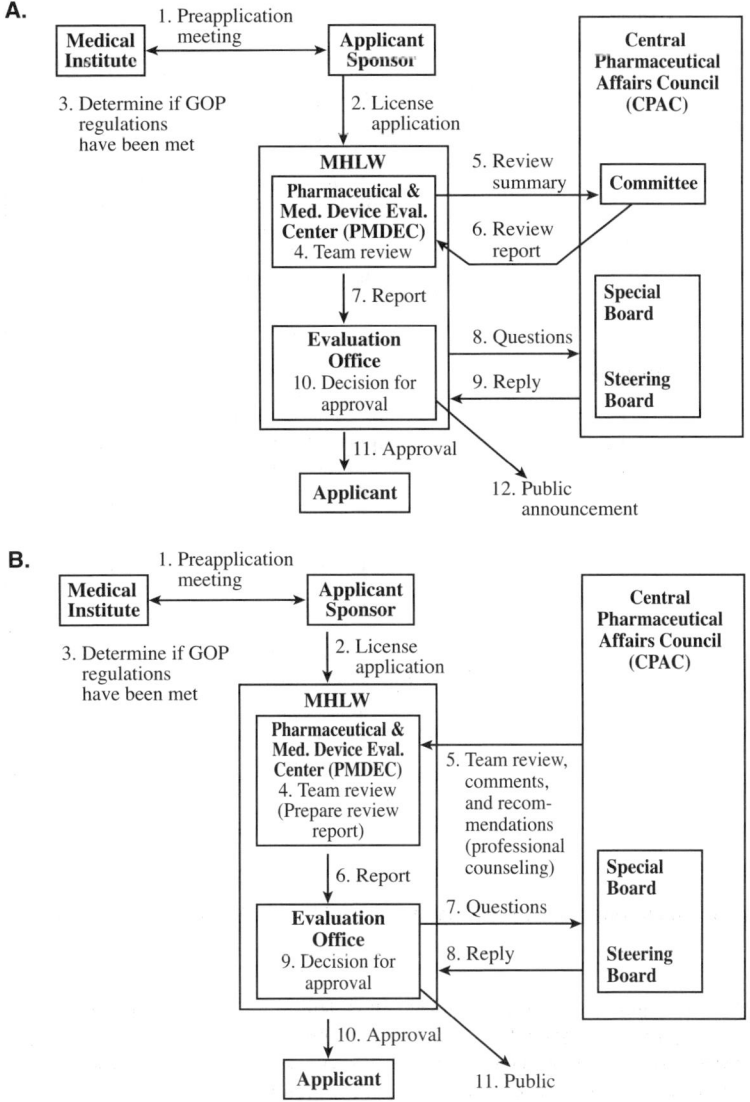

Figure 5.4   Drug evaluation and approval in Japan: (A) from July 1997 to October 1999; (B) after November 1999.

out in three phases: collection of adverse drug reaction data, reexamination of drugs, and reevaluation of drugs.

- Collection of adverse drug reaction information — During the 4 to 6 years immediately following drug approval, the manufacturer or importer of a new drug is required to conduct investigations on the use and adverse reactions of the drug and report the results to the Ministry every year. The manufacturer must report adverse reaction cases within 30 days of each incident. From these reports, the Ministry can then notify the appropriate people regarding adverse reactions that were unknown at the time of approval. Since 1972, Japan has been a member of the World Health Organization's international drug monitoring system and has reported its domestic monitoring activities on adverse drug reactions. Japan also exchanges adverse drug reaction information with the FDA and with agencies in other countries.

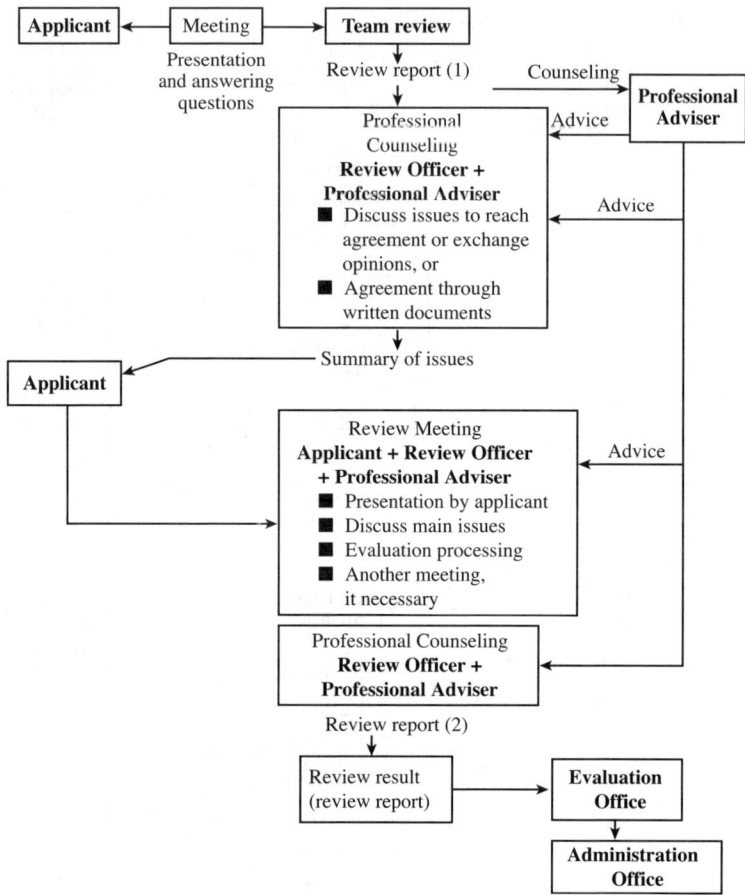

Figure 5.5 Evaluation process of the Pharmaceutical and Medical Device Evaluation Center (PMDEC).

- Drug reexamination — The drug reexamination system was established in 1980 to monitor the use of a new drug for 4 to 6 years following the postmarketing period. Postmarket reexamination of a drug focuses particularly on the elderly, children, and pregnant women. Usually, 10,000 cases or more are reviewed. Special attention is paid to drug complications involving hepatic, renal, blood, and other tissue disturbances. The period of reexamination for drugs with a new chemical entity, new combination, or new route of administration is 6 years after approval of the drug. Drugs with additional indications, new dosages, or new routes of administration must be reexamined after 4 years.
- Drug reevaluation — *First round reevaluation* is based on administrative guidance. This system was established in 1971. Between 1973 and 1989, 18,986 products were reevaluated, including 1765 substances contained in prescription drugs. As a result, 1079 prescription drugs were determined as "having no basis for indicated usefulness" based on the following: insufficient basis for efficacy, adverse drug reactions outweighed the therapeutic benefit, inadequate duration to achieve therapeutic drug levels, and inadequate dosage form. Similarly, in 1988, among 1269 combination drugs, 190 items were similarly judged. *Second round reexamination* is based on the Pharmaceutical Affairs law. Drugs subject to this reevaluation include newly developed drugs approved after October 1, 1967, and those drugs containing the same ingredients as newly developed drugs but which were exempted from the first reevaluation based on administrative guidance. In the second evaluation program, 129 formulas out of 611 items have been selected for reevaluation; one item has been judged "not useful." As of May 1988, all prescription drugs must be reviewed every 5 years.

5.4.2 Clinical Trials and Drug Evaluation in Taiwan

The island state of Taiwan, with a population of 23 million, has achieved an annual growth rate of approximately 10% from 1981 to 1991. According to the World Bank's *World Development Report 2002: Building Institutions for Markets* (Oxford University Press, 2001), Taiwan had the world's 16th largest economy in 2000. Taiwan's gross national product (GNP) was $313.9 billion, and its per capita GNP was $14,188, ranking among the highest GNPs in Asia. Taiwan's total pharmaceutical market value was $2.4 billion in 2001 and $2.6 billion in 2002, making it the fifth largest Far East country.

Health agencies in Taiwan are organized in four levels: national, city and province, county and city, and township. At the national level, the Department of Health of the Executive Yuan is the highest health authority. The department has several bureaus, including the Bureau of Pharmaceutical Affairs, the National Laboratories of Foods and Drugs, and the Narcotics Bureau. Until its modification in 1986, Taiwan's patent law protected only the manufacturing process for new drugs but not the end products. In the 1990s, the protection of intellectual property became a major issue in trade negotiations between the United States and Taiwan. Registration requirements were modified in July 1993 to protect intellectual property. Under the new regulation, sponsors must conduct a good local clinical trial with at least 40 subjects before marketing a drug in Taiwan. After approval, the applicant receives marketing exclusivity for a 7-year safety monitoring period. Sponsors applying for generic drug permits also should conduct local clinical trials during the first 5 years of the monitoring period.

Since passing its new regulations, Taiwan has demonstrated its ability to conduct clinical trials designed by multinational pharmaceutical companies. The Department of Health has encouraged local pharmaceutical companies to invest in research and development, and extensive integrated efforts have been made to develop drugs and biological products. As a result, the number of clinical trials has increased greatly.

In 1996, Taiwan established its GCP guidelines. In 2002, Taiwan revised its GCP guidelines in accordance with the ICH E6 guideline for clinical trials in a variety of medical subspecialties, including antiinfection, anticancer, cardiovascular, endocrinology, and radioactive drugs. In 2000, guidelines for herbal extracts were established. From 2001 to 2002, guidelines were established for clinical trials of drugs in special populations, such as geriatrics, pediatrics, and patients with impaired hepatic or renal function, in addition to the following guidelines:

- Guidance for Bridging Studies: Ethnic Factors in the Acceptability of Foreign Clinical Data
- Guidance for the Content and Format of Clinical Trial Reports

Since 1995, to deal with increasing demands for performing domestic clinical trials, the Department of Health, through the management of the Foundation of Medical Professionals Alliance in Taiwan, has cooperated with medical centers and professional medical associations to conduct a series of training courses on clinical trials covering the following topics:

- Clinical trials in specific diseases or specialties (heart and vascular diseases, oncology, infectious disease, endocrinology and metabolic disease, gastroenterology, neurology, and respiratory diseases)
- Clinical inspections (GCP inspections and ethnic factors)
- Clinical trials in certain classes of drugs (antiinflammatory drugs, antiinfectious drugs, analgesics, and radiological drugs)
- Statistics in clinical trials and GCP issues
- Assessment of drug safety
- Ethics
- Developing new alternative therapies
- Pharmacokinetics
- Case studies and bridging studies in oncology
- Safety evaluation for biological products

These training courses have received good feedback from physicians, pharmacists, nurses, and other participants. As of the end of 2001, 1942 clinicians, 1073 pharmacists, 151 nurses, and 1732 researchers had participated in these courses.

Good clinical practice inspections have been conducted in all registered clinical trials performed in Taiwan. In 2002, the Department of Health inspected 37 trials; of these:

- Five were accepted.
- Twelve were accepted upon further clarification.
- Four required reinspection.
- Two were dismissed.
- Fourteen were pending, awaiting supplemental information from sponsors

For carrying out effective clinical trials, Taiwan established a joint institutional review board (IRB) in March 1997. The joint IRB has improved Taiwan's competitiveness in attracting multicenter trials, including global phase IIIa trials. The goals of the joint IRB include:

- Improving the safety of study subjects in clinical trials
- Shortening the time required to obtain permission for clinical trials
- Avoiding repetition of trial applications and different application formats
- Establishing a communications network for regional IRB-related issues
- Reviewing multicenter clinical trials and phase I to III studies of new drugs

At present, 44 hospitals have participated in the joint IRB: 17 medical centers, 23 regional hospitals, and 4 specialized clinics. In 2002, the joint IRB reviewed 5 multinational phase II studies and 13 multinational phase III studies.[7]

At one time, the evaluation of new drug applications (NDAs) in Taiwan was performed by a drug advisory committee composed of external experts invited by the Bureau of Pharmaceutical Affairs. The old system could not perform independent reviews of drug applications, and it required preapproval (licensed products) from at least three major foreign governments before submission of an application. The part-time academic advisory boards was able to offer little assistance to the pharmaceutical industry in regulatory drug development. To meet the national policy of developing the pharmaceutical industry and competing in the global market, the Center for Drug Evaluation (CDE) was established as a nongovernmental, nonprofit foundation by the Department of Health in 1998 to facilitate effective NDA reviews. The CDE assists in evaluating clinical trial protocols for new drugs, herbal products, and biologics. It holds meetings with sponsors to clarify review concerns, shorten the protocol review time, and elevate the legitimate approval rate for trials. Generally, the Center reviews a protocol within about 6 weeks. At present, the CDE has 43 full-time employees and plans to have 100 employees in 5 years.

The Asia Pacific region represents a large and densely populated area, but it is also a region with small individual markets, weak regulatory authorities, primitive local drug industries, and a poor system of conducting clinical trials. Thus, the region has no independent voice in global drug evaluation processes, and its local needs in new drug development are often ignored. An independent drug review system for the Asia Pacific region is necessary to account for population differences in drug response, to promote local industry, and to meet regional needs for new drugs. To achieve this goal, the Asia Pacific region will have to establish a unified market for new drugs to provide a favorable development environment and participate in a harmonized regulatory system. It is recommended that regulatory agencies in this region pool their resources and collaborate on drug regulations for the purpose of examining issues related to clinical bridging studies, collaborate on inspections, share postmarketing monitoring, and establish joint review of new drug applications, with the eventual goal of achieving mutual recognition of new drug approvals.[8]

5.5 INTERNATIONAL CONFERENCE ON HARMONISATION[9]

The industrialized world has learned important lessons regarding the regulation of medical products through the painful experience of history. The importance of independent and thorough evaluation of medical products before their use by the public was realized at different times in different regions. In the United States, after the death of 13 children in St. Louis as a result of receiving tetanus-contaminated diphtheria antitoxin, in addition to other adverse events, the Biologics Control Act was passed in 1902. In Japan, the government began to require the regulation of all medical products for sale in the 1950s. In Europe, the thalidomide tragedy of the 1960s alerted the public to the potential harm as well as benefit of new drugs and triggered the regulation of medical products.

Because the various regulatory systems have differed with regard to basic requirements for evaluating the quality, safety, and efficacy of products, many time-consuming and expensive evaluation and testing procedures have been duplicated before new products can reach the international market. The rising costs of new drug development have fueled the urgency to harmonize regulations. The International Conference on Harmonisation (ICH) brings together the regulatory authorities of Europe, Japan, and the United States, as well as experts from the pharmaceutical industries in the three regions, in order to seek ways to eliminate redundant and duplicate technical requirements for registering new drugs and biologics. The main objective is to expedite the global development and availability of new medical products without sacrificing efficacy, safety, or quality. Cosponsors of the ICH include:

- Europe — Commission of the European Communities (CEC) and European Federation of Pharmaceutical Industries Association (EFPIA)
- Japan — Ministry of Health, Labour, and Welfare (MHLW) and Japan Pharmaceutical Manufacturers Association (JPMA)
- United States — Food and Drug Administration (FDA) and Pharmaceutical Research and Manufacturers of America (PhRMA)

In addition, the International Federation of Pharmaceutical Manufacturers Association (IFPMA) participates as an umbrella organization of the pharmaceutical industry and provides the ICH secretariat.

The ICH Technical Requirements for Registration of Pharmaceuticals for Human Use bring together regulatory authorities and experts of the United States, Europe, and Japan to discuss scientific and technical aspects of product registration. The establishment of guidelines and use of common reporting procedures reduce the potential confusion and eliminates duplicate practices. These guidelines promote:

- *Efficacy* – The guideline on the extent of population exposure emphasizes that it is necessary to assess clinical safety for medicinal products intended for long-term treatment of non-life-threatening conditions.
- *Safety* – The guideline on reproductive toxicology intends to save research time and resources and eliminate duplicate animal testing. The carcinogenicity testing procedures allow endpoints other than maximum tolerated dose (MTD).
- *Quality* – The guideline on stability testing grants assessment of new molecules under a standard set of temperature and humidity conditions.

The ICH has been successful in achieving harmonization, initially of technical guidelines and more recently on the format and content of registration applications. All sponsors agree that it is necessary to maintain this harmonization in the interest of public health and to prevent unnecessary duplication without compromising regulatory responsibilities. The ICH will continue to encourage:

- Implementation and monitoring of harmonization actions within a rapidly changing international environment, particularly with regard to common technical documents (CTDs)
- The selection of new topics for further harmonization
- A focus on the important areas of new technological advances, new innovative drugs, and post-marketing surveys

The ICH has emphasized and acknowledged the cooperation of international organizations, such as the World Health Organization, in disseminating information and providing input to non-ICH regions. A need exists to explore new approaches to the ICH model of expert working groups, particularly in areas where changing scientific information has been produced, using advanced techniques of videoconferencing and electronic communication to enhance the exchange of ideas, opinions, and information among ICH groups and with other involved parties. The ICH has focused on achieving the following objectives:

- Maintain a forum for constructive dialog between regulatory authorities and the pharmaceutical industry regarding real and perceived differences in the technical requirements for product registrations.
- Monitor and update harmonized technical requirements leading to the mutual acceptance of research and development data.
- Avoid divergent future requirements through harmonization of selected topics.
- Facilitate the adoption of improved technical research and development approaches to update regulatory activities.
- Facilitate the dissemination of information on harmonized guidelines and their use to encourage the implementation of common standards.

REFERENCES

1. DiMasi, J.A., Hansen, R.W., and Grabowski, H.G., The price of innovation: new estimates of drug development costs, *J. Health Econom.*, 835, 1–35, 2003.
2. McClellan, M.B., *The Food and Drug Administration's Strategic Action Plan — Protecting and Advancing America's Health: Responding to New Challenges and Opportunities*, U.S. Food and Drug Administration, Washington, D.C., 2003 (http://www.fda.gov/oc/mcclellan/strategic.html).
3. Chien, D.S., The role of Asia in global drug discovery and development, *Drug Inform. J.*, 37(Suppl.), 3S–9S, 2003.
4. Lee, C.J., Lee, L.H., and Lu, C.H., *Development and Evaluation of Drugs: From Laboratory through Licensure to Market*, 2nd ed., CRC Press, Boca Raton, FL, 2003.
5. Sato, T., The current status of clinical trials in Japan, *Drug Inform. J.*, 37(Suppl.), 183S–188S, 2003.
6. Tanaka, K., Morita, Y., Kawane, E. et al., Drug use investigation (DUI) and prescription-event monitoring in Japan (J-PEM), *Pharmacoepidemiol. Drug Safety*, 10(7), 653–658, 2001.
7. Wang, H.P. and Chen, S.S.Y., Clinical trials in Taiwan: regulatory achievements and current status, *Drug Inform. J.*, 37(Suppl.), 173S–177S, 2003.
8. Jao, S.H.L., Chern, H.D., and Chu, M.L., Reinventing drug regulation in the Asia Pacific region: Taiwan's experience and a vision for the region, *Drug Inform. J.*, 37 (Suppl.), 41S–48S, 2003.
9. ICH, *Past and Future*, International Conference on Harmonisation of Technical Requirements for Registration of Pharmaceuticals for Human Use, Geneva, Switzerland (http://www.ich.org).

CHAPTER 6

Decision Points in Drug Development

Lucia H. Lee, Christopher L. Wu, Benjamin R. Lee, and Chi-Jen Lee

CONTENTS

6.1 INTRODUCTION

Drug development has undergone dramatic changes in recent years. A few decades ago, it was an empirical field inadequately organized and often pushed by pharmacologists or clinicians to develop new drug products. Decision making was erratic, and development time was long. The number of failed trials was high, and many projects did not result in marketable products for therapeutic use. Today, under the influence of scientific progress, increased regulatory activities, and economic factors, the drug development process has become more complicated and rational. It is now necessary for the pharmaceutical industry to maximize returns on the huge investments that are now required to develop new drugs. Also, the quality of products and speed of manufacturing must be improved. Decision making in the various stages of preclinical research and clinical trials plays an important role.

Drug development begins with a development plan that defines the target profile of the proposed product. The main components of this target profile are indications, patient population, usage, safety, dosage, and administration. The development plan also specifies the activities that will take place during the various preclinical research and clinical trials over the lifetime of the project. To identify the time critical activities that determine the overall duration of the project, it is important to perform a critical path analysis and examine decision points.

During the drug development process, several major decision-making points can be identified. At these critical points, key results must be reviewed and evaluated to make a decision as to whether to continue the plan to meet the target profile or to stop if the goals cannot be achieved. Obviously, the quality of this decision making is a key factor in the successful development of a product. Some of the important decision points during the process of drug development include:

- Selection of a compound in the drug discovery phase for development
- Determining the desired physicochemical and pharmacokinetic characteristics of the compound
- Deciding whether or not to initiate clinical studies
- Deciding, at the end of phase II clinical trials, whether or not to conduct expensive and long-term phase III trials
- Deciding, before the end of phase III trials, whether or not to file the product license application
- Deciding on production necessary for marketing and anticipated premarketing requirements

6.2 DECISION POINTS IN PRECLINICAL STUDIES

6.2.1 Toxicity and Safety Studies

After one or more lead compounds have been selected for further development, additional preclinical studies are necessary before clinical trials can begin. The primary studies during this phase are toxicity and safety studies in animals. The goals of these studies are not only to find safely compounds and reject toxic ones but also to learn under which conditions a potentially beneficial compound can be harmful and to find out how it can be used safely in humans.

Toxicity studies are conducted in healthy animals. For small molecules, two species are used: one a rodent, such as rats or mice, and the other a nonrodent, such as a rabbit, dog, or monkey. Biotechnology-derived large-molecule compounds should be tested in a species in which they are pharmacologically active, such as the monkey. The route of administration is the same as that of the intended use in clinical trials. The primary questions to be answered by the toxicity and safety studies are what the adverse effects of the compound are and what the target organ is in the species tested. During these studies, changes in animal behavior, appearance, food intake, and body weight will be observed. Blood and urine tests are done regularly. At the end of the study, the animals are killed and a full necropsy performed, including microscopy of various tissues and organs. Other questions include determining whether the observed toxicity is reversible and whether the occurrence of toxicity can be detected in clinical trials.

Usually, the maximal doses used in toxicity studies should be much higher than the doses subsequently used in humans. At the end of these studies, the following doses should be established:

- No-effect dose, which is the highest dose that does not cause an adverse effect
- Threshold dose, which is the lowest dose that produces an adverse effect
- Maximal permissible dose
- Therapeutic index, which is the ratio between the median toxic dose (TD_{50}) and the median effective dose (ED_{50}) and which gives an indication of the safety margin

In the past, the results of toxicity and safety studies were interpreted and extrapolated to the human situation on the basis of the dose/kg or dose/m^2; however, measuring the plasma concentration of the compound and its metabolites provides a better indication of the exposure. The area under the plasma concentration–time curve (AUC) and the peak plasma concentration (C_{max}) are the most frequently used parameters for reliable extrapolation to the clinical situation. In addition, the possible dose dependency of the pharmacokinetics (PK) and time effects (e.g., a decrease in exposure over time as a result of enzyme induction) is important information for the interpretation of toxicity findings as well as for the planned clinical studies.

Another type of toxicity study is the genotoxic study, which is used to examine the possible harmful effects on genes. Usually, the following tests are conducted:

- A test for gene mutation in bacteria (Ames test)
- An *in vitro* test for chromosomal damage in mammalian cells or an *in vitro* mouse lymphoma tk assay
- An *in vivo* test for chromosomal damage using rodent hematopoietic cells

For biotechnology-derived products, it is usually not necessary to test for genotoxicity. The effect of the compound on several body functions is examined. The most relevant studies involve the possible effects on the respiratory system, the cardiovascular system, and the central nervous system. Recently, increasing interest has been paid to the effect of new drugs on electrocardiogram (ECG) parameters that have been associated with the risk for lethal arrhythmias.

6.2.2 Pharmacokinetic and Other Preclinical Studies

In addition to toxicity and safety data, the preclinical studies also investigate the pharmacodynamic (PD) and PK properties of the compound. PK studies in different animal species and some *in vitro* studies can provide information on the human PK parameters of a drug, including dose and time dependencies, protein binding, the effect of food, and cytochrome P isoenzymes responsible for metabolism, as well as the structure–activity relationship of the major metabolites. A valid assay to measure the compound and its metabolites in human blood and urine should be developed. Physicochemical properties, purity, and stability of the compound should be evaluated.[1–3]

6.3 DECISION POINTS IN CLINICAL TRIALS

Clinical trials can be divided into phases I, II, and III. Sometimes the terms *early* and *late clinical development* are used for describing these phases. Early development refers to all studies before the full development decision point, whereas late clinical development refers to all studies thereafter. Several key disciplines and issues are involved in the clinical development of new drugs: design for conducting trials, clinical pharmacology, and clinical development, as well as biostatistical analysis and data management. Drug development can be carried out successfully when close, harmonious collaboration and mutual understanding exist among various professional groups.

6.3.1 Design for Clinical Trials

Supporting evidence of the efficacy and safety of new drugs requires testing in human subjects. This is best achieved by carrying out controlled trials. The use of a placebo treatment or an established treatment is necessary as a control for comparison. The trial includes an adequate number of patients to allow a reliable projection of the results to future patients. Thus, it is necessary to include various levels of severity of diseases or different ages and sex of the high-risk population in the trial. Generally, patients are assigned to treatments at random, and allowances are made to study the effects of variables by using suitable statistical methods.

To be sure that random allocation is followed and to remove subjective bias on the part of both patient and investigator in assessing the effects of treatments, the clinical trial should be carried out blindly. A double-blind trial is one in which neither the patient nor the investigator is aware of the nature of the treatment administered. To ensure that the study remains blind, all treatments must be packaged as identical-appearing dosage forms.[4]

Laboratory determinations usually include such measures as complete blood count, liver function tests, and analyses on urine and stool specimens. The occurrence of adverse effects are recorded as ascertained by inquiry or as volunteered by the patient. It is more difficult to evaluate clinical data than laboratory animal data. Some of the contributing factors include:

- Patients do not take the medication or report for examination as directed, or they do not report for examination at stated intervals.
- Patients' use of concomitant medications can cause drug interactions.
- Incomplete data can result from patients dropping out of the study for various reasons.

These factors are more prevalent among outpatients than among hospitalized patients.

6.3.2   Phase I Studies

The main studies in phase I are single-dose and multiple-dose studies in healthy volunteers. For compounds given by continuous intravenous infusion, a single study in which different rates of the compound are infused to steady state is sufficient. The objective of both the single-dose and multiple-dose studies is to investigate the tolerability, safety, and PK/PD of the compound. At the end of phase I studies, the optimum dose range and dose regimen for the subsequent first efficacy trials in patients should be established. Various designs are used for the single-dose study:

- Sequential groups of volunteers receive, in a double-blind way, either active compound or placebo in a ratio of 6 to 3. The advantage of this design is that volunteers will receive only one dose and that adverse event reporting is not affected by experiences from previous sessions.
- In crossover studies, one or more panels of six volunteers receive several doses of active compound, with a double-blind placebo being randomly interposed. The advantage of this design is that, before giving a higher dose, the reaction to lower doses in the same subject is known, thus reducing the risk of exaggerated response. It also allows the collection of dose–response data within the same subject. Potential disadvantages are the risks of carryover between doses and subjects dropping out before the study is complete.

For the multiple-dose study design in trials, a starting dose has to be selected, together with the dosing intervals. When a maximal permissible dose is a factor, the highest dose is also determined before the start of the study. The starting dose is selected on the basis of the toxicity observations, AUC and C_{max}, and the predicted human pharmacokinetics. The dose-escalation scheme is usually a doubling or tripling of the lowest dose, depending on the expected type of toxicity and pharmacokinetics. The doses in the first human study should be flexible and adding, deleting, or repeating should be allowed when necessary. In the multiple-dose study, the compound is administered for several days, and usually a steady state has been reached at the end.

The assessment of PD parameters in phase I studies can be informative. It helps to define the starting dose for subsequent studies in patients. It also helps to build a PK/PD model that can be used as a framework for further development. Oral compounds often require a bioavailability study and a preliminary assessment of the effect of food on the PK of the compound during phase I. The information obtained will allow the choice of a proper dose for the phase II studies.

6.3.2.1   Should the First Study Be Performed in Healthy Volunteers
or in Patients and the Young or Elderly?

The potential reversibility of the preclinical toxicity findings should contribute to the decision as to whether to use healthy or patient volunteers. In principle, as healthy volunteers will not receive the therapeutic benefit, they should not be exposed to adverse events. On the other hand, many anticancer or anti-AIDS compounds are introduced into patients even though the toxic effects are predictable (but reversible). Recently, many biotechnology-derived therapeutic proteins have been introduced into clinical trials. These compounds create unique issues as to whether the first study should be administered to healthy volunteers. The important problem is that most proteins, when administered to humans, can induce antibody formation, thus raising the possibility that the antibody will react with a naturally existing protein and neutralize its biological activities.

Conducting the tolerability studies in healthy volunteers provides several advantages:

- Studying healthy subjects allows rapid enrollment and completion of the trial.
- Physiologic reserves are greater in healthy subjects than in the intended patients; if an adverse event occurs, the healthy subject would be more likely to recover without suffering long-term adverse reactions.
- Frequent measurements are more acceptable from a healthy individual who has a greater volume of blood than a patient.

On the other hand, PD effects of the drug should be measured in patients. For example, an antihypertensive drug such as nifedipine exhibits little or no effect on blood pressure in healthy individuals. In addition, the tolerability of a drug differs between healthy individuals and patients, thus favoring enrollment of patients in the initial studies; for example, many antipsychotic drugs are tolerated by patients at higher doses than by healthy individuals.

Traditionally, the first studies are conducted in young, rather than elderly people, because elderly subjects have a higher incidence of occult diseases that would put them at an increased risk if adverse events occur. They may have decreased physiological functioning in many organs that could influence their ability to eliminate the drug. In general, the tolerability of a compound should be similar in young and elderly people, provided the exposure is comparable in both groups. As a result, dosage must be modified in the elderly so equivalent exposures are observed. For some compounds, however, the tolerability is different in elderly people compared to young subjects; for example, the elderly have an increased central nervous system sensitivity compared to young subjects. For such compounds, elderly people should be enrolled in the initial studies.[5]

6.3.2.2 What Safety Parameters Should Be Followed?

When conducting tolerability studies, two types of safety issues are considered:

- The consequence of an extension of the therapeutic effects of the drug (e.g., hypotensive effects of vasodilators or prolonged bleeding time associated with antiplatelet drugs) — These effects are predictable and should be monitored. Such effects are related to the plasma concentration of the drug, so a rational dosage scheme for clinical trials can be established. A drug could have an effect on physiologic functions that becomes apparent in a patient with a compromised physiologic reserve; for example, beta-adrenergic blockers are well tolerated in terms of respiratory effects by healthy subjects but not by asthmatic patients.
- The toxicologic profile of the drug — Toxicity of a drug may include findings in parallel with the preclinical observations and those that are unexpected.

An objective of the entry-into-humans studies is to monitor for an early indication of more severe toxicity. It is important to monitor the function of the major organs identified in the toxicology studies. Furthermore, the occurrence of unexpected and unpredictable effects not related to the type of toxicity should be observed during the preclinical evaluation of the compound.

Early studies should monitor the effects of the drug on important organ systems, including cardiovascular, pulmonary, hepatic, renal, and hematologic systems, as well as other systems indicated as target organs based on the preclinical studies. The drug development models are based on rational schemes that focus on developing drugs designed to interfere with a specific biochemical process as either agonists or antagonists of metabolic pathways. The investigators need to determine how the pharmacologic properties can be measured during the first human studies and whether these effects occur at dose levels that are tolerated in humans.

6.3.2.3 Should the Drug Be Administered after the Meal or in a Fasted State?

Traditionally, the early studies are conducted with subjects in the fasted state. The most common food interactions observed are a retardation and increased variability of absorption. A fasting subject will allow for an easier quantification of the PK and PD effects of the drug. When animal studies indicate that the absorption of a drug is greater in the fed state, the initial human trials should be conducted with the subjects under fed conditions. With fat-soluble drugs, meals have significantly increased the absorption of many compounds; for example, the bioavailability of Accutane® increases twofold in the presence of food compared to the fasted state.[6]

6.3.3 Phase II Studies

Phase II is a critical phase in drug development. During this phase, it becomes clear whether the compound is worth developing further or not. The main objectives for phase II studies are, therefore, to prove efficacy and to determine the dose range for phase III studies. In addition, the safety of the compound should be further evaluated. Phase II can be conducted in one step or two (i.e., phase IIa and phase IIb). For innovative compounds, the uncertainty about efficacy and safety triggers investigators to follow a cautious approach by conducting a proof-of-concept study at phase IIa, before conducting the much larger and more expensive trials of phase IIb and III. The objective of a phase IIa study is to show that the compound has therapeutic efficacy in the selected disease. If it does, the project will proceed, whereas if it does not then the project will be discontinued or another target will be selected. The proof-of-concept study is carried out as a double-blind, two- or three-arm parallel study, with compound, placebo, and active control groups. The active control is used as an internal validation of the study and to obtain preliminary comparative information. Demonstration of positive results with the active control as well as the investigative compound and a negative result with the placebo will provide data to determine the efficacy of the product.

Selection of the dose of active treatment is critical for the success of a proof-of-concept study.[7] Depending on the available information and the type of compound, the investigator can select the adequate dose from the following:

- Maximal tolerated dose
- Dose that produces a certain pharmacologic effect
- Dose that produces a certain exposure, based on extrapolation of preclinical safety and efficacy data to the human situation

Phase IIa studies should use a sufficient number of patients for assessing clinically meaningful improvement; furthermore, they can be combined with dose-finding trials. In this case, three or four doses of investigative drug (covering a 10- to 20-fold range), placebo, and a positive control are studied, using a double-blind, parallel, fixed-dose design. If the results of such a study are positive, the project can proceed to phase III immediately. In the case of me-too-like compounds with known therapeutic activity, a phase IIa study is not necessary, and the project can proceed directly to dose-finding trials.

Today, much attention is paid to proper dose-finding, and an International Conference on Harmonisation (ICH) working group has issued a guideline for the industry entitled *Dose–Response Information To Support Drug Registration*. The main points from this guideline include:

- Dose–response data for beneficial and adverse effects are desirable for all new drugs entering the market.
- The data should be derived from properly designed trials as well as from a metaanalysis of the entire database.
- The data should be used to identify a starting dose, titration steps, and a maximal dose.
- The clinical endpoints may vary at early and late stages of development.
- A randomized, parallel, dose–response study with several doses of active treatment and placebo is the most robust design for obtaining population average dose–response data.
- Regulatory agencies and drug companies should be open to new approaches in search of dose–response data.

6.3.3.1 Determining Clinical Efficacy in a Short Period of Time

Surrogate endpoints are parameters used to track the clinical course of a disease. A positive drug effect on the surrogate endpoint should translate into a clinical benefit. The selected surrogate endpoint should be validated to predict the outcome of the disease being studied in patients. A change in the clinical status of the patient should be reflected in a change in the surrogate endpoint. To validate a surrogate endpoint, a correlation of a measurement with outcome must be demonstrated. In addition, a successful intervention should occur and both a positive clinical outcome and a correlated effect on the surrogate should also be observed. If therapeutic benefits exhibit the increase in a dose/plasma concentration–response relationship, there is strong evidence that the drug is effective. Determination of the no-effect dose is helpful in finding the initial dose to be administered to patients. If the disease requires immediate efficacy, the dose must be effective in all patients (e.g., antibiotics). On the other hand, with chronic diseases, the investigator can titrate the patient to the effective dose. Those patients exhibiting a clinical benefit with the lower dose would not require a higher dose and would be spared an increased risk of adverse events.

6.3.3.2 Dealing with Drug Interactions

It is important to determine whether drug dosage can be adapted in the presence of concomitant medication. Two interactions must be considered:

- Does the experimental drug affect the PK of a standard drug?
- Does a concomitant drug affect the PK of the experimental drug?

In general, drug interactions are considered only with drugs that have a narrow therapeutic index, such as digoxin, warfarin, and theophylline. A frequent error in drug development is that excessive dosages of prescribed drugs are administered concomitantly to treat the disease being studied rather than considering a scientific rationale and the therapeutic index.

By understanding the PK of the experimental drug, through *in vitro* metabolic studies with hepatic microsomes or liver slices, the drug interactions can be predicted. If a drug is metabolized by the cytochrome P-450 3A4 pathway, drugs such as erythromycin, cimetidine, and ketoconazole must be examined. Renal clearance of a drug with a clearance rate greater than the glomerular filtration rate implies that the drug is tubularly secreted. The possibility of drug interactions with other tubularly secreted drugs such as cimetidine or probenecid must be examined. The protein binding for drugs can also be assessed *in vitro* and the potential for displacement interactions predicted.

6.3.3.3 Information Required To Discontinue Drug Development

In the drug development process, only 10 to 20% of the new chemical entities proceeding to clinical trials are eventually approved as drugs for therapeutic use. An important objective of early drug development is to identify and eliminate compounds that will not be approved for marketing. The development project should establish the minimal criteria for the development of a compound, such as the required dosing frequency and an acceptable therapeutic ratio. Any new drug candidate that does not meet the criteria will not be considered for further development. To consider a drug for continued development, PD activity should be present at tolerable dose in the first studies. If this does not occur, no scientific rationale exists for continued development.

A further requirement is a minimal duration of PD effects that allows for an acceptable dosing frequency. For oral drugs, this will involve a duration that is long enough to allow an acceptable PD effect between doses. A typical oral drug should require administration no more than 4 times a day, and twice or once-daily dosing is more desirable. For intravenous drugs, a short half-life is desirable.

In determining dosing frequency, the PD effects should be related to the PK of the compound. As a surrogate for duration of PD effects, an acceptable kinetic profile is required. Such a profile includes a relatively long and consistent half-life. For orally administered drugs, low or unstable bioavailability makes drug development difficult. Erratic absorption with large variability is common with drugs of low bioavailability that tend to overdose in patients most of the time.

For most drugs, the occurrence of unpredictable and serious adverse reactions would cause drug development to be terminated. In making this decision, the risk–benefit ratio must be evaluated. If a fatal and nontreatable disease is the target indication, such as cancer and AIDS, drug development may be continued even in the presence of adverse events. Nevertheless, if at any time the data indicate that the drug has an undesirable risk–benefit ratio, then further development should be reassessed.

6.3.4 Phase III Studies

The main purpose of phase III studies is to confirm the findings of phase II studies and to provide evidence of a favorable risk–benefit ratio. If necessary, additional studies will be conducted to meet the regulatory requirements to support specific claims on the label. The phase III study is the largest, longest, and most expensive part of the development process. Depending on the drug, the indication, and the endpoint for efficacy, phase III studies can range in size from a few hundred to several thousand patients, whereas the duration of the studies may be 2 to 4 years of treatment. These studies are carried out as a national, multinational, or intercontinental cooperative effort. Usually, they are multicenter trials under the supervision of one or more steering committees with representatives from academia and a sponsor. Frequently, a special committee has access to all safety data and randomization codes, and this committee has the authority to stop the study if they observe evidence of injury to patients. Full compliance to good clinical practices (GCPs) as well as scientific integrity are prerequisites for the acceptance of these trials by regulatory agencies, and the pivotal trials should undergo inspection to safeguard these aspects.

The approval of a new drug depends on evidence that it improves one or more clinical endpoints related to how a patient feels, functions, or survives. In certain types of drugs (e.g., pain killers and antibiotics for acute infection), it is easy to show such effects. It is more difficult, however, for many other drugs that require large-scale studies over a long period of time. It is practical and convenient to use surrogate endpoints in drug evaluation. Surrogate endpoints are defined as biochemical markers intended to substitute for clinical endpoints. For example, an increase in serum antibody levels is accepted as a surrogate for clinical efficacy against infection. In the treatment of hypertension, the lowering of blood pressure is accepted as a surrogate for the clinical endpoint (i.e., the prevention of cardiovascular complications). In addition, changes in CD4 count or viral load as surrogate endpoints can be used in the treatment of human immunodeficiency virus (HIV) infections. Surrogate markers should be validated before being used as endpoints in clinical trials.

REFERENCES

1. Griffin, J.P., O'Grady, J., and D'Arcy, P.F., *The Textbook of Pharmaceutical Medicine*, 3rd ed., The Queens University of Belfast, U.K., 1998.
2. Drews, J., *In Quest of Tomorrow's Medicines*, Springer-Verlag, New York, 1998.
3. Graham, M.A. and Kaye, S.B., New approaches in preclinical and clinical pharmacokinetics, *Pharmacokin. Cancer Chemother.*, 17, 27, 1993.
4. Bolton, S., Design and conduct of clinical trials, in *Remington: The Science and Practice of Pharmacy*, 20th ed., Gennaro, A.R., Ed., Lippincott Williams & Wilkins, Baltimore, MD, 2000, pp. 130–131.
5. FDA, *Guideline on Studies in Support of Special Populations: Geriatrics*, U.S. Food and Drug Administration, Washington, D.C., 1994.
6. Colburn, W.A., Gibson, D.M., Wiens, R.E. et al., Food increases the bioavailability of isotretinoin, *J. Clin. Pharmacol.*, 23, 534–539, 1983.
7. ICH, *Efficacy Tripartite Guideline on Dose Response Information To Support Drug Registration*, International Conference on Harmonisation of Technical Requirements for Registration of Pharmaceuticals for Human Use, Geneva, Switzerland, 1993.

CHAPTER 7

Management of Clinical Development Costs

Mark Hovde

CONTENTS

7.1 INTRODUCTION

The research-based pharmaceutical industry is under increasing cost pressure from slowing sales and high drug development costs. Cost pressures are exacerbated because of the need for rapid cost recovery, which creates a need for expensive multicountry development programs. The amount of work involved in a single regulatory submission is increasing. These factors will continue to press the industry to consolidate and force managers of clinical trials to look for new ways to control costs without compromising time or quality.

Costs continue to increase, and clinical spending is under pressure as never before, with estimates of the cost of developing a new drug, including failures and time value of money, of $600 million to $2 billion. In contrast, the clinical work for a single, successful 4000-patient new drug application (NDA) can be bought for about $60 million. By supplier, there are three approximately equal types of spending: investigators, contract research organizations (CROs) and central labs, and internal costs. By cost driver, there are data costs, patient costs, site costs, country costs, and one-time study costs. These costs are concentrated in North America and are dominated by the therapeutic areas of cardiovascular system, central nervous system, and immunomodulation. Many of the costs are directly related to the number of procedures performed on a patient, and the trend is for more procedures per patient and greater costs across most phases and therapeutic areas. By country, costs are growing fastest in Germany, Canada, Switzerland, Norway, and Finland.

Cost, time, and quality in clinical research are intimately connected. The performance of CROs and sites plays a large role in whether a project is accomplished on time and on budget. Biotechnology firms face special challenges in managing clinical costs. Regardless of the type of sponsor, biotechnology or major pharmaceutical, it is important to closely manage the timed allocation of resources to clinical projects so redundant resources are not applied. Cost reduction results from limiting the number of countries involved, insisting on lower investigator fees where the number of patients per site is high, and focusing on English-speaking sites. Project plans can often be restructured to reduce costs. CROs leave some room to negotiate lower fees, but CROs overall are not particularly profitable and will not be able to reduce their fees much beyond 5% without severely compromising their profitability. Investigator sites also offer some room for fee negotiation, but it is important to keep in mind the total cost of running a site, not just the investigator fees, when considering potential budgets. Preferred provider relationships are of limited value. Site-management organizations can accelerate study completion and should be used when they have ready access to patients. CRO and site performance can be optimized and costs reduced with the sound selection and intelligent management of major costs, communication, roles, contract terms, and incentives.

7.2 INCREASING COST PRESSURES

An ongoing challenge facing managers of clinical development programs is the judicious management of trial costs. Costs of clinical trials are rising, while the development budgets of most large
companies are constrained as never before. The conventional wisdom is that costs can be controlled,
but only if time or reliability suffer; that is, a less costly program will take longer or will be less
likely to deliver results than a more costly program. Nevertheless, trial managers are under pressure
to reduce costs, increase quality, and reduce development timings. To do so, they have been forced
to look for new methods of trial management that improve timings and quality while minimizing
costs. This chapter explores leading practices in judicious trial cost management and concludes
with lessons for managers that should deliver immediate and sustainable improvements in trial
timings, quality, and costs.

7.2.1 Slowing Sales

Though slowing some, sales continue to grow at single-digit rates in the global research-based
pharmaceutical industry, and, perhaps as importantly, the industry continues to spend under the
assumption of continued sales growth. Large companies invest 10 to 20% of sales in research and
development (R&D), and approximately one third of this amount in a mature, research-based firm
is devoted to clinical trials and submission. Despite expensive reengineering programs, the time
required to progress a drug through the preregistration stages of clinical development has remained
stubbornly static. The Food and Drug Administration (FDA), on the other hand, has reduced the
time necessary to approve a submission from the historically high levels of the late 1990s.

7.2.2 High Drug Development Costs

Observers disagree on the exact magnitude of drug development costs. Difficulties in analyzing
the costs of drug development arise because of the long time frames involved and the number of
failed compounds that never reach market. The Center for the Study of Drug Development (CSDD)
at Tufts University has published widely on determining drug development costs using a method
that assigns a cost of capital to early investment, therefore accounting for the long time frames,
and accounts for compound failure rates using extensive major pharmaceutical survey data dating
back to the 1960s. Using the Tufts method, costs per new chemical entity (NCE) registered in the
United States are $600 to $700 million. Others have taken a simpler approach, summing the R&D
budgets of the major pharmaceutical companies for a year and dividing the total by the number
of NCEs approved in that year. This approach gives a figure between $1 billion and $2 billion
per NCE.

7.2.3 Need for Rapid Cost Recovery

These costs must be recovered in the first 7 years after approval, as the typical drug will have only
7 years left in its patent life by the time it reaches market. This implies sales of $100 to $140
million per year just to recover development costs (the substantial costs of marketing and sales,
perhaps equal to development in the aggregate, require additional sales). This means that many
drugs must be launched in multiple markets simultaneously or nearly so because usually no single
market is big enough to generate sufficient sales. Many large firms endeavor to launch in commercially critical core markets (e.g., United States, United Kingdom, France, Germany, Italy, Japan)
with no more than 6 months between the first and last approval. To achieve rapid, multiple-market
approvals, it is often necessary to pursue a multinational development program. This means that
patients will be treated in each of the core markets to support local approval and country launches.

This requirement vastly increases costs as study management, regulatory support, medical and monitoring oversight, drug distribution, handling of lab specimens, and all related infrastructure must be duplicated in each country where patients will be treated.

7.2.4 Increasing Volume of Work for New Drug Applications

The volume of development work in a single new drug application (NDA) is growing. Anecdotes in the popular press refer to 100,000-page NDAs, but in this electronic age other size parameters are perhaps more telling. The average NDA approved in the United States over the past few years has averaged 5000 to 6000 patients, although this figure varies by therapeutic area (in oncology, for example, NDAs have been approved with as few as 600 patients, while some antibiotic NDAs have exceeded 10,000 patients). Typically, each patient will have 40 to 80 case report forms (CRFs); therefore, 200,000 to 400,000 CRFs support the entire clinical database in an average NDA. Unfortunately, the industry continues to struggle with the problem of recruiting adequate numbers of patients into the trials, with the result that the average study center recruits just six to eight patients in common indications, with up to one third recruiting one or none. This means that 5000 patients will require about 700 investigator centers, each of which must be recruited, trained, equipped with study materials and investigational drug, monitored, and shut down. These centers must also be paid for the direct patient work, including their effort to recruit patients and manage the study documents and monitoring. Below are the direct costs for a typical 4000-patient NDA:

- 4000 patients and investigator fees of $6000 per patient = $24 million.
- 700 sites to set up, monitor, and close out at $1500 per visit = $12 million.
- 400,000 CRFs to enter and clean at $10 per page = $4 million.
- 35 protocols to write at $25,000 per protocol = $.9 million.
- 35 statistical analyses at $25,000 each = $.9 million.
- 35 integrated clinical statistical reports at $25,000 each = $.9 million.
- 4000 patients × 6 visits × $80 labs per visit = $1.9 million.
- 400 sites managed for 1 year each = $1.7 million.
- 35 projects managed over 7 years = $12.1 million.

The total out-of-pocket pocket costs for an NDA are, therefore, $58.4 million.

7.2.5 Pharmaceutical Industry Consolidation

The inability to generate sufficient sales to support the large cost structures of the major pharmaceutical companies has caused them to continue to consolidate. In addition, pricing pressures have become more severe in nearly all of the major markets. Rising development expenses and an inability to license sufficient numbers of new compounds and bring them rapidly to commercialization have led to earnings disappointments and continued pressure to consolidate. As a result, all of the major pharmaceutical and biotechnology companies are looking with renewed vigor at process improvement, expense tightening, and paying increased attention to the business aspects of research and development.

7.3 CLINICAL SPENDING OVERVIEW

Industry statistics from the Pharmaceutical Research and Manufacturers of America (PhRMA) show that member companies spend $35 billion a year on research and development. Of this, approximately $11 billion is spent in clinical research and approximately $24 billion is spent in nonclinical research.

7.3.1   Clinical Research Spending by Type of Supplier

Clinical research spending can be further divided into three major categories of expense based on to whom the money is paid:

- *Investigator spending* — These are fees paid directly to investigators for patient work and include finding, recruiting, consenting, screening, and entering the patient; treating the patient; managing the drug supplies; recordkeeping; dealing with the pharmaceutical company monitor; dealing with auditors; and, increasingly, managing the data entry process when electronic data capture tools are distributed to investigative sites. In total, the author estimates investigator fees to be $4 billion in the United States and Western Europe. This figure includes phase IV studies but does not include financial support for investigator-initiated studies.
- *Internal costs* — An additional $4 billion is spent by members of the Pharmaceutical Manufacturers Association on internal costs. These are costs directly associated with conducting clinical trials. Examples usually include (sometimes they are outsourced) the cost of internal medical monitors; clinical trial management systems; clinical data management systems; investigator databases; drug distribution systems; study drug formulation; acquisition of comparator medicines; project management; protocol writing; writing study reports, safety summaries, and other regulatory documents; and biostatistical analyses required to support them.
- *Contract research organizations and central laboratories* — The third major cost area in clinical spending is the expense of CROs and central laboratories. Most of the CRO spending is made up of contracted monitoring, site management, and project management, although other activities are also outsourced. Central laboratories are typically used wherever they can be used (where the lab work is not required for acute treatment of the patient). The total market for CROs and central laboratories is about $4 billion. Of this figure, central laboratories account for about $800 million.

7.3.2   Clinical Spending by Principal Cost Driver

Some managers break clinical research costs into schemes of approximately five subcategories. This is useful for thinking about the factors that drive costs and for the management of functional expense. These expenses are not collected and analyzed across the industry by PhRMA or others, so to provide perspective the author has estimated these expenses for a "typical" large pharmaceutical company. A typical top-20 pharmaceutical company spends about $1.5 billion on research and development. Using the figures above, it would spend about $500 million on clinical research. To do this work, it would employ 2000 clinical staff. It would probably have an objective of one to two major filings per year. This means it would conduct approximately 100 protocols, operate 1000 clinical research sites, treat 10,000 patients, and process 1 million CRFs. Functional costs would include:

- *Data-related costs* — Data-related costs consume about $10 million for the 1 million CRFs. These costs include data entry, data cleaning, database programming, generation and review of tables, costs for the use of patient diaries if necessary, implementation of coding conventions, translations, and electronic data capture. The key cost driver for these costs is the number of CRFs.
- *Patient-related costs* — Patient-related costs (investigator fees) would be about $60 million for the 10,000 patients. Patient-related costs are higher when a higher number of procedures is performed on each patient. The number of procedures performed on each patient varies widely by therapeutic area and disease indication. The study may also require extensive time from the study nurse or study coordinator, which also drives up patient costs. In addition, fees will be higher when the principal investigator is required to invest administrative and patient care time beyond that required for the administration of procedures in the protocol flow sheet. The key cost driver for this cost is the number of patients times the number of procedures per patient.
- *Site-related costs* — Site-related costs would be about $30 million for recruiting, initiating, training, holding investigator meetings, monitoring, and closing out each site. Regulatory audits

and laboratory setup as well as site overhead are also included here. The key cost driver for this cost is the number of investigator sites.

- *Country-related costs* — These are the costs of investigational new drug (IND) filings, country-level institutional review board (IRB) filings, and language translations. Together, these country costs create about $2 million of additional expense. The key driver for these costs is the number of countries where patients will be treated.

- *Study-related costs* — Study costs include one-time-per-study costs such as the cost of creating the protocol, the cost of drafting and creating the paper or electronic case record form, investigator brochure, project management, statistical plan, statistical report, integrated clinical statistical report, manuscript preparation (if any), interactive voice response system (IVRS) costs (if any), drug packaging and distribution, and outsourcing management. Study costs are usually less than $1 million in a phase III study.

7.3.3   Geographic Distribution of Clinical Development Expense

Clinical spending is concentrated disproportionately in North America. Of the $11 billion of estimated clinical spending in 2003, $7.2 billion was spent in North America. Of this total, about $3 billion was investigator spending, $2.2 billion was internal spending, and $2 billion was CRO and central laboratory spending. Western Europe clinical spending was estimated to be $3.4 billion. Of European spending, $1 billion was for investigators, $1.6 billion for internal spending, and $.9 billion for contract research organizations and central laboratories.

7.3.4   Therapeutic Distribution of Clinical Development Expense

Patient volume and therefore investigator spending patterns vary by therapeutic area. The largest three areas are cardiovascular, central nervous system, and immunomodulation. All of these areas show investigator spending of over $450 million per year in the United States alone. Midsized areas include gastrointestinal, antiinfective, oncology, endocrine, and hematology. Spending in these areas exceeds $100 million per year. The smallest areas are device studies, pain and anesthesia studies, respiratory, genitourinary, dermatology, and ophthalmology. All of these areas show spending under $100 million per year. Investigator spending on device studies, though small, is rapidly growing.

7.4 PROCEDURES PER PATIENT

A key driver of investigator spending, monitoring, and data entry and cleaning is the number of procedures performed on each patient. From the author's experience consulting to over 40 large pharmaceutical and biotechnology companies, of the typical phase III study performed in 1997, 51 were procedures performed on a patient. That figure currently is 68 procedures per patient, an increase of 33%. In this analysis, I have held constant factors such as therapeutic area, geographic location, patient status (whether the patient is inpatient or outpatient), and site affiliation. Procedures per patient vary by country of study. U.S. studies tend to be the most complex. Studies used only in European filings tend to be simpler when measured by procedures per patient.

7.4.1   Trends in Procedures per Patient

The number of procedures per patient has increased across all four research phases. In phase I, which is the most procedure-intensive phase, procedures per patient have climbed from 95 to 102 in the period from 1997 to today. Phase II procedures per patient have grown from 56 to 65 over the same time period. In phase IIIa, procedures per patient have grown from 51 to 67, while in phase IIIb the growth has been from 36 to 53. Finally, growth in phase IV has been the highest on a percentage basis, growing from 32 procedures per patient to 47.

7.4.2 Trends in Cost per Patient, per Visit, and per Procedure

In the United States, the cost per patient has risen 25% since 1997. This is an increase from $5000 per patient to $6255 per patient currently. The cost of an individual patient visit is up by about 9% over the same time period, from $707 in 1997 to $770 currently. Thus, the cost paid per procedure has dropped from $110 in 1997 to $93 currently. This means that today's investigator site is getting paid less for each unit of work it performs on behalf of the pharmaceutical industry. Cost per patient, the industry's standard metric for investigator fees, has grown in phases I, IIIa, IIIb, and IV, whereas phase II has shown a slight decline since 1997.

7.4.3 Investigator Fee Growth by Country

Growth in the cost of investigator fees has averaged 6.3% per year over the last decade. Investigator fees have grown the fastest in Germany, Canada, Switzerland, Norway, and Finland, at a rate of over 7.5% per year. In the middle of the pack are Italy, United Kingdom, Sweden, The Netherlands, and Belgium. The fees in these countries grew at a rate of over 4% per year over the past decade. The countries with the slowest growth rate are United States, France, Austria, and Denmark. Fees in all of these countries grew at less than 4% per year over the past decade.

7.5 COST, TIME, AND QUALITY IN CLINICAL RESEARCH PROGRAMS

Managers of clinical research programs are constantly faced with trade-offs among cost, time, and quality. The conventional wisdom says that a development program may have two, but not three, of the following attributes:

- Inexpensive, or low-cost
- Reliable, or high-quality
- Fast, or low time

Following the conventional wisdom, if your program is inexpensive and fast, it will not be reliable. If your program is inexpensive and reliable, it will not be fast. If your program is reliable and fast, it will be expensive. These trade-offs must be considered within the financial realities of a large pharmaceutical or biotechnology company. These companies do not operate in a perfect capital market. They cannot go to market and secure additional funding any time they wish. They must deliver certain profit commitments to the investment community or management will lose credibility. Typically, the R&D budget is predetermined as a percentage of sales. When this determination has been made, it is very difficult to spend significantly more than the committed amount.

To illustrate the problem of trading-off cost, time, and quality in clinical programs, consider a typical pharmaceutical company, TortoisePharm. This company has $10 billion of sales and devotes 17% of sales to R&D. The clinical department gets $600 million of the $1.7 billion budget. The clinical portfolio consists of 15 major projects, each consuming $40 million per year. Each project is expected to deliver $365 million of sales for 10 years before patent expiration, which is $1 million per day! It takes TortoisePharm 7 years to get to market following discovery and patent filing. Like many companies, the managers of TortoisePharm are besieged by vendors who would like to sell them systems to reduce development time. TortoisePharm is currently considering a program that will promise a 10% reduction in time to market. Because time to market is 7 years, this represents a reduction of .7 years, and .7 years times $365 million equals $255 million additional sales due to acceleration of each project. Project costs will rise 25% for the service provided by the vendor. This is an extra $10 million per project per year, and 6.3 years times $10 million equals $63 million to accelerate one project.

One might think that these economics are compelling: $255 million of benefit vs. $63 million of incremental cost. TortoisePharm, however, will not buy. Why not? The reason is that TortoisePharm operates a portfolio of projects, not a single project, and it must operate its portfolio within the fixed budget committed to investors. TortoisePharm would have to drop three projects if it accepted the 25% higher per-project costs from the acceleration vendor. If TortoisePharm declines to accelerate but keeps its bigger portfolio of 15 projects, it will have revenues of 15 projects times $365 million times 10 years equals $54 billion. If it accelerates but accepts a smaller portfolio, it will have revenues of 12 projects times $365 million times 10.7 years, or $46 billion. TortoisePharm is better off staying slow but supporting a larger, less expensive portfolio. TortoisePharm will win by declining to accelerate because it is looking at its portfolio as an entirety and is optimizing cost, time, and revenue together. This is true even though its projects sales of $1 million per day. Thus, cost control is a strategic issue for large pharmaceutical and biotechnology companies. Speed and quality are important, but cost ought to have an equal place in strategic planning.

7.6 SPECIAL CHALLENGES FACED BY BIOTECHNOLOGY COMPANIES

Biotechnology companies face special challenges in the planning and budgeting of their clinical trials. Consider:

- Without their own in-house study execution infrastructure, biotechs are forced to outsource not just clinical investigator activities but also nearly 100% of monitoring and data handling. Outsourced expenses can be large, with pivotal phase III trials in CNS and oncology indications often involving several hundred patients, over $5 million of investigator fees, and over $10 million of CRO and central laboratory fees.
- Biotech compounds often target novel drug indications, so few comparison studies may be available to provide benchmarks for likely costs.
- Many biotechs are venture funded. Money is often tight, and the infrastructure, management systems, and procedures that are common in large pharmaceuticals may be nonexistent. This leads to the sometimes dangerous practice of doing things on the fly, with scant documentation and weak business controls.
- Experienced full-time staff is usually in short supply.
- Often the "contracts department" is one person who has been pressed into service without prior contracting or negotiating experience.
- Biotech clinical portfolios are typically focused on only one or two scientific ideas. The entire company may depend on the success of one compound or one key trial. This leads to risk aversion and a tendency to overdesign protocols and programs "just to be sure." Vendor selection tends to favor large, established firms to minimize operational risks of failure.
- Science, not administration, is the key capability of the biotech, and it is scientists, often physicians, who usually make up the senior management. Often biotechs will allow scientists to establish and run vendor relationships, to the detriment of customary negotiation and vendor management principles.

Regardless of whether development costs occur in biotechnology or large pharmaceutical settings, all are under intense scrutiny and most major companies have expense control initiatives ongoing in all three areas.

7.7 MANAGING COSTS

In managing investigator fees, most companies use benchmarking databases to ensure that their payments are reasonable in relation to the work required from the clinical protocol. Internal costs are also under constant review. Companies continue to take a hard look at internal headcounts and the contribution of each person on the payroll. Contract research organization and central laboratory spending is also under intense review. Typically, large pharmaceutical and biotechnology companies have contracts offices that manage the request-for-proposal process, contracting and negotiation, and performance management after the contract is signed and the project is proceeding to completion. These professional contracting groups have made an enormous difference in both the quality of vendor performance and cost levels paid for it.

7.7.1 Quantity and Cost per Unit: Two Methods of Controlling Total Cost

A company willing to pursue all possible means of cost control and improved budgeting has two basic levers to control costs. The first is the quantity of activity present in the project. In clinical research, quantity can be expressed by a number of metrics that typically show up in a trial. One metric is the number of procedures performed on a patient or the number of procedures performed on all patients during the trial. A second common metric is the number of visits. The total amount of monitoring as well as that the amount of data entry and data cleaning are also useful metrics for estimating the total work volume in a project. Other metrics, more closely related to quality and quantity, include the number of protocol amendments, the number of data queries, and the number of site queries. When we consider all of the multiple dimensions of a clinical trial, it is clear that the work volume depends on many factors and could be measured in many ways.

Many interactions exist among project parameters, costs, quality, and time; for example, the more vendors involved in a project, the higher will be the administrative costs and the greater will be the range of performance in vendors. When investigators are paid less, the study will require more time to enroll and clean data. Also, the more countries involved and the higher the number of sites involved, the greater will be project management and site management costs. In addition, the performance of the contract research organization and the sites it oversees will have a large impact on costs. When performance lags, time drags, project management costs rise, oversight costs rise, and the entire project goes over budget.

The first and most effective means of cost control is to reduce the total work involved in the project. This could happen by reducing the protocol requirements for the number of procedures performed on a patient or by reducing the number of visits required of each patient. Reducing procedures or visits will reduce investigator effort, coordinator effort, data entry, and probably monitoring effort as well. Improving the quality of the protocol will probably reduce the likelihood of amendments and site queries. Any reductions in the work-driving factors in the project will ultimately lead to less reliance on outside vendors, lower costs, and a higher likelihood of timely, on-budget execution. As a result, leading-edge companies are looking at protocol design with ever-increasing scrutiny. Their goal is to minimize the protocol required to accomplish the medical and business objectives intended for the project. Some are benchmarking their protocols against designs from comparable protocols. When teams put forward protocol designs that are much more procedure intensive, visit intensive, or otherwise work intensive than comparison protocols, they are queried by reviewers and asked to defend their choices.

The second fundamental method for cost control is negotiating lower prices for the cost of each unit of work performed in the project. This is true of CRO, investigator, and central lab work. When the design has been determined and the number of units of work is fixed, the only option left for reducing costs is to reduce the cost paid per unit. This can be accomplished through benchmarking, negotiation, forcing sites to accept take-it-or-leave-it budgets, competitive bidding exercises, and the negotiation of so-called preferred provider rates with favored CROs and central labs.

7.7.2 Importance of Understanding Timings

When managing project costs it is important to understand the exact timings of the steps in the project. For example, in a typical clinical project, a project manager will be assigned at initiation and will continue to bill time to the project until the last deliverables are accepted. In contrast, the activity of site management occurs only as long as sites are open and attempting to recruit, treat, or follow-up patients. It is important to ensure that site management runs only for the time needed and that project management runs only for the time needed.

7.7.3   More Countries Mean More Cost

Smart companies seeking to control costs also seek to minimize the number of countries involved in clinical research projects. As noted earlier, registration and marketing objectives often require the inclusion of multiple countries. In addition, project managers may seek to involve nontraditional countries (e.g., Poland, Czech Republic, Thailand, South Africa) to find treatment-naïve patients who cannot be found in the West; however, it is important to minimize the number of countries if cost control is a primary consideration. Additional countries mean that travel and project management expenses will be far higher than in single-country projects. If the extra countries are in nonstandard locations such as Eastern Europe, Asia, or Latin America, then it is likely that higher costs for site support and monitoring will also be encountered. In addition, countries where investigators and site staff and patients do not speak English create the cost of translations. Country variations in clinical research practices may also introduce additional costs or delay. Will an IRB in South Korea allow children to participate in a clinical study? Can shipments of tissue samples pass unhindered from Belarus to a central lab in The Netherlands? Although investigator fees are higher in North America than elsewhere, total study costs may in fact be lower because study practices are familiar, and monitoring logistics, shipping of lab specimens, and other costs of site support and administration are far lower than in nonstandard clinical trial venues.

7.7.4   Importance of Sites Speaking English

Ideally, personnel at all sites should speak English, both the principal investigator and the coordinator. All documents and systems ought to be in English in order to minimize costs. This includes investigator meetings and materials, consent materials, IVRS, help desk, and site portal.

7.7.5   Scale Economies of Investigator Fees

Few economies of scale have been demonstrated in clinical research and in R&D programs. One economy, however, is the level of investigator fees per patient when the number of patients is increased at a site. From the author's research on the Grants Manager™ database maintained by the commercial company Fast Track Systems, doubling the number of patients handled by an individual site results in a 7% reduction in the investigator fees per patient. Therefore, if one has a choice of doing 40 patients at one site vs. 10 patients at four sites, then one would expect investigator fees per patient to fall by 14% when a single 40-patient site is used vs. the four-site scenario, as two doublings occur between 10 and 40 patients.

7.7.6   Other Considerations for Cost Reduction

Sites should also have broadband Internet and a trial portal for updates and document downloads. Where possible, the same organization should be used for the lab work and CRO work. Discounts are usually unavailable from the large CROs when they are selected to perform both tasks.

7.7.7   Restructuring the Project Plan To Reduce Costs

Some companies consider cost reduction by combining site initiation with site evaluation and the investigator meeting. Sites can be selected that permit a centralized institutional review board. It is also economical to select sites that have worked previously with the contract research organization and the central laboratory. Ideally, these will be high-performing sites from previous trials. Where possible, sites should be avoided when they are running competitive trials. Some companies, especially in Europe, have paid sites a premium in order to guarantee patient exclusivity. The source data verification policy should be considered carefully for each trial. Is it really necessary to verify all fields for all patients? Can the site gain more efficient verification if it delivers quality early on? Which fields require critical and expensive verification, and which do not? Does the project have to be done to GCP standards at all? Finally, what is driving the visit frequency? Is it a standard operating procedure to visit every 6 weeks, or does the visit happen when sufficient data have accumulated to justify a full monitoring day?

7.8 PERSPECTIVE ON CONTRACT RESEARCH ORGANIZATIONS COSTS

The CRO industry is not particularly profitable. The implications for those managing clinical trials are that CRO project fees cannot be negotiated infinitely downward. Top CROs operate at best with low-teens profitability. The reasons can be traced to the industry structure, which can be described in a five-forces analysis, and to the fact that many projects are delayed or canceled, leading to irregular utilization of CRO staff.

7.8.1 Brief History of the CRO Industry

The CRO industry was founded in the early 1970s. The first major firm was the precursor to Covance, Besselaar Associates. Covance really took off in the 1980s when good clinical practices were widely adopted. In the 1990s, large pharmaceutical companies became victims of headcount myopia. The penetration enjoyed by CROs rose from the small single digits to 35%, leading to huge growth in CRO revenues and attracting much new capital to the industry. Many new CROs were launched, leading to high rates of new company formation despite ongoing merger activity. Several CROs went public, with Quintiles going public at 80 times earnings. Flush with new capital, rollup strategies were pursued. Geographic expansion strategies were pursued, especially in the Far East and Latin America. Some of the larger CROs attempted to become one-stop shopping companies, providing assistance in preclinical and clinical development, as well as sales and marketing. At the peak of the boom, the U.K.-based contract sales organization Innovex was acquired by Quintiles at 100 times earnings. By the year 2000, growth had leveled off. Although some virtual pharmaceutical and biotech companies had no study execution infrastructure of their own (and therefore had to outsource 100%), the huge shift from no outsourcing to 30 to 50% outsourcing by the large pharmaceutical companies had been completed. The CRO industry began to grow at the underlying rate of expansion in clinical research budgets. This disappointed investors, and the sector fell out of favor. It is now much more difficult for CROs to raise capital, as they trade for market or submarket multiples. Some of the largest CROs grew so large that they began to rival their pharmaceutical counterparts in number of projects, number of NDAs processed, size of clinical staff, scope of country operations, and other key parameters. Some CROs even acquired patents and commenced their own development programs for their own portfolios.

7.8.2 Five-Forces Analysis for the CRO Industry

The five-forces analysis was pioneered by an industrial economist at Harvard Business School (Prof. Michael Porter). The author's analysis of the five forces (rivalry, potential entrants, substitutes, buyers, and suppliers) predicts that the long-term profitability of the CRO industry will be poor. Porter defines an industry as a set of products or services that are close substitutes for each other.

Most agree that little rivalry exists in the CRO industry; therefore, this factor is not contributing to reduced profitability for the industry. The key suppliers are Clinical Research Associates, data software suppliers, EDC software suppliers, safety software suppliers, and clinical trial management system software suppliers. For the most part, these suppliers do not extract high profits through high pricing to the CRO industry; therefore suppliers do not artificially suppress the profitability of the CRO industry.

Potential entrants include central laboratories, advertising agencies, temp agencies, toxicology laboratories, and startups. Because barriers to entry are low, all of these potential entrants have in fact entered the CRO industry. The presence of new firms continually seeking to enter the business has suppressed the pricing that CROs have been able to achieve.

Substitutes for clinical trials are few. Pharmacokinetic and pharmacodynamic modeling was once touted as a potential substitute for clinical trials; however, to date, applications of these technologies have been few. The promise of modeling to replace clinical trials has not been fulfilled. Until much more is learned about the functioning of the many biochemical pathways in the human body, modeling is unlikely to change the number of clinical trials performed.

The key factor that has suppressed profitability in the CRO industry is the power of the sponsor companies or buyers. Large pharmaceutical companies are capable of carrying out most studies themselves. This means that if they become dissatisfied with the prices charged by the CRO industry, they can simply back integrate. Indeed, a number of companies have announced a strategy to insource more of their clinical trial work and outsource less, although the overall trend since the 1970s has been to outsource more. Biotechnology companies have also been significant users of outsourced services, but the larger biotechnology companies have also put in place their own study execution infrastructure that has allowed them to become credible insourcers as well.

The second largest purchaser of CRO services — government — has well-tuned algorithms for determining exactly what it will pay for clinical research work performed by investigators. These algorithms generally yield investigator reimbursement that is far below that paid by the mainstream commercial industry sponsors. Similarly, the government follows rigid outsourcing procedures when it purchases CRO services. These procedures virtually guarantee that work performed from the government will not be highly remunerative. In sum, buying power exercised by sponsor companies and by the government has suppressed CRO industry profitability.

7.8.3   Response of Pharmaceutical Companies

Pharmaceutical companies responded to their growing dependence on large CROs by setting up professional contracting organizations, usually located inside R&D finance units. Budgets for contract research organizations were becoming a tens of millions of dollars expense per year. The large companies realized that they had significant exposure to outside vendor performance including operational performance and the financial stability of their vendors. Staffing for contracting groups often came from CRO proposal and business development units. And, while major pharmaceutical companies wanted the flexibility of variable project expense that CROs provided, they did not want to pay the real costs of providing it. This led to bitter and sometimes acrimonious negotiations with CROs and the perception among sponsors that CROs were expensive. Exacerbating this was the inability of major pharmaceutical companies to understand their own fully loaded costs. One large company ran an extraordinary controlled experiment to settle the issue of whether internal or external projects were more expensive. A project was subcontracted to a CRO, and careful metrics were collected on cost, time, and quality. At the same time, the same project was redundantly carried out by internal staff. The same metrics were collected. The company concluded that internal costs were slightly less than costs for CROs; however, the work was later criticized because the internal costs were calculated without allocating certain corporate overheads. Most people concluded that internal and external costs were about the same.

Global pharmaceutical companies were also strangely reluctant to understand the investments that CROs were making (and that their customers would have to pay for) in building global infrastructure to support global pharmaceutical company development projects. Ultimately, the largest CROs began to look like the pharmaceutical company clients that they were designed to help. They had the same staffing, career development, training, systems, facilities, travel budgets, benefits expense, and ultimately costs. The difference was they also had downtime because their business model was built around virtual teams, and they also faced the expense of ongoing project-level business development. On project completion, the team would be disbanded and reassigned to the next project. While it was unassigned those previously billable people became overhead, creating costs that would have to be recovered in other projects.

7.8.4   Pharmaceutical Company and CRO Business Relationships

As reliance on contract research organizations took hold, new forms of business relationships were attempted. The first model was a time and materials approach. This prevailed from the 1970s to about 1990. This method caused problems because it was difficult for the sponsor companies to link value created with charges paid. In response, some companies adopted unit-based contracting approaches. The ultimate unit in clinical trials is probably a patient's worth of locked clinical data. Some companies tried to pay only when locked data were received; however, this method led to problems also because CROs had many expenses leading up to data lock and were forced therefore to play banker to the pharmaceutical companies. As a result, in 1995 most companies moved to a modified unit-cost approach. In this approach a clinical project is broken down into about 20 activity categories. Some of them deliver real value to the pharmaceutical company, while others are just activities along the way that consume cash and must be paid for as they occur to avoid putting the CRO in a cash-negative position. A typical framework follows:

- File regulatory documents.
- Write protocol.
- Create case record forms.
- Recruit investigator sites.
- Conduct investigator meeting.
- Initiate investigator sites.
- Manage investigator sites.
- Monitor investigator sites.
- Close investigator sites.
- Manage project.
- Audit sites.
- Program database.
- Generate tables and listings.
- Write statistical plan.
- Enter data.
- Clean data
- Write statistical report.
- Write integrated clinical and statistical report.

Companies found that they could easily benchmark these activities by requiring vendors to prepare bids in this framework, leading to higher confidence that CRO fees were reasonable in relation to project requirements. Eventually, systems of this type were adopted by most major pharmaceutical and biotechnology companies.

7.8.5   Preferred Provider Relationships

The next major innovation was the establishment of preferred provider relationships, commencing in about 1995. In these arrangements certain vendors would be prequalified and would be asked to bid on an accelerated basis when a project occurred. It was hoped that preferred provider relationships would lead to increased sharing of development plans, better utilization of vendor staff, lower costs, faster projects, and higher quality. Most industry observers believe that preferred provider relationships, though positive, have failed to live up to their full promise. They are no longer considered a panacea by most contracting groups or by the senior management of CROs.

7.8.6   Using Site Management Organizations

A site management organization is often economical despite the cost of the organization itself. This is because site management organizations can reduce the time it takes to get the sites up and running through centralized administration of study documents. A shorter ramp-up time leads to lower costs of project management.

7.8.7   Maximizing the Performance of CROs

Poor contract research organization performance is a major source of budget overruns and time delays in clinical research. The first step in making sure that CRO performance is top-notch is clear project specifications. The sponsors should visit and prequalify CROs that will be asked to be involved in future projects. A timely prequalification visit before the heat of the project forces a decision that will lead to better qualification of prospective vendors. Adding information to the selection process will lead to higher quality vendor performance and ultimately lower cost vendor performance.

7.8.8   Criteria for CRO Selection

Ideally, the sponsor should choose a CRO that has delivered successful performance before. Costs of coordination, rework to standard operating procedures, and implementation of CRO deliverables in the sponsor's format will be lower when the CRO has worked with a sponsor previously. Experience with the sponsor company is a necessary, but not sufficient, condition for optimal performance. The CRO ought to have prior experience in the drug indication. Ideally, the vendor will be able to contribute protocol design and other operational choices. In addition, the CRO ought to have experience in the specific countries where the work will be performed. Experience in asthma studies in Canada is not the same as experience in asthma studies in Thailand. The CRO should be able to demonstrate that its project managers and clinical research associates are highly experienced. Having a highly experienced study staff usually leads to fewer errors and better performance. It is critical to assess the CRO knowledge of the investigator group. The more experience it has with the kind of investigator the sponsor intends to use and the more prior performance it can point to its investigator selection decisions, the higher will be the performance of the investigator group. All information on investigators should be entered into the company customer relationship management system for later reference. In addition, the central laboratory can be asked to provide metrics and validation of potential investigators.

7.8.9   Managing CRO Incentives

The incentives of CROs and sponsors are sometimes in opposition. The CRO finds that its revenues are highest when the project is large and complicated; therefore, the CRO will tend to advocate for extra activities that cause its fees to be higher. The CRO should always be required to use sponsor formats and project management systems. Sponsors should insist on writing their own protocols and designing their own CRFs, but they should always allow the CROs to comment. Where possible, the sponsor should use standard data dictionaries, safety reporting, edit checks, and coding systems. To enhance communication, the sponsor should hold at least half the project meetings at the location of the CRO.

7.8.10   Avoid Performance Penalties

Contract arrangements with CROs and investigator sites should never use performance penalties. These are rarely enforceable, especially in Europe. They lead to bad blood, and the author knows of no major company that regularly uses performance penalties. Performance bonuses paid to CROs, on the other hand, can be effective, creating a win–win situation for the vendor and sponsor. In one example, the CRO proposed a budget of $3.7 million for a project. The sponsor thought this figure was high. The sponsor used a benchmarking database and concluded that the project should cost $2.7 million. After tough negotiations, with the entire relationship on the line, the CRO agreed to total fees of $2.7 million. The sponsor at this point added a $300,000 performance bonus tied to the achievement of certain enrollment milestones. The vendor hit the milestones and earned a $300,000 bonus, thus creating a win–win for both sides. The CRO got paid $300,000 above standard rates, and the sponsor got the project accomplished on time. Performance bonuses paid to sites are generally ineffective. An exception is the performance bonus paid specifically to the study coordinator. In some cases, these bonuses lead to dramatic improvements in site performance.

7.8.11   Improving the Performance of Investigator Sites

Most trial managers agree that a competent and experienced trial coordinator is critical to a well-performing site. Sponsors should pay sites themselves and not outsource this activity. When outsourced, it is difficult to keep control of payments, and an opportunity for branding and building customer loyalty is lost. Most believe that investigators tend to prescribe more of a company's drugs after they have participated in a clinical trial; however, it is the author's view that this prescribing boost is reduced when the CRO, not the sponsor, handles the payments. Some managers of trials focus too intently on the investigator fees per patient. It is important to consider all costs of finding, setting up, and operating a site. Generally, a well-performing site, even if it requires somewhat higher investigator fees, will have far lower total costs that a poorly performing site that accepts a low budget per patient. Site performance can also be improved by the intelligent application of technology (e.g., electronic diaries), which reduces data cleaning and improves data quality.

7.8.12   Other Budgeting and Contracting Considerations

All costs should be benchmarked before final agreements are reached with investigators and other vendors. This is standard practice in most large companies. CROs should be required to bid in the sponsor company's standard format so bids may be easily compared. Three bids should be required for each project, and the bidders should know that they are in a competitive bidding situation. Centralized control of the contracting process should be enforced. This will avoid the problem of handshake deals where high rates occur because proper negotiating practice has been circumvented. If vendors go around the contracts office, they should be frozen out for some period of time. If unit costs rather than time and materials contracts are used, then change orders will be tightly controlled because the change order will involve only an adjustment to quantity and the cost change will be easy for the parties to calculate. In most CRO contracts, the sponsor can economize effort by focusing negotiating and benchmarking effort on the 20% of cost items that account for 80% of total cost. These are usually monitoring, project management, data entry, and data cleaning.

CHAPTER 8

Ethical Aspects and Good Clinical Practice

Lucia H. Lee, Christopher L. Wu, Benjamin R. Lee, and Chi-Jen Lee

CONTENTS

8.1 INTRODUCTION

Clinical trials are an important foundation for the development of new drugs and are the most critical factor during the licensure process of a new biologic. Most drugs and biological products are initially studied in healthy volunteers; subsequent studies are conducted in a much larger, diverse patient population, including those with the disease for which the product is indicated. The stages of clinical trials include phases I to IV. Further trials may be required after licensure and marketing. Although the scientific basis and concept of clinical trials are identical throughout these stages, practical differences exist among the phases. Clinical trials for chemical drugs and biological products are designed to study the efficacy and safety of the product in humans, identify the risk–benefit relationship, and examine the absorption, distribution, and metabolism of the product in healthy people as well as patients. The design of the clinical trials is based on the chemical nature of the product being tested, results of preclinical animal studies, and intended clinical uses. This is particularly relevant for biopharmaceuticals, which frequently demonstrate complex and multiple pharmacological activities. The basis for license approval depends on the adequacy and validity of the trial data available. A larger number of biotechnology-derived products are proceeding in clinical trials at various stages of their development. The progression through these phases is the usual means by which the sponsor collects the data required for evaluation and approval.

8.2 ETHICAL ASPECTS

Clinical research in healthy subjects can result in benefits for society. Ethical aspects of research include reasoned analyses of moral obligations, including (1) justice, being fair; (2) beneficence, doing good; (3) nonmalfeasance, not doing harm; and (4) respect for autonomy, allowing the individual to determine what happens to him or her.[1–4]

The moral duty of justice requires the investigators to be fair in the treatment of research subjects. Thus, the treatment of participants in clinical studies should be compensated adequately for inconvenience, discomfort, and loss of time when participating in studies. The principle of fairness also requires that healthy volunteers be studied in addition to patients. The healthy members of society should share with victims of disease the burden of helping in the development of medicines for which there is no certainty that those victims will benefit.

Beneficence requires that the research activities benefit study subjects and other people. The experience of participating in a clinical study is socially rewarding in that it involves contact with doctors, nurses, technical staff, and volunteers. It involves the opportunity of contributing to the welfare of others and medical progress. Beneficence imposes upon investigators an ethical obligation to maintain high standards in the design and execution of research. It requires that investigators be nice to volunteers and patients.

The investigators conduct research in healthy volunteers to achieve maximized benefits with low risks. The investigators should be extensively trained, experienced, and conscientious. The risk of injury to participants in research should be kept to the lowest level possible, and good safety records must be maintained. Furthermore, the respect for autonomy preserves the right of subjects to determine what should or should not be done to the them. Subjects are required to give their consent to participate in research projects. Consent must be both informed and freely given. Participants should receive a fair description of what will be done to them and what the risks of discomfort or injury are. The information has to be provided in a form that the participant can understand. The subject must also be of sufficient maturity and intelligence to understand the implications of the study.

The ethical review of research projects and obtaining informed consent from participants are important in clinical trials. The objectives of a research ethics committee are to protect the subjects who participate in the research projects, to preserve their rights, and to provide public assurance. The ethics committee evaluates and approves the protocols for clinical trials and investigators conducting such trials. The committee is responsible for evaluating the following issues regarding clinical trials:

- Is the scientific quality of the protocol properly assessed?
- Are the investigators and other persons involved in the trial competent and are the facilities adequate?
- What are the possible hazards to the trial participants and what precautions will be taken to deal with them?
- Has appropriate informed consent been obtained?
- Are adequate arrangements in place in the event of adverse reactions?
- What methods of recruitment will be used and how will the subjects be paid?

Informed consent involves the process whereby explicit information is provided to participants regarding the treatment in clinical trials. It also describes the obligation of the investigator to inform the subject about the personal benefits and risks the individual faces in the study, as well as the significance of the research for the advancement of medical knowledge and social welfare.

Certain subjects in special populations may be recruited to participate in studies. These volunteers should be recruited by a general notice rather than by direct approach, particularly in the case of students or staff within the investigator's institution. Students have been used as research subjects in the studies of pharmacology and physiology; however, consent cannot be considered freely given when volunteers are students and the investigator their professor. Students may also feel pressure not to disappoint their professor or investigator by withdrawing from the study. A solution in the case of volunteer studies is for investigators to recruit students from other institutions.

The use, by academic department or pharmaceutical companies, of their own staff as volunteers brings up ethical difficulties similar to those encountered with students. The head of a department has great control over the performance and career development of his junior staff, just as a professor does over his students. Pharmaceutical manufacturers should be careful not to exert pressures on employees to act as volunteers and should recruit subjects by general notice only to avoid the risk that the volunteer's autonomy will be compromised in the process of consent or of withdrawal from the study.

Children cannot be considered as true volunteers because of their inability to give valid consent. In some cases, the parents' consent for their children's participation may not be adequate or acceptable.

No particular ethical problem exists with regard to women volunteers; however, one issue is a concern with safety. Women with child-bearing potential should be excluded from any study that could cause harm to the individual or her future offspring. Because these risks are frequently not apparent until late in the drug development, most early studies are conducted in men.

Elderly people are recruited as volunteers if risks are low and acceptable and if the project cannot be conducted well in the young. The investigator's duty in this case is to ensure that the elderly in the study are really necessary and the risk is negligible.

8.3 GOOD CLINICAL PRACTICE REGULATIONS[5,6]

The purpose of biomedical studies involving human subjects is to improve prevention and treatment procedures and understand the pathogenesis of diseases. Medical progress and the development of effective drugs and biological products depend on clinical trials. Good clinical practice (GCP) regulations are designed to achieve these objectives:

- Ensure the quality and integrity of bioresearch and test data obtained from clinical studies submitted to the regulatory agencies.
- Protect the rights and safety of human subjects participating in clinical trials.

Good clinical practice regulations are described in several documents that define the clinical-trial-related responsibilities of the sponsor, investigator, monitor, and institutional review board (IRB). The sponsor takes responsibility for and conducts the clinical trials and may be an individual or pharmaceutical manufacturer, research institute, or private organization. Sponsors are responsible for selecting qualified investigators and monitors, informing investigators, reviewing and monitoring studies, and maintaining trial records.

Investigators, such as physicians and other professionals qualified by training and experience, conduct or supervise the clinical study. They prepare a general outline of the planned studies that specifies the duration of the study, number of subjects that will be involved, and clinical observations and laboratory tests to be performed.

The monitors are responsible for ensuring the quality and integrity of the data obtained from clinical trials, as well as the rights and safety of human subjects participating in the study. The monitor must visit the clinical site frequently to ensure that clinical trials are carried out according to the scheduled plan and that investigators have followed the specified regulations. The monitor also reviews the reports that are prepared by the investigator and submitted to the sponsor.

The function of the institutional review board is to ensure that risks to participating subjects are minimal and that subjects are adequately informed about the clinical trial and its implications for treatment. The IRB may review and address other issues, including selection bias, statistical analysis, appropriate informed consents, and confidentiality of data. The IRB committee consists of at least five persons, including physicians, pharmacologists, and administrative managers from the institution related to the sponsor or investigator.

The informed consent is designed so patients participating in a clinical trial can obtain an adequate understanding of the objective and procedures of the clinical trial. Patients participate in such trials voluntarily. The information given to the subjects must be written in lay terms and include the following key components:

- A statement explaining the objective of the study, duration of the subject's participation, and procedures of clinical trial
- Description of any possible risk, adverse reactions, discomforts, and benefits to the subject
- A statement that the confidentiality of the subject's records will be maintained
- An explanation of whether compensation and medical treatment are available if injury occurs during the clinical trial
- A statement that participation is voluntary and refusal to participate will not involve penalty or loss of benefits to the subject (subjects may discontinue their participation in the trial at any time without penalty or loss of benefits)
- A list of persons to contact for questions related to the clinical trial and trial-related injury

An investigator must obtain an informed consent bearing the signature of the subject or the subject's representative before the clinical trial is initiated.

REFERENCES

1. ABPI, *Guidelines for Medical Experiments in Non-Patient Human Volunteers*, Association of the British Pharmaceutical Industry, London, 1988.
2. Royle, J.M. and Snell, E.S., Medical research on normal volunteers, *Br. J. Clin. Pharmacol.*, 21, 548–549, 1986.
3. Vere, D.W., Ethics, in *Handbook of Clinical Drug Research*, Glenny, H. and Nelmes, P., Eds., Blackwell Scientific, Oxford, 1986.
4. Vere, D.W., The ethics of adverse drug reactions, *Adverse Drug Reaction Bull.*, 128, 480–483, 1988.
5. Lee, C.J., *Managing Biotechnology in Drug Development*, CRC Press, Boca Raton, FL, 1996, pp. 17–70.
6. Soul-Lawton, J. and Kroon, R., Good clinical practice, in *A Guide to Clinical Drug Research*, 2nd ed., Cohen, A. and Posner, J., Eds., Kluwer Academic, Boston, MA, 2000, pp. 145–186.

CHAPTER 9

Investigational New Drug Application and the Licensure Approval Process

Lucia H. Lee, Christopher L. Wu, Benjamin R. Lee, and Chi-Jen Lee

CONTENTS

9.1 INTRODUCTION

An investigational new drug is a pharmaceutical product for which effectiveness and safety in humans have not yet been demonstrated. A licensed drug used for investigational purposes in a manner that varies from the approved indication would likewise be considered an investigational new drug. In the United States, the Food and Drug Administration (FDA) helps to ensure that products approved for commercial use are pure, potent, safe, and effective. The regulatory process affects drug development at the preclinical, clinical, license application, and post-licensure stages. This chapter primarily describes the role of the FDA during the clinical and license application stages. In the United States, before a clinical research study can be initiated, a sponsor submits an investigational new drug (IND) application to the FDA for review and approval.[1] The three types of IND applications are (1) *commercial*, which pertains to clinical trials that provide supporting data for a new drug application (NDA) or biologics license application (BLA) and where licensure of the product for marketing purposes is the long-term goal; (2) *noncommercial*, which is submitted by investigators who want to use an investigational product for academic research purposes; and (3) *treatment*, which provides an early mechanism for making an unapproved drug available to people with serious or life-threatening diseases, such as cancer, for whom adequate alternative therapy is not available.

9.2 COMMERCIAL INVESTIGATIONAL NEW DRUG APPLICATIONS

A product manufacturer, academic scientist, clinician, or government agency can sponsor an IND application. The content and format of a commercial IND are the same as for a noncommercial IND, except that a person that both initiates and conducts the clinical investigation is referred to as a sponsor–investigator. The designated sponsor takes responsibility for initiating a clinical trial and for providing manufacturing, quality control, toxicology, and pharmacology information to the FDA.

9.3 INITIAL IND APPLICATION: CONTENT AND FORMAT

The content of the initial IND application includes the following information:[2]

- An IND application form (FDA Form 1571) and statement of investigator (FDA Form 1572), which specify the name, address, and contact information for the designated sponsor, investigators, and institutional review board
- The purpose and overall clinical development plan for the drug or biological product
- Chemistry, manufacturing, and quality control (CMC) information for the active moiety of the drug — for a biological product, this information includes the physicochemical characteristics, such as structure (if known), identity, purity, potency, and stability; a description of drug composition, formulation (e.g., liquid, powder), dosing regimen, and route of administration in the proposed clinical trial; and the manufacturing and quality control systems that establish the quality of the drug product
- Pharmacological and toxicological data in animal models that demonstrate that the proposed investigational product has a pharmacologic effect, without associated toxicity, at the dosing and dosing regimen proposed for human study (included with these data would be a description of the mechanisms of action and information describing the drug absorption, distribution, metabolism, and excretion)
- A study protocol, which states the clinical trial objectives, design, eligibility criteria, monitored parameters, laboratory testing and procedures, and statistical analysis plan, if applicable, as well as information describing previous human experience with the investigational product or similar products (protocols for phase I studies focus on preliminary safety evaluation in healthy participants, while phase II and III studies are more detailed, controlled studies in a target study population)[3]
- Investigator's brochure, which describes to other investigators the possible adverse reactions anticipated, based on previous human experience with the investigational product or with a similar product (a sponsor–investigator is exempt from submitting an investigator's brochure as long as the clinical trials conducted are only at a study site for which the sponsor is also the investigator, but if the sponsor–investigator decides to conduct a multicenter trial then an investigator's brochure is required when more than one principal investigator is involved in conducting the trial)

After 30-day IND review period, the regulatory agency makes a decision to permit the sponsor to begin a clinical trial according to the proposed protocol or to delay the start of a clinical trial pending corrected deficiencies or provision of additional information. Reasons for placing a phase I trial on clinical hold commonly involve the perceived exposure of human subjects to harmful effects or excessive risk, conduct of clinical trials by unqualified investigators or personnel, or inadequate presentation of potential risks in the investigator's brochure. Phase II and III studies can also be placed on clinical hold for safety reasons or study design concerns.

The sponsor is encouraged to arrange pre-IND meetings with FDA staff to discuss, prior to submitting the IND application, whether proposed pharmacology and toxicology preclinical data would provide sufficient evidence to initiate human studies; consequently, a clinical hold might be avoided when the initial IND application is submitted. The pre-IND meeting is also an opportunity for the sponsor to present the overall plan for product development and provide background information on the upcoming application and any potential manufacturing issues.

9.4 INVESTIGATIONAL NEW DRUG AMENDMENTS

9.4.1 Protocol Amendment

After an IND is approved, subsequent IND amendments can contain new study protocols or changes to previously submitted protocols:

1. *New protocol* — The new clinical study should also be supported by animal toxicity study results or other human data. The study may begin if approval by the institutional review board (IRB) was received and the protocol was submitted to the IND for FDA review.
2. *Changes in a protocol* — A protocol amendment is needed if changes to previously submitted protocols include the following types of revisions:
    - Any protocol change that significantly affects the safety of subjects (such as an increase in drug dosage, increased duration of drug exposure to study participants, or an increase in the number of subjects under study) or any change in a phase II or III protocol that significantly affects the scientific quality of the study. (The criteria for placing a study on clinical hold also apply for new or amended protocols; thus, for any study conducted under an IND, a review of protocols by a regulatory agency helps to ensure that the safety of study participants is not compromised by clinical investigation, and for phase II and III studies such a review helps to ensure that the quality of the scientific evaluation of drugs is adequate to evaluate drug effectiveness and safety.)
    - Any change in the design of a protocol, such as adding or eliminating a control group
    - The addition or removal of a test or procedure intended to monitor for adverse drug effects
3. A *protocol amendment* should be submitted when a new clinical investigator is added.

9.4.2 Information Amendment and IND Safety Reports

An information amendment contains details about new toxicology, chemistry, and other technical information. Notification of premature termination of a clinical trial would also be submitted as an information amendment. For any event that is both serious and unexpected, the sponsor must notify the FDA, in a written IND safety report, within 15 days after the sponsor initially receives the information. An event that results in an unexpected death or life-threatening experience and is associated with the use of the investigational drug should be reported to the FDA no later than 7 days after the sponsor initially receives the information. A brief summary of similar adverse events reported for the same investigational product should also be included in the safety report.

9.4.3 Annual Report

An annual report is a brief update that includes the following information:

- A brief progress report of the status of each clinical study
- A summary of the most frequent adverse events and most serious adverse experiences
- A list of subjects who died during participation in the study, with the cause of death for each subject
- A list of subjects who withdrew from the study due to an adverse event
- Updated information pertaining to the mechanism of action, pharmacological effect, dose response, and bioavailability
- A list of the preclinical animal studies completed or in progress during the past year and their major findings

- A summary of any significant manufacturing changes or foreign marketing developments made during the past year
- A description of the general investigational plan for the upcoming year

9.5 LICENSURE APPROVAL PROCESS

The primary clinical trial data submitted in support of drug or biological product approval depends on specific requirements of the regulatory agency.[4,5] In the United States, formal meetings between the sponsor and FDA representatives can be arranged at several time points in clinical development to provide greater assurance that the data and documents submitted in the license application will be adequate to support market approval. Meetings between the sponsor and FDA representatives are usually scheduled at the end of phase II/pre-phase III or in preparation for submitting a new drug license application or biologics license application.

A meeting at the end of phase II is held to discuss whether phase II study results are sufficient to proceed with plans for phase III trials, whether the design of the proposed phase III trial is adequate to demonstrate safety and efficacy, and whether additional information is necessary to comply with regulations for product approval. Agreements are commonly reached on statistical analyses. Meetings held at the end of phase II are particularly important for novel molecular entities proposed for important therapeutic gains, for drugs with toxicity problems, or for a marketed drug with a new indication. A meeting held at the end of phase III/pre-NDA meeting provides an opportunity to present a general summary of the information intended to be included in the NDA, to discuss a format for the final study reports, and to resolve any major disagreements that could affect approval of the application.

When the license application is submitted to the FDA, the review committee initially determines, within 60 days of receipt of the application, if all the essential information needed to make a conclusive decision regarding market approval has been included. If no major omission of data necessary to evaluate safety, purity and potency is found, the application is considered complete. The applicant is notified by written correspondence, and the review committee proceeds with an in-depth review of the application. A 10-month time period is usually allotted for standard review of a license application. If critical information is missing or the format of the data is poorly organized or presented to the extent that results are uninterpretable, the application would not be filed or reviewed further until the deficiencies are corrected. Only partial reimbursement of the application fee would be returned to the applicant.

During the course of the standard review period, in addition to review of the clinical data and product information, on-site inspection of the manufacturing facility is scheduled to confirm that production equipment and manufacturing procedures are in compliance with the guidelines for good manufacturing and laboratory practices. Visits to clinical study sites help to verify that the integrity of data collection is consistent with the good clinical practices and study procedures specified in the protocol. In addition, purity, potency, identity, and stability specifications are checked via several methods as part of lot-release testing for biologic products. Clinical data for a product application containing a novel component, products with particular public health importance, or those with controversial issues are usually discussed in a public forum with an advisory committee. The advisory committee is comprised of multidisciplinary experts.

In the event that a drug or biologic product is *not* approved, a formal meeting can be scheduled after a nonapproval letter to an application is issued so the FDA and the sponsor can determine what steps are necessary to remedy the deficiencies in the application.

9.6 FAST TRACK DEVELOPMENT, PRIORITY REVIEW, AND ACCELERATED APPROVAL PROCESSES

Fast track development, priority review, and accelerated approval are formal mechanisms by which regulatory processes for investigational drugs can be expedited to reduce the time required before market approval is obtained. An investigational drug intended to treat a serious or life-threatening medical condition and that potentially addresses an unmet medical need can fulfill the criteria for fast track development. Fast track development is a formal mechanism for incorporating scheduled meetings with the FDA very early in clinical development. Rather than at the end of phase II, a formal meeting is scheduled at the end of phase I to expedite the review of phase I data and discuss plans for phase II studies.

An investigational drug that fulfills the criteria for fast track development is also eligible for priority review of the license application. In contrast to a standard license application review, which requires a complete application at the time of submission, priority review allows portions of the application to be submitted to the FDA before the official review clock starts. Under priority review, the FDA can initiate early review of these portions, thus allowing more efficient application review when the review clock has begun. In addition, when all portions of the application have been submitted, the applicant informs the FDA that the license application is complete, and all data are reviewed within a 6-month time frame.

Accelerated approval can be granted for an investigational drug intended to treat a serious or life-threatening illness and which would provide therapeutic benefit to persons intolerant or not responsive to available therapy.[6] Demonstration of effectiveness is based on a determination that the drug product effect on a surrogate endpoint is reasonably likely to predict clinical benefit. Post-licensure studies, which include a control group, are required to verify the intended clinical outcome.

9.7 TREATMENT IND

The purpose of a treatment IND is to provide a mechanism to expedite public access to potentially beneficial investigational drugs for patients who are not participants in a controlled clinical trial, who have an immediate life-threatening or serious disease, and who are not responsive to available therapy.[7] The regulatory process reflects the recognition that physicians and patients are willing to accept greater risk and adverse drug effect for therapeutic products indicated for life-threatening and incurable diseases, such as advanced AIDS or cancer, than for products intended for treatment of less serious diseases. Even minimal therapeutic benefit is acceptable in light of the disease circumstances under consideration. An investigational drug can be administered under a treatment IND if the same drug is also being evaluated in controlled clinical trials under a commercial IND, and the IND sponsor is proceeding with plans for market approval within a reasonable time frame. When no prior IND exists, permission to use an investigational drug, under a compassionate use protocol, may be granted.

REFERENCES

1. FDA, 21 CFR 312.20: Investigational New Drug Application (IND), U.S. Food and Drug Administration, Washington, D.C., April 1, 2004.
2. FDA, 21 CFR 312.23–312.33: Investigational New Drug Application (IND), U.S. Food and Drug Administration, Washington, D.C., April 1, 2004.

3. Goldenthal, K.L. and McVittie, L.D., The clinical evaluation of preventive vaccines for infectious disease indications, in *Biologics Development: A Regulatory Overview*, Mathieu, M., Ed., Parexel, Waltham, MA, 1993, pp. 119–130.
4. Kessler, D.A., The regulation of investigational drugs, *N. Engl. J. Med.*, 320, 281–288, 1989.
5. Baylor, N., Midthun, K., and Falk, L.A., Role of the Food and Drug Administration in vaccine testing and licensure, in *New Generation Vaccines*, Levine, M.M., Kasper, J.B., Rappuoli, R., Liu, M.A., and Good, M.F., Eds., Marcel Dekker, New York, 2004, pp. 117–125.
6. FDA, 21 CFR 314.500–314.510: Miscellaneous Provisions, U.S. Food and Drug Administration, Washington, D.C., April 1, 2004.
7. FDA, 21 CFR 312.34–312.36: Investigational New Drug Application (IND), U.S. Food and Drug Administration, Washington, D.C., April 1, 2004.

CHAPTER 10

Clinical Trials from Phase I to Phase IV

Lucia H. Lee, Christopher L. Wu, Benjamin R. Lee, and Chi-Jen Lee

CONTENTS

10.1 INTRODUCTION

Clinical trials are an important foundation for the development of new drugs and are the most critical factor during the licensure process of a new product. Most drugs and biological products are initially studied in healthy volunteers. Subsequent studies are conducted in a much larger, diverse population, including those with the disease for which the product is indicated. Further trials may be required after licensure and marketing. These stages are known as phases I, II, III, and IV. Although the scientific basis and concepts of clinical trials are identical throughout these stages, practical differences exist among the phases. Clinical trials provide an objective method for evaluating the safety and efficacy of an experimental chemical drug or biological product. Although these studies are expensive and take time, the process has proven essential and valuable. The data from clinical trials are used to support the efficacy and safety of the product in humans, define the risk–benefit relationship of the product, and characterize the absorption, distribution, and metabolism in the intended population. The design of the clinical trials is based on the chemical nature of the product being tested, results of preclinical animal studies, any available previous human experience with related products, and intended clinical uses. Preclinical data are particularly relevant for biopharmaceutical products, as the mechanism of action of a new drug may involve complex and multiple pharmacological activities and would impact the choice of an appropriate range of starting doses.

10.2 CLINICAL TRIALS FROM PHASE I TO PHASE IV

In general, the stages of clinical evaluation are conducted sequentially, but they may overlap.

10.2.1 Phase I Trials

Subsequent to preclinical animal studies, if no serious adverse events or toxicities are identified, a drug is then evaluated in human subjects. A phase 1 study represents the initial evaluation of an investigational new drug in people. The primary objective is to assess the safety of the new drug by testing a range of doses or dosing intervals in a sequential manner. Phase I trials typically include detailed safety monitoring in a small number of healthy adult volunteers. The total number of subjects included in phase I studies is usually in the range of 20 to 80, and these studies require fewer than 12 months to complete.

Characterization of the safety profile includes an evaluation of drug absorption, distribution, excretion, and structure–activity relationships. Other objectives in phase I studies may also include determining the extent of drug metabolism; identifying interactions with other medications, the mechanism of action, and the preferred route of administration; and, sometimes, gaining early evidence on drug effectiveness. Sufficient information about the pharmacokinetics and pharmacological activities of the drug should be obtained during phase I to support the proposed choice of dose, dosing regimen, and use of the drug in subsequent studies. Conducting thorough dose-ranging and dose-response studies early in product development reduces the possibility of later failed phase II or III studies. Of drugs tested in phase I, 50 to 70% are abandoned because of problems with safety or efficacy.

A phase I trial for an experimental vaccine, in general, also involves a small number of healthy volunteers, as these individuals are at low risk for the vaccine-relevant infection or complication. One trial of a new live oral typhoid fever vaccine was conducted on a sample of only three.[1] A vaccine eventually intended for infants is first assessed in adults and then toddlers before proceeding to infants. A range of doses or dosing regimens is evaluated for each population, and, similar to a chemical drug, dose escalation proceeds in a stepwise manner. The objective of a phase I study is primarily to evaluate the safety of the new vaccine but another objective may be to assess immunogenicity. Because vaccine trials often involve healthy participants, inclusion of prespecified criteria for discontinuing immunization for individuals and the cohort is often necessary. These criteria are relatively more stringent than those for therapeutic drug trials.

The ability to mount an antibody response is age dependent but can be improved with modifications to the dosing regimen or vaccine formulation. Whereas a single dose might suffice for an adult, a vaccine regimen for an infant often consists of two or more doses in the primary immunization series. Inclusion of an adjuvant in the vaccine may also be necessary to induce adequate antibody responses in infants. Sustained antibody response can be achieved by administering a booster dose at a later age. Conjugation of a polysaccharide to a protein carrier results in a T-cell-dependent antibody response to the capsular polysaccharide. Prior to the development of conjugate vaccines, the antibody response observed in infants and young children following vaccination with an unconjugated polysaccharide vaccine was often suboptimal.[2] The presence of detectable antibody may not be indicative of a vaccine-induced immune response. In infants, antibodies measured at baseline are attributed mainly to the presence of maternally acquired antibody. In older children and adults, high levels of preexisting antibody may be due to prior natural exposure to the infectious agent or to cross-reacting antigens; consequently, the elicited antibody response may reflect secondary rather than primary responses. In a phase I trial that involved an acellular pertussis vaccine in adults, only 8 of 54 participants had confirmed seronegativity to any of the pertussis antigens prior to vaccination.[3]

10.2.2 Phase II Trials

Early phase II studies are conducted to optimize and definitively select the final formulation, dose, and dosing regimen and to evaluate drug safety in the intended target population. These studies generally enroll several hundred subjects and may include populations with the actual disease or who have risk factors for developing the disease. Although a single study can address several questions, multiple studies are often planned in order to achieve all intended objectives. Potential immunological interference and adverse safety interactions of a candidate vaccine, when coadministered with routinely recommended childhood vaccinations, are also evaluated at this stage in clinical development.

Phase II studies are generally designed as multicenter, randomized, controlled trials that address a specific hypothesis. The sample size calculations and statistical plan should be adequate to support valid conclusions about clinically important differences in reaction rates and immune responses. Optimally, a double-blind study design is implemented to avoid biased comparisons and invalid inferences. Demographic characteristics that may affect host immune response, such as age, ethnicity, and gender, are usually balanced by randomization.

In some cases, a phase II study may also serve as a pilot study to provide a preliminary estimate of drug effect to serve as a basis for planning a larger, confirmatory clinical efficacy trial. Epidemiologic information on disease incidence in the target population is also obtained in preparation for a phase III trial. Other important considerations include selecting an appropriate endpoint that is clinically relevant to changes in the disease state, is reliably measured over a prespecified time frame, and quantitatively reflects changes in drug effect. If a surrogate endpoint is chosen, laboratory assays that might be used to measure the primary outcome should be developed and validated no later than the end of phase II. Careful planning of phase II trials enables sufficient data gathering to support subsequent well-planned, scientifically valid, phase III trials. Approximately one third of new drugs will continue to be evaluated in a phase III trial.

10.2.3 Phase III Trials

The main objective of a phase III trial is to demonstrate the efficacy of a drug in the actual target population that is proven in a statistically and clinically significant manner. In general, a phase III trial is a randomized, double-blind, controlled study, a design that provides the greatest assurance that potential variables affecting disease risk are balanced and avoids possible bias in the assessment of the primary endpoints. The design maximizes the chance that a difference in disease incidence between two equivalent groups is due to a true effect of the drug being evaluated. A phase III trial has a clearly defined primary endpoint, valid case definition, and prespecified hypotheses. Clinical pharmacology, safety, and immunogenicity data from early clinical trials provide the framework for the statistical analysis plan, scientific rationale, and selection of endpoints for the phase III study. The sample size of a phase III trial, which often involves several hundred to several thousand participants, must be adequate to support rigorous hypothesis testing. The study conclusions, supported by statistically valid comparisons, provide a convincing basis for demonstrating effectiveness. Two pivotal trials are usually necessary to fulfill regulatory requirements for adequately demonstrating effectiveness of a new drug. For a new vaccine, one confirmatory trial may suffice, as study enrollment typically includes several thousand participants.

In a phase III trial, a single primary endpoint is usually proposed that pertains to reduction or prevention of disease. Multiple secondary endpoints, however, can be included. In a vaccine efficacy trial, vaccine efficacy (VE) is defined as the percentage reduction in the incidence rate of disease in vaccinated compared to unvaccinated individuals. Thus,

$$VE = 100 \times (IRU - IRV)/IRU$$

where IRU is the incidence rate in unvaccinated individuals and IRV is the incidence rate in vaccinated individuals. These incidence rates are usually calculated as the number of events per total person-time of follow-up, thus allowing for different observation times between individuals. Efficacy is usually assessed over a period of several years. Due to the large number of participants and the extended duration of an efficacy trial, detection of less common and serious adverse events might be more easily identified in a phase III trial. Monitoring for local and systemic reactions in a subset of the study population would be feasible.

Sometimes, the evidence of safety and effectiveness obtained from phase II studies is so compelling that phase III trials are not necessary. For example, in studies on the anti-AIDS drug zidovudine, one AIDS patient died while being treated with zidovudine, compared to 10 AIDS patients given placebo. Because the results were dramatically better with zidovudine as compared to the placebo, the FDA was able to approve the drug for marketing only 4 months after receiving an application from Burroughs Wellcome.[4] On average, only about 25% of new drugs achieve successful results in phase III trials.

In some cases, vaccine efficacy trials are conducted in foreign countries because the disease incidence is too low in the United States. For example, the efficacy trial of a *Haemophilus influenzae* type b (Hib) polysaccharide (PS) vaccine was conducted in Finland,[5] and the acellular pertussis vaccine trial was performed in Sweden.[6] Data obtained from foreign trials have been used to support product license applications in the United States; however, because differences in the immune response in a population may by affected by host and environmental factors, such as genetic inheritance patterns, preimmune antibody levels, epidemiologic distribution of certain disease serotypes, and nutritional status, studies comparing clinical and safety data for a foreign population to the U.S. population are usually necessary to bridge results from foreign studies.

The primary outcome can also be measured by surrogate markers, such as a change in blood pressure or cholesterol level, which can be indicators predictive of the risk for coronary artery disease. This approach is less invasive than trying to confirm the presence of arterial plaques. In situations where a protective serologic correlate has been determined or clinical effectiveness previously demonstrated, efficacy has been inferred from an immunological endpoint rather than directly measured from a clinical disease endpoint. Serologic endpoints have been used to receive approval of combination vaccines for which the individual components were already licensed or when a licensed vaccine for the same indication already existed. Immunologic endpoints were used as the primary evidence of efficacy to support the licensure of subsequent Hib polysaccharide and PS–protein conjugate vaccines after initial Hib vaccines were licensed based on data from several clinical efficacy trials. Meningococcal Y and W135 components of a tetravalent (A, C, Y, W135) meningococcal polysaccharide vaccine were licensed only on the basis of an immunologic correlate of protection. Clinical efficacy was not demonstrated for groups Y and W135 due to the low incidence of disease isolates. Efficacy was instead evaluated based on data showing that bactericidal antibodies to groups Y and W135 PSs were elicited in $\geq$90% of adults following vaccination. Significant reduction in the incidence of meningococcal disease was previously demonstrated for monovalent meningococcal A and C and meningococcal AC combined PS vaccines. When a comparative immunogenicity study is conducted in lieu of a large clinical efficacy trial, a supplemental large-scale safety study is also planned to ensure that an adequate overall database is available to characterize the adverse event profile. A phase III safety trial would include active monitoring for local and systemic adverse events, other nonserious adverse events, and serious adverse events.

When a biologic product is manufactured using recombinant DNA technology, the host organism used to express the recombinant protein antigen is frequently *Escherichia coli*. The recombinant product is subsequently extracted and purified from the host organism. Quality assurance testing is used to confirm that residual amounts of *E. coli* protein are not present in the biological product. For example, when a rDNA protein expressed in *E. coli* is used in clinical studies, the antibodies against known hypersensitivity to *E. coli*-derived protein must be excluded from the trial. Also, patients with known sensitivity to ampicillin should be excluded from the trials if the biological product was manufactured in the presence of such antibiotics. Sometimes antibody formation against the administered recombinant DNA protein may inhibit activity of the biological product. The production of neutralizing antibodies in multiple sclerosis patients treated with γ-interferon fortunately did not affect the effectiveness of the product or cause side effects.

The overall risk–benefit relationship of a product is evaluated thoroughly throughout prelicensure studies. A drug or biologic product for healthy populations favors a high potential benefit with a low risk of adverse reactions. In unusual cases, new products with less favorable risk–benefit ratios may be accepted for patients with life-threatening disease or diseases not curable by conventional treatments. For example, cancer patients tolerate products with many adverse side effects because they may provide the only chance for adjunct treatment and cure. High doses of interleukin-2 are associated with serious side effects, such as capillary leakage syndrome; however, interleukin-2 produces significant tumor regression in melanoma and renal cell carcinoma and has been used in certain patients. Because the efficacy and safety of a product are not absolute, the evaluation of its risk–benefit relationship is a critical factor in the drug development and approval process.

10.2.4 Phase IV Trials (Post-Licensure Studies)

Following licensure of the product, phase IV studies are conduct to address concerns arising during review of prelicensure data. These studies are becoming a more common requirement for license approval. Continued postmarketing surveillance is also undertaken to monitor drug efficacy and safety in a large population or in certain subpopulations (e.g., children and the elderly). When a drug is used in millions of people, detection of very rare adverse events is possible, unrecognized drug interactions with commonly administered medications may be revealed, and the incidence of nonresponders can be determined. Phase IV studies are undertaken to monitor vaccine effectiveness and to document the less frequent adverse reactions. Very rare reactions cannot be observed in phase II or III clinical trials, even with sample sizes of tens of thousands. In addition, if the vaccine is widely used, herd immunity effects will enhance the effectiveness of the vaccine. Such studies are essential for the identification of changes in the epidemiology of disease that may have implications for the vaccination program.

Following licensure approval, a manufacturer continues to routinely submit adverse event information to the FDA. Since the early 1970s, the FDA has continued to monitor the safety and quality of drugs. Physicians, pharmacists, nurses, and other healthcare professionals are asked to report adverse drug reactions to the FDA using a standard report form or by telephone if the reaction is life threatening or dangerous.

10.3 CLINICAL TRIAL DESIGN CONSIDERATIONS

10.3.1 Types of Control Groups

The optimal design for a clinical trial is a double-blind, randomized, controlled study. This design provides the greatest assurance that variables possibly affecting disease risk are balanced and avoids potential bias in the assessment of endpoints. The design also maximizes the chance that any difference in disease incidence observed between two treatment groups is due to the effects of the drug. In a double-blind study, neither the investigator nor the participant knows the treatment assignment at the time the drug is being administered. Large-scale clinical trials frequently involve more than one study site in order to recruit enough eligible participants. A multicenter trial also allows quicker subject enrollment and greater diversity among the study population. The choice of control depends on a number of factors, including preferences of the approving regulatory authority:

- A *placebo control* is a product that is identical in appearance and constituents but does not include the active components under investigation. Use of a placebo with these features, when feasible in a clinical trial, allows blinding of the treatment assignment to be maintained and optimizes reliability of the study results.
- An *active or positive control* is a comparator drug indicated for the same disease and which, in most cases, is an existing approved drug. Established efficacy for the relevant indication has already been previously evaluated for the active control, and similar effectiveness observed in the control group is expected when planning a phase III trial.

10.3.2 Blinding to Treatment Assignment

A double-blind design for vaccine trial may sometimes be modified due to the number of injections. For example, in clinical trials of diphtheria–tetanus–pertussis (DTP) and *Haemophilus influenzae* b (Hib) vaccines given separately or combined to infants in a single vaccine, group membership could not be masked. When the two vaccines were given separately, parents were not told which vaccine was administered to which arm, so an element of single blinding was maintained.[7] A further comparison, again necessarily unblinded, was also made between injection sites — all injections in the first half of the study were given in the thigh and all in the second half in the arm. In such cases, any bias due to a lack of double blinding could have been eliminated by use of a placebo; however, this was considered unethical, as both vaccines have proven beneficial.

10.4 SAFETY MONITORING AND OVERSIGHT

Informed consent is part of the process designed to protect trial participants from unnecessary risk and suffering and to protect individual rights and privacy. The investigator must explain, prior to enrollment, the purpose of the clinical trial, describe any procedures that are experimental, and provide any available information about the potential risks and benefits of participation. These elements are also described in an informed consent document. Patients have the right to refuse to participate or to withdraw from a trial at any time; however, because it is not possible to anticipate all possible adverse effects of an experimental drug, the central role of an institutional review board (IRB) is to determine whether the risks to participants in a biomedical research study are minimized and if the risks to trial participants are reasonable relative to the anticipated benefits. IRB members consist of professional personnel as well as patient advocates, lawyers, and consumer representatives. An IRB reviews the protocol, relevant background information, and the informed consent document to ensure the well-being of participants involved in a clinical trial. Assessment of risk, particularly in populations perceived to be vulnerable, frequently involves ethical considerations. Thus, large-scale trials, which are typically phase III studies, may also include formal establishment of a data safety monitoring board (DSMB) to provide further protection of study participants. The DSMB reviews accumulating safety and efficacy data while the trial is ongoing to detect early indications of dramatic benefit or harm to trial participants that might require early trial termination. Unlike the investigators and trial organizers, DSMB members are otherwise not involved in clinical trial conduct and analysis. The outcomes of DSMB discussions are considered representative of unbiased input and help to ensure the scientific validity of the trial.

The concern about possible conflicts of interest has received increased attention lately.[8,9] Because close partnerships have formed among the pharmaceutical industry, academic investigators, and government agencies, personal or financial interests may interfere with official duties and professional responsibilities; consequently, bias in the conduct of clinical studies, trial outcome, or high-level committee recommendations might occur. Everyone is accountable to ensure that data, especially from clinical trials, are scientifically robust and without ethical bias. Sometimes, informing the public about unfavorable study results places academic scientists in an awkward position. While an investigator's academic advancement depends on publishing articles, publishing unfavorable results often dissuades the pharmaceutical industry from future collaborative efforts with that investigator. On the other hand, clinical trials funded by a government agency are often considered to produce high-quality and unbiased study results.

REFERENCES

1. Bellanti, J.A., Zeligs, B.J., Vetro, S. et al., Studies of safety, infectivity and immunogenicity of a new temperature-sensitive (ts) 51-1 strain of *Salmonella typhi* as a new live oral typhoid fever vaccine candidate, *Vaccine*, 11, 587–590, 1993.
2. Gold, R., Lepow, M.L., Goldschneider, I. et al., Kinetics of antibody production to group A and group C meningococcal polysaccharide vaccines administered during the first six years of life: prospects for routine immunization of infants and children, *J. Infect. Dis.*, 140, 690–697, 1979.
3. Rutter, D.A., Ashworth, L.A.E., Funnell, S. et al., Trial of a new acellular pertussis vaccine in healthy adult volunteers, *Vaccine*, 6, 29–32, 1988.
4. Cohn, J.P., The beginnings: laboratory and animal studies, in *New Drug Development in the United States*, U.S. Food and Drug Administration, Rockville, MD, 1988, pp. 8–11.
5. Peltola, H., Kayhty, H., Virtanen, M. et al., Prevention of *Haemophilus influenzae* type b bacteremic infections with the capsular polysaccharides vaccine, *N. Engl. J. Med.*, 310, 1561–1566, 1984.
6. Ad Hoc Group for the Study of Pertussis Vaccine, Placebo-controlled trial of two acellular pertussis vaccines in Sweden: protective efficacy and adverse effects, *Lancet*, 1, 955–960, 1988.
7. Scheifele, D., Bjornson, G., Barreto, L. et al., Controlled trial of *Haemophilus influenzae* type b diphtheria toxoid conjugate combined with diphtheria, tetanus and pertussis vaccines in 18-month old children, including comparison of arm versus thigh injection, *Vaccine*, 10, 455–460, 1992.
8. Lo, B., Wolfe, L.E., and Berkeley, A., Conflict-of-interest policies for investigators in clinical trials, *N. Engl. J. Med.*, 343(22), 1616–1620, 2000.
9. Martin, J.B. and Kasper, D.L., In whose best interest? Breaching the academic-industrial wall, *N. Engl. J. Med.*, 343(22), 1646–1649, 2000.

PART III

Evaluation and Quality Assurance of Drugs and Biopharmaceuticals

CHAPTER 11

The Assessment of Pharmacokinetics in Early-Phase Drug Evaluation

Paul E. Rolan and Valeria Molnar

CONTENTS

11.1 INTRODUCTION

In modern drug development, companies wish to make rational decisions as to whether to proceed with or abandon further development based on the likelihood of the compound meeting its target profile. These decisions are made most rapidly in early-phase development, and most compounds rejected during clinical development are discarded in this phase. One of the most common reasons

Table 11.1 Descriptive Pharmacokinetic Terms

Term	Definition
C_{max}	Maximum (plasma) concentration
T_{max}	Time to maximum (plasma) concentration
AUC	Area under the plasma concentration–time curve, a measure of exposure used to measure clearance
$T_{1/2}$	(Elimination) half-life

for rejection of a drug candidate is unsuitable pharmacokinetics;[4] hence, the assessment of pharmacokinetics in early-phase drug development is strategically important. Some of the drug development issues that are likely to be answered at least in part by a thoughtful interpretation of pharmacokinetic data include the following:

1. Is the compound adequately absorbed to elicit a therapeutic effect?
2. Is the compound absorbed at a speed consistent with the desired clinical response?
3. Is there evidence of a formulation problem?
4. Does the compound stay in the body long enough to be consistent with the desired duration of action?
5. Is the within- or between-subject variability acceptable, given the likely therapeutic index of the compound? What factors contribute to the variability?
6. Is a dose range covering the plasma (or tissue) concentrations likely to be associated with a desired clinical response or give rise to safety concerns?
7. Does a relationship exist between plasma concentrations and a relevant measure of drug effect?
8. Are metabolites produced that may confound the therapeutic response or complicate the safety profile?
9. In terms of absorption, metabolism, and excretion profiles, do subsets of the target population behave differently from the general population?
10. Considering the above issues, what is a suitable dosing regimen for clinical efficacy trials?

This chapter discusses these and related issues. It also defines and discusses some of the key pharmacokinetic terms and concepts; however, for a detailed discussion of pharmacokinetic theory and analysis, the reader is referred elsewhere.[6]

11.2 BASIC PHARMACOKINETIC TERMS AND CONCEPTS

Pharmacokinetic analysis and interpretation begin with the plasma concentration–time profile of an administered drug. Several readily understood terms describe and quantitate aspects of this profile (see Table 11.1); however, description, no matter how informative, rarely enables prediction or understanding. Prediction and understanding come from the derivation of more pharmacokinetic parameters that may be less readily understood but are fundamentally important. These are listed and described in Table 11.2.

11.3 THE FUNDAMENTAL PHARMACOKINETIC PROCESSES

The four fundamental pharmacokinetic processes are absorption, distribution, metabolism, and excretion. These terms are defined in Table 11.3 and are sometimes collectively referred to by the acronym ADME. We will now discuss some aspects of how examining the ADME properties of a drug early in development can be used to address the questions posed in the Introduction as well as others.

Table 11.2 Primary Pharmacokinetic Parameters

Term	Definition	Use
Clearance	Volume of plasma cleared of drug in a unit of time; relationship between the plasma concentration and elimination rate	Determining maintenance dose to achieve a given concentration (in addition to bioavailability)
Volume	Relationship between the plasma concentration and amount of drug in the body	Determining loading dose (in addition to bioavailability)
Bioavailability	Proportion of an administered dose that reaches the systemic circulation	Determining loading and maintenance doses (except intravenous)

Table 11.3 The Pharmacokinetic Processes

Absorption	Process that gets the drug into the body (not necessarily the systemic circulation)
Distribution	Process that distributes the drug to the tissues
Metabolism	Process that changes the drug into another molecule in the body
Excretion	Process that removes the drug from the body

11.3.1 Absorption and Bioavailability

Most drugs are given orally, and it is desirable for the drug absorption to be complete, consistent, and predictable. Although it may be possible to make some prediction about the rate and extent of absorption from solubility, lipophilicity, pKa, molecular size, and animal and *in vitro* data, a study in humans will give quantitative information, as the mechanisms of drug absorption are generally complex and incompletely understood. To facilitate discussion of the underlying topic, it may be helpful here to distinguish between the terms *absorption* and *bioavailability.*

Absorption refers to the rate and extent to which the administered dose is taken into the body. If a drug is taken up into intestinal cells but then extensively metabolized, it is still regarded as having been absorbed; however, for a drug to be bioavailable, unchanged drug must reach the systemic circulation. Hence, a drug with very high first-pass metabolism might be well absorbed, but poorly bioavailable. Although, in therapeutic terms, poor absorption and poor bioavailability pose similar problems (low concentrations in the blood), it is important to distinguish the reasons for low concentrations, because there are likely to be different solutions.

Poor absorption might be approached by reformulation, changing the route of administration, or development of a prodrug; low bioavailability due to extensive presystemic metabolism might only be avoided by a change in the route of administration or chemical modification. Poor absorption is still frequently encountered in modern drug development, because the rational drug discovery process often puts more emphasis on potency and selectivity (because these programs are run by biochemists and pharmacologists) than factors likely to be associated with good absorption. This can result in lead compounds that perform very well *in vitro* but present major bioavailability or formulation problems (see discussion of this by Taylor[8] and an example by Rolan et al.[5]). In recent years, some companies have been successful in reducing the proportion of poorly absorbed candidates progressing from the discovery stage to preclinical development by the use of *in silico* and *in vitro* technologies that aim to predict the absorption of drugs in humans.[10]

Quantitative assessment of the extent of bioavailability (absolute bioavailability) is most rigorously obtained by comparison of the areas under the plasma concentration–time curves (after adjusting for dose) following intravenous and oral administration; however, even after oral administration alone, an estimate of absorption or bioavailability can be obtained in the following ways:

1. If a drug is not substantially metabolized, urinary excretion of unchanged drug may be a useful measure of absorption and bioavailability.
2. If a drug is substantially metabolized, but it is reasonable to assume that metabolites are not produced in the gut lumen, urinary recovery of the drug and metabolites *might* be a useful measure of absorption (but beware of the validity of the assumption).
3. If the "apparent" plasma clearance (dose/area under the plasma concentration–time curve, equivalent to true clearance/fraction of dose absorbed) gives an implausibly high value of clearance (e.g., greater than hepatic and renal plasma flow), it is likely that the bioavailability is low; however, this could be due to presystemic metabolism in addition to low absorption.
4. If very large variability in "apparent" clearance is observed within or between subjects, it might indicate variable absorption or bioavailability, which in turn might result in low absorption or bioavailability.

Determining whether absorption is related to the formulation or to an intrinsic property of the molecule can be achieved by comparing absorption from a solid formulation and an oral solution, ideally with an intravenous solution as a reference. An estimate of the rate of absorption can be obtained from examination of the plasma concentration–time profile. It should be remembered, however, that the time to maximum plasma concentration (T_{max}) does not reflect when absorption is complete but rather indicates the point when the rates of drug absorption and elimination are equal. Thus, two drugs with the same absorption rate may differ in T_{max} if their elimination rates differ. Assessment of the rate of absorption can also be confounded by complex or slow drug distribution; for example, the calcium-channel blocker amlodipine has a much later T_{max} than other similar drugs. This is not due to slow absorption but to partitioning in the liver membrane with slow redistribution.[11] A quantitative assessment of the rate of absorption can be obtained by analysis of plasma profiles following intravenous and oral administration.

11.3.1.1 *Effect of Food on Absorption and Bioavailability*

Food is one of the important factors under patient control that may affect the absorption and bioavailability of a drug.[12] Food can dramatically increase absorption, have no effect, or decrease absorption. Even when the extent of absorption is unaffected, the rate is often delayed due to the inhibition of gastric emptying. In addition to affecting absorption, postprandial changes in hepatic blood flow can also affect hepatic extraction and, hence, the bioavailability of some high first-pass drugs. First-time administration studies in humans are usually performed in the fasting state to avoid the possible confounding effects of food. Under such conditions, however, patients in clinical trials would need to adhere to a similar restriction, which is often impractical and may affect compliance. In order to expedite early clinical trials, then, it is advisable to study the effect of food on absorption. Often, the effect of food can be estimated from the physicochemical characteristics of a drug; for example, a poorly absorbed lipophilic drug can reasonably be expected to have improved absorption after food. For such a drug, a separate study on the effect of a high-fat meal may be appropriate. However, when it is thought that the effect of food is unlikely to be clinically important, including a single fed limb in the first ascending-dose study may be an efficient way of screening for an important food effect. A more formal and adequately powered study may still be required later for registration purposes.

11.3.2 Distribution

Few drugs work directly in the biological fluids that are readily accessible (e.g., blood, urine) for pharmacokinetic studies. Most drugs require access to tissues for their therapeutic effects; thus, understanding the rate and extent of transfer of a drug from plasma to the target tissues is essential if one is trying to predict the time course of a drug action. For example, clues from the pharmacokinetic profile may indicate that the drug is extensively distributed outside the plasma. The concentration–time profile as a log–linear plot may not exhibit a simple linear decline with a single half-life but may show several distinct decline phases with different half-lives. This *may* (but not necessarily) be due to varying rates and extents of distribution of the drug to different types of tissues. The notion of extensive distribution will come from the magnitude of volume of distribution, which can only be obtained after intravenous administration. A volume of distribution much larger than the body volume would indicate that the drug is concentrated in at least one tissue. In general, one would expect that a drug with action in the central nervous system is lipophilic and has a high volume of distribution.

11.3.3 Metabolism and Excretion (Clearance)

Both metabolism and excretion result in the disappearance of a parent compound from plasma so their consequences can be considered together in the clearance concept. Measuring clearance early in drug development can assist in making predictions regarding the factors that will affect the drug. Imagine that, for a drug that is given intravenously in a first-in-human study, negligible drug is found in the urine, and the clearance is found to be 1000 mL/min. Based on this information, we can assume that the drug is eliminated by metabolism, presumably hepatic. Because the clearance value is about two thirds of liver blood flow, the liver removes most of the drug presented to it in the blood. We could now predict that the drug would have a low oral bioavailability due to the high hepatic first-pass effect, and changes in hepatic blood flow (e.g., related to meals) might alter bioavailability. Clearance is also used to predict steady-state concentrations on repeated dosing and is a key component in establishing a dosing regimen.

11.3.3.1 *Understanding Human Metabolism of a Drug*

The three important reasons for understanding the metabolic fate of a new compound in humans as early as possible are:

- An active metabolite may be formed that may alter the clinical profile in a desired (e.g., prolongation of action) or undesired (different side-effect profile) manner. Even though *in vitro* work with human microsomes and comparison with animal data may allow prediction of whether metabolites are likely to be active, only *in vivo* data in humans will confirm or refute this question and, more importantly, quantitate the circulating concentrations.
- New metabolites may be produced in humans that were not observed in the animal toxicology studies, or they may be produced in quantities that approach or exceed those associated with toxicity in the animal studies, although the concentrations of parent drug are not toxic. In these circumstances, further toxicology studies with the metabolites may be necessary.
- With a greater increase in our understanding of the substrate specificities of different metabolic processes (in particular, cytochrome P-450 enzymes), identification of the enzymes responsible for metabolism may help predict important drug interactions or better identify classes of drugs with which the new compound is unlikely to interact. This would rationalize the selection of human drug interaction studies (see Section 11.4.3). This approach is recommended because this work can be performed *in vitro* with modest resources and can also increase the potential pool of patients in efficacy studies by allowing more concomitant medications.

Historically, metabolite identification and quantitation in humans were sought using radiolabeled studies. The rationale was that one can be confident in identifying all drug-related materials with an appropriate radiolabel; however, with the growing public sensitivity to radiation issues, the approval and adequate recruitment required for such a study are increasingly difficult to obtain and such studies tend to involve only small numbers of subjects (e.g., four to six). An alternative approach is to use an extremely low dose of radioactivity where assay sensitivity can be improved several orders of magnitude by using accelerator mass spectrometry to count the ^{14}C atoms rather than measure their radioactivity.[3] With some drugs, it may be predicted from *in vitro* work that only a very limited number of metabolites will be produced. In this case, it may be possible to quantitatively account for all drug-related material using conventional assay techniques and avoid the use of radioactivity altogether.

11.3.4 Linearity and Stationarity

The pharmacokinetics of a drug are described as showing *linearity* when the kinetic parameters that are expected to be proportional to dose (such as C_{max}, AUC) are found to be linearly proportional, and parameters that should be independent of dose (clearance, bioavailability, volume distribution, half-life) are indeed independent of dose. Linearity is desirable, as it allows extrapolation of concentrations under different dosing regimens with more confidence. Some reasons for a lack of linearity include saturable absorption, elimination, or enzyme induction. *Stationarity* relates to pharmacokinetic and pharmacodynamic properties that are independent of time. Under pharmacokinetic stationarity, clearance, half-life, etc. do not change with time. Again, this is highly desirable as it enables confident prediction of concentrations on repeated administration. Reasons for a lack of stationarity include enzyme induction or saturation of metabolism as the drug accumulates.

11.4 EXPLORING AND UNDERSTANDING SOURCES OF VARIABILITY

Drug developers, regulators, and prescribers prefer a simple dosing regimen for as many patients as possible; hence, an important part of determining the clinical and commercial success of a drug will be to assess how different sections of the target population handle the drug and whether dose modification is necessary. Following are some of the important considerations.

11.4.1 Gender

Although many gender differences in pharmacokinetics have been reported,[1] most are small and do not lead to a dose modification; however, an early search for possible gender differences in pharmacokinetics should be sought. Although outside the scope of this chapter, gender differences in pharmacodynamics are more likely to be important and should also be sought during the drug development.

11.4.2 Polymorphisms in Genes Coding for Drug-Metabolizing Pathways

Genetic polymorphisms for drug-metabolizing pathways have been extensively studied. The technology is now readily available to rapidly screen volunteers and patients for polymorphisms that might result in different drug handling. In early-phase studies, because the metabolic pathways may not be identified or their relative contributions known, it is useful to genotype subjects taking part in the pharmacokinetic studies. It should be noted that this is not done with the intention of excluding people who may be poor metabolizers for a given drug but to include such individuals to explore possible relationships between metabolism status and pharmacokinetic profile.

11.4.3 Drug Interactions

Historically, the potential and ability of a drug to elicit drug interactions were generally considered late in drug development as a labeling issue; however, it is increasingly recognized that the interaction potential of a drug may be a key determinant of its commercial success or failure. For example, the antihypertensive drug mibefradil was voluntarily withdrawn from the market as a result of increasing adverse reaction data regarding its interaction with other drugs, making it difficult to use in the clinical setting. Conversely, in a therapeutic sector (e.g., antidepressants) where the prescriber may have several alternatives and the target population has a high rate of concomitant medication use, a clean data sheet indicating little interaction potential may be an important factor for choosing the drug. During clinical development, if a large proportion of the target population is taking other medications, early exclusion of a clinically relevant interaction might allow a wider range of patients with fewer exclusion criteria to be enrolled in clinical trials. For these reasons, prediction and identification of potential drug interactions or confirming absence of such interactions has become increasingly important in the package of early-phase pharmacokinetic information.

As mentioned earlier, some ability to predict such interactions may come from *in vitro* experiments where both the drug of interest and interacting drug are studied for their ability to interact with each other. Selection and design of such studies has recently become easier with the recognition that certain well-characterized drugs may be used as probes to describe a metabolic pathway. This will allow extrapolation to a wider family of drugs that share a common elimination pathway (refer to the drug interaction table at http://medicine.iupui.edu/flockhart/). Including several probe drugs in the same study or even simultaneously (known as "cocktail" studies) has been considered; however, the issues of which probes to use, which pharmacokinetic metrics to use, and the confidence level of extrapolations that can be made from such studies are still being discussed.[9] It should also be kept in mind that the *in vitro* techniques are useful as a preliminary screen in most cases.

11.4.4 Elderly

Because the elderly constitute the majority users of many medicines, data will be required by regulators for registration unless a medication will not be used in the elderly. An important issue in early-phase development is whether to perform a separate kinetic/tolerability study in elderly volunteers before elderly patients are included in later phase clinical trials. The main reason for doing this study in early drug development is to address the safety concerns for the elderly population; however, the utility of such studies has been questioned. For example, the subjects recruited for these studies are usually in much better health than the general population they are intended to represent. Also, the elderly may differ from the young not so much in terms of mean kinetic parameters but in their greater variability. The relatively small sample size (typically 12 to 18) may not allow a good estimation of the variability within the elderly population. For these various reasons, the U.S. Food and Drug Administration (FDA) has indicated that information about the kinetics of a drug in the elderly may come from a larger group representative of the target population, which can be done in efficacy clinical trials. Although these data are useful, such studies are not always good substitutes for specific pharmacokinetic studies in elderly volunteers because the information is only available after many patients have been exposed to the drug, and clinical investigators may be reluctant to enroll patients without such data in advance. In practice, for a drug that is likely to be given to the elderly, an elderly volunteer study should be performed soon after a young healthy volunteer study to expand the potential population for efficacy studies. If elderly patients are also included in the main efficacy and safety studies, the population approach can then be used to explore the pharmacokinetic variability in this subset of the population and whether this is associated with an altered clinical outcome.

11.4.5 Ethnicity

The effects of race on pharmacokinetics or pharmacodynamics may be subtle, thus large sample sizes are required and may be sought in a sophisticated analysis of a phase III treatment population; however, a small study in volunteers of a given ethnic groups may be essential to initiate clinical trials in a particular country. Given the trend for simultaneous global drug development, an early study in Japanese volunteers, for example, known as a "pharmacokinetic bridging study," may be important for registration in Japan.

11.4.6 Renal and Hepatic Impairment

These studies are generally performed late in clinical development or may be required at a very early stage if such patients constitute a key part of the target population. The design of these studies is reasonably well covered by various regulatory guidelines.[13,14]

11.5 RELATING PLASMA CONCENTRATIONS
TO PHARMACODYNAMIC EFFECT

A critical question to be addressed after the first human study is whether the actions of the compound, both desired and undesired, and the speed of onset and duration of such actions are likely to be consistent with the desired clinical response. Speed of onset is clearly of interest for treatments that are taken intermittently for symptom relief (e.g., acute treatment for migraine, analgesics, antihistamines for hay fever). Duration of action is particularly important when the therapeutic effect must be sustained continuously (e.g., anticonvulsants). The first information on the probable time course of action often comes from the plasma pharmacokinetic profile; however, it has become increasingly evident that the kinetic profile alone may be misleading if the concentration–time and effect–time curves are substantially different. Some reasons for this observation include:

1. The effect may be delayed with respect to plasma concentration because of slow uptake into the target tissue from the plasma. A well-known example is digoxin, which exhibits a delay of several hours between peak plasma concentration and peak effect.
2. The effect may wane faster than the plasma elimination curve due to tolerance (e.g., benzodiazepines and nitrates).
3. The effect may persist despite apparent elimination from plasma. This can occur with an irreversible effect of the drug (e.g., acetylation of platelet cyclooxygenase by aspirin). Another reason is very tight binding of the drug near the receptor (e.g., salmeterol) or concentration and trapping in the target tissue (e.g., omeprazole).
4. The formation of active metabolites may also contribute to a delay in onset or prolongation of action.
5. The effect may initiate a cascade of effects (e.g., the delay in action of warfarin due to the time for depletion of clotting factors) or the delay of onset of antidepressant action presumably due to the development of important adaptive responses.

Some of these mechanisms may become apparent in animal pharmacology studies, but the clinical pharmacologist must always be aware of the possible discrepancy between concentration–time and effect–time curves. Clearly, if a relevant drug effect can also be measured in early human studies, establishing a relationship between plasma concentration and effect may be possible. If the desired clinical effect can be measured directly (e.g., blood pressure for an antihypertensive drug), the pharmacokinetic profile may not contribute greatly to the assessment of time course of action, but these circumstances are the exception rather than the rule. Because of the many causes of discrepancies between the time course of drug concentrations and effect and because it is often difficult to measure the clinical effects directly, a potentially useful approach comes from the use of biomarkers (discussed elsewhere in this book) combined with pharmacokinetic–pharmacodynamic modeling to explore the relationships between dose, plasma concentrations, and effects.

11.5.1 Pharmacokinetic–Pharmacodynamic Modeling

As was mentioned earlier, the time course of drug effect may differ from the plasma concentration–time curve for several reasons; however, some relationship between plasma drug concentration and effect is still often present even when this may not be immediately apparent because of confounding factors. Elucidating the underlying concentration–response relationship can be a powerful technique as it may enable the prediction of an effect–time course with a given dosage regimen in a special patient group or suggest the release characteristics of a novel formulation to achieve a desired effect–time profile. It may also be possible to determine whether confounding factors are present and allow deductions about possible mechanisms responsible for the observation.

The basic approach of pharmacokinetic–pharmacodynamic modeling is as follows. A study is performed in which the drug (and if appropriate, metabolite) concentration and effect are measured frequently. The effect may be the desired effect or a biomarker of the desired or undesired effect. The pharmacokinetic and pharmacodynamic data are used to build a model that may describe the time course of drug effects. A typical model would include parameters that would quantify the maximum effect and the concentration required to achieve half the maximum pharmacodynamic effect. Such a model could take into account, for example, the cascade of action displayed by warfarin. The model may subsequently be used to predict future scenarios, such as the impact of different dosing regimens on the desired or undesired effects. The model would typically be revised as information accumulated during the development of the drug. For a review of this approach, see Holford and Sheiner.[2]

The approach of pharmacokinetic–pharmacodynamic modeling has become a key tool in modern drug development. In particular, the FDA has expressed interest in seeing this form of data analysis used as a tool to rationally select dosing regimens. For some drug classes where drug effect can be easily measured accurately (e.g., neuromuscular blockers), this technique has been particularly useful.

11.6 SUMMARY: THE ROLE OF THE CLINICAL PHARMACOKINETICIST IN EARLY-PHASE DRUG DEVELOPMENT

The clinical pharmacokineticist can contribute to early-phase drug development in many ways. The most important contributions relate to examining the relationships among dose, plasma concentrations, and drug effects so the question of whether the compound and formulation meet the target profile can be addressed and, if so, an estimate can be made as to what may be the best dosing regimen or whether a different formulation might improve the clinical profile. Additional important contributions include early examination of factors likely to affect drug handling so the widest possible range of patients with the fewest restraints can be enrolled in efficacy trials. The ultimate goals are to ensure that these trials are representative of the target population and can be completed rapidly.

REFERENCES

1. Harris, R.Z., Benet, L.Z., and Schwartz, J.B., Gender effects in pharmacokinetics and pharmacodynamics, *Drugs*, 50, 222–239, 1995.
2. Holford, N.H. and Sheiner, L.B., Understanding the dose–effect relationship: clinical applications of pharmacokinetic–pharmacodynamic models, *Clin. Pharmacokinet.*, 6, 429–453, 1981.
3. Lappin, G. and Garner, R.C., Big physics, small doses: the use of AMS and PET in human microdosing of development drugs, *Nat. Rev. Drug Discov.*, 2(3), 233–240, 2003.
4. Prentis, R.A., Lis, Y., and Walker, S.R., Pharmaceutical innovation by the seven UK-owned pharmaceutical companies (1964–1985), *Br. J. Clin. Pharmacol.*, 25, 387–396, 1988.
5. Rolan, P.E., Mercer, A.J., Weatherley, B.C., Holdich, T., Meire, H., Peck, R.W., Ridout, G., and Posner, J., Examination of some factors responsible for a food-induced increase in absorption of atovaquone, *Br. J. Clin. Pharmacol.*, 37, 13–20, 1994.
6. Rowland, M. and Tozer, T., *Clinical Pharmacokinetics*, 3rd ed., Lippincott Williams & Wilkins, Baltimore, MD, 1995.

7. Sheiner, L.B., The population approach to pharmacokinetic data analysis: rationale and data analysis methods, *Drug Metab. Rev.*, 15, 153–171, 1984.

8. Taylor, J.B., Discovery of new medicines, in *The Textbook of Pharmaceutical Medicine*, Griffin, J.P., O'Grady, J., and Wells, F.O., Eds., Greystone Books, Belfast, 1993.

9. Tucker, G.T., Houston, J.B., and Huang, S.M., Optimizing drug development: strategies to assess drug metabolism/transporter interaction potential — toward a consensus, *Clin. Pharm. Ther.*, 70(2), 103–114, 2001.

10. van de Waterbeemd, H. and Gifford, E., ADMET in silico modelling: towards prediction paradise?, *Nat. Rev. Drug Discov.*, 2(3), 192–204, 2003.

11. Walker, D.K., Humphrey, M.J., and Smith, D.A., Importance of metabolic stability and hepatic distribution to the pharmacokinetic profile of amlodipine, *Xenobiotica*, 24, 243–250, 1994.

12. Welling, P.G., Effects of food on drug absorption, *Pharmacol. Ther.*, 43, 425–441, 1989.

13. FDA/CDER, *In Vivo Drug Metabolism/Drug Interaction Studies: Study Design, Data Analysis, and Recommendations for Dosing and Labeling*, Center for Drug Evaluation and Research, Center for Biologics Evaluation and Research, U.S. Department of Health and Human Services, U.S. Food and Drug Administration, Washington, D.C., 1999 (http://www.fda.gov/cder/guidance/2635fnl.htm).

14. EMEA, *Note for Guidance on the Investigation of Drug Interactions*, CPMP/EWP/560/95, European Agency for the Evaluation of Medicinal Products, London, 2003 (http://www.emea.eu.int/pdfs/human/ewp/078801en.pdf).

CHAPTER 12

Drug Interactions

Lucia H. Lee, Christopher L. Wu, Benjamin R. Lee, and Chi-Jen Lee

CONTENTS

12.1 INTRODUCTION

The use of multiple drugs is common. Serious drug–drug interactions have resulted in recent U.S. market withdrawals and the unacceptability of several new products. Many of these interactions involve mechanisms of pharmacokinetic interactions, such as altered gastrointestinal absorption, displaced protein binding, altered metabolism, and renal excretion, in addition to pharmacodynamic interactions, such as synergistic and antagonistic effects, as well as altered transport systems and effects at receptor sites, resulting in a decrease or loss of pharmacological activities or inducing adverse effects. The various methods that can be used for assessment of drug interactions include *in vitro* and *in vivo* pharmacokinetic and pharmacodynamic studies, population pharmacokinetic studies, clinical safety and efficacy studies, and postmarketing observational surveillance. Drug–herbal product interactions can also cause adverse drug reactions or loss of effectiveness and are important issues to consider in the evaluation of new drug development.

Drug–drug interactions result in modification of the pharmacological activities of one drug by the prior or combined administration of another drug. Adverse effects due to drug interactions can result in toxicity, a loss of therapeutic effect, or an unexpected increase in pharmacological activity. Serious drug interactions have caused half of the recent U.S. market withdrawals of approved drugs and have contributed to some new products not being approved. Many of these interactions involve inhibition of metabolizing enzymes or efflux transporters, resulting in increased systemic exposure of the drug and, in turn, adverse reactions. In addition, induction of cytochrome P-450 enzymes, transferases, or transporters results in diminished exposure and loss of efficacy of coadministered drugs.

In the United States, polypharmacy (i.e., multiple drug use) has become a common practice for the general public.[1] To provide optimum information for practitioners and patients via product labeling, drug development and regulatory scientists should be sure that each approved new drug is well characterized with respect to its metabolic vulnerability as a substrate as well as its potential role as an inhibitor or inducer of an enzyme or transporter in the body.

12.2 MECHANISMS OF DRUG INTERACTIONS[2]

In a drug–drug interaction, the drug for which the effect is altered (e.g., increased or decreased) is referred to as the *object drug* or the *substrate*, and the drug that induces the interaction is the *interacting drug* or *precipitant*. Drug interactions can be characterized as pharmacokinetic or pharmacodynamic. Pharmacokinetic interactions involve changes in the kinetics of the object drug, including absorption, distribution, metabolism, and excretion. Pharmacokinetic interactions alter the dose and systemic exposure relationships, as reflected in a blood or plasma drug concentration–time curve, when an interacting drug induces or inhibits the pharmacokinetics of a substrate drug. In contrast, pharmacodynamic interactions are related to the pharmacologic activity of the substrate or interacting drugs — for example, changes in the response to a drug caused by an altered exposure–response relationship. This type is the most common mechanism for drug interaction and may arise when the substrate and interacting drug affect the same physiologic system or when one drug interferes with an appropriate response to the other. These interactions may include synergism, antagonism, altered cellular transport, and effects on receptor sites.

12.2.1 Pharmacokinetic Interactions

12.2.1.1 Altered Gastrointestinal Absorption

Changes in drug absorption by the gastrointestinal (GI) tract can result from altered pH, altered bacterial flora, formation of drug chelates or complexes, drug-induced mucosal damage, or altered GI motility. These changes may produce a decrease or increase in drug absorption. Most drugs are weak acids or bases. Acidic drugs that have dissolved tend to be absorbed in the upper portion of the GI tract. In contrast, weak bases such as antacids (e.g., sodium bicarbonate) may delay and decrease absorption of certain drugs (e.g., ketoconazole). Antibiotic administration decreases intestinal bacterial flora. In approximately 10% of the patients receiving digoxin, 40% or more of an orally administered dose is metabolized by GI flora to inactive digoxin reduction products. Clarithromycin and erythromycin inhibit this process by altering GI flora in such a way that more digoxin is absorbed, so digoxin toxicity may occur. Certain drugs (e.g., tetracycline) can combine with other drugs such as iron preparations in the GI tract to form poorly absorbed complexes, thus decreasing the absorption and serum levels of both drugs; therefore, it is necessary to lengthen the time interval between administrations of the two drugs by 2 to 4 hours. Taking aluminum-magnesium hydroxide antacid with ciprofloxacin together may drastically decrease the absorption of the antibiotic by about 85%, resulting in a reduction of its pharmacologic activity.

Drugs that damage the GI mucosa may reduce the absorption of some drugs (e.g., antineoplastic drugs). Reduced GI absorption of digoxin preparations has been attributed to alterations in the intestinal mucosa induced by chemotherapy agents (e.g., cyclophosphamide, vincristine). Increased absorption can occur when the drug is retained at the site of absorption for a prolonged period of time. Moreover, changes in GI motility may increase or decrease absorption.

12.2.1.2 Displaced Protein Binding

Many drugs are reversibly bound to plasma proteins. The combined administration of two or more drugs bound to the same protein fraction may displace either drug from its binding site, thus increasing the free concentration of the displaced drug. The drug with the stronger affinity for the binding site will displace the drug with the weaker affinity (i.e., low association constant). After displacement, the drugs will be redistributed to various tissues. Drugs bound to plasma protein are pharmacologically inactive, because they are not available to the receptor sites; therefore, when the object drug is displaced from the protein-binding site, more free drug will be able to exert its pharmacological activity, and more drug will become available for metabolism and distribution to other tissues. The total plasma concentration of a drug is the sum of the bound form of the drug and the free form of the drug. Clinically important interactions may result from protein displacement if the drug has a high protein binding and is accompanied by enzyme inhibition, such as coadministration of warfarin and phenylbutazone, or when the displaced drug has a narrow therapeutic index or a rapid onset of action. Examples of drugs that are highly protein bound include phenytoin (90%), tolbutamide (96%), and warfarin (99%). Common precipitant drugs include aspirin and phenylbutazone.

12.2.1.3 Altered Metabolism

Combined administration of one drug with another may lead to an increase or decrease in the metabolic rate. These modifications may affect the intensity and duration of pharmacologic activity. The major site of drug metabolism is the liver; however, other tissues, including white blood cells, skin, lung, and GI tract, are involved in drug metabolism. The metabolizing enzymes primarily convert lipophilic drugs into more water-soluble metabolites so they are excreted more rapidly. Biochemical reactions of drug metabolism involve hydroxylation, oxidation, and reduction (phase I) and glucuronide, glycine, and sulfate conjugation (phase II). The major hepatic enzyme system consists of the microsomal P-450 oxygenases, and many forms of cytochrome P-450 (CYP) exist.[3]

Differences in the safety and efficacy of drugs may be caused by genetic polymorphisms of drug-metabolizing enzymes, drug transporters, and drug receptors. Five CYP enzymes (1A2, 2C9, 2C19, 2D6, and 3A4) are thought to be responsible for metabolizing most drugs. The CYP3A4 enzymes account for the metabolic routes in approximately 50% of these drugs, whereas CYP2C9, CYP2C19, and CYP2D6 enzymes account for another 40% of drug metabolism. Within these P-450 subfamilies, each individual enzyme is also polymorphic in nature, which brings about different degrees of drug metabolism and drug–drug interactions. For example, CYP2D6 isozyme is not present in 5 to 10% of Caucasians, who have been designated as poor metabolizers. In contrast, Asians rarely have CYP2C9 isozymes and have a frequency of the CYP2C9*3 allele of only 2 to 5%. In addition to CYP enzymes, various other metabolic enzymes such as glucuronosyl transferase, and transporters such as P-glycoprotein (P-gp), organic anion transporting peptide (OATP), and multidrug resistance protein (MRP) also play important roles in drug interactions.[4,5]

Increased metabolism due to drug interactions results from the induction of metabolizing enzymes and involves the reactions of phase I and II metabolism. For example, phenytoin induces CYP3A4 and increases the hepatic metabolism of mexiletine, thereby decreasing steady-state plasma mexiletine levels and reducting its efficacy. Similarly, theophylline and phenytoin appear to increase the metabolism of each other. When both drugs are administered concomitantly, serum drug concentrations may decrease and loss of seizure control or an exacerbation of pulmonary symptoms may occur.

Enzyme inhibition due to drug interactions may result from competition between the coadministered drugs for binding sites on the metabolizing enzyme in the liver. The onset of this interaction is more rapid than with enzyme induction, frequently occurring within hours after dosing. Enzyme inhibition is one of the most common mechanisms of metabolism-based drug interaction. The enzymes involved most often are monooxygenases, and the onset and reversal of such interactions often occur within 24 hours. The resulting increase in serum drug concentration results in augmentation of both pharmacologic and adverse effects of the object drug. For example, erythromycin and other macrolide antibiotics can inhibit the metabolism of astemizole and terfenadine, thus increasing the serum concentrations of the antihistamines as well as their cardiotoxicity. Similarly, isoniazid inhibits the hepatic metabolism of phenytoin, resulting in an increase in serum phenytoin concentrations and subsequent toxic effects.

Some drugs are metabolized extensively during the first pass through the GI tract and liver before they reach the systemic blood circulation. In these cases, drugs that increase or decrease liver blood flow will exhibit profound effects on the bioavailability of the object drug. As an example, propafenone increases plasma concentrations of both metoprolol and propranolol by decreasing first-pass metabolism and reducing systemic clearance of either drug.

12.2.1.4 Altered Renal Excretion

The renal excretion of a drug may be increased or decreased by the coadministration of another drug. Most lipophilic drugs are metabolized by the liver enzymes to form inactive water-soluble metabolites before renal excretion. Various mechanisms are involved in drug interactions that may affect renal excretion, such as competition for active tubular secretion and pH-dependent renal tubular transport. Plasma concentrations of the object drug may be increased via inhibition of renal elimination, resulting in an increase in therapeutic or toxic effects. Cyclosporine decreases etoposide renal clearance by inhibiting drug transport in the proximal renal tubule, thus increasing serum etoposide concentrations and its toxicity. Quinidine reduces the renal and biliary clearance of digoxin by 30 to 40%, thus increasing serum digoxin concentrations in about 90% of patients receiving both drugs. The passive tubular reabsorption of drugs is regulated by the concentration and lipid solubility of the drugs. An increased amount of weakly acidic drug is reabsorbed from acidic urine, whereas basic drugs are excreted. Administration of sodium bicarbonate tends to increase renal lithium clearance, thus decreasing the effectiveness of lithium. Long-term antacid therapy utilizing a combination of magnesium and aluminum hydroxide is associated with increased aspirin clearance and a 30 to 70% decrease in serum salicylate concentrations.

12.2.2 Pharmacodynamic Interactions

Pharmacodynamic interactions involve changes in the response of the subject to a drug combination without alterations in the serum concentration or pharmacokinetics of the object drug. Pharmacokinetic and pharmacodynamic drug interactions may occur simultaneously.

12.2.2.1 Synergistic and Antagonistic Effects

Drug interactions involve synergistic or antagonistic effects when the therapeutic or toxic effects of two concurrently administered drugs are greater or less than the sum or difference of their individual activity. These interactions frequently occur in drugs acting on the same site of action. Propranolol and verapamil exhibit synergistic or additive cardiovascular effects. The pharmacologic effect of fluoxetine is reversed by concurrently administered cyproheptadine. In addition, the capacity of warfarin to interfere with the activation of the vitamin-K-dependent clotting factor is reversed by the administration of vitamin K.

12.2.2.2 Altered Transport System and Effects at Receptor Sites

Certain drug interactions interfere with biochemical transport systems, limiting the access of certain drugs into cells. The serum concentration of the drug is generally unchanged unless a pharmaco-kinetic interaction occurs simultaneously. Both phenothiazines and tricyclic antidepressants inhibit the neuronal uptake of guanethidine, thus preventing the antihypertensive activity of guanethidine.

12.3 ASSESSMENT OF DRUG INTERACTIONS

Assessment of a potential pharmacokinetic drug–drug interaction relies on the available information regarding the absorption, distribution, and elimination processes for both substrate and interacting drugs. Such information allows estimation of the potential role of one or more metabolic routes of elimination in contributing to a clinically relevant drug–drug interaction. Even when a metabolic route is important to the elimination of a substrate drug and is affected by an interacting drug, additional studies may be necessary to understand whether a metabolic drug interaction has clinical impact. Various methods may be used to obtain the required information, such as *in vitro* and *in vivo* pharmacokinetic and pharmacodynamic studies, population pharmacokinetic studies, clinical safety and efficacy studies, and postmarketing surveillance. All of these approaches can produce useful information about potential and important drug interactions, and many of these approaches are described in guidelines published by the U.S. Food and Drug Administration (FDA).[6–8] In addition, strategies to assess the potential for drug metabolism and transport interactions have been discussed and described in conference proceedings.[9] Metabolic drug interactions involving CYP3A4 require special consideration because CYP3A4 is responsible for more than half of drug metabolism and occurs in the liver or wall of the GI tract. Interactions in the GI tract can affect bioavailability, as reflected in the C_{max} and AUC parameters, but cause little or no effect on half-life. Interactions in the liver may have only a small effect on single-dose C_{max} but may alter the half-life and accumulation index. Interpretation of drug–drug interaction data is complicated when a substrate drug is actively transported from the serosal to mucosal side of the GI tract by transporters such as P-gp. Like CYP3A4, these transporters are subject to inhibition or induction.

Metabolism data can provide information on the relevance of preclinical and toxicological data and permit early identification of drugs that are likely to have large pharmacokinetic variability due to genetically determined polymorphisms in drug metabolizing enzymes or drug interactions. Possible drug interactions should be examined at all stages of drug development, including:

- Preclinical *in vitro* studies of drug metabolism and drug interactions to determine which *in vivo* studies should be conducted
- Phase I and II clinical trials to assess the important potential drug interactions indicated by *in vitro* data
- Phase III and IV postmarketing population pharmacokinetic and pharmacodynamic studies to expand the range of potential interactions studied, including unexpected ones, and to allow examination of pharmacodynamic drug interactions

Recently, the Pharmaceutical Research and Manufacturers of America (PhRMA) issued guidance on *in vitro* and *in vivo* pharmacokinetic drug–drug interaction studies targeted at development and definition of a data package that will be accepted by regulatory agencies. The objective of this document is to achieve consistency in quality and predictability for drug–drug interaction studies.[10]

12.3.1 *In Vitro* Drug–Drug Interaction Studies

In vitro drug–drug interaction studies are used as the basis for design of clinical trials. The experimental procedures and documentation of data should be rigorous and reproducible, with specific analytical methods and documentation of assay procedures and results. Although a scientific approach is important for all experiments, it is most critical for negative *in vitro* observations. Positive *in vitro* findings are likely to be followed up with a clinical trial, but negative *in vitro* findings comprise the critical information in support of a claim regarding the lack of involvement of a particular enzyme or inhibition of the enzymes in the metabolism of the new molecular entity (NME).

 In vitro drug–drug interaction studies can be performed using both isotope-labeled and unlabeled chemical agents. If nonisotope compounds are used in the experiments, quantitation of metabolites should be conducted using standard bioanalytical methods (e.g., liquid chromatography/mass spectrometry). Standard assay procedures should include a standard curve range, a blank standard used to ensure that no assay interference by endogenous substances has occurred. The substrate or inhibitor drug should not interfere in the analysis of the substrate metabolite. If authentic standards of metabolites are not available, a high-performance liquid chromatography (HPLC)–radiometric approach can be used in the analysis of *in vitro* reactions.

12.3.1.1 *Cytochrome P-450 Inhibition Test*

Many drugs that are strong inhibitors of CYP enzymes are not directly involved in the clearance of the drug and could greatly affect the metabolism of coadministered drugs. The information from enzyme inhibition studies is extremely valuable, as it can allow extrapolation of the data to other compounds and evaluation of drug interactions in other organs. Inhibition of CYP activity by a drug is examined in human liver microsomal preparations. For the inhibition of enzyme-selective activities, the tissue from individual donors or recombinant CYPs can be used.

12.3.1.2 *CYP Substrates and Inhibitors*

The selection of CYP enzyme-specific substrates and inhibitors has been discussed in conference proceedings.[7]

12.3.1.3 *Inhibition Assays*

To assess whether or not a drug inhibits a particular CYP enzyme activity, changes in the metabolism of a CYP-specific substrate by human liver microsomes can be monitored for various concentrations of the drug. The potency of the inhibitor and rank order of the inhibition by different CYP enzymes can be assessed by determination of the K_i (inhibition constant) or IC_{50} value (drug concentration that reduces the metabolism of the CYP substrate by 50%). The turnover of the substrate by the test system should first be optimized; it should be linearly dependent on time, and less than 20% of the substrate should be consumed. It is better to use the lowest amount of protein (e.g., less than 0.5 mg microsomal protein per mL) in the incubation medium. In addition, it is recommended that a low percentage of organic solvent (e.g., <0.5% final [v/v]) be used to sustain CYP activity in any kinetic incubation experiment.

 A reaction time-course experiment should be performed in which the incubation is conducted at a single concentration of protein near the lowest substrate concentration anticipated to be used in subsequent experiments, as well as specific metabolite formation measured at several time points. Furthermore, the relationship between enzyme concentration and reaction velocity at an incubation time determined in the earlier experiment should be established.

12.3.2 *In Vivo* Drug–Drug Interaction Studies

Whether or not the two coadministered drugs interact in humans depends on various factors, including the relative affinities of each drug for the binding site on the metabolizing enzymes and the free drug concentrations available for binding. In addition, alternative pathways for elimination of one or both drugs tend to reduce the potential for pharmacokinetic interactions. The magnitude of increase in concentrations of a drug recipient caused by the inhibition of CYP enzymes depends on the degree of inhibition of CYP enzymes by the precipitant. Even small pharmacokinetic interactions can result in obvious adverse effects for a drug with narrow therapeutic index.

Safety data obtained from clinical trials and postmarketing surveillance are more definitive and important in assessing the effects on drug interaction. In addition, those pharmacokinetic interactions having clinical relevance should be described on the label of the drug. Accurate information regarding the clinical data on the interactions of a drug product with other drugs will help regulatory agencies and pharmaceutical sponsors to promote the effective and safe use of drugs.

To achieve greater consistency, it is important to select appropriate CYP substrates for drug interaction studies. Standardization of *in vivo* CYP substrates, doses, and sampling procedures would allow for more effective comparison in these studies. An optimum CYP substrate:

- Serves as a single CYP pathway
- Is highly sensitive to changes in activity of the specific CYP enzyme
- Is unaffected by P-gp or other transporters
- Has no adverse effects at the dose of the substrate used
- Is commercially available
- Has a measurable pharmacokinetic endpoint

The preferred *in vivo* probe CYP substrates have been reported.[10] For example, orally administered midazolam is metabolized exclusively through CYP3A and possesses all of the characteristics of an appropriate CYP substrate. In addition, the metabolism of oral midazolam relies to a comparable extent on intestinal and hepatic CYP3A, thus allowing for assessing the effects on CYP3A activity in both the GI tract and liver. Midazolam given orally can be used as a model of the CYP3A substrate to identify CYP3A inhibitors. This paradigm may be applied for evaluation of drug interactions mediated through other CYP pathways or by various transporter systems.

Three study designs are generally utilized for pharmacokinetic drug interaction studies in humans:

- Single-dose new molecular entity (NME) and single-dose CYP substrate administered in combination and each component given alone in a three-way crossover trial
- Single-dose CYP substrate followed by multiple-dose NME plus single-dose substrate, or single-dose NME followed by multiple-dose precipitant drug (inhibitor or inducer) plus single-dose NME in a sequential two-way crossover
- Multiple-dose CYP substrates and multiple-dose NME in a three-way crossover trial or two-way crossover trial.

Recently, the simultaneous administration of two or more probe substrates (cocktails) has been proposed for confirmation of *in vitro* predictions for drug interactions prior to more definitive single-substrate studies. Additional substrate mixtures — midazolam (CYP3A), dextromethorphan (CYP2D6), caffeine (CYP1A2), and omeprazole (CYP2C19) — have been developed in response to the need for other substrate interactions. Substrate mixture screening for CYP enzyme inductions is also useful when *in vitro* methods are not predictive. Another approach to characterize the possible drug interactions associated with an NME is to apply population pharmacokinetic techniques.

The active transport of drugs and their metabolites has been recognized as an important determinant in their absorption, distribution, and excretion. Many transporters in the intestine, liver, kidney, and other tissues are characterized by their structure–function relationship, tissue distribution, and regulation. P-gp is the most well-understood drug transporter with regard to its functions in regulation, tissue-specific expression, substrate specificity, and modulation by inhibitors or inducers, both *in vitro* and *in vivo*. One of the most common and serious interactions in clinical practice occurs between the narrow therapeutic index drug digoxin and other drugs that reduce its clearance. Digoxin is not extensively metabolized but is eliminated unchanged by P-gp and OATP transport in the kidney. Elevated plasma concentrations of digoxin have been observed with the antiarrhythmic agent quinidine and many other drugs. Quinidine and many of this type of drug inhibit P-gp transport, thereby inducing the increased exposure to digoxin.

12.4 DRUG–HERBAL PRODUCT INTERACTIONS

A better understanding of the interaction mechanisms and clearance pathways allows the use of similar approaches to assess the interactions between certain herbal products and drugs; however, unlike chemical drugs in which the content and interacting components are well characterized, the components responsible for drug–herbal interactions as well as contents of herbal products and other dietary supplements are complicated and unclear. For this reason, labeling requirements designed to avoid drug–herbal or drug–dietary supplement interactions are more restrictive than those for products that involve potential drug–drug interactions. Certain drug–drug interactions can be managed by adjusting the dose or dosing interval of drugs; however, drug–dietary supplement interactions may only be managed by recommending avoidance of their concomitant use when the interactions induce serious adverse effects. Recently, extensive studies were conducted in drug–herbal products interactions.[11] Due to an increased understanding of the interacting mechanisms, the various active components in herbal products, and the resulting pharmacokinetics,[12,13] it is now possible to offer more specific guidance regarding these interactions. The top five selling herbal products in the United States in 1999 were *Ginkgo biloba*, St. Johns wort, ginseng, garlic, and *Echinacea*, each claiming more than 10% market share.

12.4.1 St. John's Wort

St. John's wort is a dietary supplement widely used for depression. Although current products are evaluated based on hypericin levels, hyperforin appears to be one of the main components, as it exhibits selective serotonin reuptake inhibitor (SSRI) activity *in vitro*. Hyperforin also appears to be the more potent inducer of CYP3A enzymes.[14] It has been reported that plasma levels of indinavir, an antiviral drug for treatment of AIDS, were decreased when St. John's wort was coadministered in healthy subjects.[15] In addition, heart transplant rejection along with a decrease in plasma levels of cyclosporine were observed in patients taking St. John's wort with cyclosporine.[16] Based on these reports, the FDA issued a health advisory in 2000 recommending against the concomitant use of St. John's wort with protease inhibitors or non-nucleoside reverse transcriptase.[17] As of July 2002, 498 reports had been filed on adverse effects related to dietary supplements; of these, 42 involved interactions of St. John's wort with cyclosporine, oral contraceptives, and sildenafil.[18]

The interaction mechanisms between St. John's wort and many drugs have been investigated. Various compounds, including midazolam, caffeine, dextromethorphan, and tolbutamide, were administered to healthy human volunteers to evaluate activities of CYP3A, CYP1A2, CYP2D6, and CYP2C9. After administration for a short period, St. John's wort exhibited minimal effects on these enzymes. In contrast, long-term administration of St. John's wort selectively induced CYP3A.[19] When using fexofenadine as a substrate for P-gp transporter, administration of St. John's wort for a short period increased fexofenadine levels.[20] In addition, administration of St. John's wort for 8 weeks decreased plasma levels of norethindrone and reduced the half-life of ethinyl estradiol. More bleeding was observed in the group treated with St. John's wort compared to the controls. Midazolam clearance was markedly increased in the participants with bleeding compared to those who did not show the bleeding.[21] The labels of drugs that are substrates of CYP3A or P-gp and for which the activity of the product may be decreased by the use of this herbal product must indicate that St. John's wort, along with other known inducers such as rifampin and rifabutin, can possibly reduce the plasma levels of the drug.

12.4.2 *Echinacea*

Echinacea is frequently and widely used for the treatment of colds and other viral infections. *In vitro* studies in liver microsomes have investigated how *Echinacea* might affect the activity of the metabolizing enzymes CYP3A, CYP1A2, CYP2D6, and CYP2C9 in healthy human subjects. Administration of an *Echinacea* product did not change CYP2D6 and CYP2C9 activities; in contrast, CYP1A2 and intestinal CYP3A activities were inhibited, while hepatic CYP3A was induced.[22,23] These results indicate that the effect of *Echinacea* on various CYP3A substrates may vary, depending on the responses of intestinal vs. hepatic CYP3A activity to a given drug.

12.4.3 *Ginkgo biloba*

Ginkgo biloba is frequently used for memory improvement. *In vitro* studies have shown that *Ginkgo biloba* affects the activity of metabolizing enzymes in liver microsomes. In clinical trials, the *Ginkgo biloba* extract Egb761 showed induction of CYP2C19 with a change in the ratios of plasma AUC of a probe drug and its metabolite, omeprazole/5-hydroxymeprazole.[24] Recent studies indicated that other herbal products such as garlic supplements may also alter the pharmacokinetics of CYP3A substrates.[25] To avoid variable outcomes due to the uncontrolled use of herbal products in clinical trials, it is important to include them in the exclusion criteria for recruitment of study subjects. Participants must refrain from the use of prescription or over-the-counter medications, including herbal products, for 2 weeks prior to participation in a study.

Advances in our understanding of the mechanisms of drug interactions and the influences of genetics, gender, and environmental factors have allowed us to effectively detect, evaluate, and address the risks associated with drug–drug interactions to prevent or reduce the incidence of adverse reactions.

REFERENCES

1. Kaufman, D.W., Kelly, I.P., Rosenberg, L. et al., Recent patterns of medication use in the ambulatory adult population of the United States: the Slone survey, *JAMA*, 287, 337–344, 2002.
2. Tatro, D.S., Drug interactions, in *Textbook of Therapeutics: Drug and Disease Management*, Herfindal, E.T. and Gourley, D.R., Eds., Lippincott Williams & Wilkins, Baltimore, MD, 2000, pp. 35–49.
3. McInnes, G.T. and Brodie, M.J., Drug interactions that matter: a critical reappraisal, *Drugs*, 36, 83–110, 1988.
4. Mizuno, N., Niwa, T., Yotsumoto, Y. et al., Impact of drug transporter studies on drug discovery and development, *Pharmacol. Rev.*, 55, 425–461, 2003.
5. Lin, J.H., Drug–drug interaction mediated by inhibition and induction of P-glycoprotein, *Adv. Drug Deliv. Rev.*, 55(1), 53–81, 2003.
6. FDA, *Guidance for Industry: Drug Metabolism/Drug Interactions in the Drug Development Process — Studies In Vitro*, Center for Drug Evaluation and Research, U.S. Food and Drug Administration, Washington, D.C., 1997 (http://www.fda.gov/cder).
7. CDER MPCC/CPS In Vivo Drug–Drug Interaction Working Group, *Guidance for Industry: In Vivo Metabolism/Drug Interactions — Study Design, Data Analysis and Recommendations for Dosing and Labeling*, Center for Drug Evaluation and Research, U.S. Food and Drug Administration, Washington, D.C., 1999 (http://www.fda.gov/cder).

8. CDER MPCC/CPS Population PK Working Group, *Guidance for Industry: Population Pharmacoki-netics*, Center for Drug Evaluation and Research, U.S. Food and Drug Administration, Washington, D.C., 1999 (http://www.fda.gov/cder).

9. Tucker, G.T, Houston, J.B., and Huang, S.-M., Optimizing drug development: strategies to assess drug metabolism/transporter interaction potential — toward a consensus, *Clin. Pharmacol. Ther.*, 70(2), 103–114, 2001; *Br. J. Clin. Pharmacol.*, 52(1), 107–117, 2001; *Eur. J. Pharm. Sci.*, 13(4), 417–428, 2001.

10. Bjornsson, T.D., Callaghan, J.T., Einolf, H.J. et al., The conduct of *in vitro* and *in vivo* drug–drug interaction studies: a PhRMA perspective, *J. Clin. Pharmacol.*, 43, 443–469, 2003.

11. Huang, S.M. and Lawrence, J.L., Drug–drug, drug–dietary supplement, and drug–citrus fruit and other food interactions: what have we learned?, *J. Clin. Pharmacol.*, 44, 559–569, 2004.

12. Tucker, G.T., Houston, J.B., and Huang, S.-M., Optimizing drug development: strategies to assess drug metabolism/transporter interaction potential — toward a consensus, *Pharm. Res.*, 18, 1071–1080, 2001.

13. Bhattaram, V.A., Graefe, U., Kohlert, C. et al., Pharmacokinetics and bioavailability of herbal medicinal products, *Phytomedicine*, 9(Suppl. 3), 1–33, 2002.

14. Moore, L.B., Goodwin, B., Jones, S.A. et al., St. John's wort induces hepatic drug metabolism through activation of the pregnane X receptor, *Proc. Natl. Acad. Sci. USA*, 97, 7500–7502, 2000.

15. Piscitelli, S.C., Burstein, A.H., Chaitt, D. et al., Indinavir concentrations and St. John's wort, *Lancet*, 355, 547–548, 2000.

16. Ruschitzka, F., Meier, P.J., Turina, M. et al., Acute heart transplant rejection due to Saint John's wort [letter], *Lancet*, 355, 548–549, 2000.

17. FDA, *Public Health Advisory: Risk of Drug Interactions with St. John's Wort and Indinavir and Other Drugs*, Center for Drug Evaluation and Research, U.S. Food and Drug Administration, Washington, D.C., 2000 (www.fda.gov/cder/drug/advisory/stjwort.htm).

18. Chen, M.C., Huang, S.-M., Mozersky, R. et al., Drug Interactions Involving St. John's Wort: Data from FDA's Adverse Reaction Reporting System, paper presented at the annual meeting of the American Association of Pharmaceutical Scientists, Denver, CO, October 2001.

19. Wang, Z., Gorski, J.C., Hamman, M.A. et al., The effects of St. John's wort (*Hypericum perforatum*) on human cytochrome P450 activity, *Clin. Pharm. Ther.*, 70, 317–326, 2001.

20. Hall, H.D., Wang, Z., Huang, S.-M. et al., Effect of St. John's wort on the pharmacokinetics of fexofenadine, *Clin. Pharmacol. Ther.*, 71, 414–420, 2002.

21. Hall, S.D., Wang, Z., Huang, S.-M. et al., The interaction between St. John's wort and an oral contra-ceptive, *Clin. Pharmacol. Ther.*, 74(6), 525–535, 2003.

22. Budzinski, J.W., Foster, B.C., Vandenhoek, S. et al., An *in vitro* evaluation of human cytochrome P450 3A4 inhibition by selected commercial herbal extracts and tinctures, *Phytomedicine*, 7, 273–282, 2000.

23. Gorski, J.C., Huang, S.-M., Zaheer, N. et al., The effect of *Echinacea* on CYP3A activity *in vivo*, *Clin. Pharmacol. Ther.*, 73, 8, 2003.

24. Yin, O.Q., Tomlinson, B., and Chow, M.S., Prediction and Mechanism of Herb–Drug Interaction: Effect of *Ginkgo biloba* on Omega Zole in Chinese Subjects, paper presented at the annual meeting of the American Society of Clinical Pharmacology, Washington, D.C., April 2003 (abstract in *Clin. Pharmacol. Ther.*, P94, 2003).

25. Piscitelli, S.C. et al., The effect of garlic supplements on the pharmacokinetics of saquinavir, *Clin. Infect. Dis.*, 34, 234–238, 2002.

Assessment of Cardiovascular Drugs

PART IV

Assessment of Cardiovascular Drugs

CHAPTER 13

Antianginal Drugs

Nancy C. Pauly and Edmond Roland

CONTENTS

13.1 INTRODUCTION

The treatment of stable angina pectoris has two major aspects. The first is to reduce the risk of mortality by preventing myocardial infarction (MI) and death. The second is to reduce symptoms of angina and occurrence of ischemia, thereby improving the quality of life. Treatments to prevent MI and death due to coronary artery disease include a variety of pharmacological approaches: antithrombotic therapies, lipid-lowering agents, and angiotensin-converting enzyme inhibitors. These treatments are beyond the scope of this chapter, which describes only methods for the evaluation of antianginal or antiischemic drugs to alleviate symptoms of angina or reduce ischemia.

The purpose of this chapter is to give practical information to professionals confronted with the need to design initial trials of antianginal drugs and who have little previous experience in this field. The description of the various methods is detailed enough to serve as preparatory reading before drafting a protocol or approaching the expert in the specific field. In addition, some pathophysiologic considerations are presented to better understand the scope of application of various methods and their limitations. Obviously, patients with ischemic heart disease are the preferred test subjects for the assessment of an antianginal effect. Information derived from healthy volunteers can only be used for safety or pharmacokinetic purposes. This chapter deals with phase II and confirmatory phase III protocols.

13.2 PATHOPHYSIOLOGY OF CORONARY AND MYOCARDIAL FUNCTION IN ANGINA PECTORIS: CRITICAL ASPECTS FOR DRUG EVALUATION

Under physiological conditions, a close correlation is observed between the increase in myocardial oxygen consumption and coronary blood flow over a wide range.[1] Coronary flow is regulated by oxygen demand (momentary oxygen consumption) and by oxygen delivery. The main factors for determining the level of myocardial oxygen consumption (MVO_2) are those that use most of the energy available: heart rate, myocardial contractility, and myocardial wall tension.[1] With respect to wall tension, the components are primarily pressure development and left ventricular volume. For contractility, the major component is the velocity of fiber shortening. Unlike the situation in skeletal muscle, oxygen extraction by the myocardium is almost at a maximum level at rest; this results in a wide and constant arteriovenous oxygen difference between coronary arteries and coronary sinus in humans. The normal coronary system consists of large epicardial vessels, which normally function as passive conduits and offer little intrinsic resistance to flow.[1,2] The intramyocardial arterioles, on the other hand, alter their intrinsic tone in response to the oxygen demands of the myocardium. Because of their small diameter and well-developed media, they have the capacity to alter profoundly resistance to flow.[1,2] Through the autoregulatory system provided by these arterioles, myocardial oxygen delivery and myocardial oxygen consumption are closely linked; when MVO_2 increases, the resistance vessels dilate, thereby permitting myocardial flow to increase in proportion to the increased oxygen demands.[2,3] Ischemia is induced when the capacity of oxygen delivery can no longer meet the oxygen demand due to increasing proximal resistance in the coronary system. This situation is provoked by either an excessive increase in MVO_2 beyond a certain threshold or a primary critical reduction in the coronary lumen.[1,3]

When a large epicardial vessel is narrowed by a fixed atherosclerotic lesion, its conductance function is compromised and it now offers considerable resistance to flow. If no other alteration occurs, the increased resistance leads to a decrease in flow and thereby causes ischemia; however, ischemia-induced metabolic derangements activate autoregulatory mechanisms, resulting in arteriolar dilatation and decrease in arteriolar resistance.[1] Although this compensatory mechanism may prevent the occurrence of ischemia under resting conditions, it is not adequate to prevent ischemia when large increments in flow are required, as with exercise. When this maximal flow threshold is exceeded, myocardial ischemia and angina appear. Although the concept of fixed obstruction provides a simple explanation for the onset of angina with exercise when MVO$_2$ increases considerably, it cannot explain the onset of angina occurring at rest without any obvious increase in MVO$_2$ or the reason why the anginal threshold should vary markedly in individual patients.[1,3,4] The finding that dynamic increases in either large- or small-vessel coronary resistance can also precipitate ischemia or reduce the threshold of MVO$_2$ at which it occurs has important implications for the treatment of angina pectoris.[3] This dynamic coronary obstruction may occur within or at a distance from a stenotic segment. The product of systolic pressure and heart rate (double-product) at angina onset is a reflection of the maximal level at which the obstructed coronary artery is capable of delivering oxygen. By assessing the antianginal effect of an agent on the double-product, the indirect index of myocardial oxygen demand, two types of pharmacological intervention can be considered. An intervention that improves exercise capacity but the double-product at angina is no higher than control levels implies that the intervention produces the beneficial effect by decreasing oxygen demand at any level of external stress, and this type of pharmacological action would be more effective against fixed coronary obstruction. If exercise capacity is improved and double-product at angina increases, the implication is that the myocardium can attain a higher workload before the ischemic threshold, most probably because of an increase of myocardial flow. Such an intervention would be designed more against a dynamic coronary obstruction. A single antianginal agent can combine both types of response.

The onset of myocardial ischemia is followed by left ventricular dysfunction, electrocardiographic changes, and angina pain, in that order. In the presence of ischemia, the absence of angina pain does not mean the absence of ventricular dysfunction.[1-3] After a brief episode of severe ischemia, prolonged myocardial dysfunction with gradual return of contractile performance can occur. This condition is termed *myocardial stunning*.[1]

The first hemodynamic changes observed during exercise-induced ischemia are the slowing of isovolumic relaxation and contraction. This is followed by an abnormal increase in end-diastolic pressure due to the decrease in contractile forces and increased wall stiffness in the ischemic left ventricular wall segment. Of special importance is the relation between diastolic pressure and volume (i.e., diastolic compliance during ischemia). Several studies have clearly shown that during ischemia the immediate hemodynamic alterations may result primarily from a change in left ventricular diastolic compliance rather than left ventricular systolic pressure.[1] Thus, the increase in left ventricular end-diastolic pressure is a very early sign of ischemia. In addition, abnormalities at the level of the small coronary arteries (endocardial layers) can contribute to precipitation of myocardial ischemia, by either dynamically increasing coronary resistance following a vasoconstrictor effect or by restricting the vasodilator reserve due to a lack of flow increase required by an increase of myocardial oxygen demand (e.g., during exercise).[4] Although the abnormal coronary vasodilator reserve can be ascribed to vasoconstrictor influences modulating the tone of small coronary arteries, it is also possible that the inadequate vasodilator reserve could be due to abnormal myocardial compressive force; that is, increased left ventricular diastolic pressure might increase myocardial wall tension during diastole and thereby interfere with coronary flow.[1-3,5] This fact emphasizes the complex relationship between left ventricular function and coronary flow, particularly in the endocardial layers.[5] Furthermore, subendocardial blood flow rather than oxygen demand may be the major determinant of exercise-induced myocardial ischemia.[6] Because the majority of coronary blood flow occurs during diastole, the diastolic perfusion time may be an excellent measure of myocardial oxygen supply.[1,2,6,7]

In summary, pharmacodynamic effects that reduce myocardial oxygen consumption are (1) a decrease in preload (left ventricular diastolic pressure), (2) a decrease in heart rate, (3) a decrease in contractility, and (4) a decrease in afterload through a decrease in arterial impedance. Pharmacodynamic effects aimed at reducing the dynamic coronary obstruction are (1) spasmolytic action on coronary arteries, and (2) reduction of preload through a decrease in diastolic pressure.

13.3 METHODS FOR EVALUATION OF ANTIANGINAL DRUGS

By definition, angina pectoris is a clinical symptom that implies acute transient myocardial ischemia. The goal of therapy will be to alleviate ischemic pain through a reduction of the imbalance between oxygen supply and consumption. This chapter is primarily devoted to the evaluation of drugs for exertional angina. Methods for early evaluation of antianginal agents can be divided into two categories: (1) measurements that give the pharmacodynamic profile in humans and indirect evidence for efficacy, and (2) methods that determine direct evidence of drug efficacy.

13.3.1 Pharmacodynamic Profile in Humans

In view of the pathophysiology of angina pectoris in humans, it seems important to consider the mode of action of a potential antianginal drug as it may predict the clinical efficacy of the drug;[8] however, such studies, in general, do not provide direct evidence for antianginal efficacy. Many antianginal agents act, at least in part, by causing dilatation of the peripheral vessels;[8] therefore, when animal studies indicate that the experimental drug has vasoactive effects at concentrations comparable with the therapeutic level, initial studies in humans should include assessment of the effects of the compound on resistance in arteries and veins. While the symptoms of angina pectoris and their relief by antianginal agents can be assessed only with reference to the sufferer, a full understanding of the mechanisms of action of antianginal drugs requires an objective assessment of their circulatory effects, including those on the peripheral circulation. Such drugs can relieve anginal pain through myocardial oxygen consumption by either cardiac or extracardiac effects.[8] The cardiac effects may include contractility, heart rate, coronary flow, left ventricular function, and direct myocardial cell protection. The extracardiac effects involve the peripheral circulation by reducing preload or afterload. Preload is reduced when venous capacity rises as a result of venous dilatation and, hence, venous return and cardiac filling are decreased. In fact, reduction of preload and afterload is also a possible means of treating heart failure, so the same vasodilator drug may be of benefit in both angina and heart failure. This convergence of interests strengthens the case for adequate assessment of the peripheral actions of antianginal drugs and the valuable role played by hemodynamic studies at this stage.

13.3.1.1 Hemodynamic Studies: Right and Left Catheterization Protocols

The purpose of such a study is to gain information on the effects of the antianginal agent on basic hemodynamic parameters and, more precisely, on the cardiac loading condition. An adequate population would be patients undergoing routine right or left catheterization for chest pain and patients with normal left ventricular function who need close monitoring of their hemodynamic state — for example, after an acute myocardial infarction with signs of heart failure.

Right Heart Catheterization[9] — With the technique of flow-directed right heart catheterization, the effects of antianginal medication on cardiac output and left ventricular filling pressure can readily be quantified and even monitored at the bedside throughout the medical intervention. Pressures measured by flotation catheters must be referred to an appropriate zero point (related to the level of the tricuspid valve, which is usually located in the supine position at the upper border of two thirds of the transverse diameter of the thorax, measured from the table surface). Different types of catheters are available, ranging from the 4F end-hole latex system for single pressure recordings to the 7F double-lumen flotation catheter (Swan–Ganz type) used for double-chamber diameter pressure recordings and evaluation of cardiac output by thermodilution. With careful maintenance of the zero reference point and exact calibration, pressure may be recorded with an accuracy of ±2 mmHg under clinical conditions. Left ventricular end-diastolic pressure is reflected by the pulmonary end-diastolic pressure in wedge position (PWP), if both mitral stenosis and pulmonary hypertension are absent. Thus, PWP is a good assessment of cardiac preload, and the normal value is less than 12 mmHg. Thermodilution is the most common technique for the determination of cardiac output because of its convenience. Ice-cold water is injected into the right atrium, and the change in temperature is detected by a thermistor located 4 cm from the catheter tip, which is positioned in the main stem of the pulmonary artery.[9] The blood need not be withdrawn, in contrast to other indicator techniques such as indocyanine green. The procedure is easily carried out at the bedside by one person. The thermodilution technique meets the assumptions of Fick's law of diffusion if homogeneous temperature mixing is present. Portable computer devices providing rapid data display are commonly used for uniform sampling and calculation of the transient changes in blood temperature. To improve precision, repeated (at least three consecutive) measurements of the same conditions are advisable, and the mean value should be taken.

Left Heart Catheterization[9] — This is only acceptable if patients have an indication for coronary angiography. Left heart catheterization from the right femoral sheath may be performed with a variety of catheters. Manometer-tipped catheters, with which the transducer is placed in the cardiac chamber, are usually used to achieve the most accurate recording of pressures. The principal advantage of left heart catheterization is the facility to assess left ventricular contractility or performance through measurements of left ventricular pressures, stroke volume, and ventricular volume.

Pressure Measurements — The accuracy of the assessment of cardiac performance can be increased by adding a measurement of left ventricular end-diastolic pressure to that of stroke volume; thus, when the ventricular end-diastolic pressure is elevated and the stroke index is reduced, myocardial contractility is probably impaired. Because changes in the maximum rate of rise of ventricular pressure (peak dp/dt) are known to be highly sensitive to acute changes in contractility, measurement of ventricular dp/dt may be employed along with filling pressure in the assessment of contractility. High-fidelity catheter-tip micromanometers should be employed to obtain a reliable assessment of peak dp/dt. Peak dp/dt is largely independent of afterload and appears to be more markedly affected by changes in contractility than by preload;[9] however, the latter influence cannot be disregarded.

Quantitative Angiography — Measurements of the volumes of cardiac chambers can be made utilizing cineangiograms with contrast material injected into the left ventricle. The hyperosmolarity produced by the contrast agent increases blood volume, which begins to raise preload and heart rate within 30 seconds of the injection, an effect that may persist for as long as 2 hours. Therefore, when multiple observations in a comparable state are desired, it is essential to monitor the hemodynamics to ensure that they have returned to control levels before the angiogram is repeated. Selective injection of contrast material is essential to obtain the image of the opacified left ventricular cavity in either monoplane or biplane views. The ejection fraction (EF) is derived from planimetric measurements with the assumption that the ventricle is ellipsoidal in shape. The definition of the ejection fraction is:

$$EF\ (\%) = \frac{End\ diastolic\ volume - end\ systolic\ volume \times 100}{End\ diastolic\ volume}$$

In addition to the measurement of the global EF of the left ventricle, the ventriculogram can also assess regional EF to detect segmental wall motion abnormalities.[9] The wall motion may be normal or may show decreased inward movement (hypokinesis) or absent movement (akinesis). The presence of a hypokinetic or akinetic segment on the resting ventriculogram may not necessarily indicate fibrous scarring after infarction but may also be caused by severe underperfusion of still-viable myocardium. The regional wall motion can be readily improved after acute reduction of preload by vasodilating drugs. Pharmacologically induced venous pooling has beneficial effects on both myo-cardial oxygen supply and demand, especially when ventricular diastolic pressures are elevated. Moreover, when coronary vessels are narrowed by atherosclerotic lesions or by spasm, relaxation of normal or increased smooth muscle tone at the site of the stenosis by a vasodilating agent may increase native and collateral flow,[5] enabling critically underperfused territories to reestablish con-tractile function. Depressed regional left ventricular EF due to regional ischemia will normalize if the oxygen supply/demand ratio is normalized by any pharmacological intervention.

13.3.1.2 Quantitative Coronary Angiography

Quantitative measurement of stenosis severity could become a useful tool in the evaluation of vasoactive drugs.[10,11] Adequate geometric analysis by quantitative coronary arteriography includes dimensions of percentage narrowing, absolute diameter, and length combined into fluid dynamic equations to provide a single integrated measure of severity (i.e., flow reserve).[11] This anatomic–geometric method has been validated experimentally, completely automated, and tested for routine clinical use.[10] Both the area of stenosis and the cross-sectional area of a normal segment can dilate with infusion of vasodilators. In the presence of coronary stenosis involving primarily a single vessel, downstream flow may be maintained through collateral channels arising from neighboring relatively normal coronary arteries.[5] Thus, in the presence of coronary obstruction localized to a territory with collateral development, vasoactive agents may increase collateral flow through vasodi-lation of collateral vessels or by relaxation of normal smooth muscle tone at the site of stenosis.

The four different mechanisms for altered severity of coronary artery stenosis during changing vasomotor states of the distal vascular bed are (1) arterial smooth muscle relaxation and vasodilation of the stenotic segment, (2) vasodilatation of the coronary artery adjacent to the stenotic segment, (3) the appearance of fully developed turbulence in the stenotic segment, and (4) narrowing of the stenotic segment due to decreasing intraluminal pressure caused by arteriolar vasodilatation and decreasing distending pressure.

When performing pharmacological interventions during coronary angiography, two different approaches may be used: either repeated angiography in the same single view without altering the x-ray setting or use of multiple angiographic views.[10] In the first case, if the coronary segment is nonaxisymmetric, induced vasodilatation may accentuate asymmetry of the lumen by preferentially relaxing the nonatherosclerotic part of the arterial wall; consequently, the use of a single angio-graphic view will be misleading.[10] The effects of vasodilators are better quantified if multiple projections are obtained. This will increase the accuracy of diameter measurements and will better reflect the true luminal cross-sectional area. The attempt to visualize the vasodilation action of drugs with antianginal potency by quantitative evaluation of coronary arteriograms is often difficult, as relief of angina depends on several mechanisms.

13.3.1.3 Assessment of Coronary Flow Reserve

Coronary blood flow in an epicardial vessel can be easily and directly measured by Doppler velocity guidewire or temperature guidewire using the thermodilution method. In patients undergoing coronary angiography, the influence of a coronary stenosis on the distal arterial pressure–flow relationship is determined with sensor-tipped angioplasty guidewires that measure the poststenotic coronary flow reserve (CFR) and the pressure-derived fractional flow reserve (FFR) of the myo-cardium. The FFR is a new concept of a pressure-derived estimate of coronary blood flow.[12] CFR is derived from Doppler flow velocities and accounts for both epicardial and microvascular resis-tances. FFR is derived from pressure measurements and specifically accounts for the contribution of the epicardial artery to total coronary resistance.[12] Usually, these indices are obtained with two separate guidewires, one pressure-monitoring wire and one Doppler flow-velocity wire.[12,13] CFR can also be determined from coronary thermodilution curves;[13] therefore, a single guidewire can be used for pressure and temperature measurements, as well as determination of both CFR and FFR.[13]

The fractional flow reserve is the fraction of maximal coronary blood flow that goes through the stenotic vessel, expressed as a percentage of blood flow through the same artery in the theoretical absence of stenosis. FFR is calculated as the ratio of the absolute distal coronary and aortic pressures measured during maximal vasodilatation.[12] CFR is calculated as the ratio of maximum vasodilatation to resting coronary blood flow.[12] CFR is a useful measurement in the cardiac catheterization laboratory because it interrogates the functional status of the entire coronary arterial system, including both epicardial artery and endocardial microcirculation, whereas FFR is epicardial artery specific.[12] Determination of both FFR and CFR requires coronary measurements after maximum vasodilatation with intravenous adenosine or intracoronary papaverine. Theoretically, both parameters can yield information to discriminate between increased epicardial or microvascular resistance and their respective contribution to myocardial hypoperfusion.[12] FFR has been used as an index of the functional severity of coronary stenoses and for making clinical decisions on the need for coronary revascularization procedures.[14,15] Validation studies of these indexes have demonstrated good correlation with results of noninvasive tests of myocardial ischemia: exercise test, stress echocardiogram, and radionuclide perfusion scintigraphy.[14,15] Reported sensitivity and specificity for FFR to detect myocardial hypoperfusion are 86 to 92% and 89 to 100% respectively.[12,13] In addition, FFR may predict late clinical outcome after coronary angioplasty.[16] Therefore, CFR and FFR could serve as useful physiological endpoints for the evaluation of drug effects on coronary perfusion.

13.3.1.4 Radionuclide Methods

Radionuclide methods have demonstrated value in the evaluation of diagnosis and prognosis in patients with coronary artery disease.[17] The experience in drug evaluation with these techniques is still limited; however, they may be useful because radionuclide methods have demonstrated utility in the evaluation of patients with coronary artery revascularization, either by percutaneous coronary angioplasty or by coronary artery bypass surgery.[17] Radionuclide methods are performed at rest and when myocardial ischemia occurs under stress conditions (most often exercise test or under pharmacological stress). Two types of information can be obtained with radionuclide methods: myocardial perfusion and ventricular function.

Radionuclide Procedures for Myocardial Perfusion — Myocardial perfusion imaging can be performed with various radiopharmaceutical tracers. The greatest experience in myocardial perfusion imaging has been with the tracer thallium-201(Tl-201), but recent evidence suggests that the newer tracers Tc-99m sestamibi and Tc-99m tetrofosmin have similar diagnostic accuracy.[17] Clinical imaging can be performed using either planar or single-photon emission computerized tomography (SPECT) techniques. SPECT imaging offers the potential for improved resolution and regional localization of perfusion abnormalities and is now the technique of choice.[17] Following an intravenous injection, tracers accumulate in the myocardium very rapidly, and myocardial concentration is proportional to flow. It has been demonstrated that the quantitative analysis of tracer uptake correlates directly with the magnitude of preservation of tissue viability. The exercise images are of better quality because of a higher myocardial concentration of tracer (a result of inward coronary blood flow) and lower background activity. The presence of a perfusion defect on the initial image may represent either ischemia or scar or both. The distinction can be made by comparing the initial images with delayed images obtained 4 hours after injection. The persistence of a defect in the delayed images denotes a fixed defect. The advantages of radionuclide imaging over exercise electrocardiography (ECG) are higher sensitivity (80 to 90%) and specificity (85 to 95%), in addition to the ability to localize the disease vessels and assess the viability of the myocardium.[17]

Visual analyses of perfusion imaging or quantitative technique may be used. Quantification may improve the sensitivity of the test. The TI-201 SPECT is generally more sensitive than planar imaging for diagnosing coronary disease and localizing hypoperfused territories;[17] however, the sensitivity and specificity of exercise radionuclide images depend, to a certain extent, on the observer's interpretative ability and experience. The variability of observers in interpretation as to the presence or absence of a defect is 10%. Computer quantification of tomographic images improves the accuracy of the procedure. Excellent intraobserver and interobserver reproducibility of this method for quantifying perfusion defects has been reported, with correlation coefficients of 0.98 and 0.97, respectively.[18] Using SPECT quantitative analysis, the 95% CI for absolute change required to exceed the variability for perfusion defects is 8 to 10%.[19,20] Acquisition of SPECT data synchronized with the electrocardiographic R-wave (gated SPECT) also improves determination of radionuclide images. Exercise myocardial perfusion SPECT can be used to document reductions in myocardial ischemia with drug therapy; however, information on the correlation between radionuclide imaging improvement and clinical outcomes is limited.[17]

Assessment of Left Ventricular Performance with Radionuclide Angiography — The approach of nuclear cardiology is based on the assumption that cyclic motion of each myocardial region can be described as a set of time-dependent count rates. After radiolabeling the blood pool with a bolus of Tc-99m sestamibi or another suitable tracer, the myocardial count rate depends on the volume changes of the heart. This technique involves external imaging of the cardiac blood with an external imaging device, such as a probe or gamma scintillation camera. The simplest procedure is to show the scans in rapid sequence so the heart motion becomes visible. Two methods of radionuclide analysis of left ventricular function have been utilized.[17] In the first method, the transit of a bolus of radionuclide material is observed as it passes through the central circulation (first-pass technique). In the second method, the left ventricle is visualized using radioactive substances that circulate in the blood at steady state. This equilibrium technique requires gating of multiple R–R intervals to produce a summed, composite cardiac cycle (gated blood-pool technique). The latter is preferred for pharmacological intervention, because after one injection serial studies of EF and volume can be performed for several hours. Regional wall motion abnormalities can be detected immediately. This is of special interest for drug administration, because after injection of Tc-99m-labeled erythrocytes, the heart motion can be observed for about 5 to 7 hours; thus, improvement of regional wall motion after administration of antianginal drugs can be closely monitored. Gated SPECT perfusion imaging also allows evaluation of left ventricular performance (ejection fraction) with a correlation coefficient of approximately 0.9 with other techniques: first-pass, gated blood-pool, and contrast ventriculography.[17]

Rest and exercise radionuclide angiography is a useful technique for studying the cardiac adaptation during exercise in patients with coronary artery disease. Most patients with coronary artery disease have an abnormal ejection fraction response to exercise.[17] Radionuclide angiography permits evaluation of the regional wall motion, global systolic function, and pressure–volume relationship during both systole and diastole.[17] Reproducibility and variability in these measurements should be considered. In good laboratories, the inter- and intraindividual variability is less than 5%, but each laboratory should establish its own reproducibility results. A more important point, however, is the reproducibility of results when measurements are separated by days or weeks. Sequential studies in normal individuals and patients with coronary artery disease have shown up to 10% differences in EF, especially in subjects with normal resting EF.[17] While such variation may reflect technical limitations, it could also be due to variation in sympathetic tone. Similar variations in EF have been observed when contrast angiography is used instead of radionuclide angiography. In addition, the drug-induced changes in EF may depend on baseline EF and the presence or absence of myocardial ischemia. The latter is especially important in interpreting changes in exercise EF.

13.3.1.5 Pharmacological Stress Test

Pharmacological stress tests can be categorized into two groups: those that produce coronary vasodilatation as a mean of assessing coronary vasodilator reserve (dipyridamole and adenosine) and those that produce ischemia by increasing myocardial oxygen demand (dobutamine). This alternative form of stress is used in conjunction with radionuclide myocardial perfusion imaging, two-dimensional echocardiography, or magnetic resonance imaging.[21–25] Similar to radionuclide images, echocardiographic images are acquired on dedicated software for the analysis of regional wall motion. Because of technical difficulties associated with physical exercise on a bicycle, stress two-dimensional echocardiography is increasingly performed in conjunction with pharmacological stress test. In view of the different mechanisms of action of adenosine and dobutamine, it is not clear which pharmacological stress is best suited for which imaging modality.[21,22] If two-dimensional echocardiography is used, dobutamine is the stress agent of choice, whereas if myocardial perfusion imaging is used then either adenosine or dobutamine is an appropriate agent.[21,22,26] With dobutamine stress echocardiography, normal myocardium shows an increase of movement and thickening, while ischemia is recognized by reduced regional wall thickening and transient regional wall motion abnormalities.[23,24,26] The pharmacological stress test does not reproduce the physiological condition of physical exercise and therefore should be considered as a surrogate or second-choice stress test.[22] Moreover, proper interpretation of changes in wall motion on a stress echocardiogram requires considerable experience and expertise.[25,26] Optimal recording equipments and computer displays are essential. The pharmacological stress test has not been widely used in the assessment of antianginal drugs, although some publications have shown interesting results.[26,27]

13.3.1.6 Cardiovascular Magnetic Resonance Imaging

Cardiovascular magnetic resonance imaging (CMRI) allows noninvasive cardiac structure visualization with high spatial and temporal resolution. This new imaging technique has been valuable in the diagnosis and assessment of various cardiovascular diseases.[28] CMRI can detect myocardial ischemia by observing wall motion abnormalities induced by stress. Unlike echocardiography and radionuclide methods, CMRI is a three-dimensional modality, has no problems with imaging windows, and has high resolution and ability to depict soft tissues.[28] When dobutamine-stress CMRI was compared with dobutamine-stress echocardiography, the sensitivity was increased from 74 to 86% and specificity from 70 to 86% for detection of ischemia-induced wall motion abnormalities.[25] CMRI can evaluate ventricular function; left ventricular volumes and ejection fraction can be accurately determined.[28,29] The correlation between CMRI left ventricular function and contrast angiography or radionuclide angiography is good.[29] CMRI is also a valuable tool for assessing myocardial viability[30] and may be more accurate for the detection of subendocardial infarcts when compared to SPECT.[31] With all of these advantages, CMRI appears to be a useful tool for assessing the effects of an agent on myocardial ischemia.

13.3.2 Direct Evidence of Efficacy: Exercise Tests

Exercise testing is an established method for detecting coronary artery disease and evaluating the severity of disease and prognosis.[32,33] In addition, exercise tolerance testing is considered the primary method for establishing antianginal efficacy[34] and is widely used to evaluate anti-ischemic interventions.[32]

13.3.2.1 Exercise Test Modalities

Two types of exercise tests can be used: isometric or dynamic. Isometric exercise, defined as constant muscular contraction without movement (e.g., handgrip), imposes a disproportionate pressure load on the left ventricle relative to the body's ability to supply oxygen. Dynamic exercise, defined as rhythmic muscular activity resulting in movement, initiates a more appropriate increase in cardiac output and oxygen exchange.[35] Because a delivered workload can be accurately calibrated and the physiological response easily measured, dynamic exercise is preferred for clinical testing.[32,33,35] Using progressive workloads of dynamic exercise, patients with coronary disease can be protected from rapidly increasing myocardial oxygen demand. A maximal exercise test brings an individual to a level of intensity where fatigue or symptoms prohibit further exercise or when maximal oxygen consumption (VO_{2max}) is achieved and no further increase in heart rate occurs. Estimates of predicted maximal heart rate may be used as a guide for test termination, but these estimates should not be used as predetermined termination points in maximal testing.[33,35,36]

The maximal capacity of an individual to perform aerobic work is defined by the VO_{2max}, the product of cardiac output (CO) and arteriovenous oxygen difference (AVO_2) at exhaustion. Although VO_{2max} is measured in liters per minute, it is usually expressed per kilogram of body weight to facilitate intersubject comparisons. Functional capacity, particularly when estimated rather than measured directly, is expressed in metabolic equivalents (METS); 1 MET represents resting oxygen uptake: 3.5 mL O_2 per kilogram of body weight per minute ($mL \cdot kg^{-1} \cdot min^{-1}$). VO_{2max} is affected by age, sex, conditioning status, and disease.[33,35,36] At any age, VO_{2max} in men is 10 to 20% greater than in women.[36]

When measurement of maximal exercise capacity is intended, possibilities include the treadmill and upright bicycle ergometer. Cycle ergometer tests provide for stable ECG and blood pressure recording. Intravascular catheters may be kept in place, expired air may be collected easily, and both echocardiographic and scintigraphic observations may be made. The main disadvantages are that individuals who are not accustomed to cycling will often be unable to reach maximal heart rates due to leg fatigue. Results also depend upon complete subject cooperation in order to maintain a constant work rate in following a specific protocol. Treadmill testing permits the highest oxygen consumption rate of any common exercise device, usually 10 to 15% higher than cycle exercise.[35-37] Studies have demonstrated a consistent relationship between aerobic capacity on a treadmill and a cycle ergometer. The relationship is defined by the following formula: treadmill METS = 0.98(cycle ergometer METS) + 1.[36] Both the speed and elevation of a treadmill can be varied over a wide range of exercise intensities with excellent reproducibility.[33,35-37] External control of the work rate is attained with a minimum of subject cooperation, and treadmill exercise is generally the preferred modality in the United States. It may be more difficult to obtain exact recordings of blood pressure and the ECG at near-maximal workloads. In addition, treadmill exercise is less suitable for studies requiring a relatively immobile thorax, such as those involving indwelling vascular catheters or sensitive precordial detectors such as echocardiographs or scintillation cameras.

13.3.2.2 Test Protocols

For each subject, an appropriate cardiovascular history and examination should be performed prior to the exercise test. The subject should be tested no earlier than 2 hours after a light meal to avoid the effects of food on myocardial oxygen demand and CO. Similarly, patients should abstain from tobacco, alcohol, and caffeine for at least 3 hours prior to testing.[35,37] The subject should be informed of the indications for the test, the details of its procedure, and the potential hazards of testing and should then provide written informed consent. A 12-lead conventional resting electrocardiogram must be recorded and examined for possible contraindications (Table 3.1),[35] and the interpretation should be recorded prior to exercise. A number of different treadmill and cycle ergometer protocols are widely used.[33,35-37] Cycle ergometer protocols use an increased external work of 25 to 30 W per stage. The duration of each stage should be 2 to 3 minutes. For drug evaluation, generally, protocols with small increments in work, with work rates set to yield a test duration of approximately 10 minutes, are recommended.[37] Shorter duration may produce a nonlinear relationship between VO_{2max} and work rate, whereas durations greater than 12 minutes may cause subjects to terminate

Table 13.1 Contraindications to Exercise Testing

Recent acute myocardial infarction (less than 2 days)

High-risk unstable angina pectoris

Symptomatic severe aortic stenosis

Uncontrolled cardiac dysrhythmia

Acute myocarditis or pericarditis

Severe hypertension

Decompensated congestive heart failure

Intracardiac conduction block greater than first degree

Suspected or known dissecting aneurysm

Thrombophlebitis or pulmonary embolus

Acute systemic illness

exercise because of muscle fatigue or orthopedic factors.[35–37] The Bruce treadmill protocol is the most commonly used protocol in published studies. It has the disadvantage of large interstage increments in work.[35,36] The modified Bruce protocol with an initial zero or one-half stage is, therefore, preferable.[37] Functional capacity can also be determined with the use of the ramp protocol, in which small increments in work rate occur at fixed intervals of 30 to 60 seconds. The limitation of the ramp test is the requirement to estimate functional capacity from an activity scale and adjust the ramp accordingly.[35] This protocol may offer some advantages, including more accurate estimates of MET level, but is not widely used for drug assessment.[35,37]

Electrocardiogram tracing should be continuously displayed on a scope and then recorded on paper at least once per exercise stage and at each minute after exercise. Blood pressure should be measured before exercise, at least once during each exercise stage, and every 2 minutes after exercise until stable. Exercise is continued until termination points are reached (Table 13.2). In the post-exercise period, a complete 12-lead ECG should be recorded immediately and at 2 and 4 minutes after exercise in addition to any other leads. Post-exercise observation should continue for 6 minutes or until all exercise-induced abnormalities have disappeared. Exercise testing should be supervised by a physician trained in the procedure, and the exercise laboratory should be equipped and

Table 13.2 Indications for Stopping an Exercise Test

Angina-like pain that is progressive during exercise (stop at 3+ level or earlier on a scale of from 1+ to 4+)

Excessive degree (= 0.4 mV) of ischemic type of ST-segment depression or elevation

Ventricular tachycardia, multifocal premature ventricular contractions, or frequent (>30%) premature ventricular contractions aggravated or precipitated by exercise

Ectopic supraventricular tachycardia

Exercise-induced intracardiac block

Signs of severe peripheral circulatory insufficiency: pallor, confusion, ataxia, diminished pulse

Any significant drop (10 mmHg) of systolic blood pressure or failure of the systolic blood pressure to rise with an increase in exercise load

Excessive blood pressure rise: systolic greater than 250 mmHg, diastolic greater than 120 mmHg

Unexplained inappropriate bradycardia

Excessive fatigue or dyspnea

Failure of monitoring system

Subject requests to stop

Table 13.3 Causes of a False-Positive Exercise Test

Drug administration (digitalis, psychotropic drugs)
Left ventricular hypertrophy
Bundle branch block
Wolff–Parkinson–White syndrome
Electrolyte abnormalities
Anemia
Pericardial disorders
Mitral valve prolapse syndrome
Valvular heart disease
Hypertension

organized for patient safety measures.[35,38] The risk of exercise testing is approximately 10 myocardial infarctions or deaths per 10,000 tests in patients with coronary heart disease.[35] The more common risk can be detected by careful search for contraindications to exercise testing (Table 3.1).

13.3.2.3 Interpretation of Exercise Test

Exercise testing in clinical practice has two main objectives. The first is to provoke an identifiable clinical response, which may be a symptom such as angina pain, a change in some physiological variables including heart rate or blood pressure, or the appearance of a specific ECG abnormality, most commonly ST segment shift. The second is to determine the workload achieved at the time of the response or at the maximum effort. Some criteria for stopping a test are listed in Table 13.2. Some of these criteria constitute an abnormal response to exercise testing. These abnormal responses may or may not be a result of ischemia. Symptom-limited tests are designed to continue until the patient demonstrates abnormal signs or symptoms that necessitate termination of exercise. They are the preferred test modality in drug evaluation.[34,37]

13.3.2.4 Evaluation of ECG Data

Many different lead systems have been used for exercise testing.[33,35] A 12-lead system is usually preferred.[33,35] The normal ST-segment vector response to tachycardia and to exercise is a shift to the right and upward. The most common manifestation of exercise-induced myocardial ischemia is ST-segment depression. The standard criterion for this type of abnormal response is horizontal or downsloping ST-segment depression of 0.1 mV (1 mm) or more for 80 msec.[33,35] The probability and severity of coronary artery disease are directly related to the amount of J-junction depression and are inversely related to the slope of the ST-segment. Table 13.3 lists some of the conditions that can possibly result in false-positive responses. Digitalis, psychotropic drugs such as tricyclic agents, and other antidepressant drugs can cause exercise-induced repolarization abnormalities, especially in women. Anemia, electrolyte abnormalities, hypertension, meals, and even glucose ingestion can alter the ST segment and T wave in the resting ECG and can potentially cause a false-positive response.[35] To avoid this problem, all ECG studies should be performed after at least a 2- to 3-hour fast. This requirement is also important because of the hemodynamic stress put on the cardiovascular system by eating. After a meal, functional capacity is decreased and the ischemic threshold may vary. Left bundle branch block, left ventricular hypertrophy, and Wolff–Parkinson–White (WPW) syndrome may induce ST depression without coronary artery disease. Exercise ECG responses correspond more closely in men than in women with the presence or absence of a coronary artery disease.[32,33,35]

Development of ST-segment shift other than exactly one or two divisions of the chart paper and problems with exercise artifact distortion of the ECG have set the stage for computer enhancement of ECG evaluation. By computerized averaging of ECG complexes, artifacts may be reduced.

Recognition algorithms identify the points on the ECG to be measured. Computer analysis offers the theoretical potential of much greater precision than is possible by visual measurement of conventional ECG; however, the raw analog data should be compared with the computer-generated output to validate its accuracy. Computer processing is not completely reliable because of software limitations in handling all artifacts and inadequacy of recognition algorithms.[35] Several computer software systems have been developed, and commercial adaptations are available.

13.3.2.5 Heart Rate and Blood Pressure

The normal blood pressure response to exercise is a progressive rise in systolic pressure with little change in the diastolic pressure. In most exercise protocols, the systolic blood pressure rises about 8 to 10 mmHg per stage. A pathological fall in blood pressure during exercise is encountered occasionally; although it is an insensitive sign, it is claimed to be highly specific for severe coronary artery diseases.[32,33,35] During dynamic exercise, heart rate increases linearly with work load. The heart rate–pressure product is the most accurate noninvasive index of myocardial oxygen demand;[37] therefore, a comparison of a given treatment at this point on a patient's rating of angina pain or ST-segment depression provides an efficacy parameter.[37] A close match of the rate–pressure product between treatments is more important than the rate–pressure product *per se*. A point in exercise testing as close as possible to the functional limits of the patient is of greatest value for the determination of the treatment effect.[37]

13.3.2.6 Maximal Work Capacity

During exercise, oxygen uptake (VO_2) is directly related to the work performed. True VO_{2max} is usually defined by a leveling off of VO_2 between the final two exercise work rates and requires that maximal effort be achieved and sustained for >1 minute. In practice, the goal of testing is simply the attainment of peak VO_2 rather than VO_{2max}.[36] The average peak VO_2 of symptomatic patients taking part in clinical trials corresponds to approximately 6 METS.[32,33] It is usual to record exercise capacity in terms of minutes for treadmill tests and watts for bicycle tests; however, these values vary considerably according to the exercise modality, thus creating confusion in the interpretation of the result when data from various exercise protocols are pooled.[32,33] Therefore, exercise capacity should be expressed in METS.[33,35,36] The translation of maximal exercise duration or workload into METS has the advantage of providing a common measure of exercise performance regardless of the type of exercise test or protocol used.[33] Stages I and III of the Bruce protocol represent 3 and 10 METS, respectively. This conversion for bicycle exercise is provided by standard tables based on workload and body weight.[35,36]

13.3.2.7 Respiratory Gas Exchange Techniques

In drug studies, maximal oxygen uptake (VO_{2max}) is usually derived from treadmill time or bicycle work. Although VO_{2max} and treadmill time are closely related with correlation coefficient to a range between 0.80 and 0.90, a wide scatter around these regression lines has been observed.[35,36] Measured oxygen uptake seems to be more accurate and reproducible than treadmill time and may improve the quantification of the drug effect in clinical studies.[37] The use of gas-exchange techniques, however, is still limited due to the availability of exercise test laboratories with adequate expertise in this field.[36]

13.3.2.8 Effort Angina

For drug evaluations studies, it is preferable for patients to exhibit both subjective (angina) and objective (ST-segment shift) markers of ischemia during exercise.[37] As symptoms, patients may have angina or fatigue. Regarding assessment of fatigue, although a quantification of the patient's perceived symptoms during exercise is subjective, the use of perceived exertion scales such as the Borg scale seems to be the most useful method.[35,37] If angina occurs, the endpoint of exercise test should be the point of pain that would typically cause the patient to stop his activity or take nitroglycerin outside the laboratory setting.[37] Rating a patient's symptoms at each minute and at peak exercise is better than rating only at the end of each stage.[37,39]

13.3.2.9 *Measured Variables for Evaluation of Antiischemic Interventions and Testing Endpoints*

In asymptomatic and symptomatic coronary artery disease, the strongest independent and most consistent prognostic marker identified for mortality is the maximum exercise capacity.[32,33,35,39–41] The latter is influenced, at least in part, by the extent of resting left ventricular dysfunction and the amount of further left ventricular dysfunction induced by exercise. Maximum exercise capacity can be reported as maximum exercise duration, maximum workload achieved, and maximum MET level achieved. As discussed previously, maximum exercise capacity expressed in METS should be preferred; therefore, in clinical trials evaluating the antiischemic effects with exercise tests, maximum exercise capacity in METS should be the preferred primary clinical endpoint. Other exercise-derived measurements are valuable as secondary endpoints:[34,37]

- ST-segment depression during identical workloads, especially the highest workload reached before and after intervention
- Rate–pressure product (RPP) matched at identical workload and maximal exertion
- Exercise tolerance (watts, exercise time, METS, RPP) without angina pectoris (i.e., angina-free exercise tolerance)
- Exercise tolerance (watts, exercise time, METS, RPP) at 0.1-mV (1-mm) ST-segment depression

Several studies have incorporated multiple exercise variables into a prognostic score based on the coefficients from Cox proportional hazard models for estimating cardiovascular mortality.[33,35] The most widely used scoring scale is the Duke treadmill score, which is based on the presence of angina and ischemic ST segment depression during testing, as well as peak duration or MET level achieved.[33,35] To improve the ease of use, this treadmill score has been converted into a nomogram. The nomogram uses both times on the Bruce protocol and corresponding METS which can be calculated for other exercise test protocols.[33,35] With this score, patients are at high risk (mortality of 5% per year) if their score is –11, which generally requires both angina and significant ST-segment depression at a low level of exercise. Similarly, patients are at low risk (mortality <1% per year) if exercise capacity is >7 METS, with normal exercise ECG and no angina.[33,35] Exercise scoring systems that incorporate exercise-induced ECG changes, exercise-induced angina, and exercise capacity clearly provide superior discrimination over information obtained with only exercise ECG;[33,35] therefore, treadmill scoring systems may be interesting as measured variables for evaluation of antiischemic drugs, although they have not yet been validated for drug development.

13.4 METHODOLOGICAL ISSUES IN OPTIMIZING PROTOCOL DESIGN FOR THE EVALUATION OF ANTIANGINAL DRUGS

The objectives of the early-phase or therapeutic exploratory studies are twofold:[34]

1. Exploratory clinical pharmacology to identify some surrogate evidence for drug efficacy in angina: The various methods described in the pharmacodynamic section are relevant to address this issue.

These exploratory studies might be important when developing drugs with a completely new mechanism of action for which some clues for a beneficial effect are required before embarking on a full development program. These methods, however, are inadequate as endpoints for dose-ranging protocols and therapeutic confirmatory trials.

2. Dose determination is indeed the most important objective at this stage and can only be addressed with exercise-test protocols. Exercise testing is the most clinically relevant technique to evaluate antiischemic interventions. In addition, exercise protocols are considered by regulatory agencies as the efficacy variable most closely related to clinical benefit.

The preliminary efficacy and safety evidence accumulated in therapeutic exploratory studies is then confirmed in therapeutic confirmatory studies involving wider patient populations, longer duration of exposure, and comparison and combination with other antianginal agents.

13.4.1 Patient Selection

The quality of studies using exercise test to evaluate drug efficacy in angina patients depends heavily on careful screening of patients.[32,34,37] Patients should be symptomatic of stable-effort angina, which should be well characterized from the patients' histories. The main task is to recruit only patients with true ischemic heart disease; therefore, ischemic heart disease should be diagnosed using an acceptable objective criterion: documented past history of myocardial infarction; significant stenosis (>50%) of at least one major coronary artery on the coronary angiogram; positive symptom-limited exercise test (patients should exhibit both markers of ischemia during exercise: angina pain and 0.1-mV ST-segment depression); or positive SPECT stress test. A patient's condition should be stable; that is, over a period of at least 1 month no deterioration or improvement should have occurred. The resting electrocardiogram should be such that it does not interfere with interpretation of ST-segment changes during angina. For this reason, it is advisable to recruit only male patients in early pilot trials and to exclude patients with left bundle branch block.

Suitable study subjects should be identified by their responses to exercise testing. The primary efficacy criterion is maximal exercise capacity. An agent cannot be considered antianginal unless it increases the ischemia-free exercise level after drug administration.[34] In order to be able to demonstrate an improvement in exercise capacity, selected patients should have neither too severe a form of angina nor too mild a degree of coronary artery disease. In this respect, the best population is patients who experience chest pain within 3 to 7 minutes of beginning exercise with the Bruce protocol.[37] In addition, for purposes of being able to detect efficacy using small sample sizes, the reproducibility of the anginal pain in relationship to exercise becomes an important consideration. It has been reported that exercise capacity has a variability of 10 to 15% with serial testing on the same day and on different days.[36,37] Thus, prior to randomization, the reproducibility of exercise tolerance should be evaluated and the decision to randomize patients should incorporate one additional criterion: a reproducibility exercise test within the range of 10% with at least two exercise tests on separate days.[36,37] In contrast to a reasonably rigorous means of identifying patients with stable angina pectoris suitable for randomization for early efficacy trials, a patient population with vasospastic angina, unstable angina, or silent myocardial ischemia is more difficult to deal with. Due to the high variability and often critical condition of those patients, it is not recommended to focus early trials on this specific population when rough information on drug efficacy, dose–response relationship, and duration of effect is not yet available; therefore, evaluation of antianginal drugs in this specific setting is beyond the scope of this chapter.

In summary, the logic of the selection scheme for efficacy trials with exercise protocols is to (1) select patients who have stable angina due to myocardial ischemia, (2) demonstrate that such patients have a positive symptom-limited exercise test, and (3) demonstrate that spontaneous variation of exercise capacity to serial maximal exercise testing is less than 10%.

13.4.2 Protocol Design To Optimize Exercise Testing for Drug Investigation

Treating angina is particularly challenging, because the patient's symptoms are subjective and highly prone to improvement due to the placebo effect,[42,43] which can cause a 30 to 80% reduction in angina frequency. Even objective improvement as assessed by exercise testing has been reported with an increase in exercise performance of 14 to 49%.[44] The most unambiguous means of demonstrating efficacy at this early stage is to use a placebo control; however, such placebo-controlled trials are not always easy to implement in symptomatic patients with coronary artery disease. This difficulty could be overcome by careful selection of patients and a rather short duration of treatment, from 2 days to 2 weeks. It has been shown that assignment to a placebo group is not associated with increased adverse experience in short-term trials[45] or even in a long-term protocol.[44]

For exercise efficacy protocols, a run-in period is essential. After carefully supervised withdrawal of prior antianginal drug therapy, the patient may be started on a single-blind placebo run-in period of 1 week, which (1) allows assessment of exercise capacity and variability, and (2) allows the patient to become accustomed to the experimental procedure. Because maximal oxygen uptake is generally higher on the treadmill than on the bicycle, the treadmill is preferable for studies in which the efficacy parameters include the functional limits of the patient and objective signs of ischemia. As previously discussed, an exercise protocol with small increments in work and with work rates set to yield a test duration of approximately 10 minutes is recommended.[36,37]

Titration studies can be useful for early dose findings. It is important to start with low doses because the noneffective dose or minimum effective dose should be determined. The most common titration design is one where each patient is titrated up to a certain point according to specified rules, either forced titration or according to efficacy or safety criteria. A minimum of four different dose levels should be explored. The advantage of this design is that few patients are required. Disadvantages are possible carryover effects from one dose to another, confounding of dose and time, and problems with early withdrawals from study, thus resulting in incomplete data for some patients. The titration rules must be clearly defined in the protocol and carefully explained to investigators. Frequently, investigators titrate patients according to different criteria and no firm conclusions can be drawn from the analysis. A control group preferably on placebo is mandatory.

The parallel-group design is, in fact, the most appropriate for confirmatory dose finding. The earlier titration studies will have identified the range of a possible dose, and the confirmatory placebo-controlled studies are then carried out using only three or four doses. The duration of studies should be long enough to detect tachyphylaxis (i.e., a minimum of 2 to 4 weeks). Careful assessment of differences between results from intention-to-treat and per protocol analysis is particularly important in dose-finding studies. For parallel design protocol using a placebo-controlled group, it is usual to recruit 40 to 80 patients per group. These dose-ranging studies should be performed with patients receiving no other antianginal agents except sublingual nitroglycerin for relief of anginal pain.

Because of diurnal variability in exercise capacity and ischemic threshold (i.e., greater exercise tolerance in the afternoon than the morning), the exercise test should be performed under well-defined conditions with regard to the time of day, the period that has elapsed following administration of the drug or placebo, and the timing with respect to meals.[33,36,37] Exercise tolerance tests should be carried out, if possible, between 9:00 a.m. and 11:00 a.m. in the fasting state or at least 2 hours after a light breakfast. With frequent exercise testing, carried out on the same day or on successive days, a training effect may be observed.[37] This fact emphasizes the need for adequate randomization and for a control group.

In terms of analysis, the variables described for evaluation of exercise are recommended. The main efficacy criteria are maximal exercise capacity and changes in exercise performance, which were discussed earlier. Diary studies with counts of anginal attack rate or nitroglycerin consumption may provide supportive evidence of efficacy; however, such measurements cannot be considered hard study endpoints.

Assessment of the time–effect relationship of single as well as multiple doses of treatment is necessary. This duration-of-effect evaluation should be performed with serial exercise tolerance tests. Such designs are usually flexible and do not raise safety issues. The most appropriate is to perform exercise test prior to administration of the morning dose (trough measurement) and after drug dosing (peak measurement). Every attempt should be made to study the relationship between blood concentrations and measures of efficacy.[46] Such a study can be performed during the dose–effect, time–effect studies. The correlation or lack of correlation between blood levels and effect or time-course of blood concentrations and time-course of effect should be considered a necessary description of the clinical pharmacology of the antianginal agent.[46] A well-designed dose–response study can be considered as an adequate and well-controlled trial that provides primary clinical evidence of effectiveness for regulatory purpose.[46]

13.4.3 Therapeutic Confirmatory Studies

Therapeutic confirmatory studies are designed to confirm the preliminary efficacy and safety evidence and to provide an adequate clinical database for regulatory approval. Exercise testing remains the primary criteria for efficacy. These main therapeutic studies should be performed with a randomized, double-blind, controlled, parallel group design of at least 12 weeks' duration. An even longer duration is advisable. Because drug exposure is longer at this stage of development, the use of placebo might not be appropriate, and an active control with standard therapy is necessary. The drug in the active control group should be used at its optimum recommended dose and dosing interval. Active controlled trials raise specific issues, and to avoid possible flaws in the design of the study appropriate guidelines should be followed.[47,48] Generally, active control trials are designed to demonstrate that the efficacy of the investigational drug is not clinically inferior to the comparative agent (non-inferiority trial). The choice of the active comparator is critical. A suitable active comparator should be a widely used agent for which antianginal efficacy has been clearly established and quantified in well-designed and well-documented superiority trials (e.g., superior to an active agent or placebo controlled).[47] The non-inferiority design should be clearly prespecified in the clinical protocol. In addition, a non-inferiority margin should be determined.[47,48] This margin is the largest difference that can be judged to be clinically acceptable and should be smaller than differences observed in the superiority trials of the active comparator. The choice of non-inferiority margins should be justified clinically.[48] When the margin is set, sample size can be estimated based on power requirements. Depending on its pharmacodynamic profile, an antianginal drugs may be used as add-on therapy to other antianginal agents. Furthermore, the new agent may be efficacious in patients who remain symptomatic despite maximal treatment with other antianginal drugs. These specific situations must be addressed with specifically designed clinical trials that include a sufficient number of patients.

13.5 CONCLUSION

In the early evaluation of antianginal drugs, exercise test protocols performed in a selected population of patients are the only means to accurately determine appropriate doses and dosing intervals; however, despite great attention to detail, the assessment of a drug with a real antianginal effect could remain inconclusive during exercise testing. It is, therefore, important to follow the recommendations made to optimize exercise testing for pharmacological investigations. Other pharmacodynamic measurements may provide insights into the mechanism of drug action but cannot be selected as surrogates for dose-ranging or regulatory purposes. Although exercise capacity currently remains the primary efficacy variable for antianginal agents in therapeutic confirmatory trials, outcome variables (e.g., mortality/survival data) may also be required for regulatory purposes in the future.

REFERENCES

1. Ganz, P. and Ganz, W., Coronary blood flow and myocardial ischemia, in *Heart Disease: A Text Book of Cardiovascular Medicine*, Braunwald, E., Zipes, D.P., and Libby, P., Eds, W.B. Saunders, Philadelphia, 2001, chap. 34.

2. Schaper, W., Schaper, J., and Hoffmeister, H.M., Pathophysiology of coronary circulation and of acute coronary insufficiency, in *Clinical Pharmacology of Antianginal Drugs*, Abshagen, U., Ed., Springer-Verlag, Berlin, 1985, p. 47.

3. Collins, P. and Fox, K.M., Pathophysiology of angina, *Lancet*, 335, 94, 1990.

4. Maseri, A., Role of coronary artery spasm in symptomatic and silent myocardial ischemia, *J. Am. Coll. Cardiol.*, 9, 249, 1987.

5. Klocke, F.J., Ellis, A.K., and Canty, Jr., J.M., Interpretation of changes in coronary flow that accompany pharmacologic interventions, *Circulation*, 75(Suppl. V), V34, 1987.

6. Crawford, M.H., Exercise-induced myocardial ischemia: importance of coronary blood flow, *Circulation*, 84, 424, 1991.

7. Ferro, G., Spinelli, L., Duilio, C., Spadafora, M., Guarnaccia, F., and Condorelli, M., Diastolic perfusion time at ischemic threshold in patients with stress-induced ischemia, *Circulation*, 84, 49, 1991.

8. Kraupp, O., Pharmacodynamic principles of action of antianginal drugs, in *Clinical Pharmacology of Antianginal Drugs*, Abshagen, U., Ed., Springer-Verlag, Berlin, 1985, p. 97.

9. Davidson, C.J. and Bonow, R.O., Cardiac catheterization, in *Heart Disease: A Text Book of Cardiovascular Medicine,* Braunwald, E., Zipes, D.P., and Libby, P., Eds, W.B. Saunders, Philadelphia, 2001, chap. 11.

10. Serruys, P.W., Foley, D.P., and de Feyter, P.J., Eds, *Quantitative Coronary Angiography in Clinical Practice*, Kluwer Academic, Dordrecht, 1994.

11. Gould, K.L., Kirkeeide, R.L., and Buchi, M., Coronary flow reserve as a physiologic measure of stenosis severity, *J. Am. Coll. Cardiol.*, 15, 459, 1990.

12. Kern, M.J., Coronary physiology revisited: practical insights from the cardiac catheterization laboratory, *Circulation*, 101, 1344, 2000.

13. Pijls, N.H.J., De Bruyne, B., Smith, L. et al., Coronary thermodilution to assess flow reserve: validation in humans, *Circulation*, 105, 2482, 2002.

14. Pijls, N.H.J., De Bruyne, B., Peels, K. et al., Measurement of fractional flow reserve to assess the functional severity of coronary artery stenoses, *N. Engl. J. Med.*, 334, 1703, 1996.

15. Chamuleau, S.A.J., Menwissen, M., Van Eck-Smit, B.L.F. et al., Fractional flow reserve: absolute and relative coronary blood flow velocity reserve in relation to the results of technetium-99m sestamibi single photon emission computed tomography in patients with two-vessel coronary artery disease, *J. Am. Coll. Cardiol.*, 37, 1316, 2001.

16. Pijls, N.H.J., Klaus, V., Siebert, U. et al., Coronary pressure measurement after stenting predicts adverse events at follow-up: A multicenter registry, *Circulation*, 105, 2950, 2002.

17. Klocke, F.J., Baird, M.J., Bateman, T.M. et al., *ACC/AHA/ASNC Guidelines for the Clinical Use of Cardiac Radionuclide Imaging*, a report of the American College of Cardiology/American Heart Association task force on practice guidelines, 2003 (www.acc.org/clinical/guidelines/radio/rni_fulltext.pdf).

18. Mahmarian, J.J., Fenimore, N.L., Marks, G.F. et al., Transdermal nitroglycerin patch therapy reduces the extent of exercise-induced myocardial ischemia: results of a double-blind, placebo-controlled trial using quantitative thallium-201 tomography, *J. Am. Coll. Cardiol.*, 24, 25, 1994.

19. Mahmarian, J., Moye, L., Verani, M. et al., High reproducibility of myocardial perfusion defects in patients undergoing serial exercise thallium-201 tomography, *Am. J. Cardiol.*, 75, 1116, 1995.

20. Lewin, H.C., Haclamovitch, R., Harris, A.G. et al., Sustained reduction of exercise perfusion defect extent and severity with isosorbide mononitrate (Imdur) as demonstrated by means of technetium-99m sestamibi, *J. Nucl. Cardiol.*, 7, 342, 2000.

21. Marwick, T., Willemart, B., D'Hondt, A. M. et al., Selection of the optimal nonexercise stress for the evaluation of ischemic regional myocardial dysfunction and malperfusion, *Circulation*, 87, 345, 1993.

22. Wackers, F.J.Th., Which pharmacological stress is optimal? A technique-dependent choice, *Circulation*, 87, 646, 1993.

23. Armstrong, W.F., Stress echocardiography: introduction, history and methods, *Prog. Cardiovasc. Dis.*, 39, 499, 1997.

24. Fletcher, G.F., Flipse, T.R., Kligfield, P., and Malouf, J.R., Current status of ECG stress testing, *Curr. Prob. Cardiol.*, 23, 355, 1998.
25. Nagel, E., Lehmkuhl, H.B., Bocksch, W. et al., Noninvasive diagnosis of ischemia-induced wall motion abnormalities with the use of high dose dobutamine stress MRI: comparison with dobutamine stress echocardiography, *Circulation*, 99, 763, 1999.
26. Geleijnse, M.L., Fioretti, P.M., and Roelandt, J.R., Methodology, feasibility, safety and diagnostic accuracy of dobutamine stress echocardiography, *J. Am. Coll. Cardiol.*, 30, 595, 1997.
27. Lattanzi, F., Picano, E., Bolognese, L. et al., Inhibition of dipyridamole-induced ischemia by antianginal therapy in humans, *Circulation*, 83, 1256, 1991.
28. Pohost, G.M., Hung, L., and Doyle, M., Clinical use of cardiovascular magnetic resonance, *Circulation*, 108, 647, 2003.
29. Lethimonnier, F., Furber, A., Balzer, P. et al., Global left ventricular cardiac function: comparison between magnetic resonance imaging, radionuclide angiography and contrast angiography, *Invest. Radiol.*, 34, 199, 1999.
30. Klein, C., Nekolla, S.G., Bengel, F.M. et al., Assessment of myocardial viability with contrast-enhanced magnetic resonance imaging: comparison with positron emission tomography, *Circulation*, 105, 162, 2002.
31. Wagner, A., Mahrholdt, H., Holly, T.A. et al., Contrast-enhanced MRI and routine single photon emission computed tomography (SPECT) perfusion imaging for detection of subendocardial myocardial infarts: an imaging study, *Lancet*, 361, 374, 2003.
32. Gibbons, R.J., Abrams, J., Chatterjee, K. et al., *ACC/AHA 2002 Guideline Update for the Management of Patients with Chronic Stable Angina*, a report of the American College of Cardiology/American Heart Association task force on practice guidelines, 2002 (www.americanheart.org).
33. Gibbons, R.J., Balady, G.J., Bricker, J.T. et al., *ACC/AHA 2002 Guideline Update for Exercise Testing*, a report of the American College of Cardiology/American Heart Association task force on practice guidelines (committee on exercise testing), 2002 (www.americanheart.org).
34. CPMP, *Note for Guidance on the Clinical Investigation of Antianginal Medicinal Products in Stable Angina Pectoris*, CPMP/EWP/234/95, Committee for Proprietary Medicinal Products, European Agency for the Evaluation of Medicinal Products, London, 1996 (www.emea.eu.int).
35. Fletcher, G.F., Balady, G.J., Amsterdam, E.A. et al., Exercise standards for testing and training: a statement for healthcare professionals from the American Heart Association, *Circulation*, 104, 1694, 2001.
36. Fleg, J.L., Pina, I.L., Balady, G.J. et al., Assessment of functional capacity in clinical and research applications, *Circulation*, 103, 1591, 2000.
37. Myers, J. and Froelicher, V.F., Optimizing the exercise test for pharmacological investigations, *Circulation*, 82, 1839, 1990.
38. Rodgers, G.P., Ayanian, J.Z., Balady, G. et al., ACC/AHA clinical competence statement on stress testing: a report of the American College of Cardiology/American Heart Association/American College of Physicians–American Society of Internal Medicine task force on clinical competence, *Circulation*, 102, 1726, 2000.
39. Mark, D.B. and Lauer, M.S., Exercise capacity: the prognostic variable that doesn't get enough respect, *Circulation*, 108, 1534, 2003.
40. Myers, J., Prakash, M., Froelicher, V. et al., Exercise capacity and mortality among men referred for exercise testing, *N. Engl. J. Med.*, 346, 793, 2002.
41. Gulati, M., Panday, D.K., Arnsdorf, M.F. et al., Exercise capacity and the risk of death in women, *Circulation*, 108, 1554, 2003.
42. Benson, H. and McCallie, D.P., Angina pectoris and the placebo effect, *N. Engl. J. Med.*, 300, 24, 1979.
43. Parisi, A.F., Strauss, W.E., McIntyre, K.M., and Sasahara, A.A., Considerations in evaluating new antianginal drugs, *Circulation*, 65(Suppl. I), 138, 1982.
44. Boissel, J.P., Philippon, A.M., Gauthier, E. et al., Time course of long-term placebo therapy effects in angina pectoris, *Eur. Heart J.*, 7, 1030, 1986.
45. Glasser, S.P., Clark, P.I., Lipicky, R.J. et al., Exposing patients with chronic, stable exertional angina to placebo periods in drug trials, *JAMA*, 265, 1550, 1991.
46. FDA, *Guidance for Industry: Exposure–Response Relationships — Study Design, Data Analysis, and Regulatory Applications*, Center for Drug Evaluation and Research, U.S. Food and Drug Administration, Washington, D.C., 2003 (www.fda.gov/cder/guidance/index.htm).

47. ICH, *Statistical Principles for Clinical Trials*, E9 ICH harmonized guideline, International Conference on Harmonisation, Geneva, 1998 (www.ich.org).

48. Gomberg-Maitland, M., Frison, L., and Halperin, J.L., Active-control clinical trials to establish equivalence or noninferiority: methodological and statistical concepts linked to quality, *Am. Heart J.*, 146, 398, 2003.

CHAPTER 14

Antihypertensive Drugs

W. Stephen Waring and David J. Webb

CONTENTS

14.1 INTRODUCTION

Ischemic heart disease and stroke are the leading causes of death worldwide.[1] Cardiovascular disease accounts for about 1.5 million deaths (44% of all deaths) in the European Community each year,[2] and has been estimated to cost the American economy in excess of $128 billion annually.[3] Hypertension is a modifiable major cardiovascular risk factor[4,5] and is thought to be the single most common cause of physician visits in developed nations.[6] Blood pressure lowering is associated with a consistent and significant reduction in stroke risk[7] and, to a lesser extent, myocardial infarction.[8–10]

Uncertainty and debate over the most appropriate definition of hypertension are ongoing. Across populations, a continuous relationship exists between blood pressure and cardiovascular risk, which causes difficulty in defining a suitable arbitrary cutoff point to distinguish patients with hypertension from individuals with "normal" blood pressure. While the association between cardiovascular risk and blood pressure bears a particularly steep relationship across unusually high blood pressure values, the relationship persists, nonetheless, among individuals with "average" blood pressures. Ideally, the definition of hypertension should identify those individuals in whom blood pressure reduction could be expected to reduce cardiovascular risk. Despite recognition of a continuous association between blood pressure and cardiovascular risk, it cannot be assumed that blood pressure lowering will allow risk reduction across such a wide range of baseline blood pressure values. Trials of antihypertensive medication in the 1960s were the first to demonstrate that blood pressure lowering causes a reduction in cardiovascular morbidity and mortality. These studies had included patients with unequivocally high blood pressure, typically associated with diastolic blood pressure values of >105 mmHg.[11,12] Clinical trials have also shown clear benefits associated with blood pressure lowering in mild to moderate hypertension, although the absolute risk reduction appears to be smaller.[13] Furthermore, the continuous association between blood pressure and cardiovascular risk has led to considerable debate over the most appropriate blood pressure target, and this remains the focus of considerable interest. For example, the Gothenburg Primary Prevention study found that patients with hypertension who achieved target systolic and diastolic blood pressures of <160 and <95 mmHg, respectively, remained at significantly increased cardiovascular risk compared to age- and sex-matched normotensive controls.[14] A number of clinical studies suggest a strong relationship between the achieved blood pressure and cardiovascular risk, consistent with that predicted from epidemiological data in untreated populations. This might suggest that greatest risk reduction can be achieved by attaining the maximum tolerated blood pressure reduction; however, a number of studies have found a J-curve relationship between attained blood pressure and morbidity and mortality, suggesting a limit to the benefit that might be derived from blood pressure lowering.[15] In contrast, the comparatively small numbers of patients with very low blood pressure and the possibility that low blood pressure might be due to another pathology independently associated with increased risk are important potential confounding factors.

A plethora of guidelines concerning the diagnosis and management of hypertension has been published by a number of national and international groups, based on the best available clinical trial data.[16-19] These serve to collate information obtained from large, randomized controlled studies into clinical practice so as to achieve maximum cardiovascular risk reduction. They have been subject to frequent revisions, reflecting constant revisions and the development of our understanding of mechanisms linking hypertension to cardiovascular risk, and incorporation of data emerging from large clinical trials that provide clearer information about target blood pressures likely to achieve the greatest clinical benefit.

Despite increased choice of effective blood pressure lowering treatment and the proliferation of clinical guidelines, management of hypertension in the community remains poor. The so-called "rule of halves" was first described in the early 1970s in the United Kingdom. Community-based studies showed that only half of all patients with hypertension were identified and, of these, only half were receiving blood pressure lowering treatment. Of treated patients, only half attained adequate blood pressure control.[20-22] Unfortunately, recent studies have found that the detection, implementation of treatment, and attainment of optimal blood pressure control have not significantly improved.[23,24] From a clinical perspective, successful treatment of hypertension is highly cost effective, given the reduced burden of cardiovascular disease that is conferred.[25] From a commercial perspective, the expanding market for antihypertensive drug treatment is enormous and justifies the research and development expenditure of more than $250 million by the pharmaceutical industry for each new antihypertensive drug granted a license.[26] Recent clinical studies have shown that attainment of adequate blood pressure control requires administration of more than two different antihypertensive agents in the majority of patients. For novel blood pressure lowering drugs, their tolerability, lack of significant adverse effects, and freedom from problematic interactions with existing antihypertensive agents are of paramount importance to ensure that they might be successfully implemented into clinical practice. Despite the availability of a number of different classes of antihypertensive drugs, there remains a significant unmet clinical need in patients with hypertension.

The information gained from earlier clinical trials has had a significant impact on the design of clinical trials in the development of novel antihypertensive drugs. The earliest studies established the efficacy of chlorthalidone, reserpine, hydralazine, and beta-adrenoceptor antagonists in both lowering blood pressure and reducing cardiovascular risk.[11-13] Moreover, this group of drugs, thiazide-type diuretics in particular, has been used as a "gold standard" against which more recent blood pressure lowering agents were compared. The range of drugs available for treating high blood pressure has increased substantially over the past 20 years with the addition of calcium antagonists, angiotensin-converting enzyme (ACE) inhibitors, angiotensin receptor antagonists, and novel centrally acting sympatholytic agents. All appear effective in lowering blood pressure, but data on their individual efficacies have only recently become available from large randomized double-blind clinical trials against active comparator treatments. For example, the efficacy of sustained-release nifedipine has been established by showing a similar reduction in cardiovascular events to that achieved with diuretic therapy.[27] Similar efficacy in reducing cardiovascular endpoints has been demonstrated for other dihydropyridine calcium channel blockers and ACE inhibitors as compared to diuretic and beta-blocker treatment, the gold standard.[28] Treatment of hypertension with losartan, an angiotensin II receptor antagonist, has been shown to be at least as effective as a beta-adrenoceptor antagonist in reducing cardiovascular events.[29]

The expanding number of new antihypertensive drug classes has raised considerable interest in and speculation about the potential advantages and disadvantages of the various ancillary properties associated with each. For example, a direct vascular effect has been proposed as an important mechanism that contributes to the benefits of the ACE inhibitor treatment.[30] The increase in serum uric acid concentration conferred by diuretic treatment[31] and, conversely, the uricosuric

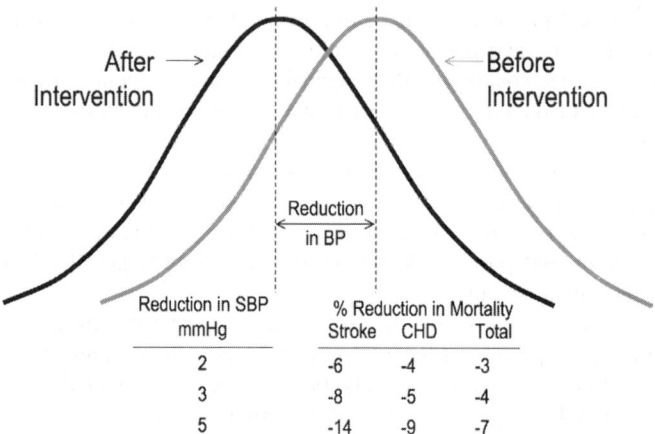

Reduction in SBP mmHg	% Reduction in Mortality		
	Stroke	CHD	Total
2	-6	-4	-3
3	-8	-5	-4
5	-14	-9	-7

Figure 14.1 Population distribution of systemic blood pressure and effects of blood pressure lowering on cardiovascular risk. (From Whelton, P.K. et al., *JAMA*, 288, 1882–1888, 2002. With permission.)

properties of losartan[32] have both been proposed as potentially advantageous therapeutic effects. Some concern has been expressed regarding the safety of doxazosin, an alpha-blocker, which reduces all-cause mortality to a similar extent as chlorthalidone in patients with hypertension but is associated with an excess incidence of heart failure.[33] One recent study has suggested that ACE inhibitor treatment might be more effective than diuretics in male patients with mild to moderate hypertension.[34] Despite this, no existing antihypertensive treatment has been consistently shown to reduce cardiovascular morbidity and mortality more than thiazide-type diuretic treatment,[35] which remains a gold standard. On balance, current antihypertensive drug classes appear equivalent in their ability to reduce all-cause mortality in the setting of comparable blood pressure reductions, which strongly suggests that improved clinical outcome is probably explained primarily on the basis of blood pressure reduction. However, recent data have suggested that important differences between classes of drugs may exist; for example, thiazide treatment appears more effective than calcium channel blockers and alpha-blockers in preventing heart failure and is more effective than ACE inhibitors in reducing composite cardiovascular events, despite a similar mortality reduction achieved by all treatment classes.[35,36] The view held by most, but not all, authorities is that the key role of antihypertensive treatment is blood pressure reduction, and that the choice of drug should be based on adverse effect profile, individual patient characteristics, and economic factors. A considerable body of clinical data that have accrued over many years demonstrates the effectiveness of existing antihypertensive treatments in reducing the incidence of stroke, myocardial infarction, and cardiovascular mortality (Figure 14.1).[37] This has significant implications for the later phases of development of novel blood pressure lowering drugs. It is necessary to demonstrate long-term therapeutic efficacy against established effective treatment, or treatment combinations, which by necessity require substantially larger numbers of patients to be studied in long-term clinical trials than might be required to demonstrate efficacy against placebo.

14.1.1 The Ideal Novel Antihypertensive Drug

The ideal antihypertensive drug should be safe and free of adverse effects that might impede patient compliance with treatment. These aspects are especially pertinent to novel antihypertensive agents because they are intended for long-term treatment in an asymptomatic patient group. Treatment efficacy should include, as a minimum, demonstration of significant lowering of systemic blood pressure. Ideally, the drug should reduce long-term cardiovascular morbidity and mortality in patients with hypertension. This might not be feasible in early development because of the large number of patients and prolonged duration of treatment required to establish efficacy in this setting. An increasing number of important surrogate markers of cardiovascular risk have been established in patients with hypertension (discussed further in Section 14.3.9), and the ideal antihypertensive drug should demonstrate favorable effects on these indices. Furthermore, the novel antihypertensive drug should ameliorate, or at least have no adverse effect on, other cardiovascular risk factors — for example, by lowering serum cholesterol or glucose concentrations.

Novel antihypertensive drugs should have peak-trough pharmacodynamic characteristics that make them suitable for once-daily administration. This will provide the greatest likelihood of patient compliance and, given that many once-daily preparations are currently available, ensure market viability of the candidate drug. The ideal antihypertensive drug should be free of interactions with other drugs likely to be coadministered, which include other antihypertensive agents, antidiabetic drugs, antiplatelets and drugs used to treat chronic heart failure. It is recognized that polypharmacy with existing antihypertensive drugs is a requisite for adequate blood pressure control in the majority of patients, and novel antihypertensive drugs prone to drug–drug interactions might have limited their clinical utility.

The pharmacokinetic and pharmacodynamic properties of a novel antihypertensive agent that emerge during phase I and II studies might identify characteristics that render it unsuitable for further development, even at this early stage. Early studies might identify pharmacodynamic characteristics of the novel antihypertensive drug suggesting a specific therapeutic role — for example, predominant lowering of systolic rather than diastolic blood pressure, indicating a potential role in the treatment of isolated systolic hypertension. Such observations require confirmation in later studies, where potential underlying mechanisms can be explored further. These findings, even during early clinical development, can allow identification of special target populations in whom the novel drug might be particularly effective.

14.2 PHASE I CLINICAL STUDIES

Phase I studies of antihypertensive drugs do not differ essentially from those dealing with other novel compounds. The key purpose of phase I investigation, and entry into human studies in particular, is to determine the safety and tolerability of new compounds or novel formulations of more established compounds. The investigator in nontherapeutic research has an obligation to ensure the safety of all research subjects,[38] which encompasses rigorous protocol design, provision of adequate research facilities, and strict adherence to good clinical practice and local standard operating procedures. The investigator must ensure that healthy subjects are recruited only after obtaining an adequate medical history, thorough physical examination, and appropriate laboratory investigations. This is primarily for the protection of subjects but also serves to exclude excess adverse event reporting due to preexisting illnesses. In the context of phase I research of a potential antihypertensive drug, it is particularly important to exclude the possibility of covert ischemic heart disease. Anticipated blood pressure lowering might compromise myocardial perfusion, which might manifest as angina or arrhythmia.

Entry-into-human studies are typically conducted using a single ascending dose design. The intended range of dosages is selected on the basis of preclinical data, using allometric modeling to estimate the expected human concentrations from those in animals. For safety, the initial dose is characteristically selected so as to give a 100- to 1000-fold lower predicted concentration of compound than the minimum effective concentration or maximum nontoxic concentrations in animal studies. Subjects will be randomly allocated to a dosing group, typically numbering eight to ten in each dose escalation step. Subjects will receive only one dose of study compound and, regardless of the dosing tier, one or two in each group will be randomly allocated to receive placebo rather than active compound. This allows early comparison of the compound and placebo-related adverse event reports. Dispensing of the compound within each dosing group is usually separated by an interval of at least 5 to 10 minutes, so if any serious adverse events emerge early then dose administration to the remainder of the group can be halted. The decision to escalate to the next dose is usually made on the basis of clinical, electrocardiogram (ECG), and laboratory safety data and, in certain cases, pharmacokinetic data relating to the compound or its metabolites.

Hemodynamic monitoring in phase I clinical trials of blood pressure lowering compounds is practically identical to that required for other new cardiovascular compounds. Resting heart rate and blood pressure should be monitored at regular intervals, where the frequency and timing of observations are likely to capture potential changes associated with the anticipated peak systemic concentrations. Similarly, regular electrocardiogram recordings are normally made so as to determine potential effects on PR and QT intervals or QRS and ST morphology. If the compound has been shown to exhibit effects on Purkinje fibers *in vitro* or animal models have suggested the potential for cardiotoxicity, more frequent and detailed analyses of the electrocardiogram may be undertaken in phase I studies, in addition to those normally proposed in later phases of drug development. Other noninvasive measurements (e.g., bioimpedance transthoracic cardiography to determine cardiac output) may be helpful, as they could give early insight into potential hemodynamic effects and influence the design of later studies. Indeed, using this technique to determine systemic vascular resistance may provide a more sensitive measure of pharmacological vasodilator effects *in vivo* than blood pressure measurement alone. For instance, bioimpedance measurements during the first human systemic studies of endothelin receptor antagonists demonstrated that a small reduction in blood pressure was accompanied by a more marked reduction in peripheral vascular resistance.[39] Later, an endothelin receptor antagonist, bosentan, was found to significantly lower systemic blood pressure in patients with essential hypertension, confirming that endothelin contributes to elevated blood pressure in this group.[40]

14.2.1 Pharmacokinetic Variables

The pharmacokinetic data obtained during single ascending dose studies can allow evaluation of the relationship between administered dose and drug exposure (determined by the area under the concentration–time curve). Furthermore, the variability in peak concentrations and drug exposure between individuals can be examined. An unpredictable relationship between dose and drug exposure and wide variability in pharmacokinetic variables between individuals are undesirable properties. Even at this early stage, such concerns may be sufficient to halt further development of the candidate antihypertensive drug. In some cases, the physicochemical properties of the compound and preclinical data might predict high pharmacokinetic variability. For example, if the compound is highly lipophilic or if animal models show a significant effect of food on gastrointestinal absorption, entry into human studies can incorporate a food-effect study arm. These exploratory data may allow undesirable kinetic properties of the drug to be established early so further development is stopped, thus avoiding unnecessary exposure of additional subjects to treatment; however, food interaction studies are often performed in subsequent studies, after preliminary pharmacokinetic data have established the doses that will be evaluated in later phase I and II studies.

14.2.2 Pharmacodynamic Data

Phase I studies may provide early insight into the blood pressure lowering efficacy of candidate antihypertensive drugs based on clinical safety observations. The lack of an obvious blood pressure effect in phase I studies should not deter further evaluation of the candidate antihypertensive agent. This is particularly important when the study population consists of young healthy subjects, who have highly effective homeostasis of blood pressure through multiple mechanisms that might be able to counter the effects of pharmacological action on a single pathway. The processes involved in the maintenance of blood pressure in hypertensive patients may be different from those in healthy subjects, and it might be argued that the response, or lack of it, in a healthy volunteer study would not reliably predict the situation in hypertensive patients. Even in elderly patients with hypertension, only around 60 to 70% showed a significant response to monotherapy with a beta-blocker, alpha-blocker, thiazide diuretic, calcium channel blocker, ACE inhibitor, or centrally acting antihypertensive agent.[41] However, drugs that are currently used in the treatment of hypertension can be described as *hypotensive* rather than *antihypertensive* because they lower blood pressure to the same proportionate level in normotensive subjects as in hypertensive patients. An additional confounding factor is that, for any proportionate reduction in blood pressure, the absolute fall in blood pressure in healthy subjects would be smaller and, therefore, more difficult to detect. A truly antihypertensive drug must have a blood pressure lowering action specific to the pathology of the hypertensive process, and this seems unlikely in a polygenic condition that is also influenced by a wide range of environmental factors.[42,43] For these reasons, detailed examination of blood pressure responses to candidate antihypertensive agents is generally reserved for late phase I or early phase II studies.

Phase I studies often incorporate specific evaluation of oral and intravenous dosing regimens, so a more complete pharmacokinetic, metabolic, and pharmacodynamic profile of the drug can be determined. This is relevant for a number of existing antihypertensive drugs; for example, the beta blocker propranolol relies on first-pass hydroxylation after oral administration to achieve its active moiety, but this does not occur after intravenous administration.[44,45] Other antihypertensive drugs are dependent on metabolic activation; for example, moxonidine and a number of ACE inhibitors require hepatic deesterification to yield the active compound.[46] The availability of an intravenous preparation in phase II can facilitate the gathering of useful information on efficacy more quickly by eliminating the considerations of bioavailability of the drug. Furthermore, a formulation suitable for systemic administration allows acute local and systemic administration in mechanistic hemodynamic studies and proof-of-concept studies in phase II and III. Intravenous formulations of drugs are of limited therapeutic potential and are generally not developed with the intention of subsequent clinical use, which might significantly limit the potentially valuable use of such compounds in academic and postmarketing research.

14.2.3 Pharmacokinetic–Pharmacodynamic Relationships

In phase I, it may be possible to identify potential dose–response relationships and evaluate pharmacokinetic–pharmacodynamic (PK–PD) relationships in subjects.[47] The drug may be active over a relatively narrow dose range, as is observed with beta-blockers and thiazide diuretics, or it may have a wider dose range, as is typically found with ACE inhibitors. Analyses of PK–PD relationships might allow early analyses of the potential mechanisms underlying a blood pressure lowering response. For example, the hypotensive effect of ACE inhibitors correlates poorly with reduction of circulating ACE activity[48] but is more closely associated with inhibition of ACE activity within tissues.[49] As such, the hemodynamic effects of an ACE inhibitor may be quite independent of its inhibition of the circulating enzyme, and its calculated circulating plasma half-life may have little bearing on its duration of action.[50] Clinical trials must consider not only the dose–response relationship of the therapeutic effects of the drug but also the relationship between overall exposure to the study drug and the incidence of adverse events; one must consider both the duration of treatment and the dose of drug administered. For example, side effects that are time related may not be apparent during the relatively short duration of most early-phase studies. Furthermore, side effects may occur across a different dose range from the therapeutic effect. For many years, what are now considered to be relatively high doses of thiazide diuretics were used both in clinical practice and in large-scale outcome trials to evaluate their effects on cardiovascular morbidity and mortality. After more than 20 years of clinical experience, it is now clear that the metabolic adverse effects of the thiazide diuretics occur at higher doses than the hypotensive effects, and that higher doses produce more adverse effects without increased antihypertensive efficacy (Figure 14.2).[51–53]

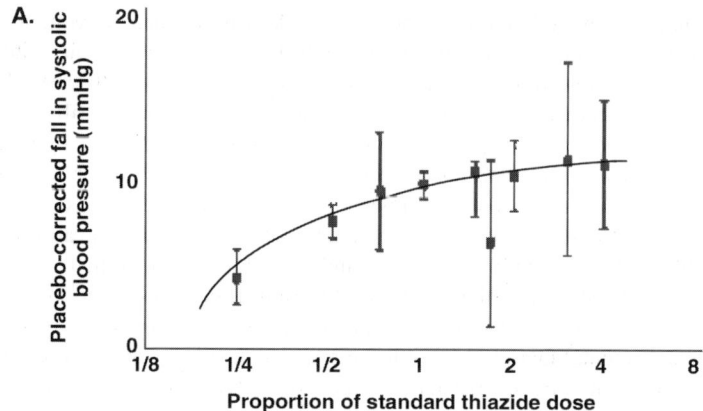

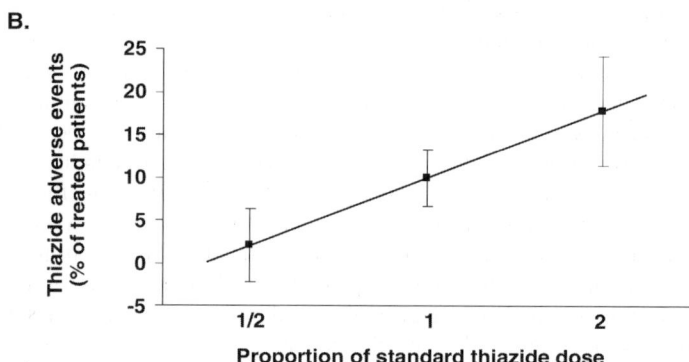

Figure 14.2 Systolic blood pressure lowering and adverse effects associated with thiazide diuretic doses. Data are presented as mean (±95% confidence intervals) placebo-corrected data with reference to the standard treatment dose (e.g., bendroflumethazide 2.5 mg daily or chlorthalidone 25 mg daily). (A) Increasing drug dose beyond standard does not significantly enhance blood pressure reduction. (B) The risk of adverse effects increases linearly with increasing thiazide drug dose. (Adapted from Law, M.R. et al., *Br. Med. J.*, 326, 1427–1435, 2003. With permission.)

14.2.4 Controlled-Release Preparations

Controlled-release formulations of antihypertensive drugs can minimize differences between peak and trough concentrations. This may limit the potential for adverse events and, when the PK–PD relationship is close, allow more predictable and gradual reduction of blood pressure. Many of these formulations result in a pharmacokinetic profile that allows once-daily dosing, which might improve patient compliance in comparison to multiple daily dose requirements. Relative bioavailability and pharmacokinetic studies are often performed early during phase I and late phase II development. A number of existing beta-adrenoceptor blockers, calcium antagonists, thiazide diuretics, ACE inhibitors, and angiotensin receptor antagonists are licensed for use as once-daily preparations. Therefore, the need to develop a once-daily formulation, if possible, is an important consideration in establishing the clinical utility of new antihypertensive drugs.

If a close PK–PD relationship exists for a particular blood pressure lowering agent, regulatory approval for a sustained-release (SR) preparation is often granted on the strength of bioequivalence data alone, between short- and long-acting formulations. Where a linear relationship exists between drug dose and clearance, it is necessary to demonstrate that the maximum plasma concentration

(C_{max}) of the SR preparation is no greater and the minimum plasma concentration (C_{min}) no less than the short-acting equivalent formulation. Whereas drugs with nonlinear elimination kinetics require bioequivalence to be established for a minimum of two doses of the SR preparation reflecting the doses from the lower and upper parts of the anticipated dose range, C_{min} should be no less than and C_{max} and the area under the concentration–time curve no more than those of the shorter-acting preparation. Where no clear PK–PD relationship exists, long-acting formulations require full pharmacokinetic and safety and efficacy characterization.

14.3 PHASE II AND PHASE III STUDIES

Subsequent development of potential antihypertensive drugs is focused on a number of issues that will influence the subsequent study phases, including demonstration of efficacy and safety in appropriate target patient groups, evaluation of pharmacokinetic and pharmacodynamic effects in the setting of renal or hepatic impairment, and interaction with vasoactive and other drugs. Foremost is the early conduct of 'proof of concept' studies to examine blood pressure lowering efficacy in patients with hypertension and, where possible, to establish a dose–response relationship. For blood pressure lowering treatment, "proof of concept" studies are often performed in phase I or early phase II development. The objectives of this type of study are to validate the relevance of preclinical efficacy to humans, to provide early evidence of potential clinical efficacy, and to rapidly eliminate potentially ineffective compounds from further development.

14.3.1 Dose-Ranging Studies

The hypotensive effects should be characterized in placebo-controlled dose-ranging studies. No fixed guidelines exist with regard to the number of doses of drug that should be studied in phases I and II. The optimal dose in clinical practice is the lowest that produces the desired therapeutic effect. Although there will be individual variation in the magnitude of the response to any given drug, it is usually not feasible to investigate more than a comparatively small number of doses. It has been suggested that at least three dose levels should be assessed against placebo during the drug development program.[54] Comparison of only one dose with placebo may allow the null hypothesis to be rejected but will not allow the construction of a dose–response relationship. Although a linear relationship might be demonstrated with two doses of active drug and placebo, it is unlikely that studying only two doses at phase III will be sufficient for registration purposes. Ideally, a dose near the bottom of the response curve, a dose near the top of the curve, a maximal dose, and a supramaximal dose would be studied early in the drug development program. Sufficient doses should be evaluated to allow determination of the early part of the dose–response relationship, as well as a dose near or at the upper end of the dose–response curve or a dose that produces less than the maximum response but beyond which side effects are unacceptable. The FDA has defined the dose producing maximal response to be that at which a two- to threefold increasing dose produces no greater effect.[55] It is not necessary to demonstrate significantly different responses between the doses studied to establish the useful dosing range of the drug, only significant difference from placebo. The objective of the dose-ranging study is to give an indication of the probable dose range in the patient population. Although dose–response data will be available from phase III and phase IV trials, it is prudent to carry out dose-ranging studies early in development (phase I or early phase II) to avoid performing phase III trials using doses that may be widely different from those that will subsequently be recommended for clinical use or the need to revise the dosing schedules of the entire clinical program at phase III or IV after accumulating data relevant to a different dose range. This has been a common problem for antihypertensive drugs in the past (usually an overestimation of the required dose).

14.3.2 Study Design Considerations

14.3.2.1 Parallel Group Design

After entering into human study, dose-ranging trials in hypertension can follow a number of designs, including parallel group, crossover, and titration models. Initial studies are performed with single drug doses, but when sufficient safety data are available multiple dose studies are required. The initial dose for multiple dose studies will be determined by the pharmacokinetic, pharmacodynamic, and safety data generated during the preceding single-dose studies. As with phase I studies, the parallel group design is that most commonly incorporated in phase II and III clinical research.[56] In order to ensure the comparability of subject groups and to avoid investigator bias, studies should be of adequate power, well controlled, randomized, and, ideally, performed double-blind. The range of doses investigated in multiple ascending-dose studies should be as wide as possible, constrained only by predetermined pharmacokinetic safety parameters and performed in a stepwise, dose-escalation manner. This approach can avoid revision of dosing schedules during the later stages of the development program. These studies most commonly use a parallel group design in which subjects are randomized to undergo multiple administrations of fixed doses of active drug.[57] The possible confounding effects of other factors can be minimized by including random allocation to placebo within each group. Furthermore, inclusion of placebo allows the magnitude of the blood pressure lowering response to be more clearly defined at each dose and is particularly important in discriminating smaller differences in effect between doses that lie close to the top of the dose–response curve. Parallel group studies allow information about a range of doses to be gathered over a short period of time but, because for the purpose of analysis each subject receives only one dose of drug, it is difficult to obtain information about individual dose–response relationships. Furthermore, relatively large numbers of subjects may be required to reach statistically significant conclusions. For these reasons, crossover or dose titration designs in which subjects receive more than one drug dose might be preferable.[58]

14.3.2.2 Crossover Study Design

Crossover study design facilitates the collection of dose–response data from all participants. In ascending-dose, multiple-dose crossover studies, all subjects will receive all or some of the treatments in a predetermined ascending dose fashion. Fewer subjects are needed than with the single-dose design. Crossover studies have distinct pharmacological advantages. Both inter- and intrasubject comparisons can be made to reduce the variability of the data. Furthermore, the statistical power of crossover studies is greater than that of parallel group studies. However, crossover studies carry with them certain inherent design difficulties. They are most easily conducted when drug effects develop and stop quickly; carryover effects from treatment are always possible, and the washout period between phases must take account of this to ensure comparability of baseline parameters between phases. Crossover studies depend on a subject's baseline blood pressure remaining constant between phases, although, in the absence of carryover effects, this will usually be the case. Inclusion of a placebo phase is essential to determine whether side effects are drug related in these early-phase studies. Crossover studies are often of relatively long duration and may be complicated by subjects dropping out, for one reason or another, before the study is complete (although all data generated by defaulters can be included in the analysis in so far as they are statistically appropriate). When such defaulters have to be replaced, it can markedly impede progress with the study. If a subject in a "first-into-humans" study experiences a clinically significant adverse event, it may become necessary to postpone completion of the study. It may be decided to abandon further investigation of the drug in humans or to investigate the effects of a lower dose on a larger number of subjects before proceeding to higher doses. Finally, the number of phases in a crossover study may be limited by the total blood loss or by the volunteers' total exposure to the study drug. Both parallel group and crossover study designs can be expanded by studying larger numbers of subjects at the maximum tolerated dose.

14.3.2.3 Dose Titration

The investigation of new antihypertensive drugs often involves a period of dose titration or escalation, with doses being increased at predetermined intervals until fixed efficacy endpoints are reached. In phase II studies, this study design can be used to study blood pressure reduction in patients with hypertension. It combines the advantages of exposing subjects to only low doses initially, but at the same time allows dose escalation to a level that is associated with a predetermined endpoint so dose–response information is obtained from all participants. Titration design involves exposing subjects to a sequence of increasing doses limited by response or adverse events and, in this manner, more closely resembles the clinical implementation of antihypertensive treatment. A significant limitation of this design, however, is difficulty in distinguishing adverse events associated with high doses from delayed effects. Time-dependent effects of antihypertensive treatment can be important because, for example, the blood pressure lowering effect of propranolol develops only slowly.[44] Administration is initially associated with a reduction in cardiac output and heart rate, but with prolonged treatment a gradual fall in peripheral resistance and blood pressure occurs. This can lead to overestimation of the dose of drug needed, so it is important that early-phase multiple-dose studies are of sufficient duration to achieve steady-state pharmacodynamic effects at each dose. Similarly, the effective dose of a drug may be overestimated because nonresponders are included in the study population. Studies of antihypertensive drugs are particularly prone to errors of this kind, because patients often have a spontaneous fall in blood pressure during research studies. This was well illustrated in the Medical Research Council trial for mild to moderate hypertension, where substantial reductions in blood pressure were observed during the first 3 months of placebo treatment.[9] The same phenomenon was also observed in early studies of captopril and probably contributed to dose-related toxicity. Indeed, these drugs were almost withdrawn from investigation before reaching clinical practice because of their side effects at high doses.[59] Studies of a similar design led to inappropriately high doses of both atenolol and chlorthalidone being employed for many years in clinical practice. Another confounding factor associated with titration study design is that the dose–response relationship is often spuriously flattened because poor responders make up a substantial proportion of subjects receiving the highest dose of any given drug;[59] therefore, the maximal drug effect and dose–response relationship are negatively skewed. The corollary to this is the situation where drugs cause greater effects after administration of the first dose, rather than subsequent doses — for example, ACE inhibitors and alpha-adrenoceptor blocking drugs.

Titration studies are most successful when the duration of the drug effect and the number of withdrawals is small. In this situation, they can provide a reasonable indication of the dose–response relationship, which can be evaluated further in subsequent studies. They offer the distinct advantage that fewer subjects are needed than in parallel group designs and are generally of shorter duration than crossover studies. As with crossover study design, data from subjects who are withdrawn before completing titration can be included in the formal data analysis.

14.3.2.4 PK–PD Analyses

As with earlier phase I data, detailed PK and PD analyses are extremely important. An all-or-nothing dose–response relationship might indicate that supramaximal doses of drug are being studied and suggest that lower doses should be included in the range. This phenomenon was originally observed with hydralazine[60] and explains the lack of relationship between hypotensive responses and doses of beta-adrenoceptor antagonist used in many studies.[61] The doses of many antihypertensive drugs commonly employed in clinical practice are much lower than in earlier years. Generally, antihypertensive drugs have been launched at doses that have subsequently been found to be too high. This may have arisen by conducting studies that were of insufficient duration to allow the full antihypertensive effect of the drug to develop or unnecessarily high doses have been selected on the basis of forced titration studies. The dose, timing, and frequency of administration and duration of treatment will be determined on the basis of preclinical data, pharmacokinetic variables obtained from phase I and II studies, and the need to observe the duration of response in multiple-dose studies. The latter is particularly important to address possible rapid development of tolerance to the pharmacodynamic effects of the drug, so-called tachyphylaxis, which is a recognized characteristic of a number of vasoactive drugs, such as nitrates.

14.3.3 Cardiovascular Outcome Measurements

Although a close relationship between blood pressure and cardiovascular risk has been identified across populations, global cardiovascular risk is determined by a number of factors that may be influenced to a different extent by different antihypertensive treatments. Although the benefits of existing antihypertensive treatments appear to be conferred primarily by blood pressure lowering, this is a highly contentious topic and subject to extensive ongoing research. Many current antihypertensive drugs achieved licensing approval on the basis of blood pressure lowering efficacy, alongside evidence of safety and tolerability. Current requirements for phase III safety evaluations of drugs for chronic use suggest that at least 1500 patients should have been exposed to the investigational drug, including 300 to 600 exposed continuously for at least 6 months and 100 or more exposed to continuous treatment for at least 1 year.[62] Larger numbers of patients than this are recommended, in view of the very asymptomatic nature of the disease and prolonged duration of hypertension treatment that is required. The aim of phase III research is to further characterize the efficacy and safety of the compound, with particular interest in cardiovascular morbidity and mortality. The study design should typically incorporate an active comparator treatment, often a thiazide diuretic, and requires predefined outcome measures that reflect cardiovascular risk — for example, the incidence of stroke, heart failure, ischemic heart disease, hospitalization due to cardiovascular disease, cardiovascular mortality, total mortality, and composite cardiovascular endpoints. As in earlier development, the study population should reflect the demographic characteristics of the target population and be sufficiently large as to allow examination of the effects in important patient subgroups. The available data on cardiovascular morbidity and mortality obtained in phase III studies is carefully considered by licensing authorities, alongside preclinical data and results from phase I and II studies. A novel antihypertensive drug is only considered acceptable if there is no suggestion from phase III studies of a potentially detrimental effect on cardiovascular risk factors or clinical outcomes.

14.3.4 Placebo or Active Comparator?

In order to establish the efficacy of any novel antihypertensive drug, studies using both active and placebo comparator drugs are usually required.[62] This might raise potential concerns regarding the safety of withdrawing or withholding active treatment from patients with established hypertension; however, a recent metaanalysis of small short-term studies of placebo treatment involving 6409 patients with hypertension found that short-term discontinuation of antihypertensive treatment does not pose a significant risk.[63] The risks of placebo treatment in longer term studies are recognized and should be avoided. In these situations, patients may usefully be included as part of a factorial trial, receiving the study drug and an established therapy.[64] The reference drug in factorial trials should always be selected with respect to efficacy (superior to others) and safety (largest amount of clinical data available). Often, in trials of antihypertensive drugs, the reference drug is a thiazide diuretic and, given that nondiuretic antihypertensive agents are likely to be coadministered with diuretics in clinical practice, the interaction with thiazides should be considered at an early stage

Table 14.1 Classification of Untreated Adult Blood Pressure

Category	Systolic Blood Pressure (mmHg)	Diastolic Blood Pressure (mmHg)
Optimal	<120	<80
Prehypertension	120–139	80–89
Hypertension:[a]		
Stage 1	140–159	90–99
Stage 2	160	100

[a] Based on the average of two or more readings taken at each of two or more visits after initial screening.

Source: Adapted from the Seventh Report of the Joint National Committee on Detection, Evaluation, and Treatment of High Blood Pressure.[16]

in the drug development program. The use of a reference drug can be particularly important in estimating the frequency of adverse effects in clinical trials. Many common symptoms, such as headache, lethargy, and cough, can occur with placebo as well as with drugs of different classes. For example, in patients discontinuing ACE inhibitor treatment due to cough, angiotensin receptor blocker treatment is associated with cough in around one third of patients but occurs in around three quarters of patients in whom ACE inhibitor treatment is reintroduced. The incidence of cough associated with the angiotensin receptor blocker is similar to that due to hydrochlorothiazide and substantially lower than that associated with reexposure to ACE inhibitor but is still not negligible.[65] The inclusion of hydrochlorothiazide as a comparator in this study suggests that cough associated with angiotensin receptor blockade is nonspecific. It can also be useful to include a reference drug of the same class as the trial drug to compare their antihypertensive effects; the inclusion of such a reference drug offers a measure of assay sensitivity in clinical studies, allowing the distinction to be made between an ineffective drug and an ineffective (i.e., null hypothesis) study. Another strategy is to perform placebo-controlled, randomized withdrawals from both arms of a study comparing the new drug to the standard agent from the same class; this is particularly useful in studies of patients with severe hypertension.

14.3.5 Statistical Considerations in Hemodynamic Studies

In early-phase studies, the number of subjects should be chosen on the basis of power calculations so sufficient numbers of subjects are included to allow a statistically meaningful conclusion to be drawn from the results. Analysis of crossover study design should exclude possible carryover effects, and analysis of titration trials should take into account that not all subjects may have received the higher dosages. Specific maneuvers can increase the power of early phase studies; for example, salt depletion increases the likelihood of a hemodynamics response, and ambulatory blood pressure monitoring avoids observer bias and might decrease measurement variability.

14.3.6 Appropriate Selection of Subjects

The chosen study population should reflect the etiology and type of hypertension for which the drug is intended. Generally, studies for early evaluation of safety and efficacy of potential antihypertensive drugs are conducted in patients with mild to moderate essential hypertension in whom both systolic and diastolic blood pressure are elevated. Before participation in studies, hypertensive patients should be adequately characterized according to the severity of their hypertension (Table 14.1) and the presence or absence of left ventricular hypertrophy. Assessment of the grade of

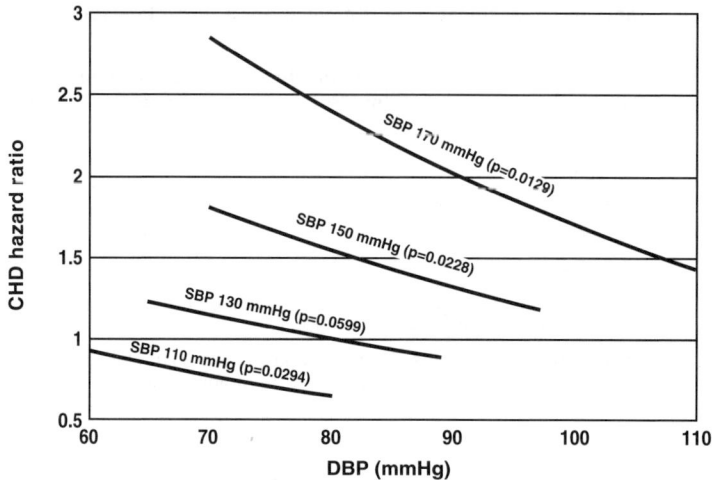

Figure 14.3 The impact of systolic and diastolic blood pressure on coronary heart disease risk based on the Framingham cohort. Coronary heart disease risk increases with increasing systolic blood pressure. At any given systolic pressure, falling diastolic blood pressure (and hence widened pulse pressure) are associated with increased risk. (From Franklin, S.S. et al., *Circulation*, 100, 354–360, 1991. With permission.)

hypertension is of particular importance so subjects recruited to studies incorporating a parallel group design will have greater comparability between groups. While the majority of patients studied are likely to have mild-to-moderate hypertension, a number of patients with severe hypertension should also be studied. There is no specific guidance as to the numbers required to be studied, but these should probably be in proportion to the anticipated prevalence of severe hypertension in the target population. In some cases, the safety, pharmacokinetic variables, and pharmacodynamic responses to treatment might be better addressed by conducting a dedicated study in patients with severe or accelerated hypertension.

14.3.6.1 Special Patient Groups

Patients with secondary causes of hypertension should be excluded from studies or studied as a separate subgroup, because the underlying mechanisms are often different from those in essential hypertension and might attenuate or exaggerate the responses to a novel hypotensive drug. It would seem reasonable to specifically exclude a secondary cause of high blood pressure in young patients (<30 years), those whose blood pressure remains uncontrolled on two drugs, and those with accelerated hypertension or hypertension of sudden onset.

Isolated systolic hypertension has emerged as a major risk factor for cardiovascular events, particularly stroke, and is characterized by elevated systolic blood pressure but normal diastolic blood pressure. Recent evidence indicates that systolic blood pressure and pulse pressure might be more important risk predictors than diastolic blood pressure alone (Figure 14.3).[66] Early studies in patients with hypertension focused heavily on diastolic blood pressure reduction and showed unequivocal benefits of blood pressure lowering treatment; however, it is likely that the systolic blood pressure response to treatment was greater than that of diastolic blood pressure, so treatment could be expected to have lowered pulse pressure. Historically, the progressive increase in systolic blood pressure and consequent widening of pulse pressure were thought to be normal phenomena associated with aging; however, two large randomized placebo-controlled studies in elderly patients with isolated systolic hypertension have provided unequivocal evidence that lowering systolic blood pressure causes a significant reduction in cardiovascular morbidity and mortality.[67,68] Isolated systolic hypertension is believed to be a manifestation of increased large arterial stiffening due to a combination of structural and functional large vessel abnormalities.[69] In view of the proposed differences in underlying etiology and the likelihood that this group may form a substantial proportion of the ultimate target population, patients with isolated systolic hypertension require investigation in a dedicated study.

Hypertension and diabetes mellitus often coexist, and both cause an important and synergistic increase in cardiovascular risk. Early drug development should address the efficacy and safety of novel antihypertensive treatment in subgroups of patients with coexistent diabetes. This would ideally involve examining the potential effects of the study compound on insulin resistance or its impact on the effectiveness of insulin or oral antihyperglycemic agents. Additionally, the effects of the study compound on triglyceride and total and low-density lipoprotein (LDL) cholesterol concentrations should be evaluated, as the effects of elevated lipid concentrations contribute more to overall cardiovascular risk in patients with diabetes than nondiabetic individuals.

The efficacy of novel antihypertensive agents should be evaluated in patients with chronic renal impairment. This group is characterized by severe hypertension and often requires treatment with multiple antihypertensive agents to gain adequate blood pressure control. In patients with impaired renal blood flow, ACE inhibitors and angiotensin receptor antagonists can precipitate acute renal impairment; therefore, the risk of treatment of this group of patients may be increased depending on the proposed mechanism of action of the novel compound. Renal impairment may have a significant influence on pharmacokinetic variables, depending on the extent to which the drug is cleared by renal excretion; therefore, dosage or frequency of administration might require adjustment in this context. Special consideration should be given to patients with chronic renal failure who require continuous ambulatory peritoneal dialysis or hemodialysis in order to determine the extent to which either treatment is capable of clearing the study compound from the systemic circulation.

Consideration should be given to investigating the effects of any novel antihypertensive agent in other special subgroups depending on the target patient population. Specifically, the treatment of hypertension in pregnancy should be considered from the perspective of effectiveness and safety. Teratogenicity or genotoxicity in preclinical studies might preclude further development of the drug for use in women of child-bearing potential.

14.3.6.2 Gender

Conducting phase I studies of candidate antihypertensive drugs with male subjects is associated with a number of potential advantages. Studies of antihypertensive drugs in premenopausal women can be complicated by changes in pharmacokinetics and pharmacodynamics associated with the menstrual cycle, a complication avoided entirely by enrollment of only male subjects. Furthermore, studying only male subjects in phase I development avoids concerns regarding the potential for teratogenicity, which is unlikely to have been established until the viability for further drug development has been demonstrated in early clinical safety studies.

Men and women exhibit significant differences in pharmacokinetic and pharmacodynamic responses;[70–72] therefore, exclusion of women from early phases of clinical research is an important design weakness,[73,74] and such variation might be detected only in later stages of drug development. Women constitute a large proportion of the target population for new antihypertensive agents, although the most significant increase in cardiovascular risk occurs after the menopause. Drug absorption, metabolism, and excretion in women are all influenced by the menstrual cycle, pregnancy, and menopause.[75] For example, propranolol is metabolized more slowly in women than men, possibly because estrogens are capable of influencing hepatic metabolism of the drug.[75] Similarly, side effects may differ between men and women; for example, cough is a significantly more frequent complication of angiotensin-converting enzyme inhibitor treatment in women,[76] a finding that became apparent only in wider therapeutic use several years after license approval and which might have been detected earlier if more women had been included in phase I and II clinical trials. Overall, observations in male subjects may not be directly relevant to women, and the clinical utility of treatments only studied in men has been questioned.[77] It is essential, therefore, that women be included in early phase II and III studies, and both genders should be enrolled in a balanced way. This view is endorsed by the Food and Drug Administration, the National Institutes of Health, and the Institute of Medicine.[78,79]

14.3.6.3 Age

Most phase I studies will have recruited healthy young subjects, typically 18 to 40 years old, to minimize the effects of comorbid disease on safety and pharmacokinetic evaluation. Hypertension, though, is predominantly a disease of older adults, and the associated cardiovascular risks increase substantially with advancing age, particularly the risk of stroke.[80-84] The proportion of elderly people in developed nations is rapidly rising,[85] and this is likely to be accompanied by an increasing prevalence of hypertension. The need to reduce cardiovascular morbidity and mortality associated with hypertension has increased the focus on elderly patients as a high-risk group likely to derive greater benefit from adequate blood pressure control than younger patients. Elderly patients are likely to form a significant proportion of patients who will ultimately receive treatment with the novel antihypertensive agent. With this in mind, it is crucial to include patients who are >60 years old and preferably also those ages 70 to 90 years in phase II and III studies at an early stage, either by way of age-stratified forced randomization or by performing dedicated subgroup studies. It is essential to characterize the safety profile, pharmacokinetics, and dose–response relationship in elderly patients, and the numbers studied should be sufficiently high to reflect the proportion of elderly patients in the target population. This is particularly important because the pathophysiological changes that accompany advancing age are known to influence pharmacokinetic and pharmacodynamic responses in a nonuniform manner.[86-88] There is international consensus that the influence of age on responses to antihypertensive compounds should be studied extensively in elderly subjects and that they should be enrolled early in the process of drug development, even as early as phase I studies.[89,90]

14.3.6.4 Race

Race may have an important influence on drug efficacy and metabolism[91] which has led to important differences in the response to a number of existing antihypertensive agents. For example, beta-adrenoceptor antagonists and ACE inhibitors have been found to be less effective in people of Afro–Caribbean race, whereas the response to thiazide diuretics is comparatively greater in this group.[92-95] Drug acetylation is subject to genetic polymorphism. "Rapid" and "slow" acetylator phenotypes are determined by Mendelian inheritance of an autosomal recessive gene and exert a significant influence on the metabolism of a number of drugs, including hydralazine. The proportion of rapid acetylators varies between populations, reflecting the genetic basis, and is present in around 40% of the U.K. population, 95% of Eskimos, and 10% of Japanese. Other more subtle forms of genetic polymorphism appear to cause differences in the response to drugs between races. For example, it is generally accepted that in many therapeutic areas, the Japanese require smaller doses of medication than Western counterparts.[56] Overall, it appears that ethnic variations influence drug kinetics and response to a lesser extent than interindividual variation in general;[56] however, it is important to exercise care in extrapolating clinical trial findings between racial groups,[91] and phase

II and III studies should aim to include subjects from a variety of ethnic backgrounds so as to reflect the anticipated target population.

14.3.7 Important Confounders in Hemodynamic Studies

14.3.7.1 Concomitant Medications

A number of over-the-counter preparations (e.g., sympathomimetics found in cough and decongestant preparations) are capable of causing increased systemic blood pressure.[96] Additionally, non-steroidal antiinflammatory drugs cause salt and water retention[97] and block prostaglandin production. They are capable of increasing baseline blood pressure and attenuate the blood pressure lowering effect of diuretics and ACE inhibitors. Nonsteroidal antiinflammatory preparations should be avoided for at least 2 weeks before study participation and for the duration of studies of antihypertensive drugs. Paracetamol does not cause any recognized hemodynamic effects and, if required for analgesia and allowed by the study protocol, might not be expected to have a significant confounding effect. Acute administration of vitamin C has been shown to reduce blood pressure in patients with established hypertension;[98] therefore, the use of vitamin supplementation prior to and during studies of antihypertensive compounds should be avoided.

Caffeine can produce an acute pressor effect,[99] and its abrupt withdrawal is associated with increased frequency of headache, anxiety, and irritability.[100,101] No consensus has been reached regarding caffeine intake in studies of antihypertensive medication, but abstinence for 24 hours before study participation and for the duration of the study might be a reasonable precaution.

Excessive alcohol consumption is associated with a pressor effect in both normotensive[102,103] and hypertensive subjects.[104] Alcohol withdrawal, too, is associated with a pressor response[105] and may be associated with disruptive behavior during the in-house phase of clinical trials. Importantly, regular alcohol consumption is capable of inducing mixed-function oxidase and might cause important pharmacokinetic interactions with the study compound. Subjects should be carefully screened so those who regularly consume alcohol to excess (typically 21 and 14 units per week for men and women, respectively) are excluded from early-phase studies. In general, alcohol should be avoided for at least 48 hours before study participation and for the duration of the study.

Smoking has an acute hypertensive effect, mediated, at least in part, by increased levels of circulating catecholamines,[106] which may have a confounding effect in studies of drugs acting through the adrenergic system. Additionally, variability in ambulatory blood pressure measurements is greater among smokers, and this is increased further by smoking cessation.[107] To minimize this effect, heavy smokers should probably be excluded from phase I and early phase II studies. Self-reporting of smoking habits is generally accurate,[108] but formal measurement of plasma or salivary cotinine concentrations provides a sensitive and specific test that can be used at screening to corroborate the subject smoking history.[109,110] Illicit smoking during studies can be confirmed using inexpensive and simple methods, for example, the Smokelyzer® (Bedfont Technical Instruments, Upchurch, Kent, England) measures the carbon monoxide concentration of expired air.

Illicit drug use has a number of important implications in studies involving hemodynamically active agents. These may arise as a result of the pharmacological effects of the drug (e.g., the pressor effects of cocaine and amphetamine derivatives) or may be due to the hemodynamic effects of withdrawal (e.g., tachycardia and hypertension caused by opiate discontinuation). Marijuana lowers blood pressure and impairs cerebral autoregulation, which may increase the risks of postural hypotension;[111] furthermore, acute marijuana use causes increased heart rate and impairs psychomotor performance for up to 24 hours.[112] Anabolic steroids are associated with increased systemic blood pressure and cause hypokalemic metabolic alkalosis. Subjects should be examined for evidence of illicit drug use at screening and, in some instances, during predose assessment and at random time points during in-house and nonresident study phases.

14.3.7.2 Diet

Diet plays an important role in modifying the pharmacokinetics of many compounds and should be highly standardized in early-phase clinical studies. Gastric absorption is generally favored by an empty stomach, but the absorption of highly lipophilic drugs is aided by a fatty meal. Food has little effect on the absorption and bioavailability of captopril[113,114] or enalapril,[115] but the bioavailability of atenolol is reduced by about 20%.[116] However, food increases the bioavailability of propranolol and metoprolol by 30 to 80%[116,117] and labetalol by 40%[118] by altering the extent of first-pass metabolism. First-pass metabolism of felodipine and other dihydropyridine calcium antagonists is inhibited by grapefruit juice,[119] an effect that may be relevant to trial design because study medication is often consumed at breakfast time. Dietary salt intake is of particular importance when considering the design of studies involving novel antihypertensive agents. Salt depletion activates the renin–angiotensin system and may sensitize subjects to the hypotensive effects of renin inhibitors, ACE inhibitors, and angiotensin receptor antagonists.[120–122] Indeed, salt depletion may be a valuable strategy to maximize the pharmacodynamic effects of such drugs in healthy subjects[120] in whom the effects of antihypertensive drugs are normally small. By increasing the magnitude of the hypotensive response, salt depletion can increase the power of a study to detect an effect of treatment. Conversely, subjects on high salt diets will have a reduced response to these drugs but may be more sensitive to the effects of diuretics. The effect of food on drug bioavailability and bioequivalence is often studied using a single-dose, two-period, two-treatment study design; more detailed guidance on the regulatory requirements of food interaction studies is available from the FDA.[123]

14.3.8 Assessment of Efficacy: Blood Pressure Reduction

The goal of treating hypertension is to reduce cardiovascular morbidity and mortality attributable to high blood pressure. A number of large morbidity and mortality studies have demonstrated significant benefits associated with blood pressure reduction in response to a number of antihypertensive drugs, including thiazide diuretics, beta-blockers, calcium channel blockers, and ACE inhibitors. Blood pressure lowering has usually been accepted as a valid surrogate endpoint for reduction of cardiovascular morbidity and mortality. Despite this, demonstration of effective blood pressure lowering in proof-of-concept studies and dose-ranging studies alone provides a comparatively simplistic primary endpoint for antihypertensive efficacy. The difficulties arising from reliance on surrogate endpoint markers are discussed in detail elsewhere.[124,125] Even if a definite blood pressure lowering effect is proven in phase II and III studies, a new antihypertensive agent might be considered acceptable by the regulatory authorities only if there is no suspicion of a detrimental effect on cardiovascular morbidity and mortality. If evidence of a potentially deleterious effect emerges from preclinical or clinical data (e.g., unfavorable changes in lipid profile), this will require detailed characterization by means of additional laboratory or clinical studies.

14.3.8.1 Blood Pressure Measurement

Measurement of blood pressure represents the minimum investigation necessary to characterize the hemodynamic effects of new antihypertensive drugs. Although supine or sitting blood pressures are acceptable as evidence of efficacy,[55] postural effects should be characterized by erect and supine measurements as evidence of safety. The mercury sphygmomanometer is the gold standard measurement technique. If unavailable, alternative devices must be calibrated in proportion to a reference mercury sphygmomanometer. Blood pressure measurement techniques should be in accordance with current recommendations, such that both systolic and diastolic pressure are recorded using Korotkov phase I and V, respectively, and measurements determined to the closest 2 mmHg. While it is acknowledged that phase IV more closely resembles invasive diastolic pressure measurements, phase

V (disappearance of sound) is more reproducible. Two or more readings, separated by at least 2 minutes, should be obtained.

Automated devices are gaining increasing popularity because they minimize observer bias and may reduce the tendency for a "white-coat effect" that may occur with repeated measurements. If an automated device is incorporated in clinical studies, this should be validated according to recognized criteria as specified in current guidelines — for example, the European Society of Hypertension international protocol for validation of blood pressure-measuring devices in adults.[126] Consideration should be given to special circumstances in which the validity of automated and semiautomated devices is less robust, such as during exercise or in the setting of atrial fibrillation or other arrhythmia. The same device should be used for all subjects in any given study and preferably between studies so data are directly comparable. It is particularly important that automated blood pressure measurement devices are used in accordance with the manufacturer's recommendations and that these are calibrated as appropriate.

Direct measurement of intraarterial blood pressure has been used in a number of phase II studies. This technique allows accurate determination of true blood pressure and has been used to investigate dose–response relationships, 24-hour efficacy, and hemodynamic changes during physical exercise; however, the invasive nature of the technique increases potential risks to study subjects. Furthermore, interpretation of the results might be difficult because intraarterial blood pressure measurements are not undertaken in routine clinical practice, and prognosis has characteristically been determined from sphygmomanometer measurements.

14.3.8.2 Ambulatory Blood Pressure Measurement

Twenty-four-hour ambulatory blood pressure monitoring is increasingly being recognized as an important research tool.[127] It eliminates observer bias during blood pressure measurements and avoids the potential for the "white-coat effect."[128] Twenty-four-hour ambulatory blood pressure recordings performed every 30 minutes correspond closely with simultaneous intraarterial recordings[129] and are highly reproducible.[130] An added advantage of this technique is that no placebo response is observed in clinical trials;[131,132] therefore, ambulatory blood pressure monitoring might simplify the conduct of trials of antihypertensive drugs by negating the need for a placebo group.[133] It has been suggested that ambulatory blood pressure monitoring offers a precision that allows valid conclusions to be drawn using smaller numbers of subjects than might be required in trials using manual blood pressure measurement,[131,134] and the routine use of ambulatory blood pressure recording in clinical trials of antihypertensive drugs has been strongly advocated.[135] However, this remains controversial, and some studies have found that this technique may not necessarily economize on cohort size.[136] The role of 24-hour ambulatory monitoring has become increasingly established in routine clinical practice, and it is able to distinguish patients with sustained hypertension from those with transient high recordings. The effects of antihypertensive treatment on the 24-hour blood pressure profile are likely to become more readily applicable to patient treatment.

Although the time course of the dose–response relationship can be examined using ambulatory blood pressure monitoring equipment, current guidelines urge cautious interpretation of blood pressure measurements recorded by ambulatory monitoring.[19] An important aspect of antihypertensive drug efficacy is the trough-to-peak response ratio, which is calculated as the percentage of the maximum decrease in blood pressure detectable at the end of the dose interval.[137] The FDA has adopted the trough-to-peak ratio as an important criterion in the evaluation of new antihypertensive drugs,[55] and, ideally, new antihypertensive agents or formulations should have a trough-to-peak ratio of at least 50 to 60%. This stipulation aims to improve the safety of new antihypertensive drugs by ensuring that drug-induced blood pressure fluctuations are minimized and the risks of symptomatic hypotension are reduced. This variable provides additional information to allow the most appropriate dosing interval to be selected so as to allow predictable control of blood pressure between doses. Ambulatory blood pressure monitoring might be a particularly useful method for determining trough-to-peak pharmacodynamic responses to antihypertensive agents. A potential limitation of this technique is underestimation of blood pressure in comparison to conventional measurements by sphygmomanometry. This is estimated to be around 12 and 7 mmHg for systolic and diastolic pressures, respectively; however, the extent to which ambulatory and conventional office measurements differ is thought to vary significantly between individuals.[19] In phase II and III studies, this effect can be minimized by incorporating a crossover or titration design, rather than parallel group design, whereby the ambulatory blood pressure responses can be compared between doses within the same individuals.

14.3.8.3 Systemic Hemodynamic Responses

It is important that early-phase studies are designed to yield maximum information about the systemic hemodynamic responses to novel antihypertensive compounds and confirmation of the mechanisms underlying the blood pressure reduction. This can be achieved, at least in part, by observing the effect of the study drug on cardiac output, systemic vascular resistance, and vascular resistance within a localized vascular bed. Accurate determination of cardiac output involves invasive vascular procedures that allow detailed assessment of the effect of the study drug on these variables. Such methods, however, are technically demanding, time consuming, and associated with potential hazards to subjects in view of their invasive nature. Development and validation of a number of comparatively noninvasive techniques has allowed additional hemodynamics measurements to be incorporated into the design of phase II and III studies more readily;[39,138–140] for example, transthoracic bioimpedance is a validated technique that allows cardiac output to be estimated quickly, reliably, and noninvasively.[140] Transthoracic bioimpedance measurements allow effective assessment of drug-induced changes in cardiac output from baseline, and the responses can be compared between drug doses and placebo. Furthermore, cardiac index can be calculated to allow standardization of measurements between subjects. Simultaneous measurement of blood pressure allows systemic vascular resistance to be derived:

$$\text{Cardiac index} = \text{Cardiac output} \div \text{body mass index}$$
$$\text{Systemic vascular resistance index} = \text{Mean arterial pressure} \div \text{cardiac index}$$

14.3.8.4 Large Arterial Compliance

The arterial pulse waveform is a composite of the primary waveform propagated from the proximal large arteries and reflected waveforms from the peripheral arterial tree. Both the morphological characteristics of the arterial pressure waveform and the velocity of arterial waveform conduction are dependent on large arterial compliance. Loss of normal large arterial compliance, so-called *large arterial stiffening*, is a characteristic pathological finding in patients exposed to any one of a number of major cardiovascular risk factors.[69] Large arterial stiffening is associated with a number of important hemodynamic consequences, including raised central systolic blood pressure and reduced central diastolic blood pressure. Large arterial stiffening is a mechanism believed to contribute to risk in the setting of cardiovascular risk factors and makes an important contribution to the development of isolated systolic hypertension.[141] Furthermore, certain agents (e.g., caffeine) have a more profound effect on central blood pressure than peripheral blood pressure by influencing functional large arterial compliance.[142] The effects of antihypertensive agents, therefore, may be underestimated by measurement of brachial artery pressure alone (Figure 14.4). Pulse waveform analysis provides a reliable noninvasive measure of large arterial stiffness and central blood pressure and may be a more sensitive indicator of hemodynamic responses to novel antihypertensive compounds. The prognostic value of pulse waveform analysis has recently been established in patients with end-stage renal failure.[143] The prognostic value of large arterial stiffness is currently being

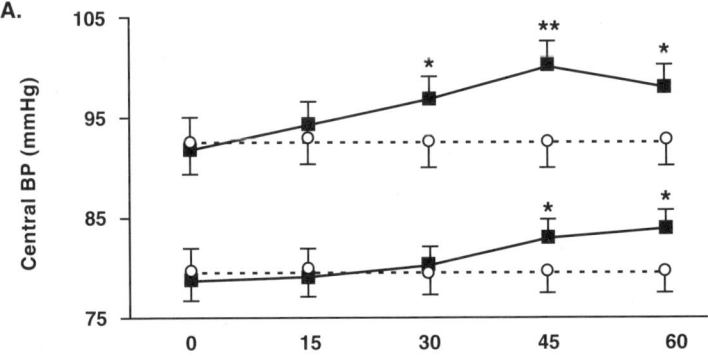

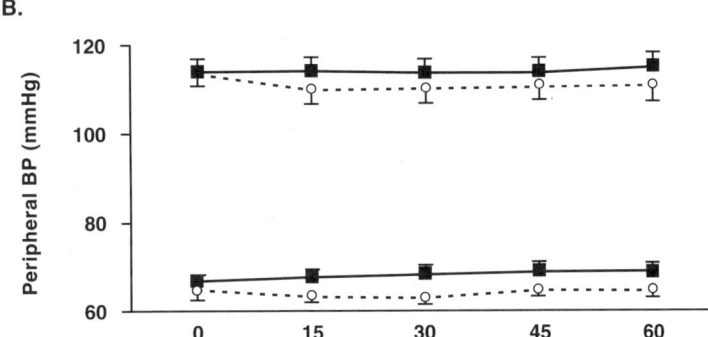

Figure 14.4 Effects of acute caffeine administration on central and peripheral blood pressure. Central blood pressure was measured using pulse-wave analysis, and peripheral blood pressure was measured at the brachial artery 0, 15, 30, 45, and 60 min after oral administration of 300 mg caffeine (■) or matching placebo (O) in healthy subjects. (A) Effects on central blood pressure. (B) Effects on peripheral blood pressure. Data are shown as mean ± SEM; $^*p < 0.05$ and $^{**}p < 0.01$ vs. placebo. (Adapted from Waring, W.S. et al., *Am. J. Hypertens.*, 16, 919–924, 2003. With permission.)

assessed in a number of large clinical trials involving patients with hypertension, diabetes, and hypercholesterolemia. Measurement of pulse waveform analysis may contribute to our understanding of the long-term consequences of large arterial stiffening in patients with hypertension and the potential impact of antihypertensive therapy.[144]

14.3.9 Assessment of Efficacy: Surrogate Risk Markers

14.3.9.1 Endothelial Function

The endothelium is a monocellular layer of tissue situated on the inner aspect of the blood vessels that provides a nonthrombogenic interface between the circulation and structural elements of the cardiovascular system.[145] The endothelium serves to maintain the structural integrity of blood vessels. In addition to its structural role, the endothelium plays a pivotal role in regulating cardiovascular function through the liberation of a number of factors that influence underlying vascular tone, thrombogenesis, and platelet adhesion.[146] For example, endothelium-derived nitric oxide is formed by the action of nitric oxide synthase and causes smooth muscle relaxation and vasodilatation, inhibits platelet aggregation and myointimal hyperplasia, and reduces local vascular inflamma-tion.[146,147] Endothelial function can be determined by examining the vasodilator responses to endot-helium-mediated, nitric-oxide-dependent mediators (e.g., acetylcholine).[138] Loss of normal endothe-lium-dependent blood flow responses, so-called *endothelial dysfunction*, is thought to be an important early step in the development of atherosclerosis. Animal models have shown that pharmacological inhibition of nitric oxide synthase by L-arginine analogs, such as L-NMMA, causes accelerated development of atherosclerosis, whereas administration of L-arginine to enhance local nitric oxide bioavailability retards the development and progression of atherosclerosis.[148]

Endothelial dysfunction is a characteristic finding in the presence of any one of a number of major cardiovascular risk factors, including hypertension, diabetes mellitus, hypercholesterolemia, and regular smoking.[149,150] Recent studies have shown that endothelial dysfunction is an independent predictor of increased cardiovascular risk in patients with hypertension and established atheroscle-rotic disease.[151–153] Moreover, treatments proven effective in reducing cardiovascular risk have been shown to allow restoration of endothelial function — for example, blood pressure lowering in patients with hypertension and cholesterol lowering in patients with hypercholesteremia.[154,155] For this reason, endothelial function has become increasingly established as a surrogate marker of future cardiovascular risk and might provide useful insight into the potential impact of risk factor inter-ventions on long-term outcomes.

Several techniques are available that allow assessment of endothelial function by utilizing localized administration of endothelium-dependent and endothelium-independent, nitric-oxide-mediated vasodilators. These involve localized administration of vasoactive drugs to isolated veins, arteries, or resistance vascular beds and are comparatively safe because the locally administered doses are significantly less than those required to achieve systemic responses (typically 0.1 to 1.0% of systemic dose). An attractive feature of localized drug administration is that systemic concen-trations are usually negligible, thereby avoiding the potential confounding effects that might oth-erwise be mediated through other organs or neurohumoral activation. These techniques can allow *in vivo* proof of concept with regard to mechanisms of action suggested by preclinical experiments and can replace or at least complement the use of animal models.

Changes in dorsal hand vein size can be measured by the Aellig technique. In healthy subjects under resting conditions, hand veins have no endogenous tone and can be used to assess the effects of novel vasoactive drugs on venous capacitance *in vivo*.[156,157] Furthermore, dorsal hand veins can be preconstricted in a controlled manner by local administration of norepinephrine, thus allowing the effects of vasodilator agents to be examined.[158,159] The hand vein can be excluded from the systemic circulation by proximal occlusion, thereby minimizing the potential risks associated with systemic drug exposure.

Beyond examining isolated blood vessels, venous occlusion plethysmography allows potential drug effects to be examined in an isolated vascular bed. The effects of intrabrachial drug infusion can be studied in the isolated forearm vascular bed, which is primarily representative of the effects on resistance vessels *in vivo*. This technique is highly reproducible[160] and has been used extensively as a cardiovascular research tool. Significantly lower amounts of drug are administered than required for comparable systemic concentrations to be achieved, so the technique avoids con-founding systemic effects and allows blood flow in the noninfused limb to serve as a contempo-raneous control.[138] The forearm vessels have intrinsic tone under resting conditions, so the effects of both vasodilators and vasoconstrictors can be assessed and blood flow responses observed in the forearm vascular bed are representative of those in other major sites contributing to systemic vascular resistance.[138] This technique has recently been employed in a study comparing the vascular effects of nebivolol and atenolol, two relatively cardioselective beta-adrenoceptor antagonists capable of achieving similar reductions in systemic blood pressure. A recent study has shown that oral nebivolol treatment, but not atenolol, allows restoration of endothelial function in the forearm vascular bed of patients with essential hypertension, determined by local blood flow responses to intrabrachial acetylcholine administration (Figure 14.5).[161] This finding suggests that nebivolol

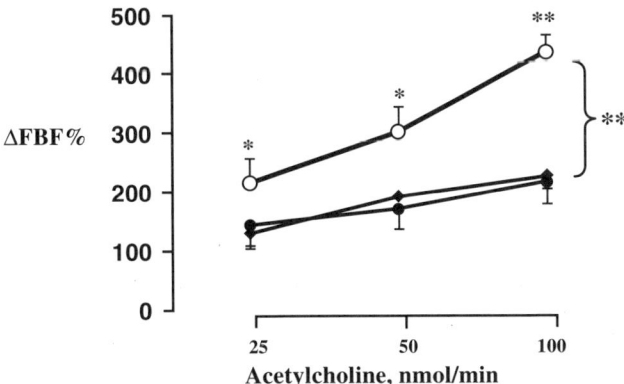

Figure 14.5 Effect of intraarterial administration of acetylcholine on forearm blood flow in patients with hypertension. Data are expressed as mean ± SEM percentage change from baseline blood flow after oral administration of placebo (♦), nebivolol (○), and atenolol (●) therapy. Values are mean ± SEM; *$p < 0.05$ and **$p < 0.001$ for differences between treatments. (From Tzemos, N. et al., *Circulation*, 104, 511–514, 2001. With permission.)

might be capable of reducing the progression of atherosclerosis through mechanisms in addition to blood pressure lowering, but this hypothesis requires confirmation in large clinical trials. Nonetheless, this observation suggests that antihypertensive drugs, even within the same class, might differ significantly in their ability to restore endothelial function, despite similar reductions in blood pressure, and important differences might exist in their effect on long-term cardiovascular risk reduction.

The effects of intrabrachial drug administration on forearm blood flow have been used to study the vasodilating properties of a number of antihypertensive drugs including ACE inhibitors, potassium channel activators, endothelin-converting enzyme inhibitors, and endothelin receptor antagonists.[162–164] For example, administration of enalaprilat (the active metabolite of enalapril) was shown to antagonize the vasoconstrictor effects of exogenous angiotensin I but not angiotensin II in the human forearm vascular bed, thereby giving proof of concept by demonstrating evidence of ACE inhibition *in vivo*.[162] Similarly designed studies have shown that losartan inhibits the vasoconstrictor responses to both angiotensin I and II, whereas enalapril inhibits the vasoconstrictor responses to angiotensin I alone, thereby providing proof of concept that losartan causes vasodilatation due to blockade of angiotensin II receptors, whereas enalapril is capable only of inhibiting the enzymatic conversion of angiotensin I to angiotensin II.[165]

Studies of localized hemodynamic drug actions have provided new insights into vascular physiology. For instance, vasoconstrictor responses to L-NMMA administration indicate that nitric oxide synthase activity contributes to resting vascular tone in resistance vessels,[166,167] and, conversely, vasodilator responses to the endothelin A-type receptor antagonist BQ-123 indicate that endothelin mediates vasoconstrictor effects under normal resting condition.[168] Studies involving localized drug administration predicted the pressor response to systemic L-NMMA[169] and the hypotensive response to systemic doses of endothelin antagonist in humans.[39] Furthermore, intrabrachial administration of phosphoramidon, a mixed endothelin-converting enzyme and neutral endopeptidase inhibitor, was found to cause a substantial increase in forearm blood flow.[170] This effect might have been due to either decreased formation of vasoconstrictors (angiotensin II and endothelin-1) by endothelin-converting enzyme or decreased breakdown of the vasodilator, atrial natriuretic peptide, by neutral endopeptidase. Somewhat unexpectedly, intrabrachial administration of thiorphan, a relatively selective neutral endopeptidase inhibitor, has been shown to cause vasoconstriction in the forearm vascular bed. These observations indicate that the vasodilator response to phosphoramidon is caused by predominant endothelin-converting enzyme inhibition. A vasoconstrictor response to neutral endopeptidase inhibition was not envisaged from preclinical data but is consistent with the failure of this class of compounds to lower blood pressure in patients with hypertension.[171] Implementation of these *in vivo* mechanistic studies in phase II development might have obviated the need for an extensive, and ultimately unsuccessful, development program for these candidate antihypertensive agents.

The hemodynamic effects of novel antihypertensive drugs might be more fully understood by using a combination of investigational techniques. The effects of drugs on human arteries and veins *in vivo* have been compared in the forearm vascular bed and isolated dorsal hand vein, respectively, giving rise to the concept of arteriovenous selectivity in the site of action. For example, prazosin and organic nitrates have been shown to exert predominant hemodynamic effects on the venous system, whereas hydralazine and nifedipine act primarily as arterial vasodilators.[172,173] These methods can be included in phase I and phase II clinical trials so concepts can be transferred more rapidly between the laboratory and clinic, thereby promoting greater cohesion between basic and clinical research.

14.3.9.2 Microalbuminuria

Conventionally, dipstick urinalysis has allowed detection of urinary protein at concentrations that accompany more than 300 mg albumin excretion per day. The normal range for urinary albumin excretion is less than 30 mg/day, and the term *microalbuminuria* has been coined to describe the excretion of between 30 and 299 mg/day.[174] The presence of microalbuminuria has been shown to predict complications in patients with diabetes mellitus and is an independent risk factor for cardiovascular disease in such patients.[175,176] Among people who do not have diabetes mellitus, microalbuminuria is also predictive of atherosclerotic vascular disease risk.[177] In unselected populations, microalbuminuria has been found to be a significant prognostic indicator of future cardiovascular disease risk and, in those patients with established coronary artery disease, it is an important marker of increased mortality.[178] Microalbuminuria has also been shown to be a powerful indicator of increased cardiovascular risk among patients with established hypertension.[179–182] Microalbuminuria is thought to be a manifestation of blood-pressure-mediated end-organ damage, and a recent study has shown a linear relationship between microalbuminuria and cardiovascular risk among patients with hypertension and left ventricular hypertrophy.[180] The association between microalbuminuria and cardiovascular risk appears particularly strong for men.[182]

The underlying pathophysiology appears due to increased transcapillary escape of albumin; endothelial dysfunction and altered extracellular matrix are believed to play an important role in patients with diabetes and hypertension.[181] Increased vascular permeability allows low-density lipoprotein to traverse dysfunctional endothelium and accumulate in the subendothelial environment which contributes to atherosclerotic plaque development. Microalbuminuria is a sensitive early marker of renal dysfunction in patients with hypertension and, therefore, provides insight into the biological consequences of hypertension *in vivo*. Microalbuminuria is a valuable surrogate marker of cardiovascular risk in patients with hypertension, and it serves to identify those patients who might benefit most from aggressive blood pressure lowering. Moreover, microalbuminuria in patients with hypertension might be a useful therapeutic target in clinical practice, and this hypothesis is currently under investigation. Consideration should be given to its inclusion in the design of studies investigating novel antihypertensive agents.

14.3.9.3 Intima-Media Thickness

Arterial intima-media thickness assessed by carotid ultrasonography is an important predictor of future atherosclerosis in patients with essential hypertension. Carotid artery intima-media thickness correlates closely with Framingham risk scores, which are based on a number of independent cardiovascular risk factors.[183] It is regarded as a highly sensitive measure of target organ damage in response to sustained high blood pressure.[184] Arterial intima-media thickness measurements are significantly higher among treated patients with hypertension than healthy controls, perhaps reflecting inadequacy of blood pressure control or the vascular effects of coexistent risk factors.[185] Amelioration of major cardiovascular risk factors (e.g., reducing cholesterol concentrations in patients with hypercholesterolemia) allows restoration of carotid intima-media thickness;[186] thus, arterial intima-media thickness is a dynamic measure that responds to amelioration of risk factors. Antihypertensive treatment has been found to delay the progression of arterial intima-media thickness in patients with mild to moderate hypertension.[187] Potentially important distinctions exist between the effects of different antihypertensive agents on intima-media thickness. For example, calcium channel antagonists have been found to be more effective in suppressing the progression of vascular changes in patients with hypertension than thiazide-type diuretics and ACE inhibitors, despite similar blood pressure reduction.[188,189] These findings suggest that different types of antihypertensive agent might be more or less protective against end-organ damage for any given blood pressure reduction; however, the implications of these differences on long-term progression of end-organ damage and cardiovascular risk require evaluation in large prospective studies.

14.3.9.4 C-Reactive Protein

Scientific evidence shows that assay of C-reactive protein (CRP) adds to the predictive ability of other established risk factors for cardiovascular disease, particularly when applied to patients with intermediate risk determined by the Framingham Coronary Risk Score. On the basis of these data, the Centers for Disease Control and Prevention and the American Heart Association have recently emphasized the importance of CRP as an independent marker of risk that may help direct further evaluation and therapy in the primary prevention of cardiovascular disease.[190] This consensus statement has suggested that an increased serum level of CRP in intermediate-risk patients should prompt aggressive treatment of this group so as to achieve maximum reduction of cardiovascular risk.

Elevated CRP serum levels are associated with abnormal endothelial vascular reactivity in patients with coronary artery disease (CAD). In 60 male patients with angiographically documented CAD, an elevated CRP serum level was a statistically significant independent predictor of a blunted response to acetylcholine-induced forearm blood flow.[191] Forearm blood flow response to acetylcholine was inversely correlated with CRP levels.

Raised CRP concentrations are an independent predictor of cardiovascular disease, stroke, death from cardiac causes, and diabetes.[192–194] Furthermore, high serum CRP concentrations are associated with the phenotypic features of the metabolic syndrome, including abdominal obesity, reduced levels of high-density lipoprotein cholesterol, high blood pressure, elevated fasting plasma glucose, and elevated plasma triglyceride concentrations.[195] High serum CRP concentrations were shown to be predictive of high cardiovascular risk, even after correcting for the presence of other features associated with the metabolic syndrome.[190]

Current research indicates that high serum CRP concentrations are an important indicator of increased cardiovascular risk in unselected populations, individuals with insulin-resistance syndromes, and patients with type 2 diabetes. Because inflammation is believed to play a role in the early development and progression of atherosclerosis, measurement of CRP concentrations might identify those patients with hypertension who are at greatest cardiovascular risk. Alleviation of inflammation, as a novel therapeutic target, might be a desirable property for a novel antihypertensive agent, in addition to blood pressure lowering alone. Currently, it is not clear whether amelioration of vascular inflammation as a primary treatment objective might allow restoration of vascular function, and this hypothesis is subject to ongoing research.

Table 14.2 Numbers of Healthy Volunteers and Patients Exposed to New Active Substances at the Time of Marketing (1987–1989)

Volunteers	Median	Range
Healthy volunteers	67	41–742
Efficacy studies	1120	43–4906
Safety database	1528	43–15,962

Source: Rawlins, M.D., *J. R. Coll. Phys.*, 29, 41–49, 1995. With permission.

14.3.10   Safety Considerations

The principal investigator is bound by the Hippocratic principle *primum non nocere* (first do no harm), which has been enshrined in local codes of practice and in international guidelines.[38,196,197] Tolerability and safety data should be collected from the first drug administration to humans onward. No requirements have been established in terms of the minimum number of healthy volunteers who should be exposed to a drug for safety assessments but, by the end of the drug development program, data should eventually be available from in excess of 1500 hypertensive patients (see Table 14.2).

14.3.10.1 Hypotension

Details of hypotension, both symptomatic and asymptomatic, and the relation to drug dosage and time of administration should be recorded. Special attention should be paid to the orthostatic hypotension and the occurrence of first-dose hypotension. Depending on the mechanism of action and the PK–PD relationship, delayed hypotension should be anticipated.

14.3.10.2 Other Hemodynamic Effects

Special consideration should be given to the possibility of rebound hypertension, particularly after multiple dose administration is discontinued. Furthermore, the occurrence of symptoms attributable to systemic vasodilatation (facial flushing, peripheral edema, and headache) should be carefully documented. Coronary steal effects associated with systemic vasodilatation may provoke angina or myocardial infarction and, if suspected, should be studied specifically. Impotence is a commonly reported adverse effect with a number of existing antihypertensive drugs and should be given specific consideration.

14.3.10.3 Electrocardiogram

All changes in the heart rate, with particular attention to tachycardia, QT prolongation and pro-arrhythmic changes, and effects on QRS duration should be carefully documented. The ECG should be examined at frequent intervals throughout the study, with particularly close monitoring at peak plasma concentrations and at the time of maximal blood pressure lowering.

14.3.10.4 Concomitant Risk Factors

Special attention should be paid to the effects of the study compound on glucose, triglyceride, and total and high-density lipoprotein cholesterol concentrations. If an effect on these variables is apparent, it should be studied in detail and the dose–response relationship examined.

14.3.10.5 Withdrawal of Antihypertensive Treatment

As cardiovascular risk is related to the severity of hypertension, important ethical considerations are raised by the withdrawal of treatment from patients with more severe hypertension. In general, drug withdrawal should not be contemplated for individuals in whom severe hypertension might be anticipated. Furthermore, the withdrawal period should be long enough to allow adequate washout of pharmacodynamic effects but sufficiently short to minimize the potential risks associated with exposure to uncontrolled hypertension. In general, a 4- to 6-week washout period might be acceptable in patients with mild to moderate hypertension, in the absence of any compelling indications for treatment continuation. An alternative approach is randomized placebo-controlled studies of withdrawal of one agent, where blood pressure has initially been adequately controlled on a combination of drugs. This design allows assessment of the contribution of individual anti-hypertensive agents to blood pressure control by observing the subsequent increase in blood pressure.

14.4 PHASE IV STUDIES

Phase I to III studies of new antihypertensive agents should be designed so as to collect sufficient appropriate clinical data to substantiate a license application to the regulatory authorities. Ideally, studies will have been performed in sufficient numbers of patients with hypertension with regard to sex, race, age, associated diseases, and medications so as to be reflective of the intended treatment population. Phase I to III studies should provide detailed data regarding the safety, tolerability, and blood pressure lowering efficacy of the candidate antihypertensive drug. Furthermore, data should be available from rigorously conducted proof-of-concept studies using optimal study design and methods to sufficiently characterize the mechanism of drug action. Phase III studies will have provided additional safety data related to cardiovascular outcomes in subjects exposed to treatment for at least one year. At the time of licensing application, several thousand patients might have been exposed to the compound.[198] In addition to enabling the requirements for regulatory submission to be met, data collected during phase I to III investigations are vital in forming the basis of subsequent large phase IV clinical trials. These might often be initiated before license approval, and the key goal of these studies is to prove effectiveness of the novel drug in reducing cardiovas-cular morbidity and mortality to at least the same extent as existing gold standard treatments. The mechanisms of action of the new antihypertensive drug and responses observed in particular patient subgroups might guide the conduct of phase IV studies toward particular types of antihypertensive intervention — for example, targeting postmenopausal female patients, patients with isolated systolic hypertension, or patients with coexistent diabetes mellitus. The choice of patient population might confer the need for special additional investigations to confirm the potential mechanism of action identified during earlier study phases; for example, pulse wave velocity measurements might be utilized to examine the drug effects on large arterial compliance in selected patient subgroups.

A key feature of phase IV studies is that they seek to establish therapeutic usefulness in long-term prospective cardiovascular risk reduction. In order to demonstrate that a new antihypertensive drug is capable of reducing the incidence of cardiovascular events, the selection criteria used to define the patient population and the duration of follow-up must be chosen so as to give a sufficiently high baseline rate of cardiovascular events. Because the study subjects must reflect the intended treatment population, there is limited flexibility in the extent to which high-risk patients can be selected; therefore, phase IV studies in hypertension usually require recruitment of large patient numbers, often at least several thousand, and prolonged follow-up for perhaps 5 to 10 years. The design of the phase IV study in hypertension is subtly distinct from that of the preceding phase III investigation, in which the primary aim is to establish long-term safety and identify only substan-tially greater differences in morbidity or mortality that might merit further investigation.

Several important confounding factors are unique to phase IV studies, particularly the need to control for time-dependent effects given that studies are often conducted over a period of years. Additionally, recruitment of very large patient numbers necessitates multicenter study design, and careful attention must be paid to ensure that regional variations in routine clinical practice are taken into consideration, such as different concomitant medications and criteria for diagnosing incident cardiovascular events. The potential effects of these factors are minimized by centrally controlled randomization and incorporating a double-blind parallel group design. More important confounding factors include concomitant use of additional antihypertensive therapy, dropouts, and use of the study medication or comparator in the crossover limb. These factors tend to limit the power of phase IV studies to detect differences between two antihypertensive treatment limbs using intention-to-treat analysis and require inclusion of even larger subject numbers. It is noteworthy that the majority of phase IV studies of antihypertensive medication that have involved an active comparator study arm have failed to detect a significant advantage or disadvantage in terms of cardiovascular outcome.

The quality and quantity of useful data generated in phase I and II studies will be governed by the quality of their design. Well-designed early-phase studies have major implications in terms of both safety and cost for the drug development program: They can lead to the speedy withdrawal of ineffective or dangerous drugs from investigation, can characterize the target population most likely to benefit from the new therapy, and can facilitate the rapid progress of registration applications for more promising compounds. Well-designed, carefully conducted early-phase studies are a prerequisite for good phase III and IV studies and can save time and money later in the drug development program.

REFERENCES

1. Schwartlander, B., Global burden of disease, *Lancet*, 350, 141–142, 1997.
2. WHO, *Health for All Indicators*, Regional Office for Europe, World Health Organization, Copenhagen, 1993.
3. CDC, *Heart and Stroke Facts*, Vital Health Statistics, Series 10, Data from the National Health Interview Survey, National Center for Health Statistics, Centers for Disease Control and Prevention, Hyattsville, MD, 1983.
4. Framingham Study, Systolic versus diastolic blood pressure and risk of coronary heart disease, *Am. J. Cardiol.*, 27, 355–346, 1971.
5. Kannel, W.B., Role of blood pressure in cardiovascular disease: the Framingham Study, *Angiology*, 26, 1–14, 1975.
6. Alderman, M.H., The 1994 model of hypertension management, *Curr. Opin. Nephrol. Hypertens.*, 3, 241–244, 1994.
7. Dollery, C.T., Risk predictor, risk indicator and benefits in hypertension, *Am. J. Med.*, 82(Suppl. 1A), 2–8, 1987.
8. Roberts, W.C., The hypertensive diseases: evidence that systemic hypertension is a greater risk factor to the development of other cardiovascular diseases than previously suspected, *Am. J. Med.*, 59, 523–532, 1975.
9. Medical Research Council Working Party, Medical Research Council trial of treatment of mild hypertension: principal results, *Br. Med. J.*, 291, 97–104, 1985.
10. Collins, R. et al., Blood pressure, stroke and coronary disease, *Lancet*, 335, 827–838, 1990.
11. Veterans Administration Cooperative Study Group on Antihypertensive Agents, Effects of treatment on morbidity in hypertension: results in patients with diastolic pressures averaging 115 through 129 mmHg, *JAMA*, 202, 1028–1034, 1967.
12. Wolff, F.W. and Lindeman, R.D., Effects of treatment in hypertension: results of a controlled study, *J. Chron. Dis.*, 19, 227–240, 1965.

13. Veterans Administration Cooperative Study Group on Antihypertensive Agents, Effects of treatment on morbidity in hypertension: results in patients with diastolic blood pressures averaging 90 through 115 mmHg, *JAMA*, 213, 1143 1147, 1970.

14. Anderson, O.K. et al., Survival in treated hypertension: follow-up study after two decades, *Br. Med. J.*, 317, 167–171, 1998.

15. Hansson, L. et al., Effects of intensive blood-pressure lowering and low-dose aspirin in patients with hypertension: principal results of the hypertension optimal treatment (HOT) randomised trial, *Lancet*, 351, 1755–1762, 1998.

16. Chobanian, A.V. et al., Seventh report of the Joint National Committee on Prevention, Detection, Evaluation, and Treatment of High Blood Pressure, *Hypertension*, 42, 1206–1252, 2003.

17. Ramsay, L.E. et al., Guidelines for the management of hypertension: report of the third working party of the British Hypertension Society, *J. Hum. Hypertens.*, 13, 569–592, 1999.

18. World Health Organization/International Society for Hypertension, Guidelines for the management of hypertension, *J. Hypertens.*, 17, 151–158, 1999.

19. Cifkova, R. et al., Practice guidelines for primary care physicians: 2003 ESH/ESC hypertension guidelines, *J. Hypertens.*, 21, 1779–1786, 2003.

20. Hart, J.T., The management of hypertension in general practice, *J. R. Coll. Gen. Pract.*, 25, 160–192, 1975.

21. Heller, R.F., Detection and treatment of hypertension in an inner London community, *Br. J. Prev. Soc. Med.*, 30, 168–171, 1976.

22. Kurji, K.H. and Haines, A.P., Detection and management of hypertension in general practices in northwest London, *Br. Med. J.*, 288, 903–906, 1984.

23. Smith, W.C.S. et al., Control of blood pressure in Scotland: the rule of halves, *Br. Med. J.*, 300, 981–983, 1990.

24. Burt, V. et al., Trends in the prevalence, awareness, treatment, and control of hypertension in the adult U.S. population: data from the health examination surveys, 1960 to 1991, *Hypertension*, 26, 60–69, 1995.

25. Bulpitt, C.J. and Fletcher, A.E., Cost-effectiveness of the treatment of hypertension, *Clin. Exp. Hypertens.*, 15, 1131–1146, 1993.

26. Vagelos, P.R., Are prescription drug prices high?, *Science*, 252, 1080–1084, 1991.

27. Brown, M.J. et al., Morbidity and mortality in patients randomised to double-blind treatment with a long-acting calcium-channel blocker or diuretic in the International Nifedipine GITS study: Intervention as a Goal in Hypertension Treatment (INSIGHT), *Lancet*, 356, 366–372, 2000.

28. Dahlof, B. et al., STOP-Hypertension 2: a prospective intervention trial of "newer" versus "older" treatment alternatives in old patients with hypertension, Swedish Trial in Old Patients with Hypertension, *Blood Press.*, 2, 136–141, 1993.

29. Dahlof, B. et al., Cardiovascular morbidity and mortality in the losartan intervention for endpoint reduction in hypertension study (LIFE): a randomized trial against atenolol, *Lancet*, 359, 995–1003, 2002.

30. HOPE study investigators, The HOPE (Heart Outcomes Prevention Evaluation) study: the design of a large, simple randomized trial of an angiotensin-converting enzyme inhibitor (ramipril) and vitamin E in patients at high risk of cardiovascular events, *Can. J. Cardiol.*, 12, 127–137, 1996.

31. Reyes, A.J. and Leary, W.P., The ALLHAT and the cardioprotection conferred by diuretics in hypertensive patients: a connection with uric acid?, *Cardiovasc. Drugs Ther.*, 16, 485–487, 2002.

32. Wurzner, G. et al., Comparative effects of losartan and irbesartan on serum uric acid in hypertensive patients with hyperuricaemia and gout, *J. Hypertens.*, 19, 1855–1860, 2001.

33. ALLHAT Collaborative Research Group, Major cardiovascular events in hypertensive patients randomized to doxazosin vs. chlorthalidone: the Antihypertensive and Lipid-Lowering Treatment To Prevent Heart Attack Trial (ALLHAT), *JAMA*, 283, 1967–1975, 2000.

34. Wing, L.M. et al., A comparison of outcomes with angiotensin-converting-enzyme inhibitors and diuretics for hypertension in the elderly, *N. Engl. J. Med.*, 348, 583–592, 2003.

35. ALLHAT Officers and Coordinators for the ALLHAT Collaborative Research Group, Major outcomes in high-risk hypertensive patients randomized to angiotensin-converting enzyme inhibitor or calcium channel blocker vs. diuretic: the Antihypertensive and Lipid-Lowering Treatment To Prevent Heart Attack trial, *JAMA*, 288, 2981–2997, 2002.

36. Antihypertensive and Lipid-Lowering Treatment To Prevent Heart Attack Trial Collaborative Research
     Group, Diuretic versus alpha-blocker as first-step antihypertensive therapy: final results from the Anti-
     hypertensive and Lipid-Lowering Treatment to Prevent Heart Attack Trial (ALLHAT), *Hypertension*,
     42, 239–246, 2003.

37. Whelton, P.K. et al., National High Blood Pressure Education Program Coordinating Committee,
     Primary prevention of hypertension: clinical and public health advisory from the National High Blood
     Pressure Education Program, *JAMA*, 288, 1882–1888, 2002.

38. ABPI, *Guidelines on Good Clinical (Research) Practice*, Ref. 413/96/6600M, Association of the British
     Pharmaceutical Industry, London, 1996.

39. Haynes, W.G. et al., Systemic endothelin receptor blockade decreases peripheral vascular resistance
     and blood pressure in humans, *Circulation*, 93, 1860–1870, 1996.

40. Krum, H. et al., The effect of an endothelin-receptor antagonist, bosentan, on blood pressure in patients
     with essential hypertension: bosentan hypertension investigators, *N. Engl. J. Med.*, 338, 784–790, 1998.

41. Prisant, L.M. and Moser, M., Hypertension in the elderly: can we improve results of therapy?, *Arch.
     Intern. Med.*, 160, 283–289, 2000.

42. Williams, R.R. et al., Are there interactions and relations between genetic and environmental factors
     predisposing to high blood pressure?, *Hypertension*, 18(Suppl.), I29–I37, 1991.

43. Lever, A.F. and Harrap, S.B., Essential hypertension: a disorder of growth with origins in childhood?,
     J. Hypertens., 10, 101–120, 1992.

44. Borchard, U., Pharmacokinetics of beta-adrenoceptor blocking agents: clinical significance of hepatic
     and/or renal clearance, *Clin. Physiol. Biochem.*, 8(Suppl. 2), 28–34, 1990.

45. Mehvar, R. and Brocks, D.R., Stereospecific pharmacokinetics and pharmacodynamics of beta-adren-
     ergic blockers in humans, *J. Pharm. Pharm. Sci.*, 4, 185–200, 2001.

46. White, C.M., Pharmacologic, pharmacokinetic, and therapeutic differences among ACE inhibitors,
     Pharmacotherapy, 18, 588–599, 1998.

47. Meredith, P.A. et al., An individualised approach to optimising long-term antihypertensive therapy using
     concentration-effect analysis, in *The In Vivo Study of Drug Action*, van Boxtel, C.J, Holford, N.H.G.,
     and Danhof, M., Eds., Elsevier Science, Amsterdam, 1992.

48. Brunner, H.R. et al., Does pharmacological profiling of a new drug in normal volunteers provide a
     useful guideline to antihypertensive therapy?, *Hypertension*, 5, 101–7, 1983.

49. Unger, T., Azizi, M., and Belz, G.G., Blocking the tissue renin–angiotensin system: the future corner-
     stone of therapy, *J. Hum. Hypertens.*, 14(Suppl. 2), S23–S31, 2000.

50. Cohen, L. and Kurtz, M.D., Angiotensin converting enzyme inhibition in tissues from spontaneously
     hypertensive rats after treatment with captopril or MK421, *J. Pharmacol. Exp. Ther.*, 220, 63–69, 1982.

51. Berglund, G. and Andersson, O., Low doses of hydrochlorothiazide in hypertension: antihypertensive
     and metabolic effects, *Eur. J. Clin. Pharmacol.*, 10, 177–182, 1976.

52. Carlsen, J.E. et al., Relation between doses of bendrofluazide, antihypertensive effect and adverse
     biochemical effects, *Br. Med. J.*, 300, 975–978, 1990.

53. Law, M.R. et al., Value of low dose combination treatment with blood pressure lowering drugs: analysis
     of 354 randomised trials, *Br. Med. J.*, 326, 1427–1435, 2003.

54. ICH, Dose–response information to support drug registration, International Conference on Harmonisa-
     tion of Technical Requirements for the Registration of Pharmaceuticals for Human Use, Geneva, 1993.

55. EAEM, ICH Principles Document for Clinical Evaluation of New Antihypertensive Drugs, draft con-
     sensus document, European Agency for the Evaluation of Medicinal Products, London, 2000
     (http://www.emea.eu.int/pdfs/human/ich/054100en.pdf).

56. Baber, N., International conference on harmonisation of technical requirements for registration of
     pharmaceuticals for human use, *Br. J. Clin. Pharmacol.*, 37, 401–404, 1994.

57. Ménard, J., Bellet, M., and Serrurier, D., From the parallel group design to the crossover design, and
     from the group approach to the individual approach, *Am. J. Hypertens.*, 3, 815–819, 1990.

58. Sheiner, L.B. et al., A simulation study comparing designs for dose ranging, *Stat. Med.*, 10, 303–321,
     1991.

59. Ménard, J., Critical assessment of international clinical development programmes for new antihyper-
     tensive drugs, *J. Hypertens.*, 11(Suppl.), S39–S46, 1993.

60. Cameron, H.A. and Ramsay, L.E., The lupus syndrome induced by hydralazine: a common complication
     with low dose treatment, *Br. Med. J.*, 289, 410–412, 1984.

61. De Mey, C., Inverse PK/PD: estimation and differentiation of bioavailability from effect kinetics — observations with beta-adrenoceptor antagonists, *Int. J. Clin. Pharmacol. Ther.*, 35, 453–457, 1997.

62. ICH Steering Committee, *Principles for Clinical Evaluation of New Antihypertensive Drugs*, International Conference on Harmonisation of Technical Requirements for Registration of Pharmaceuticals for Human Use, Geneva, 2000 (http://www.fda.gov/cder/guidance/3774dft.pdf).

63. Al-Khatib, S.M. et al., Placebo-controls in short-term clinical trials of hypertension, *Science*, 292, 2013–2015, 2001.

64. Garbe, E. et al., Clinical and statistical issues in therapeutic equivalence research, *Eur, J. Clin. Pharmacol.*, 45, 1–7, 1993.

65. Stergiou, G.S. and Skeva, I.I., Renin–angiotensin system blockade at the level of the angiotensin converting enzyme or the angiotensin type-1 receptor: similarities and differences, *Curr. Top. Med. Chem.*, 4, 473–481, 2004.

66. Franklin, S.S. et al., Is pulse pressure useful in predicting risk for coronary heart disease? The Framingham heart study, *Circulation*, 100, 354–360, 1999.

67. SHEP Cooperative Research Group, Prevention of stroke by antihypertensive drug treatment in older persons with isolated systolic hypertension: final results of the Systolic Hypertension in the Elderly Program (SHEP), *JAMA*, 265, 3255–3264, 1991.

68. Staessen, J. et al., Randomised double-blind comparison of placebo and active treatment for older patients with isolated systolic hypertension: the Systolic Hypertension in Europe (Syst-Eur) Trial investigators, *Lancet*, 350, 757–764, 1997.

69. Oliver, J.J. and Webb, D.J., Noninvasive assessment of arterial stiffness and risk of atherosclerotic events, *Arterioscler. Thromb. Vasc. Biol.*, 23, 554–566, 2003.

70. Schaefer, B.M. et al., Gender, ethnicity and genetics in cardiovascular disease. Part 1. Basic principles, *Heart Dis.*, 5, 129–143, 2003.

71. Schwartz, J.B., The influence of sex on pharmacokinetics, *Clin. Pharmacokinet.*, 42, 107–121, 2003.

72. Drici, M.D. and Clement, N., Is gender a risk factor for adverse drug reactions? The example of drug-induced long QT syndrome, *Drug Saf.*, 24, 575–585, 2001.

73. Weijer, C., Selecting subjects for participation in clinical research: one sphere of justice, *J. Med. Ethics*, 25, 31–36, 1999.

74. Horton, R., Trials of women, *Lancet*, 343, 745–746, 1994.

75. Walle, T. et al., Pathway-selective sex differences in the metabolic clearance of propranolol in human subjects, *Clin. Pharmacol. Ther.*, 46, 257–263, 1989.

76. Webb, D.J. et al., Cough associated with captopril and enalapril, *Br. Med. J.*, 295, 272, 1987.

77. Merkatz, R.B. et al., Women in clinical trials of new drugs: a change in Food and Drug Administration Policy, *N. Engl. J. Med.*, 329, 292–296, 1993.

78. Caschetta, M.B. et al., FDA policy on women in drug trials, *N. Engl. J. Med.*, 329, 1815, 1993.

79. Mastroianni, A.C. et al., Eds., *Women and Health Research: Ethical and Legal Issues of Including Women in Clinical Studies*, Institute of Medicine, Washington, D.C., 1994.

80. Bobrie, G. and Potter, J.F., The elderly hypertensive population: what lies ahead of us?, *J. Renin Angiotensin Aldosterone Syst.*, 3(Suppl. 1), S4–S9, 2000.

81. Lakatta, E.G. and Levy, D., Arterial and cardiac aging: major shareholders in cardiovascular disease enterprises. Part I. Aging arteries: a "set up" for vascular disease, *Circulation*, 107, 139–146, 2003.

82. Nawrot, T. et al., Isolated systolic hypertension and the risk of vascular disease, *Curr. Hypertens. Rep.*, 5, 372–379, 2003.

83. Miall, W.E., The epidemiology of hypertension in old age, in *Arterial Disease and the Elderly*, Stout, R.W., Ed., Churchill-Livingstone, Edinburgh, 1984, pp. 154–174.

84. Sear, J.W. and Higham, H., Issues in the perioperative management of the elderly patient with cardiovascular disease, *Drugs Aging*, 19, 429–451, 2002.

85. Anderson, R. et al., *The Coming of Age in Europe: Older People in the European Community*, Age Concern England, London, 1992.

86. Bressler, R. and Bahl, J.J., Principles of drug therapy for the elderly patient, *Mayo Clin. Proc.*, 78, 1564–1577, 2003.

87. Noble, R.E., Drug therapy in the elderly, *Metabolism*, 52(10, Suppl. 2), 27–30, 2003.

88. Turnheim, K., When drug therapy gets old: pharmacokinetics and pharmacodynamics in the elderly, *Exp. Gerontol.*, 38, 843–853, 2003.

89. International Conference on Harmonisation of Technical Requirements for the Registration of Pharmaceuticals for Human Use, Studies in support of special populations: geriatrics, *Fed. Reg.*, 58(72), 21082–21083, 1993.

90. FDA, *Guideline for the Study of Drugs Likely To Be Used in the Elderly*, U.S. Food and Drug Administration, Washington D.C., 1989.

91. Kaplan, N.M., Ethnic aspects of hypertension, *Lancet*, 344, 450–452, 1994.

92. Gibbs, C.R., Beevers, D.G., and Lip, G.Y., The management of hypertensive disease in black patients, *Q. J. Med.*, 92, 187–192, 1999.

93. Anderson, P.J. et al., Comparison of the pharmacokinetics and pharmacodynamics of oral doses of perindopril in normotensive Chinese and Caucasian volunteers, *Br. J. Clin. Pharmacol.*, 39, 361–368, 1995.

94. Jamerson, K. and DeQuattro, V., The impact of ethnicity on response to antihypertensive therapy, *Am. J. Med.*, 101(Suppl.), S22–S32, 1996.

95. Materson, B.J. et al., Single-drug therapy for hypertension in men: a comparison of six antihypertensive agents with placebo, *N. Engl. J. Med.*, 328, 914–921, 1993.

96. Johnson, D.A. and Hricik, J.G., The pharmacology of alpha-adrenergic decongestants, *Pharmacotherapy*, 13(Suppl.), S110S–S115, 1993.

97. Armstrong, E.P. and Malone, D.C., The impact of nonsteroidal anti-inflammatory drugs on blood pressure, with an emphasis on newer agents, *Clin. Ther.*, 25, 1–18, 2003.

98. Duffy, S.J. et al., Treatment of hypertension with ascorbic acid, *Lancet*, 354, 2048–2049, 1999.

99. Freestone, S. and Ramsay, L.E., Effect of beta-blockade on the pressor response of coffee plus smoking in patients with mild hypertension, *Drugs*, 25, 141–145, 1983.

100. Griffiths, R.R. et al., Human coffee drinking: reinforcing and physical dependence producing effects of caffeine, *J. Pharmacol. Exp. Ther.*, 239, 416–425, 1986.

101. Galletly, D.C. et al., Does caffeine withdrawal contribute to post-operative headache?, *Lancet*, i, 1335, 1989.

102. Klatsky, A.L. et al., Alcohol consumption and blood pressure: Kaiser Permanente multiphasic health examination data, *N. Engl. J. Med.*, 196, 1194–200, 1977.

103. Potter, J.F. et al., The pressor and metabolic effects of alcohol in normotensives, *Hypertension*, 8, 625–631, 1986.

104. Potter, J.F. et al., Alcohol raises blood pressure in hypertensive patients, *J. Hypertens.*, 4, 435–441, 1986.

105. Bannon, L.T. et al., Effect of alcohol withdrawal on blood pressure, plasma renin activity, aldosterone, cortisol and dopamine beta-hydroxylase, *Clin. Sci.*, 66, 659–663, 1984.

106. Cryer, P.E. et al., Norepinephrine and epinephrine release and adrenergic mediation of smoking associated haemodynamic and metabolic events, *N. Engl. J. Med.*, 295, 573–577, 1967.

107. Stewart, M.J. et al., Cardiovascular effects of cigarette smoking: ambulatory blood pressure and blood pressure variability, *J. Hum. Hypertens.*, 8, 19–22, 1994.

108. Patrick, D.L. et al., The validity of self-reported smoking: a review and meta-analysis, *Am. J. Public Health*, 84, 1086–1093, 1994.

109. Etzel, R.A., A review of the use of saliva cotinine as a marker of tobacco smoke exposure, *Prev. Med.*, 19, 190–197, 1990.

110. Pre, J., Les marqueurs du tabagisme, *Pathol. Biol.*, 40, 1015–1021, 1992.

111. Matthew, R.J. et al., Middle cerebral artery velocity during upright posture after marijuana smoking, *Acta Psychiatr. Scand.*, 86, 173–178, 1992.

112. Heishman, S.J. et al., Acute and residual effects of marijuana: profiles of plasma THC levels, physiological, subjective, and performance measures, *Pharmacol. Biochem. Behav.*, 37, 561–565, 1990.

113. Ohman, K.P. et al., Pharmacokinetics of captopril and its effect on blood pressure during acute and chronic administration and in relation to food intake, *J. Cardiovasc. Pharmacol.*, 7(Suppl.), S20–S40, 1985.

114. Salvetti, A. et al., Influence of food on acute and chronic effects of captopril in essential hypertensive patients, *J. Cardiovasc. Pharmacol.*, 7(Suppl.), S25–S29, 1985.

115. Swanson, B.N. et al., Influence of food on the bioavailability of captopril in healthy subjects, *J. Pharm. Sci.*, 73, 1655–1657, 1984.

116. Melander, A. et al., Enhancement of the bioavailability of propranolol and metoprolol by food, *Clin. Pharmacol. Ther.*, 2, 108–112, 1977.

117. McLean, A.J. et al., Reduction of first pass hepatic clearance of propranolol by food, *Clin. Pharmacol. Ther.*, 30, 31–34, 1981.

118. Daneshmend, T.K. and Roberts, C.J.C., The influence of food on the oral and intravenous pharmacokinetics of a high clearance drug: a study with labetalol, *Br. J. Clin. Pharmacol.*, 14, 73–78, 1982.

119. Bailey, D.G. et al., Grapefruit juice and drugs: how significant is it?, *Clin. Pharmacokinet.*, 26, 91–98, 1994.

120. Webb, D.J. et al., Reduction of blood pressure in man with H142, a potent new renin inhibitor, *Lancet*, 2, 1486–1487, 1983.

121. Hodsman, G.P. et al., Factors related to the first dose hypotensive effect of captopril: prediction and treatment, *Br. Med. J.*, 284, 832–834, 1983.

122. Doig, J.K. et al., Dose-ranging study of angiotensin type 1 receptor antagonist losartan (DUP 753/82K954) in salt deplete man, *J. Cardiovasc. Pharmacol.*, 21, 732–738, 1993.

123. FDA, *Guidance for Industry: Bioavailability and Bioequivalence Studies for Orally Administered Drug Products — General Considerations*, U.S. Food and Drug Administration, Washington, D.C., 2002 (http://www.fda.gov/cder/guidance/4964dft.pdf).

124. Friedman, L. et al., *Fundamentals of Clinical Trials*, 2nd ed., PSG Publishing, Littleton, 1984.

125. Moleur, P. and Boissel, J.-P., Definition of a surrogate endpoint, *Control. Clin. Trials*, 8, 304, 1987.

126. O'Brien, E. et al. and Working Group on Blood Pressure Monitoring of the European Society of Hypertension, International protocol for validation of blood pressure measuring devices in adults, *Blood Press, Monit.*, 7, 3–17, 2002.

127. Raftery, E.B., Understanding hypertension: the contribution of direct ambulatory blood pressure monitoring, in *Ambulatory Blood Pressure Monitoring*, Weber, M.A. and Pickering, G.W., Eds., Springer-Verlag, New York, 1983, pp. 105–116.

128. Stewart, M.J. and Padfield, P.L., Blood pressure measurement: an epitaph for the mercury sphygmomanometer?, *Clin. Sci.*, 83, 1–12, 1992.

129. Di Rienzo, M. et al., Continuous versus intermittent blood pressure measurements in estimating 24-hour average blood pressure, *Hypertension*, 5, 264–269, 1983.

130. James, G.D. et al., The reproducibility of ambulatory, home and clinical pressures, *Hypertension*, 11, 545–549, 1988.

131. Conway, J. et al., The use of ambulatory blood pressure monitoring to improve the accuracy and reduce the numbers of subjects in clinical trials of antihypertensive agents, *J. Hypertens.*, 6, 111–116, 1988.

132. Mutti, E. et al., Effect of placebo on 24-h non-invasive ambulatory blood pressure, *J. Hypertens.*, 9, 361–364, 1991.

133. O'Brien, E. et al., Ambulatory blood pressure measurement in the evaluation of blood pressure lowering drugs, *J. Hypertens.*, 7, 243–248, 1989.

134. Casadei, B., Use of ambulatory blood pressure monitoring in pharmacological trials, *J. Hum. Hypertens.*, 5, 1–4, 1991.

135. O'Brien, E. et al., Ambulatory blood pressure monitoring in the evaluation of drug efficacy, *Am. Heart J.*, 121, 999–1006, 1991.

136. Staessen, J.A. et al., Clinical trials with ambulatory blood pressure monitoring: fewer patients?, *Lancet*, 344, 1552–1556, 1994.

137. Rose, M. and McMahon, F.G., Some problems of antihypertensive drugs studies in the context of the new guidelines, *Am. J. Hypertens.*, 3, 151–155, 1990.

138. Wilkinson, I.B. and Webb, D.J., Venous occlusion plethysmography in cardiovascular research: methodology and clinical applications, *Br. J. Clin. Pharmacol.*, 52, 631–646, 2001.

139. Webb, D.J., The pharmacology of human blood vessels, *J. Vasc. Res.*, 757, 1–26, 1995.

140. Thomas, S.H.L., Impedance cardiography using the Sramek–Bernstein method: accuracy and variability at rest and during exercise, *Br. J. Clin. Pharmacol.*, 34, 467–476, 1992.

141. O'Rourke, M.F., Arterial mechanics and wave reflection with antihypertensive therapy, *J. Hypertens.*, 10(Suppl.), S43–S49, 1994.

142. Waring, W.S. et al., Acute caffeine intake influences central more than peripheral blood pressure in young adults, *Am. J. Hypertens.*, 16, 919–924, 2003.

143. Blacher, J et al., Impact of aortic stiffness on survival in end-stage renal disease, *Circulation*, 99, 2434–2439, 1999.

144. Mackenzie, I.S., Wilkinson, I.B. and Cockcroft, J.R., Assessment of arterial stiffness in clinical practice, *Q. J. Med.*, 95, 67–74, 2002.

145. Wu, K.K. and Thiagarajan, P., Role of endothelium in thrombosis and hemostasis, *Annu. Rev. Med.*, 47, 315–331, 1996.

146. Ganz, P. and Vita, J.A., Testing endothelial vasomotor function: nitric oxide, a multipotent molecule, *Circulation*, 108, 2049–2053, 2003.

147. Vallance, P. et al., Nitric oxide synthesised from L-arginine mediates endothelium-dependent dilatation in human veins *in vivo*, *Cardiovasc. Res.*, 23, 1053–1057, 1989.

148. Cooke, J.P. and Dzau, V.J., Derangements of the nitric oxide synthase pathway, L-arginine, and cardio-vascular diseases, *Circulation*, 96, 379–382, 1997.

149. Panza, J.A., Endothelial dysfunction in essential hypertension, *Clin. Cardiol.*, 20(Suppl. 2), 26–33, 1997.

150. Drexler, H., Endothelial dysfunction: clinical implications, *Prog. Cardiovasc. Dis.*, 39, 287–324, 1997.

151. Perticone, F. et al., Prognostic significance of endothelial dysfunction in hypertensive patients, *Circulation*, 104, 191–196, 2001.

152. Modena, M.G. et al., Prognostic role of reversible endothelial dysfunction in hypertensive postmeno-pausal women, *J. Am. Coll. Cardiol.*, 40, 505–510, 2002.

153. Chan, S.Y. et al., The prognostic importance of endothelial dysfunction and carotid atheroma burden in patients with coronary artery disease, *J. Am. Coll. Cardiol.*, 42, 1037–1043, 2003.

154. Taddei, S et al., Antihypertensive drugs and reversing of endothelial dysfunction in hypertension, *Curr. Hypertens. Rep.*, 2, 64–70, 2000.

155. Vita, J.A et al., Effect of cholesterol-lowering therapy on coronary endothelial vasomotor function in patients with coronary artery disease, *Circulation*, 102, 846–851, 2000.

156. Aellig, W.H., Clinical pharmacology, physiology and pathophysiology of superficial veins, parts 1 and 2, *Br. J. Clin. Pharmacol.*, 38, 181–196, 189–305, 1994.

157. Hand, M.F. and Webb, D.J., Assessment of the effects of drugs on the peripheral vasculature, in *Clinical Measurement in Drug Evaluation*, Nimmo, W.S and Tucker, C.T., Eds., John Wiley & Sons, Edinburgh, 1995, pp. 135–150.

158. Haynes, W.G. et al., Direct and sympathetically mediated venoconstriction in essential hypertension: enhanced response to endothelin-1, *J. Clin. Invest.*, 94, 1359–1364, 1994.

159. Robinson, B.F., Assessment of the effects of drugs on the venous system in man, *Br. J. Clin. Pharmacol.*, 6, 381–386, 1987.

160. Roberts, D.H. et al., The reproducibility of limb blood flow measurements in human volunteers at rest and after exercise by using mercury-in-silastic strain gauge plethysmography under standardized con-ditions, *Clin. Sci.*, 70, 635–638, 1986.

161. Tzemos, N., Lim, P.O., and MacDonald, T.M., Nebivolol reverses endothelial dysfunction in essential hypertension: a randomized, double-blind, crossover study, *Circulation*, 104, 511–514, 2001.

162. Benjamin, N. et al., Local inhibition of converting enzyme and vascular responses to angiotensin and bradykinin in the human forearm, *J. Physiol.*, 412, 543–555, 1989.

163. Webb, D.J. and Collier, J.G., Influence of ramipril diacid on the peripheral vascular effects of angiotensin I, *Am. J. Cardiol.*, 59, 45D–49D, 1987.

164. Haynes, W.G. and Webb, D.J., Venoconstriction to endothein-1 in humans: the role of calcium and potassium channels, *Am. J. Physiol. Heart Circ. Physiol.*, 265, H1676–H1681, 1993.

165. Cockcroft, J.R. et al., Comparison of angiotensin-converting enzyme inhibition with angiotensin II receptor antagonism in the human forearm, *J. Cardiovasc. Pharmacol.*, 22, 579–584, 1993.

166. O'Kane, K.P.J. et al., Local L-NG-monomethyl arginine attenuates the vasodilator action of bradykinin in the human forearm, *Br. J. Clin. Pharmacol.*, 38, 311–315, 1994.

167. Vallance, P. et al., Effects of endothelium-derived nitric oxide on peripheral arteriolar tone in man, *Lancet*, ii, 997–1000, 1989.

168. Haynes, W.G. and Webb, D.J., Contribution of endogenous generation of endothelin-1 to basal vascular tone, *Lancet*, 344, 852–854, 1994.

169. Haynes, W.G. et al., Inhibition of nitric oxide synthesis increases blood pressure in healthy humans, *J. Hypertens.*, 11, 1375–1380, 1993.

170. O'Connell, J.E. et al., Candoxatril, an orally active neutral endopeptidase inhibitor, raises plasma atrial natriuretic factor and is natriuretic in essential hypertension, *J. Hypertens.*, 10, 271–277, 1992.

171. Worthley, M.I., Corti, R., and Worthley, S.G., Vasopeptidase inhibitors: will they have a role in clinical practice?, *Br. J. Clin. Pharmacol.*, 57, 27–36, 2004.

172. Collier, J.G. et al., Comparison of effects of tolmesoxide (RX71108), diazoxide, hydrallazine, prazosin, glyceryl trinitrate and sodium nitroprusside on forearm arteries and dorsal hand veins of man, *Br. J. Clin. Pharmacol.*, 5, 35–44, 1978.

173. MacAllister, R.J. et al., Relative potency and arteriovenous selectivity of nitrovasodilators on human blood vessels: an insight into the targeting of nitric oxide delivery, *J. Pharmacol. Exp. Ther.*, 273, 154–160, 1995.

174. Bennett, P.H. et al., Screening and management of microalbuminuria in patients with diabetes mellitus: recommendations to the Scientific Advisory Board of the National Kidney Foundation from an ad hoc committee of the Council on Diabetes Mellitus of the National Kidney Foundation, *Am. J. Kidney Dis.*, 25, 107–112, 1995.

175. Mogensen, C.E., Microalbuminuria predicts clinical proteinuria and early mortality in maturity-onset diabetes, *N. Engl. J. Med.*, 310, 356–360, 1984.

176. Viberti, G.C. et al., Microalbuminuria as a predictor of clinical nephropathy in insulin-dependent diabetes mellitus, *Lancet*, i, 1430–1432, 1982.

177. Yudkin, J.S., Forrest, R.D. and Jackson, C.A., Microalbuminuria as predictor of vascular disease in non-diabetic subjects, Islington Diabetes Survey, *Lancet*, ii, 530–533, 1988.

178. Yuyun, M.F. et al., A prospective study of microalbuminuria and incident coronary heart disease and its prognostic significance in a British population: the EPIC–Norfolk study, *Am. J. Epidemiol.*, 159, 284–293, 2004.

179. Pontremoli, R. et al., Microalbuminuria: a marker of cardiovascular risk and organ damage in essential hypertension, *Kidney Int. Suppl.*, 63, S163–165, 1997.

180. Wachtell, K. et al., Albuminuria and cardiovascular risk in hypertensive patients with left ventricular hypertrophy: the LIFE study, *Ann. Intern. Med.*, 139, 901–906, 2003.

181. Pontremoli, R. et al., Microalbuminuria is an early marker of target organ damage in essential hypertension, *Am. J. Hypertens.*, 11, 430–438, 1998.

182. Romundstad, S. et al., Microalbuminuria and all-cause mortality in treated hypertensive individuals: does sex matter? The Nord–Trondelag Health Study (HUNT), Norway, *Circulation*, 108, 2783–2789, 2003.

183. Kieltyka, L., Framingham risk score is related to carotid artery intima-media thickness in both white and black young adults: the Bogalusa Heart Study, *Atherosclerosis*, 170, 125–130, 2003.

184. Takiuchi, S. et al., Diagnostic value of carotid intima-media thickness and plaque score for predicting target organ damage in patients with essential hypertension, *J. Hum. Hypertens.*, 18, 17–23, 2004.

185. Zizek, B. and Poredos, P., Dependence of morphological changes of the carotid arteries on essential hypertension and accompanying risk factors, *Int. Angiol.*, 21, 70–77, 2002.

186. Nolting, P.R., Regression of carotid and femoral artery intima-media thickness in familial hypercholesterolemia: treatment with simvastatin, *Arch. Intern. Med.*, 163, 1837–1841, 2003.

187. Terpstra, W.F. et al., Effects of nifedipine on carotid and femoral arterial wall thickness in previously untreated hypertensive patients, *Blood Press. Suppl.*, 1, 22–29, 2003.

188. Stanton, A.V. et al., Effects of blood pressure lowering with amlodipine or lisinopril on vascular structure of the common carotid artery, *Clin. Sci.*, 101, 455–464, 2001.

189. Simon, A. et al., Differential effects of nifedipine and co-amilozide on the progression of early carotid wall changes, *Circulation*, 103, 2949–2954, 2001.

190. Pearson, T.A. et al., Markers of inflammation and cardiovascular disease: application to clinical and public health practice, *Circulation*, 107, 499–511, 2003.

191. Fichtlscherer, S. et al., Elevated C-reactive protein levels and impaired endothelial vasoreactivity in patients with coronary artery disease, *Circulation*, 102, 1000–1006, 2000.

192. Ridker, P.M. et al., C-reactive protein and other markers of inflammation in the prediction of cardiovascular disease in women, *N. Engl. J. Med.*, 342, 836–843, 2000.

193. Lindahl, B., Markers of myocardial damage and inflammation in relation to long-term mortality in unstable coronary artery disease, *N. Engl. J. Med.*, 343, 1139–1147, 2000.

194. Freeman, D.J. et al., C-reactive protein is an independent predictor of risk for the development of diabetes in the West of Scotland Coronary Prevention Study, *Diabetes*, 51, 1596–1600, 2002.

195. Ridker, P.M. et al., C-reactive protein, the metabolic syndrome, and risk of incident cardiovascular events: an 8-year follow-up of 14,719 initially healthy American women, *Circulation*, 107, 391–397, 2003.

196. Medical Research Council, Medical Research Council: responsibility in investigations on human subjects, *Br. Med. J.*, 2, 178–180, 1964.

197. Declaration of Helsinki, Recommendations guiding doctors in clinical research (revised version, 1975), in *Law and Medical Ethics*, Mason, J.K. and McCall-Smith, R.A., Eds., 3rd ed., Butterworths, Edinburgh, 1991, pp. 446–449.

198. Rawlins, M.D., Pharmacovigilance: paradise lost, regained or postponed?, *J. R. Coll. Phys.*, 29, 41–49, 1995.

CHAPTER 15

Drugs for Treatment of Stroke

Mariola Soehngen, Wolfgang Soehngen, and Yasir Al-Rawi

CONTENTS

15.1 INTRODUCTION

To introduce the topic of stroke, it is best to start with the statements included in a brochure from the National Institute of Neurological Disorders and Stroke (NINDS), *Stroke: Hope Through Research*:

> More than 2400 years ago the father of medicine, Hippocrates, recognized and described stroke — the sudden onset of paralysis. Until recently, modern medicine has had very little power over this disease, but the world of stroke medicine is changing and new and better therapies are being developed every day. Today, some people who have a stroke can walk away from the attack with no or few disabilities *if they are treated promptly*. Doctors can finally offer stroke patients and their families the one thing that until now has been so hard to give: hope. In ancient times stroke was called *apoplexy*, a general term that physicians applied to anyone suddenly struck down with paralysis. Because many conditions can lead to sudden paralysis, the term apoplexy did not indicate a specific diagnosis or cause. Physicians knew very little about the cause of stroke and the only established therapy was to feed and care for the patient until the attack ran its course. The first person to investigate the pathological signs of apoplexy was Johann Jacob Wepfer. Born in Schaffhausen, Switzerland, in 1620, Wepfer studied medicine and was the first to identify postmortem signs of bleeding in the brains of patients who died of apoplexy. From autopsy studies he gained knowledge of the *carotid* and *vertebral arteries* that supply the brain with blood. He also was the first person to suggest that apoplexy, in addition to being caused by bleeding in the brain, could be caused by a blockage of one of the main arteries supplying blood to the brain; thus stroke became known as a *cerebrovascular disease* ("cerebro" refers to a part of the brain; "vascular" refers to the blood vessels and arteries). Medical science would eventually confirm Wepfer's hypotheses, but until very recently doctors could offer little in the area of therapy. Over the last two decades basic and clinical investigators, many of them sponsored and funded in part by the National Institute of Neurological Disorders and Stroke (NINDS), have learned a great deal about stroke. They have identified major risk factors for the disease and have developed surgical techniques and drug treatments for the prevention of stroke. But perhaps the most exciting new development in the field of stroke research is the recent approval of a drug treatment that can reverse the course of stroke if given during the first few hours after the onset of symptoms. Studies with animals have shown that brain injury occurs within minutes of a stroke and can become irreversible within as little as an hour. In humans, brain damage begins from the moment the stroke starts and often continues for days afterward. Scientists now know that there is a very short window of opportunity for treatment of the most common form of stroke. Because of these and other advances in the field of cerebrovascular disease stroke, patients now have a chance for survival and recovery.

While we concur with most of the above statements, we would like to stress that we strongly advocate expanding the time window for treatment because in many patients hope persists beyond the first hours after stroke onset. Due to the logistics and sometimes subtle symptoms at onset, most patients will never make it to a hospital within the current time window of 3 hours; however, we acknowledge that in any case, the earlier, the better.

This chapter is intended to describe some of the reasons why drug development programs for (acute ischemic) stroke have failed and what may be solutions to overcoming this dramatic lack of treatment options for the several million stroke victims around the world. The authors would like to thank the current and past members of the PAION development team for their contributions to the deliberation of this document. The debate on stroke treatment and drug development for stroke treatment resembles the dispute over the nature of acute myocardial infarction that those who went to medical school more than 20 years ago may recall. While recombinant tissue plasminogen activator (rt-PA) trials were ongoing there was still a broad group of supporters of the "vasospasm" theory. Right now, the dispute is centered around the question of how long after stroke onset we can initiate meaningful drug intervention. While more than 50% of the crowd will claim that there is no hope beyond 1 to 3 hours after onset, we and others believe in the individual "tissue clock" of each patient. This new paradigm is not widely favored, as it necessitates a restructuring of the way stroke patients are treated and classifying stroke as an emergency that requires immediate and adequate imaging in order to make an informed treatment (or no treatment) decision. Another dispute in the stroke community is reflected by the endless search for a "one-drug-fits-all" stroke treatment, which is a result of the blockbuster mentality of large pharmaceutical companies, healthcare providers, and stroke physicians. We want to stress that we do not believe that such a drug exists or will ever exist. In the era of growing knowledge of the human genome, the "one-drug-fits-all" approach may be substituted by an individualized treatment paradigm. It has been speculated that some of the stroke drugs that were stopped after a negative phase II or even phase III program suffered from the application of this approach, which is why we strongly advocate a careful and restrictive patient selection. All trials that went for the blockbuster approach eventually failed, and stroke is far away from having evidence-based medicine available.

15.1.1 Medical Need

The two major advances in stroke over the last decade have been the advent of stroke units and the availability of the first causal treatment for acute ischemic stroke, alteplase. The establishment of stroke units is on the agenda of many societies, as the burden of stroke on society and healthcare systems is growing due to the aging population in the developed world. It is estimated that in the United States alone stroke induces costs of more than $35 billion per year. While the progress due to these advances has made a major contribution to the care of stroke patients, it is without dispute that still no satisfactory treatment options exist for this debilitating condition.[1] The only causal treatment approved for this indication is alteplase, available in the United States, Canada, and European Union; however, the use of alteplase is restricted, first by the need to administer it within 3 hours of symptom onset[2] (although most patients arrive later than 3 hours after stroke onset) and, second, by the risk of cerebral bleeding complications.[2,3] Such risk was found to be particularly high in postmarketing surveillance studies of alteplase.[3] The increasing off-label use of alteplase is one of the strongest indicators for the huge medical need in this indication. On the other hand, all available data suggest that a reperfusion strategy is what is needed most in order to widen the treatment options for stroke.

15.1.2 Epidemiology

Stroke is a common cause of death and also an important cause of severe disability in people living in their own homes. It has been estimated that stroke causes over 4.4 million deaths in the world each year (3 million of these in developing countries) and, thus, is the second most important single cause of death (after ischemic heart disease).[4,5] In most Western populations, 0.2% (20 per 10,000) of the population per year suffer a stroke,[6] of whom one third die over the next year, one third remain permanently disabled, and one third make a reasonable recovery. Despite the high incidence of stroke events, the number of patients meeting a potential label (i.e., the patient population as defined by inclusion and exclusion criteria) treatable with a given drug may be low for the reasons described below.

The World Health Organization (WHO) definition of stroke is "rapidly developing clinical signs of focal (or global) disturbances of cerebral function, with symptoms lasting 24 hours or longer or leading to death, with no apparent cause other than of vascular origin." It is estimated that among patients hospitalized for stroke, 54 to 87% experienced ischemic stroke, 10.5% intracerebral hemorrhages, and 3.4% subarachnoid hemorrhages.[7] Several conditions and lifestyle factors have been identified as risk factors for stroke. These include systemic arterial hypertension, myocardial infarction, atrial fibrillation, diabetes mellitus, high cholesterol levels, carotid artery disease, smoking, and alcohol abuse. Satisfactory management of these risk factors is known to lead to a reduction in the incidence of stroke in asymptomatic people.[8] The symptoms associated with acute ischemic stroke are not always obvious, and patients often do not recognize immediately that they have experienced a stroke; consequently, hospitalization is still often delayed by several hours after stroke onset. This is worsened even more by the lack of urgency given to stroke patients, which is why in almost all countries major stroke programs now are underway and stroke units are being established.

15.1.2.1   Europe

Our research indicates that in principle the overall numbers of stroke for the United States and EU do not differ significantly. When we began our stroke program, we assessed whether stroke could be regarded as an orphan drug disease if one used an exact patient definition. The statement that stroke is an orphan drug disease may sound provocative; however, the authors believe that this is the best way to look at drug development in a therapeutic arena dominated by both nihilism and a search for the golden egg that has led to a vicious cycle of failure. On the other hand, some assume that stroke is probably underreported and underdiagnosed because currently no treatment options exist and no attention has been paid to diagnosing light or minor strokes.[9] When we began to explore the opportunity to extend the limited treatment window of rt-PA with a magnetic resonance imaging (MRI)-based approach, only a limited number of centers in the world could perform the necessary imaging in an acute setting. This situation has changed over time, and perfusion computed tomography (CT) is making a dramatic difference; nevertheless, we performed an in-depth epidemiology analysis for the EU in order to evaluate the possibility of an orphan drug application. The following data are the results of our search. Orphan drug status is granted if the prevalence of a disease is below 5 in 10,000 in the European community compared to a definition of "affecting less than 200,000 Americans" in the United States. For an acute condition such as acute ischemic stroke, the incidence must be set equal to the prevalence, as in such a setting acute treatment cannot generally be extended to those who have suffered the event (stroke) in the past. Table 15.1 illustrates how a thrombolytic drug (and other drugs) can become an orphan drug candidate if one would only target those who have viable penumbra (a perfusion-weighted imaging [PWI]/diffusion-weighted imaging [DWI] mismatch and other criteria). For an orphan drug application, one has to define a condition that describes exactly the future targeted patient population. The methodology to arrive at these numbers is described below.

Sources for Incidence Data on Stroke — Regarding the frequency of incidence of acute ischemic stroke, four data sources can be distinguished: population-based studies, population-based registries, hospital registries, and data from secondary literature such as health insurance reports. We used several approaches to get the best estimate of stroke incidence in the EU. The first approach was to contact all official epidemiological institutes of the EU countries in order to get the most up-to-date stroke attack rates and incidence data from nationwide registries. The second approach was a comprehensive literature search. This search focused on publications of population-based studies and registries. Data from hospital registries were only incorporated when no other sources were available, as hospital registries generally do not include outpatients and are often selection biased. Expert opinions are regarded as the lowest level of evidence and were only included in the analysis when no other references were available.

Table 15.1 Analysis of Incidence Data on Stroke in Europe

Country	Case Definition	Incidence/10,000
Austria	—	No data available[a]
Belgium	Total stroke	No data available[a]
Denmark*	Total stroke	19 (1990)
	Total stroke	19.9 (male); 16.6 (female) (1991)
Finland	Total Stroke	20.1 (male); 23.9 (female) (1990)
France*	Total stroke	14.5 (1985)
	Total stroke	10.0 (1995–1997)
Germany	Total stroke	13.4 (1994–1996)
	Total stroke	13.6 (1995–1997)
	Total stroke	13.6 (1997)
	Total stroke	20.0 (2000)
Greece	—	No data available[a]
Ireland	—	No data available[a]
Italy*	Total stroke	22.8 (1994–1998)
	Total stroke	15.5 (1986–1989)
Luxembourg	—	No data available[a]
Netherlands	—	No data available[a]
Portugal	—	No data available[a]
Spain	Total stroke	18.3 (1968–1996)
Sweden	Total stroke	22.5 (1989)
United Kingdom	Total stroke	12.5 (1995–1997)

[a] Accessed data not comparable in terms of published criteria.[12]

Data from Official Stroke Registries — In order to get the most up-to-date information on stroke epidemiology, we tried to access data directly from official stroke registries. Within the scope of the provided data, we asked for the criteria or parameters of registration and partly received documents (e.g., as to whether or not the recommendations of the National Institute of Health Stroke Scale [NIHSS] had an effect on the data collection or whether the modified Rankin scale [MRS] was included in the registration process to investigate neurological deficits). The overall output was disappointingly low, which reflects the unsatisfactory availability of data on stroke incidences in the EU. Except for some Scandinavian countries (Finland and Sweden), no validated national stroke registries were established; hence, it was necessary to investigate stroke incidence in all other mentioned countries on a regional basis or even on a hospital basis. Due to the current data protection regulations, these national stroke registries are not publicly accessible. Some countries have national databases for all hospital admittances, but the case definitions in these statistics are very imprecise. Even if the International Classification of Diseases (ICD) codes are used for identification of stroke causes (e.g., ischemic or hemorrhagic stroke), the ICD code does not routinely include a differentiation between first-ever and recurrent stroke. Moreover, it includes no details about the diagnostic methods used. For these reasons, registered cerebrovascular diseases in accordance to the ICD code in Austria, Denmark, Luxembourg, Portugal, and the Netherlands were of no value for the purpose of this evaluation.

Published Epidemiological Data on Stroke — This comprehensive literature search focused on publications of population-based studies and registries. For the reasons mentioned above, data from hospital registries were only incorporated when no other sources were available; expert opinions were not taken into account for the final incidence analysis. They were only compared to the data from other sources and discussed in this context. Population-based studies and registries have the advantage that they provide very precise data on the frequency of a disease in the study population, depending on the criteria for case ascertainment. Especially in the epidemiology of stroke, data accuracy critically hinges on case definition. A review of Malmgren et al.[10] published in 1987 found only 9 of 65 studies with incidence rates (all types of stroke combined) that could be compared reasonably. Until recently, most epidemiological studies were based primarily on "total stroke," in some cases with separate analysis of the clinical syndrome of spontaneous subarachnoid hemorrhage. Even though the increased availability of CT scanning or MRI has improved diagnostic possibilities, it remains difficult to get timely scans of all patients to exclude primary intracerebral hemorrhage.[11] In their comprehensive review, Sudlow and Warlow[12] discussed the difficulty of comparing stroke rates in different parts of the world and at different points in time. They defined standard criteria for almost "ideal" and comparable stroke incidence studies. These criteria included the definition of stroke, a complete community-based case ascertainment including strokes managed outside the hospital, and a standard data presentation. Moreover, they suggested an approach for measuring and comparing the incidence of the pathological types of stroke. Few of the published epidemiological studies on stroke fulfill these criteria. From a total of 35 studies published by the end of 1994, only 11 were selected according to the methods described.[6] Out of these, six studies were performed in Europe: the Oxfordshire Community project,[13] the Dijon registry,[14] Italian registries in Valle d'Aosta[15] and Umbria,[16] the Danish study in Fredericksberg,[17] and an unpublished study in Söderhamn (Sweden). Data from these studies were chosen as the basis for epidemiological evaluation of stroke incidence in this primary market research model. The results are marked with an asterisk (*) in Table 15.1. Moreover, we tried to identify the most reliable sources for other European countries. According to the analysis of Sudlow and Warlow, age- and sex-standardized annual incidence rates of subjects ages 45 to 84 years were similar in most places. Moreover, the distribution of different types — when these were reliably distinguished — did not differ significantly between studies. This is perhaps not surprising, given that all the populations studied have a similar lifestyle and are predominantly Caucasians.

15.1.2.2   United States

In the United States, data on stroke incidence are seemingly easier to obtain; however, the figures still vary from 500,000 to more than 700,000 stroke victims annually. According to the most recent statistics from the American Heart Association (AHA), the age-adjusted incidence rates are 16.7, 13.8, 32.3, and 26.0 per 10,000 for white males, white females, black males, and black females, respectively. Hospital discharges total more than 900,000 each year, which includes restroke (an estimated 200,000 per year). Although stroke is the third leading cause of death in the United States today, the current understanding of its etiology and variations (among groups and over time) seems to be insufficient. Stroke remains a challenging disease for several reasons. For example, distinguishing among cerebral infarction subtypes is a problem, and most publications (as in Europe) lack sufficient clarity about subtype. The numbers on hemorrhage vs. infarction are not always correct, as many asymptomatic transformations that occur in the natural cause of disease may lead one to classify from an ischemic stroke to a hemorrhagic stroke. Furthermore, the influence of several confounding factors has become apparent, including gender, geographic region (the stroke belt in the southern states of the United States), socioeconomic status, and ethnicity. The situation is complicated even more by a number of social factors such as availability of medical care. These factors may have a major impact on the design of clinical trials for stroke (i.e., stratification for ethnicity).

15.1.2.3   Japan

In Japan, the epidemiology is difficult to assess because the only "public" information is written in Japanese; however, the following figures have been confirmed by several Japanese companies. Total stroke incidence is approximately 200,000, of which more than 15% (in some cases up to

30%) are thought to be hemorrhagic. The estimates for recurrent stroke seem to be somewhat higher than those in the rest of the world. As of this writing, we have been unable to identify if these discrepancies are a result of reporting or of diagnosing differences (e.g., transitory ischemic attacks [TIAs] being counted as strokes) and if they are real. It is of special interest that the incidence of hemorrhagic strokes is significantly higher in Japan vs. the rest of world. It can be hypothesized that this is due to the fact that asymptomatic hemorrhagic transformations that occur during hospital stays in Japan (usually longer than in the Western world) are counted as hemorrhagic strokes.

15.1.2.4 Rest of the World

Figures for the rest of the world (RoW) are best taken from a publication of WHO in which stroke is listed as the number three disease with one of the highest burdens in any society.[4,5]

15.1.2.5 Conclusions

Assessments of the actual stroke rate that can be treated with a given drug and its specific profile may vary greatly. Based on our own primary and secondary research, we estimate the incidence of stroke (this excludes recurrent strokes) in the developed world to be 2.3 million per year. For planning, we suggest that the target group for each drug should be defined on the following parameters:

- Time to treatment window
- Stroke severity
- Hemorrhagic stroke vs. ischemic infarction
- Availability of suitable imaging within 24 hours (e.g., almost no 24-hour service is available in the United Kingdom)
- Other specific criteria (e.g., blood pressure, heart conditions, comedication)

When one completes such an exercise, it becomes obvious that almost no drug imaginable could target the entire population. In our case of a thrombolytic stroke, utilizing a 9-hour time window, this exercise reduced the 2.3 million target population to approximately 600,000.

15.1.3 Current Treatment Options

The current treatment of stroke consists of four main approaches. The first, *general management*, describes what has to be done for every patient in order to provide an optimal physiological basis upon which specific therapeutic treatment strategies can be built. General management of stroke patients comprises respiratory and cardiac care, fluid and metabolic management, blood pressure control, and treatment of elevated intracranial pressure if present. Table 15.2 shows the pharmacological substances (selection) used when treating patients with acute stroke.

The second approach of stroke treatment is the use of *specific therapy* directed at different aspects of stroke pathogenesis. Because stroke is primarily caused by acute local or embolic vascular occlusion, one technique is recanalization. Thrombolytic therapy with intravenous alteplase given within 3 hours after stroke onset to patients with acute ischemic stroke significantly improves the outcome after stroke.[2] The use of intravenous alteplase has changed the way acute ischemic stroke is approached; however, intravenous alteplase carries a considerably higher risk of intracerebral hemorrhage compared to placebo.[2] Current marketing experience in the United States shows that only a very limited number of stroke patients have access to alteplase due to this early time window and the bleeding risk, which makes physicians reluctant to use it;[2,3] therefore, intravenous alteplase as a treatment for acute ischemic stroke remains far from being optimal.[18–20]

The third main approach of stroke treatment is *prophylaxis and treatment of complications*, which may be either neurological (such as secondary hemorrhage, space-occupying edema, or seizures) or symptomatic medical treatment (such as infection, decubital ulcers, or pulmonary embolism prophylaxis).

Table 15.2 Drugs for Treatment of Stroke

Generic Name	Mode of Action	Adverse Reactions	Precautions/Remarks
Alteplase	Thrombolytic	Bleeding events: major bleeding, symptomatic intracranial bleeding	NIHSS >25, extended early changes of a major infarction; for use by experienced physician only; requires continuous observation of patient
Heparin	Anticoagulant	Bleeding: skin, mucosa, gastrointestinal, urogenital	Renal/liver impairment, uncontrolled high blood pressure; specific indications only (cardiac source with high risk of reembolism, arterial dissection high-grade a. stenosis). For thrombolytic therapy, administer only after 24-hour post-thrombolytic therapy unless a high risk of deep vein thrombosis exists.
Low-molecular-weight heparin (LMWH) and heparinoid (dalteparin, nadroparin, tinzaparin, danaparoid)	Anticoagulant	Bleeding: skin, mucosa, gastrointestinal, urogenital	Renal/liver impairment, uncontrolled high blood pressure. For thrombolytic therapy, administer only after 24-hour post-thrombolytic therapy unless a high risk of deep vein thrombosis exists.
Aspirin	Antiplatelet	Bleeding: gastrointestinal and other	Do not administer if thrombolytic therapy is planned or administer only after 24-hour post-thrombolytic therapy.
Clopidogrel	Antiplatelet	Bleeding	Do not administer if thrombolytic therapy is planned or administer only after 24-hour post-thrombolytic therapy.
Dipyridamole	Antiplatelet	Bleeding	Do not administer if thrombolytic therapy is planned or administer only after 24-hour post-thrombolytic therapy.
Mannitol	Osmotic diuretic	Fluid and electrolyte imbalance	Use in cases of cerebral edema.
Furosemide	Diuretic	Fluid and electrolyte imbalance, orthostatic hypotension, tinnitus	Use in cases of cerebral edema.
Corticosteroids	Antiinflammatory	Fluid and electrolyte imbalance, peptic ulcer	Use in cases of cerebral edema.

The fourth approach is early *rehabilitation*. Although this aspect does not change the neurological deficit, it helps victims to become ambulatory and largely independent. Of importance is the fact that most patients are able to live at home and do not require nursing-home care.

The prevention of stroke is aimed at reducing the risk of stroke in asymptomatic people at risk. This is termed *primary prevention* and consists of modification of life behaviors (e.g., less smoking and lower intakes of salt, alcohol, and fat). This is achieved by public health education. In *secondary prevention*, the use of drug therapy such as antiplatelet agents (e.g., aspirin, ticlopidine, dipyridamole) and anticoagulants (e.g., heparin) are used to reduce the risk of occurrence or recurrence of ischemic events.

It is important to note that general management, prophylaxis, and treatment of complications as well as rehabilitation form the basic treatment, which leads to a response rate (i.e., significant reduction of disability) of approximately 20% in placebo-controlled studies, when the response is measured 90 days after stroke.

15.2 THE FUTURE OF STROKE TREATMENT

Quite intensive research and development are being conducted to improve stroke therapy. So many clinical trials have failed in acute stroke despite promising preclinical data that efforts today are aimed at finding new ways to attack this debilitating disease. The NINDS has published an overview in its brochure *Stroke: Hope Through Research* (http://www.ninds.nih.gov/index.htm) detailing the areas in which stroke research and development are being undertaken. In addition to studying the mechanisms of stroke, the influence of risk factors, and the different types of strokes and their impact on therapy, various treatment options are being looked at with regard to their effectiveness in treating different subtypes of strokes. Further, the class of neuroprotectives must be mentioned, as well as newer generations of thrombolytics, medical devices, anticoagulants, and advanced imaging methods to determine the correct subtype of a stroke and allow patients access to the optimal therapy for their specific medical conditions.

While research and development activities have been undertaken on the above-mentioned targets, most of them did not render positive clinical results that would have allowed filing of a new drug application (NDA); therefore, the Stroke Therapy Academic Industry Roundtable (STAIR) III has suggested targeting primarily combinations of the above interventions, as the complex stroke pathophysiology would most probably necessitate such an approach.[21] This is a complicated endeavor as most of the stroke therapies are still under development and most probably will not be able to show efficacy on their own. The classical way of bringing a drug to market as a monotherapy and trying combinations with other drugs (ideally also on the market already) may not work in the special situation of treating acute stroke (and might not work in other multimodal diseases that are thus far untreated as well). The STAIR III[21] consensus paper recognizes imaging methods as the primary target of future development activities to identify patients who might be treated after some time delay (with regard to the onset of stroke symptoms). In parallel, agents that have the potential to treat patients in later time windows should be evaluated (preferably in combination). Treatments such as stem cell therapy, nerve growth factors, antileukocyte agents, and modulation of antiapoptotic pathways are considered to have the potential in very late time windows (e.g., >6 hours after the onset of stroke symptoms). Agents from the neuroprotective field and newer fibrinolytics and anticoagulants with a specific safety profile are being regarded to potentially target the earlier time window of 3 to 6 hours. Medical devices might be applied within this time window as well and even later if they show sufficient safety in clinical trials. Transcranial magnetic stimulation (TMS) is used to enhance the rehabilitation efforts by influencing the plasticity of the brain. Although this targets the rehabilitation period (i.e., days or weeks) after an acute stroke, it seems to be advantageous to start such a therapy as early as possible as well.[22,23]

Just as what has happened when developing therapies for acute myocardial infarction (with quite a similar pathophysiology when compared to stroke), it seems logical to begin an acute stroke treatment with a causative therapy, such as reperfusion, in order to remove the clot that caused the condition and free the way for other agents to access the damaged area in the brain. The subject of ongoing academic discussion, when to add a neuroprotective compound (i.e., before or after thrombolysis) may depend on the mechanism of action of a particular drug and the pharmacokinetics of the respective drug. If the drug is interfering with some early changes in stroke (e.g., radical scavenging), then it should be administered as early as possible. If it interferes with late events (e.g., leukocyte infiltration), it could be administered later. If the drug has a short half-life, it should be given as a continuous infusion beginning around the pathophysiologically sensible time point. A drug with a long half-life could be given in a shot as soon as the patient enters the hospital, especially when the drug has a good safety profile and will not interfere with a potential thrombolysis. While the above describes the current hypotheses, the authors suggest that any concurrent treatment to reperfusion therapy should be initiated as soon as possible.

Thrombolysis so far seems to be effective and safe only in the time window of 0 to 3 hours, which led to the approval of rt-PA for acute ischemic stroke; however, newer drugs such as desmoteplase have shown a positive risk–benefit ratio in the late time window of 3 to 9 hours.[24,25] These drugs could offer new ways to treat patients who come to the hospital late. Furthermore, the data show that the ischemic tolerance of the brain seems to be substantially longer than anticipated (as patients coming in late after an acute stroke had the same potential to benefit from therapy when compared to early-arriving patients).

Combining neuroprotective drugs with such newer thrombolytics might have three (or even more) effects. First, the neuroprotective drug might exert its efficacy, which so far could not be shown in any clinical trial convincingly. Second, the safety profile of the thrombolytic might be improved (e.g., the bleeding rate might be reduced).[26] Third, the time window of both drugs might be prolonged through positive additive effects. This is a hypothesis, but preclinical studies hint that such a scenario might well work. It requires an alliance of academia, regulatory agencies, and industry and the ultimate will to improve stroke treatment through unconventional methods while maintaining the patients' safety.

Other methods would be added as needed and driven by the medical situation; for example, catheters to remove clots could be used before thrombolysis (in the case of exceptionally long clots) or as an adjunct to thrombolysis (in case of unresponsive or organized clots). Safe anticoagulants could be coadministered in order to prevent early reocclusion of an opened artery or to prevent further clot growth in case no thrombolysis would be performed. Stem cell therapy might have its place if the damaged brain area was too big to find compensation of its function through other (neighboring) areas. TMS could be used as a routine method to enhance the rehabilitation process and shorten this cost-intensive phase.

Finally, as we can see it today in acute myocardial infarction treatment, stroke treatment of the future would be a whole portfolio of treatment methods that would have additive effects and should be prescribed as needed (not all patients are fit for thrombolysis, and good thrombolysis responders might not need any rehabilitation at all). The aim is to coordinate all available resources and efforts to improve the very unsatisfactory condition of stroke treatment today.

15.3 PRECLINICAL DEVELOPMENT

While rt-PA is the only approved drug for use in humans for the treatment of acute ischemic stroke, hundreds of drugs have demonstrated proof of concept in animal models. We, therefore, recommend cautiously extrapolating any findings in animals to the expected findings in humans. A particular warning would also apply to drawing conclusions from animal studies regarding time windows. This caution goes for both limited and extended time windows. In our own program, we have not been able to show that the drug protects the brain of animals for more than 2 to 3 hours, but we can show that patients benefit if treated beyond 6 hours. The authors even believe that the use of primates will not change the picture. The main reason is that the real pathophysiology in humans cannot be mimicked closely enough even in the most sophisticated animal model. From our perspective, a model is needed that has some form of a clot involved and has penumbra (reduced blood flow) as defined by Heiss.[27] In 1983, Heiss defined the ischemic penumbra as a region of tissue receiving blood flow above the threshold for loss of morphological integrity and below the threshold for functional integrity. Fisher and colleagues have shown that the penumbra in rats only exists for some 30 minutes (M. Fisher, pers. comm.). In a recent paper, Hillis and colleagues[28] showed that the penumbra can be present for several days in patients who have an elevated blood pressure, which seems to be the survival mechanism for the human brain. It seems unclear if such a model can be established in a suitable animal model at all; therefore, we recommend minimizing animal studies to show the effectiveness of a drug in principle and moving on to patients with the best available imaging methodology, which currently is MRI. In a few years, other technologies may become available that are similar to perfusion CT and others that can give the same qualitative and quantitative measurements.

15.3.1 Basic Preclinical Development

Before beginning clinical development of any given substance, nonclinical safety studies are required according to international standards (e.g., ICH M3 guideline, http://www.ich.org) to support use of the drug in humans. A stroke compound must comply with such standards, and literally no differences exist in the basic preclinical development when compared to compounds targeting other indications. It has to be kept in mind that a preclinical program has to promote safe and ethical development of a drug and forms the basis of first administration in humans. As such, preclinical activities focus on efficacy (pharmacodynamics) and safety (toxicity and pharmacokinetics) in at least two species in the basic preclinical program. Furthermore, it is common sense that the program should be structured in such a way as to minimize the unnecessary use of animals, which results in considerably smaller preclinical packages prior to phase I activities; however, these programs must be defined in such a way that they allow good extrapolation with regard to safety and efficacy in humans. Although the exact preclinical requirements differ slightly throughout the world, they agree on basic principles.

First of all is the emphasis on the safety evaluation of a given compound. At a minimum, before moving to phase I development activities, two acute toxicology studies in two different species as well as two repeated dose toxicology studies in two different species (usually rats and mice in both cases) are required for regulatory authorities and investigational review boards (IRBs). The aim of such studies is to test increasingly high dosages in acute situations to define the upper tolerance level as well as to study which organs are affected by the (overdosed) substance. In the repeated dose situation, it is more important to study the subacute to long-term effects of the substance with lower (tolerable) dose levels and the influence on various organ systems, which can differ from the acute setting. The length of the repeated dose toxicology studies varies depending on the length of the intended use in humans and is detailed in the above-mentioned ICH guideline; for example, for a single-dose study in humans, the minimum duration of the repeated dose toxicology study should be 2 weeks before beginning phase I and II activities. Such studies are also used to evaluate the pharmacokinetics to obtain information on the fate of the drug in the body. Furthermore, the standard battery of genotoxicity studies (ICH S 2B guideline, http://www.ich.org) must be accomplished before beginning phase I and II studies. Such standard packages generally consist of three studies characterizing the potential drug effect on the individual genes as well as chromosome aberrations. These studies are performed *in vitro* and in at least one *in vivo* model. In summary, the preclinical toxicology program should allow the researcher to determine the potential toxic effects that might be observed during the future clinical trials.

Another important question that must be addressed before any clinical study is initiated is pharmacodynamic validation (efficacy). In other words, does the drug do in the body what it is expected to do? Indication-specific animal models are generally used to answer this question; for the medical condition of stroke, specific stroke models have been developed and are being used internationally.

Naturally, in parallel to the clinical development program, more preclinical studies will be conducted in order to characterize the substance further; however, they usually are not mandatory before moving to phase I. Such studies will consist of further pharmacodynamic models as well as safety pharmacology studies to evaluate the influence of more physiological dosages (when compared to the above-mentioned toxicology studies) on the various main organ systems. Additional toxicology studies, such as reproduction toxicology, carcinogenicity, and local tolerance, to name just a few, will be performed depending on the nature of the drug, its risk profile, and the intended human use.

Finally, we should mention that the basic preclinical requirements might be different for a biotechnology-derived substance. Depending on the profile of such a substance, it might not be possible to perform pharmacodynamic studies in animals, as the drug might not have a target in an animal model (e.g., a human antibody or a human protein); therefore, it would not be necessary to initiate these studies because the results (if any) would be useless. Furthermore, a protein drug will not exert any effects in the genotoxicity tests. A protein generally does not enter the cell nucleus, so these tests might be superfluous. In such situations, the ultimate aim is to test the drug under development as quickly as possible in a human model — that is, design a fast into-humans program under internationally accepted conditions. In this context, even a reduced preclinical program with sound basic pharmacology and the above-mentioned toxicology studies might be sufficient to generate the necessary data for a safe start in phase I. At the very least, the data must hint at what dosages to use in phase I and what basic safety profile might be expected. The ICH S 6 guideline (http://www.ich.org) provides further guidance on how to handle these situations, and it is highly advisable to discuss any abbreviated program with regulatory authorities at an early time point.

15.3.2 Stroke Models

Recent recommendations from the Stroke Therapy Academic Industry Roundtable (STAIR)[29] group include the following guidelines for preclinical development. A dose–response study should be performed in animal models, and the timing of experimental treatment should approximate the time window of therapeutic opportunity. In other words, the time course of cerebral infarction has been described in animals and humans, so experimental therapy should be initiated at times after the onset of ischemia that correspond to the likely initiation of thrombolytic treatment in the clinic or at least within the time window available for clinical treatment. It is generally accepted that the best efficacy in humans is realized with early thrombolytic treatment (preferably within 1 to 3 hours, but perhaps up to 9 hours with newer thrombolytics) after the onset of ischemia. The time course of cerebral infarction in rats, as outlined by Chopp and colleagues,[30] shows that in rat focal ischemia models the time window for beneficial therapy is shorter than in humans. Chopp et al.[30] demonstrated complete infarction of the area at risk in rats within 2 to 4 hours. In addition, it may be possible to extend this time window with neuroprotectant treatment.[31] It is also important to distinguish between permanent artery occlusion vs. reperfusion models because of the substantial differences between the two models in the temporal evolution of the lesions, pattern of neutrophil infiltration, and chronology of microvascular occlusion. Thus, neuroprotective drugs should be evaluated in both reperfusion and permanent occlusion models.

With regard to the experimental principles of animal testing, the STAIR group[29] recommends avoiding the use of mice (except transgenic models) and gerbils. They recommend starting with rats for initial experiments and then possibly proceeding on to cats or nonhuman primates. The wealth of preclinical literature supports these recommendations.

Physiological monitoring, whenever possible, should be performed to keep confounding variables to a minimum (e.g., blood pressure, pAO_2, $pACO_2$, body temperature, and blood glucose). It is important to monitor physiological parameters during the experimental procedures to identify any confounding differences between treatment and control groups. Induction of hypothermia is protective.[32] In addition, blood pressure, relative oxygenation of the blood, and blood glucose concentration each could affect the size of resulting cerebral infarct. Infarct volume and functional responses should be determined. Functional recovery should be assessed acutely (1 to 3 days) and over a longer term (7 to 30 days). Some functional tests include paw placing, reaching, and spontaneous limb use. Cognitive tests such as the Morris water maze[33] may be useful. Many animal studies have relied on infarct size after only a day or two. It has been shown in at least one study that treatment may remain without effect on infarct size and still improve recovery of function when measured weeks later.[34] Consider using a thrombotic model such as autologous clot embolism in the middle cerebral artery (MCA) with reperfusion induced by a thrombolytic agent. Alternatively, one could use a permanent MCA occlusion if thrombolytic therapy will not be used. A markedly reduced infarct volume has been obtained in female compared with male rats in middle cerebral artery occlusion (MCAO) models and models of myocardial infarction. This finding has been attributed to differences in circulating estrogens exerting glucocorticoid effects. For first experiments, it might be best to use only males in order to eliminate unnecessary variability.

Table 15.3 Parallels Between Treatment for Acute Myocardial Infarction and Acute Cerebral Ischemia/Infarction

Early reperfusion after arterial occlusion is protective, measured by infarct size and recovery of function.

A critical species-specific time window exists for thrombolytic therapy to be optimally effective.

A critical species-specific time window exists for (myocardial- or neuro-) protective activity.

Clinically, the development of critical care centers with the ability to administer a thrombolytic intravenously as early as possible is seen as necessary in order to obtain ultimate benefits of early reperfusion.

Preclinical studies have shown a plethora of agents that are protective when used during permanent occlusion or in combination with thrombolytic therapy.

Reperfusion itself is shown to contribute to injury (reperfusion injury) as evidenced by protection with agents that inhibit inflammatory cell adhesion or inhibitors of reactive oxygen species (ROS), including scavengers and enzymes capable of metabolizing these ROS.

15.3.2.1 Similarities Between Stroke and Acute Myocardial Infarction

Many similarities exist between myocardial infarction and stroke with respect to preclinical and clinical development histories (see Table 15.3). The process of myocardial infarction involves a blockage of blood flow to the myocardium via a clot in a coronary artery. With the development of ischemia and subsequent reperfusion with thrombolytic agents, activation of endothelial adhesion molecules occurs and an accumulation of neutrophils within the damaged tissue is observed. Protection by blocking neutrophil adhesion molecules has been demonstrated.[35,36] In addition, a time window of therapy[37] was described for this beneficial therapy, similar to that described later for the brain. The process of cerebral infarction follows similar pathological processes. With occlusion of a cerebral artery, activation of endothelial cell adhesion molecule expression and the accumulation of neutrophils are also associated with the process of cerebral infarction. Moreover, the depletion of neutrophils has been shown to reduce the size of cerebral infarct,[30] as was shown in the heart in the early 1980s.[38] In addition, experiments have demonstrated protection by blocking the neutrophil adhesion molecule CD11b/CD18 in the heart[39,40] and in the brain.[41]

Clinical experience in myocardial infarction and stroke demonstrates a number of parallels between the two diseases. It was determined very early in the 1980s that critical care centers for the treatment of acute myocardial infarction with thrombolytics were needed. With the use of early thrombolytics, such as streptokinase and then t-PA, monitoring of coagulation during treatment was considered absolutely necessary, especially when combined with anticoagulants such as heparin. With the development of even more fibrin-selective fibrinolytic agents, the daily use of these agents outside of the hospital has become more practical. For stroke, a need for critical care centers for the treatment of acute stroke with thrombolytics has also been recognized. The advent of more reliable diagnostic imaging systems (such as MRI) using perfusion- and diffusion-weighted imaging has made the diagnosis of acute stroke and estimation of cerebral infarct size more accurate.[42-45]

In both the heart and the brain, the microvasculature becomes plugged during reperfusion. This has been attributed at least in part to neutrophil aggregates. Evidence supporting this hypothesis includes experiments involving antiadhesion therapy for neutrophils or depletion of neutrophils from the animal before infarcting the heart or the brain, protected against the no-reflow phenomenon. The possibility also exists that anticoagulants may help in preventing this no-reflow phenomenon. Anticoagulants are used routinely for the treatment of myocardial infarction but have been avoided in the treatment of cerebral infarction. This is probably due primarily to the risk or perceived risk of intracranial hemorrhage; however, new and safer anticoagulants may eventually be employed for the clinical treatment of cerebral infarction.

Table 15.4 Recommended Small Animal Models

Model	Problem
Two-vessel occlusion–reperfusion with hypotension. This model involves occlusion of the two common carotid arteries and reducing blood pressure to 50 mmHg by partial exsanguination. This results in extensive destruction of pyramidal neurons and CA1 cells of the hippocampus.	Difficult to make sure that blood pressure remains at 50 mml Ig.
Four-vessel occlusion model of forebrain ischemia. This model employs electrocautery of vertebral arteries, with placement of an occluding device around each common carotid artery. The occluder device is then exteriorized ventrally at the neck. On the next day, the carotid arteries are occluded. This model results in hippocampal destruction.	Even in the most experienced hands only 50% of experimental animals survive the procedure.
Bilateral forebrain compression ischemia model. This model uses infusion of artificial CSF into the cisterna magna to elevate pressure above arterial pressure. Reflex hypertension is prevented by ganglionic blockers.	This is not a model of stroke; more of a closed-head injury model of ischemia.
Graded unilateral hemispheral ischemia. This model uses temporary unilateral carotid occlusion and mechanical elevation of CSF pressure to 40–45 mmHg.	This is more of an injury model than a model of stroke.
Global ischemia by neck tourniquet. Pressure cuff (600–700 mmHg) is used around the neck to produce global brain ischemia. Blood withdrawal counters reflex cardiovascular responses and increases blood pressure.	This is not a stroke model; it is more like a global ischemia model of delayed cardiorespiratory resuscitation.
Decapitation	This model is not an *in vivo* model of ischemia, thus is not a model of stroke.
Global ischemia in the rat by occlusion of the great vessels in the thorax	Global ischemia is not a model of stroke.
Levine preparation of hypoxia-ischemia. Wistar rats are used with a unilateral carotid ligation; 24 hours later the animals are placed into a hypoxic chamber for a defined period of time.	Pathophysiologically, this is not very similar to stroke.
Focal ischemia. MCA occlusion is a good model of thromboembolic stroke. Rats with spontaneous hypertension (SHR rats) are more susceptible to infarction. An advantage is that this model results in reproducible infarct size and neurological deficits when performed by skilled scientists.	These animals exhibit homogeneous infarcts. Clinical cerebral infarction patients, overall, have very heterogeneous infarcts.

15.3.2.2   Small-Animal Models for Experimental Stroke

Ginsberg[46] has reviewed some of the many different small-animal models that have been employed over the years for the preclinical study of stroke. Table 15.4 mentions a few of these models and discusses why they are or are not ideal for pharmaceutical preclinical development.

15.3.2.3   Recommended Animal Models for Preclinical Development of Drugs for Stroke Treatment

The most widely used and most accepted preclinical animal models for cerebral ischemia are the various versions of rat focal ischemic models. Middle cerebral artery (MCA) occlusion and reperfusion is widely accepted as a good model to use to test agents that will be administered as adjunctive treatment with thrombolytic agents. This model can also be used as a permanent occlusion model. Some neuroprotective compounds have shown efficacy in this model even without reperfusion.

- *Rat MCA occlusion by electrocautery for permanent occlusion.*[47–49] This model was useful for showing the protective effects of neuroserpin on infarct size assessed after 72 hours of regional ischemia. Advantages of this model include the relative ease of performing the surgery and the relative ease of performing behavioral and cognitive functional recovery tests with rats, as well as the relative affordability of using large enough groups of animals to see a treatment effect.

- *Rat MCAO model with the use of a small piece of suture inserted into the lumen of the middle cerebral artery.*[50,51] The suture can be removed mechanically after a period of ischemia and the brain reperfused for a specified amount of time. Phillips and colleagues[52] used this model to assess the protective effect of a proteasome inhibitor on infarct size and accumulation of inflammatory cells within the infarct tissue. In addition, they used this model to determine the time window of optimal therapy after reperfusion by treating with drug at reperfusion, or after 2 or 4 hours of reperfusion. Again, the advantages include cost and ability to perform functional recovery. Table 15.4 provides a list of potential behavioral, functional, and cognitive tests of recovery.
- *Rat MCAO embolic occlusion model.*[31,53–55] An autologous fibrin-rich clot is formed *in vitro* and then placed into the MCA via the carotid artery. This model is useful for using a thrombolytic agent alone or in combination with other agents. Others have used this model in a similar fashion but have formed clots in many different ways. It has been shown that the fibrin composition of the clot is important in determining the relative ease of fibrinolysis. Neuroprotection (e.g., with excitatory amino acid antagonists[56] in an embolic stroke model in rats with delayed thrombolytic treatment) was shown to be measurable by infarct sizes. In addition, a rat embolic stroke model with fibrin-rich microemboli[57] showed protection with citicoline when combined with thrombolytic therapy.
- *Hemorrhagic stroke.* To study the effects of drugs on hemorrhagic stroke, two models may be of interest. These include an *in vitro* model of exacerbation of neuronal injury by hemoglobin[58] and an *in vivo* model of intracranial hemorrhage in the rat described as the double-blood model.[59] The latter model uses injection of whole blood directly into the ventricles of the brain. The effects of free-radical scavengers may be studied in these models, due to the known role of hemoglobin in promoting free-radical species production. Although neither of these two models is really a model of stroke, they may be useful to test for protective effects of new agents on blood-induced injuries that occur sometimes with cerebral infarction.
- *Rabbit embolic stroke models.*[60–67] Rabbits have been used extensively as embolic stroke models in a similar fashion as the rat models; however, rabbit behavioral and functional recovery tests are less common than with rats and mice.
- *Primate models.* Baboons[68–72] have been used to study cerebral infarction. It has been suggested that neurological recovery from small infarcts in baboons is very similar to recovery seen with small infarcts in humans. Of course, the relative costs of experiments with baboons have to be considered when planning experiments; they might be used for the last preclinical efficacy experiment before beginning human tests. Also, species specificity of agents may be a consideration inasmuch as baboons are genetically closer to humans than rats. Squirrel monkeys may be used to follow small infarcts and recovery.[73] Cynomolgous monkeys may also be used for cerebral infarction studies. Marmosets[74–77] are another small animal model and also a primate species.

15.3.2.4 *Choices of Animal Models*

We recommend starting with a combination of permanent and transient occlusion models in the rat. The intraluminal suture model seems to be one of the most reproducible and most easily controlled. This would be useful as a starting model for studying potential neuroprotective agents to be employed in the clinic alone or in combination with thrombolytics. The surgical cautery of the MCAO model is probably the next most reproducible. The embolic model of MCAO is the least reproducible of the three choices above; however, a recent review of models[78] shows that with very careful surgical and clot preparation, reproducibility can be obtained. Moreover, individual laboratories form their clots using very different protocols and produce clots that may have very different morphology and fibrin content; thus, the procedure used for thrombus preparation is important with respect to the mechanisms of action of the agent to be tested. Some have criticized the focus of preclinical assessment on infarct size rather than clinical outcome, which is thought to be measured by behavioral recovery. For the rat, the tests shown in Table 15.5 have been recommended.[79,80] These should be performed acutely (days 1 to 3) and on a longer time scale (7 to 30 days).

We recommend evaluation of the following prerequisites when considering the various experimental stroke models:

Table 15.5 Neurobehavioral Tests for Function in Rodents

Test	Description
Cylinder test[81]	Uses a Plexiglas® cylinder (18 cm diameter × 30 cm height) that is big enough for the rat to fit into and stand on its rear paws. This test allows one to quantify the use of both limbs and assess if a limb is not being used normally.
Forepaw placement dysfunction tests[82]	Measures the ability of the rat to walk across a wire mesh. Each paw placement requires the rat to bear weight on the paw. The test measures the number of "foot-faults" for each forepaw.
Forelimb and hind-limb placing tests[83]	Measure tactile and proprioceptive-stimulation-induced paw placing.
Reaching tests[84]	Measure normal reaching tasks; with cerebral infarction in one hemisphere, deficits on one side in reaching can be seen.
Balance beam and beam walking tests[85]	Measures deficits in normal balance and walking.
Elevated body swing test[86]	Involves elevating the rat by the tail and measuring the tendency of the rat to turn in one direction or the other. Normal, healthy rats do not exhibit a bias one way or the other, but those with unilateral cerebral infarction tend to turn more toward the side contralateral to the infarct.
Morris water tank test[33]	Measures cognitive ability by placing a rat in a water tank with a submerged platform that the rat can learn to find. A series of trials records the attempts to swim toward the platform on days 7 and 14 after the induction of stroke.

- What is the species specificity of the drug candidate?
- Are the pharmacokinetics known?
- Is the pharmacodynamic profile for the drug known?
- Are surrogate markers available to allow measurement of the potential efficacy *ex vivo* or *in vivo*?
- Is the time course of the drug effect known? (This may or may not coincide with pharmacokinetics.)
- Is the time window of therapy known?
- Should coagulation be monitored? Does the drug have effects on coagulation?
- Should inflammation be monitored? Acute phase reactants, white cell counts, platelet counts?
- Are the mechanisms of action expected to result in any toxicities?
- Are any other toxicities to be expected?

15.3.2.5 *Conclusions*

The use of animal models for experimental stroke is necessary to determine whether a drug candidate has a potential to provide benefit to patients. These experiments, when performed in a careful, reproducible manner can give important information for determining clinical doses, optimal timing of therapy, and indications of potential toxicities to watch for in clinical trials. We recommend the use of one or more rat model. One may want to test for neuroprotection with and without reperfusion. In addition, if one has an agent that affects coagulation, testing in a thrombolytic reperfusion model would be appropriate. The rat is also very easily used for determining pharmacokinetics and toxicity.

15.4 DECISION TO MOVE TO PHASE I

In the 1980s and early 1990s, the decision to move to phase I development was usually based on much larger preclinical data packages than the programs are today. One of the reasons for such a change is the fact that biotechnology-derived substances were introduced in the 1990s, and such drugs required special programs due to the specific substance characteristics. As described in Section

15.3, quite a few biotechnology products do not have a target in an animal model (because they target a human receptor that is not available in the animal); therefore, ultimately the efficacy and safety of the product can only be tested in the human model.

Another reason for cutting preclinical development programs is the fact that these programs began to be designed more in accordance with the budgets (thus, initiatives were taken to perform development activities more rationally). Also, animal models allow drawing only very limited conclusions with regard to humans. The size of the program before initiating phase I does not have to be exorbitant; a well-defined and standardized dataset should be sufficient to prepare for the first administration in humans. Finally, it became apparent that the predictability of animal models was largely overestimated. In the case of stroke, the number of drugs that have a significant effect in animals and virtually no effect in humans is astounding. The ICH initiative produced a set of guidelines dealing with this topic (ICH M3 and S6 guidelines, www.ich.org).

Investigational substances have to be studied as early as possible in humans (i.e., phase I), as this is the only way to determine whether or not a substance is safe and shows some pharmacodynamic effects in humans. The first human study should be stopped as early as possible in order to act ethically (not exposing further humans to a potentially unsafe or ineffective substance) and to save the budget for other more promising drug candidates in the pipeline.

The design of fast-into-humans programs (i.e., performing the bare minimum of preclinical development activities before first administration of the substance in humans) depends on the drug (the program will be more extensive if the drug candidate is a small molecule than a protein) and the indication (the more severe the indication and higher the medical need, the smaller the program might be). Stroke and a number of biotechnology-derived programs justify such programs. Ultimately, the design of such an approach must be discussed with IRBs and regulatory authorities.

Before the first administration of a drug candidate in humans, a careful risk–benefit ratio analysis must be performed, usually by a predefined decision-making group of researchers who are responsible for the preclinical and early clinical development of the drug or an independent data monitoring committee (IDMC), according to the ICH E6 guideline. These researchers will include a pharmacologist, toxicologist, and production/analytics expert, as well as the phase I and II clinical developer and clinical safety expert. A consensus decision will be reached on how to move on in the development of the drug candidate. According to the ICH E6 guideline, this is also the latest time point to write an investigator brochure (IB), which will give guidance to the clinical developer and form the basis for the regulatory authority as well as the IRB in granting or rejecting approval with regard to initiation of phase I.

Particularly for the fast-into-humans process, the first steps in phase I are very cautious and very well controlled. Very low dosages are used as starting doses, and the volunteers (or patients depending on the indication) are monitored very carefully. Decisions to move to higher dosages are made on the basis of data generated in the phase I trial, but such decisions will have more validity as compared to decisions primarily based on preclinical data. A drug with an unfavorable pharmacokinetic profile (e.g., drug is not absorbed intestinally or has a very short or too long half-life), an unacceptable safety profile (drug-induced adverse events, which are not tolerable and do not allow further development of the drug), and suboptimal pharmacodynamics (e.g., drug cannot be dosed high enough to reach sufficient plasma levels in the brain to exert its neuroprotective action) can be studied in such an early clinical phase, and the decision can be made whether to continue the drug development for this specific candidate at all. Such a decision can be made then on the basis of human and hard data.

15.4.1 Phase I: Basic Development

Phase I clinical studies represent the first administration of an investigational compound in humans. These trials do not generally have a therapeutic focus but rather concentrate on the evaluation of safety parameters, tolerance limits, and pharmacokinetic analyses. After finalization of the relevant pharmaceutical and preclinical studies as well as identification of the starting dose in humans and a (positive) risk–benefit evaluation, in most cases the first phase I studies are performed in young and healthy volunteers. Although male volunteers are generally the primary study population, female volunteers should be recruited in some phase I studies; however, effective contraception has to be required to prevent potential harm to a fetus. The reason for the inclusion of female volunteers is the fact that the female organism might react differently to a specific compound under investigation in terms of safety profiles (different adverse events) or pharmacokinetic profiles (e.g., different half-life due to greater accumulation in fat tissue of a drug).

Although phase I studies are generally performed in healthy volunteers, a good rationale might exist to perform such studies directly in patients; for example, with regard to cancer, the pharmacological treatments being used are not well tolerated, and it is unethical to use them in healthy young people. Another reason for an early evaluation of patients in phase I studies is to evaluate pharmacodynamic parameters that are altered in patients but not necessarily in healthy volunteers. If the influence on pharmacodynamics is a factor for deciding on further development of the drug candidate, it may be worthwhile to perform phase I studies in patients (see also the comments on fast-into-humans programs above).

Dosages to be used in humans can be calculated from preclinical data. Several mathematical models are available for determining how to approach the starting dose and define the steps to increase the dose. After each dose step, a decision is made as to whether to increase the dose depending on the (primarily safety) parameters measured. While general safety parameters (blood pressure, heart rate, body temperature, respiratory frequency, etc.) are one piece of the equation, other parameters that might be influenced by the specific drug under development are as important. These might be coagulation parameters, such as in case of an anticoagulant or thrombolytic; special markers for a drug that is known to influence one body system in the preclinical situation, such as using troponin as a marker for cardiac toxicity or transaminases for liver toxicity; or pharmacodynamic parameters that reflect the fully established drug effect with the safety parameters remained uninfluenced (which would indicate a rather wide therapeutic window).

The spontaneous reporting of adverse events by volunteers as well as structured interviews by the phase I investigator give further evidence of how the dose under evaluation is being tolerated. These reports are one parameter for deciding to increase the dose to the next dose level. Adverse events can be evaluated very carefully with regard to their causal relationship in the phase I setting, as the phase I study is so experimental in nature that reexposure of the drug can be performed (if ethically possible) and the dose can be increased or decreased to allow assessment of the relationship between the drug and adverse events (which is nearly impossible in most cases in later stages during drug development).

The ratio of adverse events (and other changes of safety parameters) and dosage is a valuable decision point for the dose selection in phase II, where in most cases patients will receive the drug for the first time (after the evaluation of the drug effect in healthy volunteers) and it has to be kept in mind that a patient might not tolerate the dosages to the same extent as a healthy person. Additionally, the treatment schemes of most drugs require multiple dosing (per day or over a period of time); it has to be taken into account that a single dose might be better tolerated but multiple dosing might require lower dosages overall. To evaluate the relationship between single doses and multiple doses, multiple dosing can be tested in the phase I setting if the drug is intended to be administered more than once in the patients. As such, the phase I studies (single-dose and repeated-dose administration) resemble the preclinical toxicology studies (acute toxicity and repeated-dose toxicity), which serve as a good paradigm for evaluating the safety profile (although different dose levels are used as compared to the preclinical studies).

When studying the safety of an investigational drug candidate in phase I studies, the pharmacokinetic profile of the drug is being evaluated as well. Frequent blood draws ensure the evaluation of the plasma-level profile reflecting the fate of the drug in the systemic circulation. Peak plasma levels (C_{max}), trough levels (C_{min}), half-life (the time required for the plasma level to drop to 50%

of its original value, $t_{1/2}$), and area under the plasma concentration curve (AUC) are some important parameters that will guide the clinical developer in planning the conduct of later stage clinical trials. Measuring pharmacokinetic parameters provides data on absorption (A; the percentage of drug dose administered that is available in the circulation is called *bioavailabilty*), distribution in the body (D; to which compartments the drug travels), metabolism of the drug to active and inactive metabolites (M), and excretion (E; through which excretion pathways the drug travels). All of these parameters in turn can be influenced by a number of other parameters: gender, age, organ function, enzyme activity, intake of other medications, time of the day, and food, to name a few. This ADME profile is an important characteristic that will be used throughout development of the drug and will be the basis for discussion with IRBs and authorities during the drug development process.

After single- and multiple-dose phase I studies, phase II studies can begin, provided the risk–benefit evaluation is positive. Depending on the drug, however, it might be necessary to perform one or more phase I studies before the phase II decision can be made. For example, if the drug has to be taken orally and it has sufficient bioavailability, it might be necessary to analyze whether or not concomitant intake of food influences the pharmacokinetics of the drug. The efficacy in phase II and III studies might well depend on the food effect of the drug. If the drug is not absorbed sufficiently under fed conditions, the drug intake must be done before meals or even under fasted conditions. Other phase I studies might be necessary (e.g., if the target patient population experiences significant liver or kidney function disturbances). It might be worthwhile to evaluate early whether such organ malfunctions have an influence on the pharmacokinetics and require a dose adaptation as a consequence. Finally, the frequent intake of special concomitant medication in the target patient population might raise the issue of potential drug interactions between the drug candidate and concomitant medication. Sometimes this drug–drug interaction can be excluded on the basis of theoretical knowledge, or it is known that special pharmacological classes interact (such as thrombolytics and anticoagulants); in such cases, the appropriate safety measure can be taken when performing clinical trials (e.g., excluding a potentially unsafe concomitant medication or requesting a dose change).

Some additional phase I studies may be undertaken in parallel (except in the cases described above) with phase II and III development. The phases of drug development (preclinical, phase I, phase II, and phase III) overlap considerably today, which makes it possible to address new findings in a phase II or III study by performing an additional phase I or preclinical study in parallel. Such programs are referred to as *bridging studies* and are common during the drug development (e.g., adding other ethnic patient groups to the program or switching the production process of a bio-technology-derived drug or protein).

The size of phase I studies is small compared to later stage clinical studies. A typical size is $n = 18$ to 24 for a single- or multiple-dose phase I study. Other studies, such as drug–drug interaction studies or bridging studies, will usually be bigger depending on the number of parameters to measure or questions to answer; however, $n = 100$ volunteers or patients is usually not the case in a phase I setting. It is advisable to interact with regulatory agencies very early in the development process in order to discuss the planned phase I studies as well as the framework of the total development program. It should not be forgotten at this stage that such an overall development program is a "working document" and will grow and be adapted according to the data generated over time.

15.4.2 Phase I: Specific Studies for Stroke Compounds

Taking the above-mentioned basic phase I development program into account, no specific phase I studies are required for the indication stroke by current guidelines. Stroke is such a severe and life-threatening situation that most questions that occur during the drug development process can only be answered in the phase II and III study setting when treating actual patients, because no healthy volunteer setting can mimic such a situation. The drugs that have been tested in humans have the following characteristics that may be detected in carefully designed phase I studies: agitation, sedation, hypotension, coagulation disturbances, disturbance of the immune system, and QTc prolongation, to name some of the most important ones.

The stroke patient population does offer some targets for phase I studies; for example, phase I studies in the elderly population might be necessary if a particular question is not better addressed in a phase II or III setting. This population might have multiple organ malfunctions that would influence the pharmacokinetics of the drug, and if this issue cannot be better addressed in the ongoing phase II and III studies then some phase I work would be necessary. Furthermore, these patients are usually taking multiple concomitant medications. It is generally assumed that medication classes such as antihypertensives, antidiabetics, or antirheumatics will not have a significant influence on the drug candidate on a theoretical or pharmacological basis. By carefully monitoring safety signs in the ongoing clinical development, additional drug interaction studies may be performed later if needed. Stroke patients have one big risk: intracerebral bleeding, either as the primary cause of stroke (hemorrhagic stroke) or as a secondary incident after a primary ischemic event. Everything must be done either to prevent such serious adverse events or to limit the aftermaths of them; therefore, special care must be taken in the coadministration of a medication that can induce or prolong bleeding. Today, stroke patients will not receive anticoagulants within the first 24 hours if they have received alteplase or other agents that interfere with the coagulation system. So, if pharmacological knowledge (e.g., a thrombolytic and an anticoagulant are hyperadditive with regard to their bleeding potential) does not allow such interactions to be ruled out, it will be necessary to perform phase I interaction studies, observe the phase II and III study population very carefully (if such a wait-and-see approach is ethically acceptable), or prohibit the use of a potentially dangerous comedication in the clinical study setting (by mention in the exclusion criteria of the study protocol). For some of these interactions, validated animal models may be useful to reduce unnecessary exposure to humans.

By seeking advice from IRBs and regulatory agencies, sponsors can receive additional input on how to enhance the safety profiles of their compounds. For a totally new (e.g., biotechnology-derived) compound with unknown properties and a poorly characterized target in the human body, development must be performed under very well-defined conditions with close supervision by safety experts (preferably by an independent data monitoring committee, as well) and close evaluation of potential safety signs. Interim data must be analyzed in depth by the experts involved, including all relevant preclinical and clinical investigators, to allow the broadest possible view and interpretation of the results as well as drawing the best conclusions as to how to proceed.

15.5 PHASE II AND III DEVELOPMENT

15.5.1 Risk–Benefit Assessment

15.5.1.1 Justification of Clinical Trials

Three parties are primarily involved in the process of assessment of benefits and risks of clinical trials: the investigator, the ethics committee and institutional review board, and the participating subject. In some countries (e.g., Canada, Japan, Sweden, United Kingdom, and United States), the health authorities are intensively involved in reviewing clinical trials and could ultimately put them on hold or reject them even if they were already approved by the ethics committee and institutional review board.

Possible risk to participating subjects represents the main ethical concern for clinical trials in general, and particularly for the indication of stroke as most patients are highly vulnerable, rendering assessment of the risk–benefit ratio a rather complicated procedure. The investigator holds the main responsibility for assessment of risks and is required to analyze their significance in terms of degree, duration, and permanence of potential harm to participants — physically, psychologically, socially, and economically.[87] The main components of these subjective analyses are based on reviewing available data and interaction with opinion leaders as well as nonexperts. The acuteness of stroke and its onset of treatment renders the prospective involvement of stroke patients not feasible; nevertheless, consulting previous stroke patients, especially those who participated in stroke trials, may be considered. As a next step, and when the risks cannot be reduced, the investigator needs to justify the risks and describe ways to limit them. It should be noted that stroke as a disease entity is associated with a number of complications, such as bleeding, edema, and progression of symptoms. These represent normal risks related to the disease itself and should be considered whenever assessing risks for potential investigations in this indication. After the investigator has analyzed the risks, it is the duty of the ethics committee and institutional review board to decide whether these risks are tolerable and whether or not the trial should be approved.[87]

The decision of either the investigator or the ethics committee and institutional review board will not only be guided by the evaluation of risks but also by the potential benefit to participants, which should be analyzed using an approach similar to the one used in the analysis of risks. A number of factors may determine possible benefits to a trial participant; among others, these include the hypothesis to be tested (e.g., noninferiority vs. superiority), the trial phase (e.g., proof of concept vs. confirmatory), trial design (e.g., placebo-controlled vs. comparator controlled), and trial procedures (e.g., intravenous vs. intraarterial thrombolysis). At the end, the participating subject is the one to weigh the potential risks against the possible benefits and either consent or decline participation.[87]

Due to the nature of stroke, consent may not be obtained from potential participants, so it will be the responsibility of the investigator alone or the investigator and the patient's representative to decide on whether exposing the patient to the risks of the trial would be justifiable.[87]

15.5.1.2 *Application of Clinical Trial Data to Medical Practice*

In most cases, stroke is a disease of the elderly population, who often find it difficult to understand information regarding the risks and benefits of any therapy that could be used to treat their condition. To date, thrombolytic therapy seems to be the only therapy with beneficial effect in acute ischemic stroke patients, as this therapy is directed toward the cause of an acute event: the obstructing clot. However, care should be taken when extrapolating data from clinical trials to real life;[88] a thorough evaluation of the individual patient condition should be performed, and easily understandable information on the risks and benefits should be made available to the patients to allow them or their representatives to make informed decisions regarding their treatment.[88] A number of limitations make it unlikely for clinical trials in stroke to be able to provide relevant data for many therapeutic decisions made in the course of daily practice. First, the design of these trials, their rationale, and detailed results may be known only to the experts who have been directly involved in planning the trials. Second, trials are not conducted in such a way as to simulate daily therapeutic decision making by physicians.[89] Third, many times it is impossible to apply the general results of clinical trials to individual patients. Fourth, the quality of many individual trials limits the usefulness of metaanalyses of the resulting data. Treatment decisions for individual patients are complicated and require the consideration of a number of factors, one of them being clinical trial data.[89] Other factors — detailed knowledge of stroke and its subtypes, the cause of the stroke, the patient's individual condition and concomitant diseases, existing risk factors, and the physician's previous experience with similar conditions — should be considered. In addition, it is of utmost importance to optimize and homogenize stroke trials by recruiting clinical neurologists and neuroradiologists to address clinically relevant therapeutic dilemmas with regard to making evidence-based therapeutic decisions.[89]

15.5.2 Trial Design

15.5.2.1 Dose-Finding Aspects

Stroke dose-finding trials are usually phase II trials (although sometimes these may be considered as phase I trials) that explore the safety and efficacy of a particular treatment in stroke patients. These trials are necessary to define the safety profile of that particular therapy as well as the dose range for efficacy.[90] Generally, these trials follow a dose-escalating design starting with a dose in the range of the dose administered to healthy volunteers that showed signs of minimal activity at the laboratory level (e.g., increase in fibrin degradation products in the case of thrombolytic agents). The escalation to higher doses is usually guided by safety complications, although preliminary indications of efficacy should also be considered. Subsequent to these trials, larger phase IIb dose-ranging trials may be performed where a number of doses from the dose-escalating trial are tested to define an optimal dose (or dose range) to be used in subsequent confirmatory phase III trials. In general, the phase II trials are not sufficiently powered to confirm efficacy. Even at this stage of drug development, it is advisable to conduct placebo-controlled, blinded, randomized trials. Although the phase I and II parts of a drug development program may not be able to adequately address all of the issues, as much information as possible should be obtained before proceeding to phase III, and the clinical selection criteria (e.g., onset of symptoms to treatment, age, stroke severity) should be selected assuming that similar groups of patients will be treated in phase II and phase III.[90]

15.5.2.2 Efficacy Endpoints

Three key elements should be addressed when designing a phase III clinical trial: (1) mechanism of action for the investigational drug, (2) onset-to-treatment time window, and (3) dose of the drug. A thrombolytic agent dissolving a clot should not be administered to patients where no perfusion deficit or arterial occlusion exists. Similarly, patients with white matter ischemia should not be given a neuroprotective drug that works only on the gray matter. The definition of the onset-to-treatment time window should be based on a careful analysis of the pathophysiological condition supplemented by preclinical findings and human data supporting the pharmacodynamics. Whenever the phase III clinical trial demonstrates clinical benefit within a short time window, subsequent trials could be performed to determine whether expanding the time window in appropriately selected patients is efficacious. In general, it is most likely that earlier therapy is associated with improved clinical outcome. The definition of the dose of drug to be investigated in a phase III trial is also based on the tolerability, safety, and efficacy of the agent in preclinical and phase I and II clinical studies.[90]

A number of assessment scales have been developed to assess the neurological status of the patient. These include, among others, the National Institutes of Health Stroke Scale (NIHSS), modified Rankin scale (MRS), Barthel index, and Scandinavian Stroke Scale. Early use of these scales in clinical development will help generate data that can be used to estimate more precisely the sample size required to detect a drug effect in confirmatory trials.[90]

Ischemic damage on a biological level can be determined by measuring the extent of cytotoxic edema by diffusion-weighted MRI or by infarct size on CT scan. The presence of a mismatch between the diffusion lesion and the overall hypoperfused area on perfusion-weighted MRI (perfusion lesion > diffusion lesion) may help to define the extent of penumbra and select patients with the best chances to benefit from treatment. Moreover, the evolution of ischemic lesion volume on diffusion-MRI at baseline to T2 lesion volume on day 30 may show drug effect in small sample size studies. This concept is being explored in a number of trials (http://www.strokecenter.org/trials), including the DWI Evaluation for Understanding Stroke Evolution (DEFUSE), the Echo Planar Imaging Thrombolytic Evaluation Trial (EPITHET), the Desmoteplase in Acute Stroke (DIAS) trial, and the Stroke Evaluation for Late Endovascular Cerebral Thrombolysis with MR (SELECT MR) trial.[21] Preliminary results suggest that it could be a superior tool for the selection of patients for inclusion and evaluation in stroke trials. Recent results from the DIAS trial showed strong correlation between the imaging endpoints (difference between T2 lesion volume at 30 days and baseline DWI lesion) and clinical outcome at 90 days.[24,25] Other markers of ischemic injury may be plasma levels of various substances released into the circulation from injured brain (e.g., neuron-specific enolase).

Ultrasound, MR angiography, or CT angiography may provide surrogate markers of *in vivo* drug activity by measuring rates of recanalization for thrombolytic therapy. Generally, surrogate measures should be easy to perform, reproducible, and sensitive to changes induced by therapeutic intervention and should not interfere with other treatments or assessments. An ideal surrogate marker of drug activity may accelerate drug development and reduce cost.[21] The DIAS trial showed that in patients with PWI/DWI mismatch, favorable clinical outcome was associated with reperfusion up to 9 hours after stroke onset.

The definition of endpoints and the time of their measurement are important issues for phase III trial design. In previous trials, measures of impairment, disability, and handicap have been used. In the NINDS trial, a global endpoint was chosen where a responder was a patient achieving 0 to 1 on NIHSS, 0 to 1 on MRS, 1 on the Glasgow Outcome Scale, and 95 to 100 on the Barthel index at 90 days. In the European Centre for Analysis in the Social Sciences (ECASS) II trial, the primary outcome measure was the proportion of patients who achieved a modified Rankin scale score of 0 to 1 at 90 days. The Glycine in Antagonist Neuroprotection (GAIN) trials of a glycine antagonist used the Barthel index as an outcome measure, implementing a trichotomized analytical approach (see http://www.strokecenter.org/trials).[90] Ninety days after stroke onset is typically used as the time to measure outcome. An earlier time for evaluating the primary endpoint of the trial may help to avoid confounding effects unrelated to the study drug (e.g., late medical complications, recurrent stroke, or imbalances in the use of prolonged rehabilitation services) that might affect the long-term outcome of stroke.[21,91]

15.5.2.3 Randomization and Control Groups

The advantage of a randomized trial over an observational study is the ability to demonstrate causality. "Randomly assigning the intervention can eliminate the influence of confounding variables."[92] Randomization should be performed via a randomization center to ensure central allocation of trial treatment. The randomization center will be called for patients fulfilling clinical and imaging selection criteria and having given informed consent. Information such as patient's age, weight, baseline NIHSS score, imaging performed, and time from onset must be given, and the randomization center will then identify a treatment for the patient. Accordingly, the study physician, nurse, or pharmacist will prepare the corresponding treatment for administration.[92] With the exception of rt-PA in the first 3 hours after onset of stroke, no other treatment for acute stroke events is available; hence, all trials investigating new potential treatments in time windows longer than 3 hours use placebos as comparators. If it is not a thrombolysis trial, the investigators also use placebo in the early time window; the problem is that randomization to rt-PA is not controlled in many cases.

"Some stroke patients and their families express reservations about participating in clinical trials investigating therapies for acute stroke,"[93] fearing that they will do worse in the trial than if treated conventionally and thereby reflecting concerns about the risks associated with the investigative drug. Moreover, many patients fear that by participating in the trial they may be deprived of some component of routine care. The placebo effect has been noted in many areas of clinical research, and it is not unreasonable to expect a placebo response (benefit) in trials of new stroke therapies because of additional medical and nursing attention integral to the design of those trials.[93] At the end, it is the responsibility of ethics committees and institutional review boards to prohibit clinical trials in which placebo patients are denied a therapy known to be effective. Generally, it should be ensured that all patients participating in stroke studies are guaranteed optimal known medical therapy.

15.5.3 Assessment Procedures

15.5.3.1 Validation of Clinical Tests and Measures

Several reliable and well-validated scoring systems have been developed. The National Institute of Health Stroke Scale is the most widely used scale to assess stroke severity and subsequent stroke outcome. It is a 42-point scale that provides a means to measure neurologic deficits and contains 15 items, including level of consciousness, language function neglect, visual fields, eye movements, facial symmetry, motor strength, sensation, and coordination (Table 15.6). The examination can be performed quickly, and the NIHSS score can be assessed by neurologists and non-neurologists; however, the examiner should be experienced in acute stroke treatment and certified in administering the NIHSS. Patients with NIHSS score of up to 6 or 7 have a mild stroke, 8 to 14 indicates moderate stroke, and a severe stroke usually scores higher than 15.

The NIHSS has been used extensively in clinical trials to measure stroke outcomes and has been validated and standardized to reduce interobserver error. The NIHSS was designed for anterior-circulation ischemic stroke evaluation and might underestimate the severity of deficit for posterior-circulation strokes, because posterior-circulation symptoms, such as vertigo or difficulty in swallowing, are not included on the NIHSS. A standardized grading system for posterior-circulation strokes is not currently available. The Barthel index (BI) of activities of daily living and the modified Rankin scale (MRS) have been the most commonly used disability outcome measures. A written examination certifies examiners in administering the BI, whereas no certification procedure is currently in place for the MRS, which is the most commonly used global assessment of stroke outcome (note: a certification test for MRS is in development). Both the MRS and BI have been shown to be reliable and valid for use in stroke. They are familiar to the stroke neurology community, are adaptable for use in patients with acute stroke, and can be used to compare outcomes. The BI is used for functional evaluation to measure activities of daily living. The BI is a 10-item scale on which disability is assessed by various aspects of self-care. Patients who score 100 (maximum score) on the BI are fully independent. They are continent, can feed and dress themselves, get out of bed, walk more than 1 block, and perform activities of daily living. The MRS is used to measure overall functional disability and handicap after a stroke. It is a six-point scale on which a patient is rated from 0 (no symptoms) to 5 (severe disability). A score of less than 2 on the MRS is considered a favorable outcome with minimal or no disability.[92]

15.5.3.2 Clinical Laboratory Data

A clinical cardiovascular examination and a 12-lead ECG should be performed in all stroke patients. Cardiac abnormalities are prevalent among patients with stroke, and the patient can have an acute cardiac condition (e.g., acute myocardial infarction, cardiac arrhythmias, atrial fibrillation) that requires urgent treatment. Cardiac monitoring often can be conducted after stroke to screen for serious cardiac arrhythmias.[91]

"Several blood tests should be performed to identify conditions that may mimic or cause stroke or may influence the acute treatment,"[91] including blood glucose, electrolytes, complete blood count, prothrombin time, activated partial thromboplastin time, and renal and hepatic function studies. Hypoglycemia may mimic the symptoms and signs of stroke, and hyperglycemia is associated with unfavorable outcomes. Determination of the platelet count and the prothrombin time/international normalized ratio (INR) are required prior to administration of thrombolytic agents. A toxicology screen, blood alcohol level, and pregnancy test should be obtained if the physician is uncertain about the patient's history or their use is suggested by findings on examination. Arterial blood gas levels should be obtained if hypoxia is suspected.[91]

Examination of the cerebrospinal fluid is indicated if the patient has symptoms suggestive of subarachnoid hemorrhage and a CT does not demonstrate blood. Electroencephalography may be

Table 15.6 NIH Stroke Scale

Test Item	Score	
1a. Level of consciousness	0	Alert
	1	Not alert, but arousable with minimal stimulation
	2	Not alert, requires repeated stimulation to attend
	3	Unresponsive (coma)
1b. LOC questions	0	Answers both correctly
	1	Answers one correctly
	2	Both incorrect
1c. LOC commands	0	Performs both tasks correctly
	1	Performs one task correctly
	2	Both incorrect
2. Gaze (only horizontal eye movement)	0	Normal
	1	Partial gaze palsy
	2	Total gaze palsy
3. Visual field	0	No visual field loss
	1	Partial hemianopia
	2	Complete hemianopia
	3	Bilateral hemianopia (blind including cortical blindness)
4. Facial palsy	0	Normal symmetrical movement
	1	Minor paralysis (flattened nasolabial fold, asymmetry on smiling)
	2	Partial paralysis (total or near total paralysis of lower face)
	3	Complete paralysis of one or both sides (absence of facial movement in the upper and lower face)
5. Motor function — arm (right and left)	0	Normal (extends arms 90 or 45° for 10 seconds without drift)
5a. Right arm	1	Drift before 10 seconds
5b. Left arm	2	Some effort against gravity
	3	No effort against gravity
	4	No movement
	9	Untestable (joint fused or limb amputated)
6. Motor function – leg (right and left)	0	Normal (hold leg in 30° position for 5 seconds)
6a. Right leg	1	Drift before 5 seconds
6b. Left leg	2	Some effort against gravity
	3	No effort against gravity
	4	No movement
	9	Untestable (joint fused or limb amputated)
7. Limb ataxia	0	No ataxia
	1	Present in one limb
	2	Present in two limbs
8. Sensory	0	Normal
	1	Mild to moderate sensory loss
	2	Severe total sensory loss
9. Language	0	No aphasia
	1	Mild to moderate aphasia
	2	Severe aphasia
	3	Mute or global aphasia
10. Dysarthria	0	Normal
	1	Mild to moderate
	2	Severe
	9	Intubated or other physical barrier
11. Extinction and inattention	0	Normal
	1	Mild (inattention or extinction to bilateral simultaneous stimulation in one of the sensory modalities)
	2	Severe hemi-inattention or hemi-inattention to more than one modality

Note: The scores from each item are added together. The 9's are not included in the total score.

helpful for evaluating patients in whom seizures are suspected as the cause of the neurological deficits or in whom seizures could have been a complication of the stroke. Seizure is a relative contraindication for the use of rt-PA in acute ischemic stroke.[91] In acute ischemic stroke patients, the values for a number of blood parameters, including leukocytes, platelets, erythrocyte relative-cell transit time, and erythrocyte sedimentation rate, were found to increase. The same applies to fibrinogen levels and plasma viscosity. In addition, high leukocyte counts and glucose levels have been found to be more frequent in patients who died within 30 days after stroke onset in hemorrhagic stroke. An increased risk of fatal brain edema in acute ischemic stroke is associated with, among others, early CT hypodensity involving >50% of the MCA territory, involvement of additional vascular territories, and increased baseline leukocyte count. Patients presenting with such risk factors may be in need of special attention and aggressive treatment.[94–96]

15.5.4 Patient Population

As phase III trials are intended to confirm the results of phase II trials, comparable patient populations should be considered for both phases. Age limits adopted for stroke trials range between 18 and 85 years; however, biological age is being considered by many neurologists whenever recruiting stroke patients in clinical trials.[90] Besides age, baseline stroke severity represents another important element. In this respect, patients with moderate strokes, defined as scoring 7 (or 8) to 14 (some extending that up to 20), could show the best clinical responses. Mild strokes usually have a higher spontaneous recovery rate, whereas severe strokes show a small therapeutic effect. Nevertheless, aiming to prevent worsening of the neurological status of mild stroke patients, many neurologists still treat mild stroke cases. Age and stroke severity are often used as stratifying parameters that are considered in the randomization schemes for stroke trials.[90]

In drug development programs, irrespective of the indication, the influence of age, race, gender, and concomitant diseases on the drug effect should be taken into account. This influence is especially important for stroke drugs, and a careful analysis of these confounding factors should be conducted. Although comprehensive study of the effect of gender, race, and age is usually performed in phase III trials, where large patient populations are included, influences of gender and race are usually addressed in phase I trials with potential differences in pharmacokinetics and pharmacodynamics being evaluated. The ultimate goal is to assess the risk–benefit ratio in these subgroups, and whether this may necessitate adjustments of the dose regimen or imply excluding some of these subgroups.[90]

The use of imaging selection criteria to identify subgroups of patients with the potential to benefit from thrombolytic therapy is being investigated in a number of trials in time windows reaching up to 9 hours after stroke onset. MR-PWI and -DWI and perfusion CT are being used to approximately identify potentially salvageable brain tissue at risk (penumbra). This concept, if proven, might change the current approach for thrombolytic therapy as well as other interventional stroke therapies from a generalized ticking clock to an individualized tissue clock.

15.5.5 Statistical Considerations

Most clinical trials in acute stroke have failed to show positive treatment effects, and the reasons for this have been explored. It was found that the inappropriate choice of cutpoints for analysis of the outcome scales is an important contributing factor. Different primary endpoints have been used in acute stroke trials, among which the NIHSS, the Barthel index, and the modified Rankin scale have been the most commonly used outcome measures. Endpoints used have included primarily dichotomized, and sometimes trichotomized, single-outcome measures. Global endpoints with multiple outcome measures were adopted in some stroke trials (e.g., NINDS).[97]

Functional outcome scores have usually been dichotomized as favorable vs. unfavorable, although little consensus exists on the optimal cutpoint. The most commonly used endpoint in clinical trials has been the BI cutpoint of 60, at which a patient is thought to be capable of independence from full-time care. The MRS has been used less frequently, although outcomes of ≤2 (no to slight disability) and ≤1 (no to no significant disability) have been utilized. A trichotomized BI endpoint has also been used. Its use has been driven by the fact that patients tend to cluster at the extreme ends of the U-shaped distribution of BI outcomes (0 and 95–100). Hence, any cutpoint selected between these two ends will have a small number of patients in the adjacent categories. In order to allow both mildly and moderate to severely affected patients to contribute to the significance test, a second cutpoint can be added and a trichotomized analysis performed.[97]

Another approach is to use a global endpoint, simultaneously incorporating outcome measures from different domains such as handicap and activities of daily living. This makes sense as no single outcome measure describes all dimensions of recovery from stroke. The statistical power of a global endpoint should be greater than or equal to that of an individual endpoint. In this regard, the significance test considers patients achieving the predefined outcome on each scale included in the global endpoint. Another approach is the global test statistical approach. This type of analysis was used in the second part of the NINDS rt-PA trial and evaluated treatment effects on four outcome scales: MRS, BI, Glasgow Outcome Scale, and NIHSS. Although each individual scale showed a significant difference, the global test showed the most robust treatment difference between rt-PA and placebo patients.[97]

The considerable heterogeneity in stroke severity renders many patients uninformative when using an endpoint with a fixed cutpoint. Although the normalization of the patient condition after stroke remains the main goal of clinical trials, stroke experts agree that baseline stroke severity should be taken into consideration when defining the endpoints to be reached. Accordingly, grouping patients according to baseline stroke severity (primarily using the NIHSS) and defining cutpoints according to group should be considered. For example, when using the MRS as an outcome measure, the following endpoint might be defined: NIHSS scores of 0, 0–1, and 0–2 for baseline stroke severities of up to 7, 8–14, and 15, respectively.[98] An MRS of 0 represents a fully independent, symptom-free patient, and an MRS of 2 indicates that the patient is unable to carry out all previous activities but is able to look after his or her own affairs without assistance, thereby representing a significant improvement and favorable outcome, especially for patients with severe stroke events. Patient-specific endpoints would give a more realistic assessment of a treatment effect and allow all patients to contribute to the results of the trial. In general, better choices of endpoints strengthen trial power or allow reduced sample sizes without loss of statistical power.[97]

15.5.6 Practical Study Conduct

Setting up a clinical trial in acute stroke is a rather complicated procedure and faces a number of challenges. It is generally recommended to include experienced academic centers in such trials in order to ensure the generation of sound and reliable data; however, this might be achieved at the expense of recruitment of patients. On the other hand, investigators with limited experience in clinical trials may be more likely to become concerned by a small clustering of adverse events at their site, which can be disruptive to recruitment.[90] As imaging is an essential part of many acute stroke trials, early involvement of the neuroradiologist in the study setup is mandatory. Successful conduct of a trial requires good cooperation between the neurologists and neuroradiologists. A lack of such cooperation could result in failure of the trials. It is extremely important to have an active study coordinator or nurse who assumes the responsibility for coordinating the various trial activities among the participating parties (neurologist, neuroradiologist, pharmacist, and laboratory staff) at an investigative site. Multiple site visits prior to and after trial initiation should be conducted to ensure good understanding of the trial procedures and compliance to the study protocol, in addition to keeping the investigative team aware of the trial.

A number of trial committees should be put in place. These should include at least a steering committee and an independent data monitoring committee. Other committees, such as an imaging committee and publication committee, might also be needed. The steering committee should ideally be composed of participating investigators, independent experts with experience in clinical trial and sponsor representatives. It should support the sponsor in interactions with the individual sites for issues related to study design and execution, safety, and interim analyses, as well as with the ethics committees and regulatory bodies. The independent data monitoring committee (IDMC, or safety committee) must ensure that patients are not being put at excessive risk. As part of their analyses, the safety committee may have occasion to review data on treatment allocation. The results of these analyses should be kept separate from the steering committee, sponsor, and investigators to avoid introducing bias into the trial.[90]

If an international study is planned, it is strongly recommended to contact major regulatory agencies in advance and seek scientific advice with regard to coordinating and unifying the study design. Significant variations in practice patterns between countries, especially with regard to approaches to studying acute stroke (e.g., time to presentation, use of specialty care, availability of specific brain imaging techniques), should be taken into consideration.[90] Ultimately, only trials that are carefully planned and well organized have the potential to be successful.

15.5.7 Future Goals of Clinical Trials To Evaluate Stroke Treatment

Only one thrombolytic trial (NINDS rt-PA trial) has led to marketing approval, and none of the neuroprotective trials has been successful. The failure of most clinical trials in acute stroke represents a big challenge. Among the reasons for such failures are the lack of preclinical data to support the time window chosen for the efficacy trial and rapid movement to the pivotal trial without an in-depth understanding of side-effect profiles, subtypes of stroke, or subpopulations of patients most likely to benefit from the drug being tested. In addition, the lack of efficacy of neuroprotective agents tested could probably be attributed to two additional reasons. First, neuroprotective strategies could have failed because of a lack of concurrent effective reperfusion; the approach of combining thrombolysis with neuroprotection was shown to be effective in animal stroke models. Second, most neuroprotective compounds target only a fraction of the ischemic cascade pathways. Combinations of agents are likely to be more effective than single interventions; however, single agents that target multiple aspects of the ischemic cascade are available for evaluation, and using them would avoid many of the problems inherent in testing drug combinations. Other factors such as blood pressure, temperature, and glycemic status could also substantially affect ischemic lesion evolution and must be addressed.[21]

Based on the above considerations, the likelihood of success may be enhanced initially by using surrogate endpoints such as diffusion/perfusion MRI and perfusion CT for proof-of-concept phase II studies. In addition, different multimodal approaches such as combined reperfusion and neuroprotective strategies, combinations of neuroprotective agents targeting differing portions of the cascade, and incorporation of physiological strategies (e.g., hypothermia) should be considered.[21]

Future trials of acute stroke therapies must incorporate new research tools (e.g., new study designs) and respond to changes in regulations, healthcare systems, and stroke population. This will allow faster and more cost-effective conduct of trials, generating more detailed data. Outcome measures should incorporate all possible outcomes that are important to patients, and their timing should be defined carefully to exclude variability. Finally, appropriate study population selection requires the attainment of a correct balance between generalizability (representing major stroke subtypes and a broader population) and homogeneity (a narrower selection of patients, concentrating on those with the best potential to benefit from therapy).

15.6 NEW DRUG AND BIOLOGICS LICENSE APPLICATIONS

Having performed state-of-the-art development for a given stroke compound, all data gathered to that point are collected, summarized, and interpreted in the so-called *common technical document* (CTD), previously known as the *dossier*. This data package is submitted to regulatory authorities for evaluation of the quality, safety, and efficacy of the candidate drug. The application for the regulatory approval procedure is a new drug application (NDA), for a drug under development that is a small molecule, or a biologics license application (BLA), for a drug that is a biologic substance. The CMC (chemistry, manufacturing, control) requirements for preclinical and clinical studies are defined as follows:

- Numerous guidelines exist for the regulatory process. A number of these guidelines have already been adopted by the International Conference of Harmonisation (ICH), which means they are valid for Japan, the United States, and Europe. Additionally, individual regions may have their own guidelines with more specific requirements for what studies must be conducted and data obtained for the CTD.
- In addition to these guidelines, the sponsor of a development program must check published evidence of necessary development activities which may include published studies (regarding endpoints, sample sizes, patient definition, etc.), consensus documents (such as those issued by neurologist associations or stroke consortia), recommendations from opinion leaders in the field, and scientific information for a given compound (e.g., properties of the drug or substance class identified by specific pharmacological or interaction studies).
- Finally, having made a decision on how to define the development program for a specific stroke product, the sponsor interacts with authorities early in the development program to receive all necessary input and reach a decision on the NDA or BLA. Such meetings are generally granted in the form of pre-IND or end-of-phase II meetings (with the FDA), scientific advice meetings (with EU authorities), or formal meetings (with KIKO, the Japanese authority). The planned development program should be presented at these meetings, and the sponsor should seek advice as to whether this program will be sufficient, in principle, to fulfill the necessary requirements.

The sponsor then develops a state-of-the-art study program. Naturally, such a program extends over several years and evolves over time due to newly published evidence, further development of guidelines, and changing requirements due to a growing (data-based) knowledge base; therefore, it is advisable for sponsors to maintain close contact with authorities during the entire development process.

Having gathered all necessary data, the sponsor compiles the CTD and submits it to initiate the approval process. The CTD format and formal approval process (structure and timelines) are defined in the relevant guidelines. If the data provided show compelling evidence that the drug candidate meets the quality demands and is safe and effective, a market authorization will be granted. The United States and Japan have one approval procedure, while the European Union has two different approval procedures (i.e., a centralized procedure and a mutual recognition procedure, which is not described here in detail; refer to the appropriate EU guidelines). An investigational biological (stroke) candidate will generally be processed by the centralized procedure in the EU on the same day. This central approval procedure will be extended to small molecules in the near future, provided the development program targets neurodegenerative diseases (such as stroke); therefore, in Europe, it is anticipated that stroke programs will be able to use the central registration procedure beginning in the year 2005.

Finally, it should be kept in mind that, when the clinical studies have been conducted, considerable time should be budgeted for the evaluation, report writing, and CTD generation process which depends heavily on the length of the follow-up period of the trial. A year can be spent on completing these tasks after the last patient has been treated in the final clinical trial for a development program.

Approval times in the EU and United States range from a minimum of half a year to several years, depending on data quality and questions the authorities might have. In Japan, reports on registration and review times suggest that the process takes at least a year and, in some cases, several years. The speed of the approval process is also influenced by several factors — for example, if the drug under review is a lifesaving compound, if it satisfies a huge unmet medical need with compelling evidence of efficacy and safety, or if it has some kind of fast-track status (a procedure only defined in the United States).

15.7 PHASE IV DEVELOPMENT

Phase IV clinical studies are performed in order to expand the safety database after receiving market approval for the drug. The clinical program (phases I to III) is considerably smaller in scale than the anticipated number of patients who will be exposed to the drug when it is on the market. Furthermore, the conditions in a clinical trial are somewhat artificial as the design of the clinical study aims at a well-defined patient population in order to evaluate the safety and efficacy of the drug. Such a patient population, however, is not the reality in the marketplace, so additional postmarket data must be gathered.

Generally, stroke drug development programs are not huge, especially when developing a thrombolytic or medical device (trials will be larger for neuroprotectives or anticoagulants), so the safety database might be insufficient to judge on the safety profile without ambiguity. In this case, regulatory approval might be granted on the basis of a limited safety database but with the requirement that phase IV studies must be conducted to enhance the existing knowledge, especially with regard to the safety profile, under market conditions (i.e., less well-defined conditions). Additionally, because sponsors are responsible for their drug and liable for its deficiencies, it is in the best interests of every sponsor to conduct sound phase IV studies, which will serve to provide the required risk–benefit evaluations and reassure the public with regard to the safety and efficacy of the product.

The design of phase IV studies can be determined by referring to relevant guidelines and current knowledge about the pharmacological class, specific compound, and indications and by discussions with authorities (e.g., in the application process). The design of phase IV studies usually focuses on safety and is less sophisticated than the phase II and III studies. Prescribers might pay less attention to the labeling of the drug and might be more liberal in deciding when and how to prescribe the drug. The patient might have easier access to the drug (provided it is not an emergency care product) but might not follow the instructions for administering it. Also, patients can be on a number of concomitant medications that might give rise to unforeseen drug–drug interactions.

ACKNOWLEDGMENTS

The authors would like to thank Ms. Dagmar Schwarz for her excellent technical assistance in writing the manuscript, Dr. Paul Simpson for his support in the scientific background of the preclinical models, and Mr. Christian Sachara for his input regarding the statistical section.

REFERENCES

1. CPMP, *Points To Consider on Clinical Investigation of Medicinal Products for the Treatment of Acute Stroke*, Committee on Proprietary Medical Products, European Agency for the Evaluation of Medicinal Products, London, 2001.
2. National Institute of Neurological Disorders and Stroke rt-PA Stroke Study Group, Tissue plasminogen activator for acute ischemic stroke, *N. Engl. J. Med.*, 333, 1581–1587, 1995.
3. Katzan, I.L., Furlan, A.J., Lloyd, L.E. et al., Use of tissue-type plasminogen activator for acute ischemic stroke: the Cleveland area experience, *JAMA*, 283, 1151–1158, 2000.
4. Murray, C.J. and Lopez, A.D., Mortality by cause for eight regions of the world: Global Burden of Disease Study, *Lancet*, 349, 1269–1276, 1997.
5. Murray, C.J. and Lopez, A.D., Global mortality, disability, and the contribution of risk factors: Global Burden of Disease Study, *Lancet*, 349, 1436–1442, 1997.

6. Sudlow, C.L. and Warlow, C.P., Comparable studies of the incidence of stroke and its pathological types: results from an international collaboration, International Stroke Incidence Collaboration, *Stroke*, 28, 491–499, 1997.

7. Williams, G.R., Jiang, J.G., Matchar, D.B., and Samsa, G.P., Incidence and occurrence of total (first-ever and recurrent) stroke, *Stroke*, 30, 2523–2528, 1999.

8. Gorelick, P.B., Sacco, R.L., Smith, D.B. et al., Prevention of a first stroke: a review of guidelines and a multidisciplinary consensus statement from the National Stroke Association, *JAMA*, 281, 1112–1120, 1999.

9. Elkind, M.S., Stroke in the elderly, *Mt. Sinai J. Med.*, 70, 27–37, 2003.

10. Malmgren, R., Warlow, C., Bamford, J., and Sandercock, P., Geographical and secular trends in stroke incidence, *Lancet*, 2, 1196–200, 1987.

11. Warlow, C.P., Epidemiology of stroke, *Lancet*, 352(Suppl. 3), SIII1–SIII4, 1998.

12. Sudlow, C.L. and Warlow, C.P., Comparing stroke incidence worldwide: what makes studies comparable?, *Stroke*, 27, 550–558, 1996.

13. Bamford, J., Sandercock, P., Dennis, M. et al., A prospective study of acute cerebrovascular disease in the community: the Oxfordshire Community Stroke Project 1981–86. 1. Methodology, demography and incident cases of first-ever stroke, *J. Neurol. Neurosurg. Psychiatry*, 51, 1373–1380, 1988.

14. Lemesle, M., Milan, C., Faivre, J., Moreau, T., Giroud, M., and Dumas, R., Incidence trends of ischemic stroke and transient ischemic attacks in a well-defined French population from 1985 through 1994, *Stroke*, 30, 371–377, 1999.

15. Carolei, A., Marini, C., Di Napoli, M. et al., High stroke incidence in the prospective community-based L'Aquila registry (1994–1998): first year's results, *Stroke*, 28, 2500–2506, 1997.

16. Ricci, S., Celani, M.G., Guercini, G. et al., First-year results of a community-based study of stroke incidence in Umbria, Italy, *Stroke*, 20, 853–857, 1989.

17. Jorgensen, H.S., Plesner, A.M., Hubbe, P., and Larsen, K., Marked increase of stroke incidence in men between 1972 and 1990 in Frederiksberg, Denmark, *Stroke*, 23, 1701–1704, 1992.

18. Brott, T., Thrombolysis for stroke, *Arch. Neurol.*, 53, 1305–1306, 1996.

19. Grotta, J., Should thrombolytic therapy be the first-line treatment for acute ischemic stroke? t-PA: the best current option for most patients, *N. Engl. J. Med.*, 337, 1310–1313, 1997.

20. Caplan, L., Mohr, J.P., Kistler, J.P., and Koroshetz, W., Thrombolysis: not a panacea for ischaemic stroke, *N. Engl. J. Med.*, 337, 1307–1310, 1997.

21. Fisher, M., Recommendations for advancing development of acute stroke therapies: Stroke Therapy Academic Industry Roundtable 3, *Stroke*, 34, 1539–1546, 2003.

22. Franzini, A., Ferroli, P., Servello, D., and Broggi, G., Reversal of thalamic hand syndrome by long-term motor cortex stimulation, *J. Neurosurg.*, 93, 873–875, 2000.

23. Stefan, K., Kunesch, E., Cohen, L.G., Benecke, R., and Classen, J., Induction of plasticity in the human motor cortex by paired associative stimulation, *Brain*, 123, 572–584, 2000.

24. Hacke, W., *The DIAS Study: Results of a Phase II, MRI-Based Dose Finding Study of Desmoteplase in Acute Stroke*, ISC, San Diego, CA, 2004.

25. Warach, S., *Early Reperfusion Related to Clinical Response in DIAS: Phase II, Randomized, Placebo-Controlled Dose Finding Trial of IV Desmoteplase 3–9 Hours from Onset in Patients with Diffusion-Perfusion Mismatch*, ISC, San Diego, CA, 2004.

26. Grotta, J., Combination Therapy Stroke Trial: recombinant tissue-type plasminogen activator with/without lubeluzole, *Cerebrovasc. Dis.*, 12, 258–263, 2001.

27. Heiss, W.D., Flow thresholds for functional and morphological damage of brain tissue, *Stroke*, 14, 329–331, 1983.

28. Hillis, A.E., Wityk, R.J., Beauchamp, N.J. et al., Perfusion-weighted MRI as a marker of response to treatment in acute and subacute stroke, *Neuroradiology*, 46(1), 31–39, 2004.

29. Stroke Therapy Academic Industry Roundtable (STAIR), Recommendations for standards regarding preclinical neuroprotective and restorative drug development, *Stroke*, 30, 2752–2758, 1999.

30. Zhang, R.L., Chopp, M., Chen, H., and Garcia, J.H., Temporal profile of ischemic tissue damage, neutrophil response, and vascular plugging following permanent and transient (2H) middle cerebral artery occlusion in the rat, *J. Neurol. Sci.*, 125, 3–10, 1994.

31. Morris, D.C., Zhang, L., Zhang, Z.G. et al., Extension of the therapeutic window for recombinant tissue plasminogen activator with argatroban in a rat model of embolic stroke, *Stroke*, 32, 2635–2640, 2001.

32. Chen, H., Chopp, M., and Welch, K.M., Effect of mild hyperthermia on the ischemic infarct volume after middle cerebral artery occlusion in the rat, *Neurology*, 41, 1133–1135, 1991.

33. Morris, R., Development of a water maze procedure for studying spatial memory in the rat, *J. Neurosci. Meth.*, 11, 47–60, 1984.

34. Kawamata, T., Alexis, N.E., Dietrich, W.D., and Finklestein, S.P., Intracisternal basic fibroblast growth factor (bFGF) enhances behavioral recovery following focal cerebral infarction in the rat, *J. Cereb. Blood Flow Metab.*, 16, 542–547, 1996.

35. Simpson, P.J., Mickelson, J., Fantone, J.C., Gallagher, K.P., and Lucchesi, B.R., Reduction of experimental canine myocardial infarct size with prostaglandin E1: inhibition of neutrophil migration and activation, *J. Pharmacol. Exp. Ther.*, 244, 619–624, 1988.

36. Simpson, P.J., Mitsos, S.E., Ventura, A. et al., Prostacyclin protects ischemic reperfused myocardium in the dog by inhibition of neutrophil activation, *Am. Heart J.*, 113, 129–137, 1987.

37. Simpson, P.J., Fantone, J.C., Mickelson, J.K., Gallagher, K.P., and Lucchesi, B.R., Identification of a time window for therapy to reduce experimental canine myocardial injury: suppression of neutrophil activation during 72 hours of reperfusion, *Circ. Res.*, 63, 1070–1079, 1988.

38. Romson, J.L., Hook, B.G., Kunkel, S.L., Abrams, G.D., Schork, M.A., and Lucchesi, B.R., Reduction of the extent of ischemic myocardial injury by neutrophil depletion in the dog, *Circulation*, 67, 1016–1023, 1983.

39. Simpson, P.J., Todd III, R.F., Fantone, J.C., Mickelson, J.K., Griffin, J.D., and Lucchesi, B.R., Reduction of experimental canine myocardial reperfusion injury by a monoclonal antibody (anti-Mo1, anti-CD11b) that inhibits leukocyte adhesion, *J. Clin. Invest.*, 81, 624–629, 1988.

40. Simpson, P.J., Mickelson, J.K., Fantone, J.C. et al., Sustained limitation of myocardial reperfusion injury by a monoclonal antibody that alters leukocyte function, *Circulation*, 81, 226–237, 1990.

41. Chopp, M., Zhang, R.L., Chen, H., Li, Y., Jiang, N., and Rusche, J.R., Postischemic administration of an anti-Mac-1 antibody reduces ischemic cell damage after transient middle cerebral artery occlusion in rats, *Stroke*, 25, 869–876, 1994.

42. Thijs, V.N., Adami, A., Neumann-Haefelin, T., Moseley, M.E., Marks, M.P., and Albers, G.W., Relationship between severity of MR perfusion deficit and DWI lesion evolution, *Neurology*, 57, 1205–1211, 2001.

43. Kidwell, C.S., Saver, J.L., Villablanca, J.P. et al., Magnetic resonance imaging detection of microbleeds before thrombolysis: an emerging application, *Stroke*, 33, 95–98, 2002.

44. Kidwell, C.S., Saver, J.L., Mattiello J. et al., Thrombolytic reversal of acute human cerebral ischemic injury shown by diffusion/perfusion magnetic resonance imaging, *Ann. Neurol.*, 47, 462–469, 2000.

45. Kidwell, C.S., Saver, J.L., Carneado, J. et al., Predictors of hemorrhagic transformation in patients receiving intra-arterial thrombolysis, *Stroke*, 33, 717–724, 2002.

46. Ginsberg, M.D. and Busto, R., Small-animal models of global and focal cerebral ischemia, in *Cerebrovascular Disease: Pathophysiology, Diagnosis and Management*, Ginsberg, M.D. and Busto, R., Eds., Blackwell Science, Malden, MA, 1998, pp. 14–35.

47. Slivka, A., Murphy, E., and Horrocks, L., Cerebral edema after temporary and permanent middle cerebral artery occlusion in the rat, *Stroke*, 26, 1061–1066, 1995.

48. Tamura, A., Graham, D.I., McCulloch, J., and Teasdale, G.M., Focal cerebral ischaemia in the rat. 1. Description of technique and early neuropathological consequences following middle cerebral artery occlusion, *J. Cereb. Blood Flow Metab.*, 1, 53–60, 1981.

49. Yepes, M., Sandkvist, M., Wong, M.K. et al., Neuroserpin reduces cerebral infarct volume and protects neurons from ischemia-induced apoptosis, *Blood*, 96, 569–576, 2000.

50. Longa, E., Weinstein, P.R., Carlson, S. et al., Reversible middle cerebral artery occlusion without craniectomy in rats, *Stroke*, 20, 84–91, 1989.

51. Kohno, K., Back, T., Hoehn-Berlage, N. et al., A modified rat model of middle cerebral artery thread occlusion under electrophysiological control for magnetic resonance investigations, *Magn. Reson. Imaging*, 13, 65–71, 1995.

52. Phillips, J.B., Williams, A.J., Adams, J., Elliott, P.J., and Tortella, F.C., Proteasome inhibitor PS519 reduces infarction and attenuates leukocyte infiltration in a rat model of focal cerebral ischemia, *Stroke*, 31, 1686–1693, 2000.

53. Wang, C.X., Yang, Y., Yang, T., and Shuaib, A., A focal embolic model of cerebral ischemia in rats: introduction and evaluation, *Brain Res. Brain Res. Protoc.*, 7, 115–120, 2001.

54. Wang, C.X., Yang, T., and Shuaib, A., An improved version of embolic model of brain ischemic injury in the rat, *J. Neurosci. Meth.*, 109, 147–51, 2001.

55. Overgaard, K., Thrombolytic therapy in experimental embolic stroke, *Cerebrovasc. Brain Metab. Rev.*, 6, 257–286, 1994.

56. Sereghy, T., Overgaard, K., and Boysen, G., Neuroprotection by excitatory amino acid antagonist augments the benefit of thrombolysis in embolic stroke in rats, *Stroke*, 24, 1702–1708, 1993.

57. Andersen, M., Overgaard, K., Meden, P., and Boysen, G., Effects of Citicoline combined with thrombolytic therapy in a rat embolic stroke model, *Stroke*, 30, 1464–1471, 1999.

58. Wang, X., Asahi, M., and Lo, E.H., Tissue type plasminogen activator amplifies hemoglobin-induced neurotoxicity in rat neuronal cultures, *Neurosci. Lett.*, 274, 79–82, 1999.

59. Al-Senani, F.M., Shirzadi, A., Strong, R., Elliott, P., Grotta, J.C., and Aronowski, J., Inhibition of proteasome reduces iNOS expression and behavioral dysfunction after intracerebral hemorrhage in rat, *Neurology*, 66(Suppl. 3), A368, 2001.

60. Lapchak, P.A., Araujo, D.M., Song, D., Wie, J., and Zivin, J.A., Neuroprotective effects of the spin trap agent disodium-[(*tert*-butylimino)methyl]benzene-1,3–disulfonate *N*-oxide (generic NXY-059) in a rabbit small clot embolic stroke model: combination studies with the thrombolytic tissue plasminogen activator, *Stroke*, 33, 1411–1415, 2002.

61. Lapchak, P.A., Araujo, D.M., Song, D., and Zivin, J.A., The nonpeptide glycoprotein IIb/IIIa platelet receptor antagonist SM-20302 reduces tissue plasminogen activator-induced intracerebral hemorrhage after thromboembolic stroke, *Stroke*, 33, 147–152, 2002.

62. Lapchak, P.A., Chapman, D.F., and Zivin, J.A., Pharmacological effects of the spin trap agents *N-t*-butyl-phenylnitrone (PBN) and 2,2,6,6-tetramethylpiperidine-*N*-oxyl (TEMPO) in a rabbit thromboembolic stroke model: combination studies with the thrombolytic tissue plasminogen activator, *Stroke*, 32, 147–153, 2001.

63. Chapman, D.F., Lyden, P., Lapchak, P.A., Nunez, S., Thibodeaux, H., and Zivin, J., Comparison of TNK with wild-type tissue plasminogen activator in a rabbit embolic stroke model, *Stroke*, 32, 748–752, 2001.

64. Clark, W.M., Madden, K.P., Rothlein, R., and Zivin, J.A., Reduction of central nervous system ischemic injury in rabbits using leukocyte adhesion antibody treatment, *Stroke*, 22, 877–883, 1991.

65. Carter, L.P., Guthkelch, A.N., Orozco, J., and Temeltas, O., Influence of tissue plasminogen activator and heparin on cerebral ischemia in a rabbit model, *Stroke*, 23, 883–888, 1992.

66. Hamilton, M.G., Lee, J.S., Cummings, P.J., and Zabramski, J.M., A comparison of intra-arterial and intravenous tissue-type plasminogen activator on autologous arterial emboli in the cerebral circulation of rabbits, *Stroke*, 25, 651–656, 1994.

67. Russell, D., Madden, K.P., Clark, W.M., and Zivin, J.A., Tissue plasminogen activator cerebrovascular thrombolysis in rabbits is dependent on the rate and route of administration, *Stroke*, 23, 388–393, 1992.

68. Garcia, J.H. and Kamijyo, Y., Cerebral infarction: evolution of histopathological changes after occlusion of a middle cerebral artery in primates, *J. Neuropathol. Exp. Neurol.*, 33, 408–421, 1974.

69. Branston, N.M., Symon, L., Crockard, H.A., and Pasztor, E., Relationship between the cortical evoked potential and local cortical blood flow following acute middle cerebral artery occlusion in the baboon, *Exp. Neurol.*, 45, 195–208, 1974.

70. Spetzler, R.F., Selman, W.R., Weinstein, P. et al., Chronic reversible cerebral ischemia: evaluation of a new baboon model, *Neurosurgery*, 7, 257–261, 1980.

71. Del Zoppo, G.J., Copeland, B.R., Harker, L.A. et al., Experimental acute thrombotic stroke in baboons, *Stroke*, 17, 1254–1265, 1986.

72. Young, A.R., Touzani, O., Derlon, J.M., Sette, G., MacKenzie, E.T., and Baron, J.C., Early reperfusion in the anesthetized baboon reduces brain damage following middle cerebral artery occlusion: a quantitative analysis of infarction volume, *Stroke*, 28, 632–638, 1997.

73. Nudo, R.J., Wise, B.M., SiFuentes, F., and Milliken, G.W., Neural substrates for the effects of rehabilitative training on motor recovery after ischemic infarct, *Science*, 272, 1791–1794, 1996.

74. Marshall, J.W., Cross, A.J., Jackson, D.M., Green, A.R., Baker, H.F., and Ridley, R.M., Clomethiazole protects against hemineglect in a primate model of stroke, *Brain Res. Bull.*, 52, 21–29, 2000.

75. Marshall, J.W., Cross, A.J., and Ridley, R.M., Functional benefit from clomethiazole treatment after focal cerebral ischemia in a nonhuman primate species, *Exp. Neurol.*, 156, 121–129, 1999.

76. Marshall, J.W., Duffin, K.J., Green, A.R., and Ridley, R.M., NXY-059, a free radical-trapping agent, substantially lessens the functional disability resulting from cerebral ischemia in a primate species, *Stroke*, 32, 190–198, 2001.

77. Marshall, J.W. and Ridley, R.M., Assessment of functional impairment following permanent middle cerebral artery occlusion in a non-human primate species, *Neurodegeneration*, 5, 275–286, 1996.

78. Krueger, K. and Busch, E., Protocol of a thromboembolic stroke model in the rat: review of the experimental procedure and comparison of models, *Invest. Radiol.*, 37, 600–608, 2002.

79. Roof, R.L., Schielke, G.P., Ren, X., and Hall, E.D., A comparison of long-term functional outcome after 2 middle cerebral artery occlusion models in rats, *Stroke*, 32, 2648–2657, 2001.

80. Stroemer, R.P., Kent, T.A., and Hulsebosch, C.E., Enhanced neocortical neural sprouting, synaptogenesis, and behavioral recovery with D-amphetamine therapy after neocortical infarction in rats, *Stroke*, 29, 2381–2395, 1998.

81. Schallert, T., Hernandez, T.D., and Barth, T.M., Recovery of function after brain damage: severe and chronic disruption by diazepam, *Brain Res.*, 379, 104–111, 1986.

82. Hernandez, T. and Schallert, T., Seizures and recovery from experimental brain damage, *Exp. Neurol.*, 102, 318–324, 1988.

83. DeRyck, M.R.J., Borgers, M., Wauquier, A., and Janssen, P.A.J., Photochemical stroke model: flunazarine prevents sensorimotor deficits after neocortical infarcts, *Stroke*, 20, 1383–1390, 1989.

84. Kolb, B., Cote, S., Ribeiro-da-Silva, A., and Cuello, A.C., Nerve growth factor treatment prevents dendritic atrophy and promotes recovery of function after cortical injury, *Neuroscience*, 76, 1139–1151, 1997.

85. Feeney, D.M., Gonzalez, A., and Law, W.A., Amphetamine, haloperidol, and experience interact to affect rate of recovery after motor cortex injury, *Science*, 217, 855–857, 1982.

86. Borlongan, C.V., Elevated body swing test: a new behavioral parameter for rats with 6-hydroxy-dopamine-induced hemiparkinsonism, *J. Neurosci.*, 15, 5372–5378, 1995.

87. Alves, W.A. and Macciocchi, S.N., Ethical considerations in clinical neuroscience: current concepts in neuroclinical trials, *Stroke*, 27, 1903–1909, 1996.

88. Dudley, N., Be careful when extrapolating trial data to real life, *Br. Med. J.*, 327, 812, 2003.

89. Caplan, L.R., Evidence based medicine: concerns of a clinical neurologist, *J. Neurol. Neurosurg. Psychiatry*, 71, 569–576, 2001.

90. Stroke Therapy Academic Industry Roundtable (STAIR) II, Recommendations for clinical trial evaluation of acute stroke therapies, *Stroke*, 32, 1598–1606, 2001.

91. Adams, Jr., H.P., Adams, R.J., Brott, T. et al., Guidelines for the early management of patients with ischemic stroke: a scientific statement from the Stroke Council of the American Stroke Association, *Stroke*, 34, 1056–1083, 2003.

92. Higashida, R.T. and Furlan, A.J., Trial design and reporting standards for intra-arterial cerebral thrombolysis for acute ischemic stroke, *Stroke*, 34, 109–137, 2003.

93. Libman, R., Bhatnagar, R., Ding, L., Kwiatkowski, T., and Barr, W., Placebo treatment in acute stroke trials: benefit or harm to patients?, *Stroke*, 31, 355–357, 2000.

94. Kasner, S.E., Demchuk, A.M., Berrouschot, J. et al., Predictors of fatal brain edema in massive hemispheric ischemic stroke, *Stroke*, 32, 2117–2123, 2001.

95. Szikszai, Z., Fekete, I., and Imre, S.G., A comparative study of hemorheological parameters in transient ischemic attack and acute ischemic stroke patients: possible predictive value, *Clin. Hemorheol. Microcirc.*, 28, 51–57, 2003.

96. Wiszniewska, M., Mendel, T., and Czlonkowska, A., Prognostic factors in the acute phase of hemorrhagic stroke, *Neurol. Neurochir. Pol.*, 36, 647–656, 2002.

97.   Young, F.B., Lees, K.R., and Weir, C.G., Strengthening acute stroke trials through optimal use of
      disability endpoints, *Stroke*, 34, 2676–2680, 2003.
98.   Abciximab Emergent Stroke Treatment Trial (AbESTT) investigators, Emergency administration of
      abciximab for treatment of patients with acute ischemic stroke: results of a randomized phase 2 trials,
      Stroke, 36, 880–890, 2005.

PART **V**

Assessment of Respiratory Drugs

CHAPTER 16

Antiasthmatic Drugs

Lucia H. Lee, Christopher L. Wu, Benjamin R. Lee, and Chi-Jen Lee

CONTENTS

16.1 INTRODUCTION

Asthma is a chronic inflammatory disease with associated bronchospasm. The inflammation results in airflow obstruction from constriction of the bronchial smooth muscle and swelling of the bronchial mucosa. Persistent inflammation is a primary cause of the increased bronchial hyperresponsiveness. The swelling of the bronchial mucosa is due to edema and cellular infiltration with eosinophils as well as mast cells, polymorphonuclear leukocytes, macrophages, and lymphocytes. Type 1 (IgE-mediated) immune responses play an important role in the development of asthma in children and many adults. In adults, allergic factors may be more difficult to identify. Exposure to cigarette smoke, aerosols, or cold, dry air; exercise; upper respiratory infections; and occupational exposure to provocative substances may trigger asthma. Specific trigger factors include airborne and ingested allergens such as house dust, mite, animal hairs, pollens, fungal spores, and various foods. Allergens and infections produce predominantly inflammation, whereas the nonspecific triggers result in bronchoconstrictions.

As a result of the inflammatory changes in the bronchial mucosa, asthma patients show an abnormal bronchoconstrictive response to histamine challenge. This abnormal response, known as bronchial hyperreactivity, is used to identify potential asthmatic subjects in epidemiological studies and to measure the effects of treatment. The clinical symptoms of asthma include wheeze, shortness of breath, cough, chest tightness, disturbance in sleep, and limited ability to carry out normal daily activities. These subjective symptoms are associated with measurable changes in airflow.

Medical treatment is directed toward reversing or preventing bronchospasm, inflammation, and edema, as well as eliminating muscle plugs and correcting hypoxemia. The duration of treatment is guided as much by the patient's response to drug therapy as by the severity of symptoms. During the process of remission, the extent of treatment is determined by the symptoms that interfere with daily functions and the results of pulmonary function tests.

Inflammatory mediators and chemotactic factors released by the mast cells and eosinophils contribute to bronchospasm. Mediators include histamine, histamine-releasing factor, interleukins, chemotactic factors, platelet-activating factor, prostaglandins, and leukotrienes. Studies on early- and late-phase asthmatic reactions have used allergens as the asthmatic stimulus. The early-phase asthmatic response to a stimulus occurs within 10 to 20 minutes after exposure and spontaneously recovers after 60 to 90 minutes. This response is caused by mast-cell-releasing mediators inducing smooth muscle contraction, increasing capillary permeability, and stimulating the release of chemotactic factors to the lung. In contrast, the late-phase asthmatic response is primarily inflammatory and begins 3 to 4 hours after exposure to an allergen; it may persist for 12 hours. This response begins with the influx of inflammatory cells into the lung.[1–3]

16.2 ANTIASTHMATIC DRUGS AND THEIR MECHANISMS OF ACTION

The goals of antiasthmatic drugs are prevention of bronchospasm as well as long-term control of bronchial hyperresponsiveness and inflammation. Usually, long-term continuous treatment is necessary. Observation over several months is required to determine that intermittent treatment is sufficient. The bronchodilators include beta agonists, which stimulate beta$_2$-adrenergic receptors, increase intracellular cyclic adenosine monophosphate (cAMP), and inhibit the release of inflammatory mediators. Anticholinergic drugs relieve bronchospasm by blocking parasympathetic cholinergic impulses at the receptor level. Antihistamines prevent or abort mild allergic asthmatic symptoms, particularly in children. Agents with antiinflammatory activities include cromolyn sodium, which prevents the release of mediator substances and blocks respiratory neuronal reflexes, and corticosteroids, which decrease inflammation and edema. (See Table 16.1.)

The main considerations for drug selection in asthma patients are the severity and status of the disease. The availability of agents with different mechanisms of action and adverse reactions, as well as the availability of inhalers, nebulizers, and prolonged-release preparations, are also important factors in selection. Airway inflammation is a critical element in all cases of asthma. The aggressive and early therapy with inhaled corticosteroids, cromolyn sodium, and other antiinflammatory agents should be considered for maintenance in patients with moderate and severe asthma.[4–6]

16.2.1 Antiinflammatory Corticosteroids

Steroids inhibit the response to inflammation and decrease bronchial hyperreactivity. These drugs prevent the synthesis or action of inflammatory mediators, resulting in the decreased release of mediators from mast cells.[7] Corticosteroids inhibit late-phase asthmatic reactions but have little effect on immediate hypersensitivity. Steroids reduce the formation of mucus and edema. They also stabilize lysosomal membranes, reduce mast and basophil histamine stores, and restore the responsiveness of leukocytes and bronchial smooth muscle to beta agonists.[8,9]

Glucocorticoids act by entering a target cell and binding to intracellular cytoplasmic steroid receptors, resulting in conformational changes termed *activation*, and by binding to DNA at sites known as glucocorticoid response elements (GREs). GRE binding controls the transcription of

Table 16.1 Antiasthmatic Drugs

Drug	Activities and Remarks
Antiinflammatory Corticosteroids	
Prednisone	Inhibits the response to inflammation and decreases bronchial hyperreactivity (oral dose: adults, 30–60 mg; children, 1–2 mg/kg/day)
Hydrocortisone sodium succinate	200–300 mg intravenous injection
Methyl prednisolone	40–80 mg intravenous injection
Dexamethasone	Long-acting but causes severe withdrawal symptoms
Antiallergy and Antihistamines	
Cromolyn sodium	Used only to prevent asthma attacks; reduces bronchial hyperresponsiveness but has no adrenergic, antihistaminic, or antiinflammatory actions and no bronchodilator activity
Chlorpheniramine	H_1-receptor blocker; induces bronchodilator activity
Terfenadine	Second-generation H_1 antihistamine, nonsedating
Astemizole	Second-generation H_1 antihistamine, nonsedating
Cetirizine	Second-generation H_1 antihistamine, nonsedating
Loratadine	Second-generation H_1 antihistamine, nonsedating
Beta-Adrenergic Agonist	
Epinephrine	Adrenergic bronchodilator that stimulates $beta_2$-receptors; now obsolete and not used
Isoproterenol	Potent bronchodilator but short acting; duration, 1–2 hr
Isoetharine	Peak effect, 15–60 min; duration, 2–3 hr
Metaproterenol	Peak effect, 30–60 min; duration, 3–4 hr
Terbutaline	Peak effect, 60 min; duration, 4 hr
Albuterol	Peak effect, 30–60 min; duration, 4–6 hr
Bitolterol	Peak effect, 30–60 min; duration, 5 hr
Pirbuterol	Peak effect, 60 min; duration, 5 hr
Xanthine Drugs	
Theophylline	Mechanism involves increase in cellular level of cAMP, intracellular calcium transport, and inhibition of adenosine receptors; also inhibits inflammatory mediators
Dyphylline	Much less potent than theophylline and rarely used
Methyl prednisolone	40–80 mg; much less potent than theophylline and rarely used
Dexamethasone	Long-acting but causes severe withdrawal symptoms
Others	
Anticholinergic agents (e.g., atropine, ipratropium)	Reduce bronchospasm; side effects include central nervous system stimulation, mydriasis, dry mouth
Calcium channel blocking agents (e.g., verapamil, diltiazem)	Selectively inhibit calcium ion influx, suppressing smooth muscle excitation

specific genes. Glucocorticoids act at multiple sites and block multiple tissue responses to bio-chemical stimuli. They prevent the initiation of reactions leading to the production of prostaglandins and leukotrienes that inhibit phospholipase A_2. Glucocorticoids increase the number of beta-agonist receptors on cell membranes.

Systemic corticosteroids are the most effective antiasthmatic drugs available. Because of adverse effects, however, their long-term use is restricted to patients who do not respond adequately to beta-adrenergic drugs, theophylline, cromolyn sodium, inhalant corticosteroids, or combinations of these drugs. Administration of oral corticosteroids (e.g., prednisone) for acute asthma prevents status asthmaticus and avoids hospitalization. The daily dose of oral prednisone for adults is 30 to 60 mg, and for children it is 1 to 2 mg/kg/day. The short-term intravenous administration of a corticosteroid is necessary in acute severe asthma. Hydrocortisone sodium (200 to 300 mg), methylprednisolone (40 to 80 mg), or the equivalent is administered intravenously over 20 to 30 minutes every 4 to 6 hours. Long-term steroids (e.g., dexamethasone) should not be used to treat asthma because of the subsequent severe withdrawal symptoms, such as fever, myalgia, and joint pain. Moreover, they can suppress the hypothalamus–pituitary–adrenal (HPA) axis. To avoid adrenal crisis before axis responsiveness returns after therapy, doses of corticosteroids must be reduced gradually over weeks to months. Once the disease symptoms are in remission, alternative therapy is used to minimize adverse effects.

16.2.2 Antiallergy and Antihistamine Drugs

Antiallergy and antihistamine drugs block various inflammatory reactions in the late-phase asth-matic response and diminish or inhibit bronchial hyperresponsiveness. Cromolyn sodium is used only to prevent asthma attacks. It reduces bronchial hyperresponsiveness but has no adrenergic, antihistaminic, or corticosteroid-like actions and little bronchodilator activity. It is as effective as theophylline in children with chronic asthma.[10] Although cromolyn has been used primarily in children, it is also effective as an antiasthmatic agent in adults. It prevents allergic asthma in patients experiencing frequent wheezing, seasonal or occupational asthma, animal- or exercise-induced asthma, and asthma not responsive to beta-adrenergic drugs and theophylline.[11] Cromolyn causes minimal adverse reactions.

Antihistamines (H_1-receptor antagonists) act by competitively antagonizing the effects of his-tamine at receptor sites; they do not block the release of histamine and hence offer only relief of allergic symptoms. After oral administration, effects are apparent within 15 to 30 minutes and persist for 4 to 6 hours. Indications for the clinical use of antihistamines vary considerably. The majority of these agents are effective for perennial and seasonal allergic rhinitis, vasomotor rhinitis, and allergic conjunctivitis.

Intravenously administered chlorpheniramine, a first-generation H_1-receptor blocker, produces bronchodilation in asthma patients.[12] Nonsedating second-generation H_1 antihistamines that have shown effectiveness in asthma therapy include terfenadine (note that Seldane® has been withdrawn from the market due to adverse reactions), astemizole (Hismanal®), cetirizine (Reactine™), and loratadine (Claritin®).

16.2.3 Beta-Adrenergic Agonists

Beta-agonists rapidly reduce bronchoconstriction. These drugs also increase the rate of mucociliary clearance. Expectoration is improved as a result of enhanced bronchodilation. Epinephrine stimu-lates beta$_2$-receptors, but also has beta$_1$- and alpha-adrenergic (vasoconstrictor) activity. It is useful for the immediate management of acute bronchospasm in children. Ephedrine is now obsolete and not used. Isoproterenol is a potent bronchodilator but short acting, and has marked beta$_1$-receptor activity. Adrenergic agents with greater specificity for beta$_2$-receptors than beta$_1$-receptors include isoetharine (Bronkometer®, Bronkosol®), metaproterenol (Alupent®, Metaprel®), terbutaline (Brethaire®, Brethine®), albuterol (Proventil®, Ventolin®), bitolterol (Tornalate®), and pirbuterol (Maxaire®). These drugs are effective when administered by metered-dose inhaler. The investigational drugs procaterol and fenoterol are also selective beta$_2$ agonists, and their efficacy is comparable to that of albuterol.

16.2.4 Xanthine Drugs

The mechanism of action of theophylline involves an increase in the level of cAMP in selective cell compartments, modulation of intracellular calcium transport, and inhibition of adenosine receptors.[13] Theophylline increases the contractility of diaphragmatic muscle and enhances its resistance to fatigue. It also inhibits the release of inflammatory mediators. The respiratory center is stimulated because the hypoxic drive is increased. It is used to treat status asthmaticus, to prevent attacks, or to minimize symptoms during the process of remission. Another xanthine, dyphylline, is much less potent than theophylline and is rarely used. An investigational xanthine, enprofylline, produces significant bronchodilation in asthma patients and is safer than theophylline.[14]

16.2.5 Others

Anticholinergic drugs such as atropine reduce bronchospasm. An anticholinergic agent is used when inhaled beta-adrenergic agonist or theophylline is ineffective or when cough is prominent. Anticholinergic drugs are much less useful than beta$_2$ agonists in treatment of asthma. Calcium channel-blocking agents such as verapamil (Calan®, Isoptin®), diltiazem (Cardizem®), and nifedipine (Adalat®, Procardia®) selectively inhibit calcium ion influx across the cell membrane, thereby suppressing calcium-dependent smooth muscle excitation. The secretion of histamine and other mediators is initiated by movement of calcium into mast cells. Calcium antagonists have prevented exercise-induced asthma.

16.3 ASSESSMENTS OF ANTIASTHMATIC DRUGS

Asthma patients exhibit variable airway obstructions. Airflow limitation is caused by both inflammatory edema and muscle bronchoconstriction. Measurement of airway function thus forms an important part of the evaluation of antiasthmatic drugs. In short-term experiments in humans, the following functions are measured:

- Large airway functions — peak expiratory flow rate (PEFR), forced expiratory volume (FEV), and forced vital capacity (FVC)
- Small partial expiratory flow rate (pEFR)

In longer term experiments, those measurements that can be repeated frequently (e.g., FEV, PEFR) are used. In some cases, more complicated measures of airway function are needed.[15]

The initial studies include characterization of the absorption, distribution, metabolism, and excretion of the drug candidate and its single- and repeated-dose tolerance in healthy subjects. These are followed by bronchial challenge studies to examine the ability of the compound to block or attenuate the bronchoconstricting effects of various agents, including inhaled antigen, exercise, sulfur dioxide, sodium metabisulfite, adenosine monophosphate, bradykinin, histamine, and methacholine. Testing with these agents is useful to explore the pharmacologic profile of the compound and to investigate the protective effect of different dose ranges and duration. The following subjects are selected for such experiments:

- Adult asthmatic patients with baseline pulmonary functions as measured by FEV exhibiting ±20% their normal value
- Pulmonary function that does not fluctuate over the period of the experiment by more than ±10%
- No other disease and no viral or other respiratory infection within 6 weeks

Each challenge is conducted under the same conditions in the same environment and at the same time each day. The entire experiment involves four challenges (two controls, active treatment preceding challenge, and placebo treatment challenge) and is conducted in a short period of 3 to 7 days between each challenge. Patients are kept under observation throughout the period of the experiment, and resuscitation equipment should be available to deal with any respiratory or cardiovascular emergency. Patients are kept in the laboratory until their pulmonary function has returned to normal values for at least 60 minutes.

The short-term therapeutic trial (4 to 6 weeks) involves an experiment that determines the therapeutic potential of an antiasthmatic drug. These trials are conduced under defined conditions in selected patients. Trials to establish the efficacy of a new drug and to compare a new drug with existing treatments must be of longer duration (3 to 12 months). These trials involve a randomized, double-blind, parallel group design in which the group treated with the new drug (X) is compared to a group treated with the control (Y or placebo). The test treatment period is a minimum of 28 days and is preceded by a baseline period of at least 14 days. During the baseline period, patients continue to take their existing therapy. The baseline period is preceded by a run-in period during which existing therapy may be altered in order to induce a defined level of symptoms. During early trials it is not appropriate to use the crossover type of trial design because of the difficulty in interpreting changes in a disease with inter- and intrapatient variability.

The selection of homogeneous patients for early trials is important. In these studies, women of child-bearing age are excluded and the trials are carried out in men. The disease state of asthma changes with age, with non-allergic mechanisms playing an important role with increasing age. Asthma that begins in adult life is different from that which begins in childhood. Patients are, therefore, selected within a narrow age range (not more than 20 years). For asthma that has begun in childhood, the age range of 20 to 40 years is suitable. If patients with late-onset asthma are selected, an age range of 35 to 55 years is more suitable. It is preferable to select either all allergic patients or all nonallergic patients. The presence of allergy is confirmed by either skin tests or specific IgE antibody response. Patients with persistant asthma symptoms are preferable to those with seasonal asthma only.

16.3.1 Pulmonary Function Tests

Pulmonary function tests are conducted each time the patient visits the clinic, testing two to three times daily. The baseline of the test can be used to categorize the extent of asthma symptoms and to measure the effectiveness of treatment. Full spirometry is carried out in each visit. During the baseline period, the pulmonary function tests should not vary by more than 10%, and all patients should be within a 20% range of predicted normal values, such as within 80 to 100% or 60 to 80% of predicted normal. Current international guidelines define the categories of asthma patients as follows:

- Mild asthma — FEV_1 or PEFR > 80% predicted normal values with a diurnal variability of < 20%
- Moderate asthma — FEV_1 or PEFR 60 to 80% predicted normal values with a diurnal variability of 20 to 30%
- Severe asthma — FEV_1 or PEFR < 60% predicted normal values with a diurnal variability of > 30%

All pulmonary function tests are standardized according to international standards.[16,17]

During the baseline period and throughout the trial, patients are asked to measure and record their peak expiratory flow rate on three occasions each day: (1) immediately after rising in the morning, (2) between 4:00 and 6:00 p.m., and (3) on going to bed. The mean daily peak expiratory flow rate should not vary by more than ±10% during the baseline period, and all patients should fall within a 20% range of predicted normal values.

16.3.2 Extent of Asthma Symptoms

After recovering to normal lung function, asthma patients may still exhibit symptoms of cough and wheeze. Daily measurement on the patient's asthma symptoms is important in the evaluation of antiasthma drugs. The following scales have been devised and used for evaluating asthma symptoms:

Scale	Asthma Symptoms
Daytime asthma	
0	No symptoms occur during the daytime
1	Occasional wheeze or breathlessness quickly relieved by bronchodilator aerosol
2	Wheezing or short of breath most of the day that does not interfere with usual activities
3	Wheezing or short of breath most of the day that interferes to some extent with usual activities
4	Serious asthma; cannot go to work or school or engage in usual activities
Night-time asthma	
0	No symptoms occur at night
1	Awake once at night because of wheezing or cough; awake for less than an hour and does not need to use a bronchodilator aerosol
2	Awake once at night because of wheezing or cough; awake for less than an hour but needs to use a bronchodilator aerosol to get back to sleep
3	Awake once for more than an hour or awake more than once because of wheezing or cough
4	Awake for most of the night because of wheezing or cough

All asthmatic patients have reactive airways that can be measured by the response of a histamine or methacholine dose. This reactivity is also reflected in a response to a single dose of an inhaled bronchodilator. Patients should be within the same broad range of bronchial reactivity and all exhibit reversibility to an inhaled bronchodilator of 15%.

16.3.3 Study Design and Conditions

For evaluating a new member of an existing class of compounds (e.g., corticosteroid), efficacy and safety may be established by substituting the new drug for an established member of that class. Patients are selected based on those who are currently maintained on the existing drug, and the new compound is substituted on a double-blind, randomized basis. All patients fit within a defined range of entry criteria with respect to symptom severity, pulmonary function, existing therapy, and use of rescue medicine. Their asthma should be stable without severe symptoms or change of therapy for at least 3 months.

Symptom severity is based on mean extent scores during the baseline period or on scores that are >1 on at least 4 days of the last week of the baseline. Pulmonary function is defined on the basis of reference to predicted normal and diurnal variation recorded during the baseline and rescue bronchodilators on the basis of daily usage during the final week of the baseline.

For evaluating a new class of compounds, it is necessary to establish efficacy using a placebo control. In these cases, it is essential to demonstrate the effectiveness of the compound as compared with the placebo by selecting patients who exhibit marked symptom severity and low pulmonary function. For many patients in clinical trials, a run-in period can be used during which a proportion of existing medication is removed in order to produce asthma symptoms. This is a difficult ethical decision, but such designs can be considered adequate and the risk small provided stable, well-controlled patients are selected who are informed, have immediate access to emergency services at any time, and are within easy reach of the hospital. The run-in period is no longer than 4 weeks, and patients are checked weekly. Patients then enter a baseline period at that level of treatment.

The following criteria can be used for patients entering into the test treatment period:

- Mean daily score for day or night asthma of 1.5 or greater over 7 days
- Mean morning PEFR over 7 days 10 to 20% lower than that over the last 7 days of the baseline period
- 10 to 20% increase in the total daily use of inhaled beta$_2$ agonist

Changes in scores greater than these criteria are considered unsuitable asthma, and these patients should be removed from the trial. When the entry criteria are established, the selection of patients should comply with these criteria. During the baseline period, the patients should get used to the measurements of disease state to provide the baseline values for the test treatments. At least two clinic visits should be made for baseline pulmonary function, reversibility, and bronchial hyperactivity tests. In addition, blood and urine samples should be taken for baseline values.

During assessment of asthma symptoms, patients should keep a daily record of the severity of their symptoms, noting two to three symptoms on a scale of 0 to 4. Patients should record their peak expiratory flow rate two to three times a day. All patients should use the same peak flow meter. In addition, patients should record their use of inhaled bronchodilators each day, including the 24-hour total and number of doses used between rising in the morning and during the night. Data analysis on efficacy should demonstrate an improvement in the efficacy variables for the drug under evaluation as compared to a placebo or active drug.

REFERENCES

1. DeKorte, C.J., Current and emerging therapies for management of chronic inflammation in asthma, *Am. J. Health Syst. Pharm.*, 60(19), 1949–1959, 2003.
2. Aronson, N., Lefevre, F., Piper, M. et al., Management of chronic asthma, *Evid. Rep. Technol. Assess. (Summ.)*, 44, 1–10, 2001.
3. Legg, J. and Warner, J., Asthma: the challenging face of drug therapy, *Indian J. Pediatr.*, 67(2), 147–153, 2000.
4. Guidelines for the Diagnosis and Management of Asthma: National Heart, Lung, and Blood Institute National Asthma Education Program Expert Panel Report, *J. Allergy Clin. Immunol.*, 88, 425–534, 1991.
5. Barnes, P.J., New drugs for asthma, *Nat. Rev. Drug Discov.*, 3(10), 831–844, 2004.
6. Hansel, T.T. and Barnes, P.J., Novel drugs for treating asthma, *Curr. Allergy Asthma Rep.*, 1(2), 164–173, 2001.
7. Norn, S. and Clementsen, P., Bronchial asthma: pathophysiology mechanisms and corticosteroids, *Allergy*, 43, 401–405, 1988.
8. Mcfadden, E.R., Jr., Corticosteroids and cromolyn sodium as modulators of airway inflammation, *Chest*, 94, 181–184, 1988.
9. Nelson, R.P. and Lockey, R.F., Treatment of asthma with glucocorticosteroids, *South. Med. J.*, 81, 761–769, 1988.
10. Bernstein, I.L., Cromolyn sodium, *Chest*, 87(Suppl.), 68S–73S, 1985.
11. Summers, R. and Smith, L., Asthma management: new perspectives, improved options, *Postgrad. Med.*, 76, 209–221, 1984.
12. Popa, V.T., Bronchodilating activity of H$_1$-blocker, chloropheniramine, *J. Allergy Clin. Immunol.*, 59, 54–63, 1977.
13. Trophy, T.J., Action of mediators on airway smooth muscle: functional antagonism as a mechanism for bronchodilator drugs, *Agents Action Supp.*, 23, 37–53, 1988.
14. Boe, J. et al., Efficacy of enprofylline, new bronchodilating xanthine, in acute asthma, *Ann. Allergy*, 59, 155–158, 1987.

15. Tattersfield, A.E. and Keeping, I.M., Assessing changes in airway caliber-measurement of airway resistance, *Br. J. Clin. Pharmacol.*, 8, 307–319, 1979.
16. American Thoracic Society, Lung function testing: selection of reference values and interpretational strategies, *Am. Rev. Resp. Dis.*, 144, 1202–1218, 1991.
17. Quanjer, Ph.H., Tammeling, G.J., Cotes, J.E. et al., Standardized lung function testing, *Eur. Resp. J.*, 6, 1–99, 1993.

PART VI

Assessment of Central Nervous System Drugs

CHAPTER 17

Anxiolytics and Hypnotics

Graham R. McClelland and Georges Moroz

CONTENTS

17.1 INTRODUCTION

In recent years, drugs used to treat anxiety disorders (anxiolytics) and sleep disorders (hypnotics) have received a great deal of attention from regulatory authorities, the legal profession, the media, and consequently the general public. This interest has been primarily directed at the benzodiazepine class of drugs and the physiological and psychological effects that may occur after stopping treatment. Anxiety and insomnia remain the two most common disorders of the central nervous system (CNS) encountered by primary care physicians.

The anxiolytic and hypnotic market has long been dominated by benzodiazepines. The advantages of benzodiazepines include useful and rapid efficacy, few somatic side effects, and safety in overdose.[1] Most of the benzodiazepines have been on the market for several years, are no longer protected by patent, and are subject to generic competition; consequently, the cost of treatment is relatively low. Any new treatment faces the difficult task of having to demonstrate a significant improvement in safety or efficacy compared with the benzodiazepines in order to achieve a price that would enable the recouping of research and development costs. Five elements have substantially altered both drug development and clinical practice over the last 10 years:

- The recognition of a fundamental epidemiological, clinical, and pharmacological overlap between anxiety disorders and depressive disorders. While the anxiolytic potential of the tricyclic antidepressants and monoamine oxidase inhibitors was already noticed in the 1960s, the marketing of safer and better tolerated serotonergic or serotonergic–noradrenergic antidepressants in the 1990s has resulted in a widening of the clinical use of antidepressants in anxiety disorders and in an almost systematic study of antidepressants in anxiety indications during both the premarketing and postmarketing phases of drug development.
- The use of high-potency benzodiazepines (alprazolam, clonazepam, and lorazepam) in specific anxiety indications, mainly panic disorder, first advocated in the early 1980s, has continued expanding, in some cases as a combination treatment with serotonergic antidepressants.
- Non-benzodiazepine GABA-ergic hypnotics interacting with the GABA–benzodiazepine receptor complex, such as zolpidem and zaleplon, have been marketed in recent years and have competed with benzodiazepines in the treatment of insomnias.
- Compounds with novel mechanisms of action are being investigated. Some aim at a dual antidepressant–anxiolytic effect (e.g., CRF antagonists and substance P antagonists). Others are GABA-ergic drugs that selectively target the alpha peptidic subunits of the GABA-A receptor so as to achieve a purely hypnotic or anxiolytic effect with minimal cognitive side effects.
- CNS neuroimaging is emerging as a tool for the selection of molecules with a psychotropic potential and for the selection of doses.

Sedation, sleep, and general anesthesia are generally regarded as being part of the same continuum of CNS depression, and because hypnotics are capable of producing such a CNS depression they are occasionally indicated for the treatment of anxiety. Most important is the substantial overlap of drugs used in the treatment of depression and most anxiety disorders (particularly panic and phobic disorders). These overlaps and continuities notwithstanding, this chapter concentrates on the development of drugs for which the initial target indication is that of anxiety or sleep disorders.

Sleep disorders (dyssomnias) have been classified in many ways. The six general headings used by the *Diagnostic and Statistical Manual* (DSM-IV) produced by the American Psychiatric Association[2] and by the World Health Organization in the International Classification of Diseases (ICD-10)[3] are as follows:

- Insomnias (disorders of initiation and maintaining sleep)
- Hypersomnias (disorders of excessive somnolence)
- Narcolepsy (excessive daytime sleepiness and cataplexy)
- Breathing-related sleep disorder
- Circadian-rhythm sleep disorder
- Parasomnias (behavioral or physiological dysfunctions associated with sleep, sleep stages, or partial arousals, such as nightmares, terrors, and sleepwalking)

Hypnotics are suitable for study in the treatment of insomnia only.

The DSM-IV manual lists many disorders under the general heading of anxiety disorders — generalized anxiety disorder, panic disorder, agoraphobia, social anxiety disorder, simple phobia, posttraumatic stress disorder, and obsessive–compulsive disorder. Most of these clinical entities are considered in Section 17.6 of the chapter. The treatment of simple phobias and posttraumatic stress disorder primarily involves nondrug, psychological treatments; anxiolytics may, however, provide useful supportive treatment.

This chapter describes the investigations that must be performed in the early clinical evaluation of new anxiolytics (particularly for the treatment of generalized anxiety disorder, panic disorder, social anxiety disorder, and obsessive–compulsive disorder) and hypnotics, in both healthy, non-patient volunteers and patients.

17.2 PHARMACOKINETICS AND METABOLISM: HEALTHY VOLUNTEERS

The ideal hypnotic for the treatment of most insomnias would be a drug that produces a rapid onset of sleep, promotes the maintenance of sleep for a short period, and then allows an immediate return to the normal awake state; however, at present no such compound is available. Generalized anxiety disorder, panic disorder, and some insomnias, such as insomnia related to psychiatric disorders, may require a different pharmacodynamic profile, involving a prolonged anxiolytic action but with minimal daytime sedation. Pharmacokinetic data are, therefore, particularly valuable in the early clinical evaluation of these drugs, with the desired pharmacokinetic profile being dependent on the particular disorder. Most new regimens for the treatment of anxiety or insomnia should have a rapid onset of action and consequently will have to possess a rapid rate of absorption. Measurement of plasma concentrations will reveal distribution to the highly vascular tissues. The brain is a highly vascular organ, so hypnotics and anxiolytics should be able to cross the blood–brain barrier with ease. Thus, plasma concentration should parallel brain concentration.

After absorption, the drug is distributed to the poorly vascular tissues, such as voluntary muscle, and then eliminated by metabolism and excretion. The duration of pharmacodynamic activity is generally determined by the drug concentration in the brain, with the therapeutic effect ceasing when the concentration falls below a threshold. If this threshold is passed during the distribution phase, then the pharmacodynamic effect of a single dose will be short. If the threshold is passed during the elimination phase, then the pharmacodynamic effect should parallel the elimination half-life. Another pharmacokinetic variable, important in the early volunteer studies, is the possibility of accumulation. Hypnotics and anxiolytics are often taken for periods of days, if not weeks; therefore, drugs with a long residence time or half-life will accumulate.

Plasma drug concentrations are not always predictive of the incidence or severity of residual daytime impairment.[4] For example, temazepam has an elimination half-life of approximately 10 hours, yet a 20-mg oral dose has been reported to cause no residual sequelae after an overnight ingestion.[5] To date (see Kunsman et al.[6]), no strong correlation between the impairment or trend toward impairment indicated in these studies and the level of drug or metabolites in body fluids has been established for temazepam or other benzodiazepines. Thus, pharmacokinetic data on the parent compound can provide valuable supporting information in early volunteer studies, but they cannot replace the use of sensitive, objective, pharmacodynamic assessments.

The formation of active metabolites may be particularly important to both the duration of drug effect and the possibility of accumulation. Flurazepam, for instance, has a plasma half-life of 2 to 3 hours; however, its active metabolite N-desalkyl flurazepam has a half-life of approximately 100 hours.[7] In his *Handbook of Clinical Pharmacokinetic Data*, Jack[8] shows that half of the anxiolytics and hypnotics currently in use have active metabolites; therefore, it is important to identify potential active metabolites by performing a [14]C (mass balance) study and develop assays to quantify plasma concentrations of active metabolites very early in development. The elimination half-life is a parameter that can have clinical relevance, particularly for the use of high-potency benzodiazepines in anxiety. The long (estimates ranging from 20 to 80 hours) half-life of clonazepam may account for the good tolerability and absence of rebound observed during gradual discontinuation.[9]

17.3 PHARMACODYNAMICS: HEALTHY VOLUNTEERS

It is difficult to extrapolate from healthy volunteers to patients with most psychotropic drugs, as the intended therapeutic effect is often difficult to identify by an action in an unimpaired subject. Hypnotics are probably the easiest of psychotropic drugs to study in normal subjects, as the intended therapeutic action (sedation) can be observed and quantified, whereas the assessment of anxiolytic properties is more difficult.

17.3.1 Anxiolytic Effect

It is possible to subject healthy volunteers to an anxiety-provoking stimulus, but the repeated administration of such a stimulus, as is required in most well-controlled volunteer studies, leads to desensitization (e.g., a changing baseline). Such stimuli that have been utilized include riding a ferris wheel,[10] anticipation of pain,[11] watching anxiety-provoking movies,[12] and simulated public speaking.[13] More recently, the fear-potentiated startle paradigm (based on the increase in amplitude of the startle reflex during anticipation of an aversive stimulus) has been used.[14] It enables the evaluation of an anxiolytic from two points of view: antiaversive effect and possible sedative effect. Pharmacological stimuli should be more reproducible, with lactic acid, cholecystokinin, and pentagastrin having been used as models of anxiety in healthy volunteers, and the anxiety thus generated being prevented by treatment with potential anxiolytics.[15] Assessment of CNS function in healthy volunteers, in the very first study in humans, can provide very useful early information. In addition, the later use of pharmacological models of anxiety may also provide vital data on the dose–response curve and allow the prediction of doses to be investigated in the first patient efficacy studies.

17.3.2 Psychomotor and Cognitive Functions

It is important that the objective and subjective measurements of CNS function be sensitive and reproducible. Many tests have been used to assess sedation in humans. A review by Hindmarch[16] lists the most commonly used ones. It is inappropriate to use only one or two tests that measure a restricted range of CNS functions. A full battery of tests, including assessment of alertness, cognitive function, reaction times, and memory, should be employed to cover the range of functions.[6,17] Some of the main categories include reaction times, tracking tasks, critical flicker fusion, rapid visual information processing, and short-term memory scanning tasks.

Some tasks are more sensitive than others to different psychotropic drugs. McClelland and Jackson[18] studied a range of psychotropic drugs using a broad battery of tests and found that the three drugs studied with hypnotic or anxiolytic properties (amylobarbitone, ethanol, and oxazepam) correlated well with one another but could be differentiated clearly from other classes of psychotropics. The objective tests most sensitive to these hypnotics were choice reaction time, a rapid information processing task, and a manipulative motor task; the least sensitive tests were digit span and elapsing time estimation.

One particularly valuable method to study the time course of anxiolytic or hypnotic drug activity in healthy volunteers is saccadic eye movement.[19] This technique is particularly useful for studying the time of onset of drug effect, as continuous testing for an hour or more is possible, as demonstrated with intravenous diazepam and lorazepam.[20]

Subjective assessments, particularly visual analog scales (e.g., subjects mark a point that represents their current feeling on a 10-cm horizontal line with opposite adjectives at either end), are often as sensitive to sedative drug effects as objective measures.[21] It is therefore important to include subjective measures in any test battery.[16] The time course of the subjective effects usually parallels the objective effects.[22] These objective and subjective measures of CNS function are clearly useful in providing information on the onset and duration of effect. They can also be used to produce dose–response curves such that the minimum effective dose is established. Another advantage of using a test battery is that any new potential psychotropic drug can be compared with previously studied standard drugs.

17.3.3 Electroencephalography and Other Electrophysiological Assessments

The computer-analyzed (or quantitative) electroencephalogram (EEG) has been used to study psychotropic drugs following the pioneering work of Fink and Itil.[23,24] Several workers have now confirmed that the EEG can be useful when classifying psychoactive drugs by their action on the different EEG frequencies[25] and studying the time course of CNS effects.[26] The EEG profile of anxiolytics and hypnotics is a decrease in alpha waves (8 to 12 Hz), an increase in delta waves (0 to 4 Hz), and slow beta activity. For some psychotropic drugs, such as nomifensine, the EEG changes do not correlate with pharmacokinetics;[27] however, the work by Saletu and coworkers[27] on nomifensine and benzodiazepines showed that psychometric measures correlated with the EEG rather than the pharmacokinetics. This emphasizes the relative importance of the pharmacodynamic assessment of psychotropic drugs. The P300 component of the auditory evoked potential is known to be a useful indicator of cognitive function[28,29] and has been shown to be a more sensitive index of the effects of midazolam than standard psychomotor tests.[30]

17.3.4 Sleep Studies

Sleep studies in healthy volunteers with both new potential hypnotics and anxiolytics can provide useful data prior to patient studies. The relative homogeneity of the normal volunteer population and possibly reduced trial-related anxiety levels mean that studies of hypnotics on sleep can be performed with fewer subjects than in an insomniac patient population. Situational insomnia can be reliably induced in such studies by artificial means — for example, by playing records of traffic noise. Such reproducibility is a potentially valuable method of studying the dose–response curve of a hypnotic in one form of insomnia. Sleep studies should include basic measures such as onset of sleep, speed of awakening, number of night-time awakenings, and the volunteers' subjective assessments of sleep quality. Subjective measures that are particularly useful include visual analog scales, such as the Leeds Sleep Evaluation Questionnaire.[31] EEG recordings can provide objective measures of the onset and offset of sleep and its overall architecture — that is, time spent in each of the four slow-wave sleep stages as well as the amount and latency of rapid eye movement (REM) sleep.

17.3.5 Mode of Action

Information on the possible mode of action of new hypnotics can be gained during early clinical studies by using specific pharmacological tools. Flumazenil is a specific benzodiazepine receptor antagonist with little, if any, intrinsic activity in normal subjects.[32] Flumazenil can be used to prevent or reverse the effects of a new hypnotic or anxiolytic and thus reveal any central benzodiazepine receptor agonistic activity.

17.3.6 Neuroreceptor Occupancy Studies

The use of radiotracers with positron emission tomography (PET) to measure receptors or transporters is increasingly an element in the development of psychotropic drugs.[33] The high sensitivity of this technique, which can measure proteins in the nanomolar to picomolar range of concentrations, opens the possibility of gaining insights into the mechanism and locus of action of therapeutic drugs. Furthermore, it enables the measurement of receptor occupancy as a function of dose and route of administration, which could in turn lead to predictions of a therapeutic dose range or of a dosing interval. Two factors limit the use and interpretation of *in vivo* molecular imaging: (1) Appropriate radioligands to label the receptor or transporter of interest are not always available, and (2) the relationship between what is measured and the therapeutic effect is not fully established for most neurochemical systems (the dopaminergic and serotonergic systems are the best studied with regard to that kind of correlation).

17.3.7 Functional Magnetic Resonance Imaging

Blood oxygenation level-dependent functional magnetic resonance imaging (BOLD fMRI) activation in the amygdala and associated structures during an emotion face assessment task has recently been used to characterize the effect of an anxiolytic (lorazepam) in healthy volunteers.[78] The intake of lorazepam dose-dependently attenuated the BOLD-fMRI signal in the amygdala, a structure considered critical in the processing of emotions. These results suggest that this type of neuroimaging may become a useful tool in the early phase development of new anxiolytic compounds.

17.3.8 Normal Elderly

Insomnia is more commonly reported in the elderly than the young;[34] thus, the elderly are twice as likely to be receiving a hypnotic.[35] In addition, aging is associated with an increased sensitivity to, and prolongation of, activity of most psychotropic drugs.[35] It is therefore important to compare the pharmacokinetics and pharmacodynamics of new hypnotics and anxiolytics in normal elderly and young subjects.

17.3.9 Safety

The standard monitoring of hematology, blood chemistry, the cardiovascular system, adverse events, and routine physical examinations should be included in all studies with new hypnotics and anxiolytics. Other areas that require specific investigation for new drugs include the existence of any "hangover" effect (i.e., impaired performance the morning after night-time administration) and even the existence of any impairment of performance when wakened during the night. Such studies should employ a battery of tests of performance similar to those used in the acute measurement of volunteers. Ataxia is a common side effect of hypnotics and anxiolytics and may be related to an increase in potentially hazardous falls, particularly in the elderly.[36,37] Body sway can be measured objectively by various methods, such as a balance platform, and is very sensitive to the effects of alcohol and benzodiazepines.[38] The inclusion of an objective measurement of body sway in early volunteer studies may, therefore, determine the extent of this undesirable side effect. Respiration is affected by hypnotics and anxiolytics. Mechanisms include a direct depressant effect via the CNS, and a reduction of resting tone of the airway muscles. The most vulnerable time for an adverse effect to occur is during sleep when arterial oxygen concentrations are lowest. It is, therefore, advisable to include the noninvasive measurement of respiration and oxygenation during early sleep studies in the laboratory. Specific studies of a possible induction or inhibition of hepatic drug-metabolizing enzymes may be necessary where chemical, pharmacological, or clinical evidence suggests that such an interaction could occur (see Section 17.3.10).

17.3.10 Tolerance, Rebound, and Withdrawal

Many hypnotics and anxiolytics seem to produce pharmacological tolerance with repeated administration and rebound actions upon withdrawal. This has led to many regulatory authorities requiring that these drugs be restricted to use for no more than 2 to 4 weeks. Studies to investigate such potential problems can be performed in normal subjects; however, even the positive effects of hypnotics are not always clearly shown in normal subjects,[39] let alone any possible tolerance or rebound.[40] An explanation provided by Lee and Lader[40] for their inability to demonstrate rebound with the benzodiazepines (quazepam and triazolam) was that such effects are difficult to demonstrate in normal subjects in contrast to insomniacs. The use of standardized, validated, sensitive rating scales such as those developed by Merz and Ballmer[41] and Rickels et al.[42] might provide valuable information on withdrawal potential in volunteers.

17.3.11 Interaction Studies

Hypnotics and anxiolytics are commonly taken with other drugs, particularly in the elderly. It is likely that they will have an additive effect with other drugs having a sedative action and with alcohol; however, interactions between hypnotics or anxiolytics and drugs other than alcohol and psychotropics are uncommon and of little clinical significance.[35] The main interaction study that must be performed is with alcohol, so the extent of any interaction can be determined. Given the importance of coprescription, interaction with benzodiazepines should be assessed for antidepressants used as anxiolytics; conversely, for hypnotics and pure anxiolytics, interaction with the widely prescribed selective serotonin reuptake inhibitors (SSRIs) should be studied. A number of psychotropic drugs are substrates of important cytochrome P-450 (CYP) isoforms, particularly CYP2D6 and CYP3A4. This creates a potential for interaction with inhibitors or inducers of these enzymes and with other substrates. Given the possible impact on safety and the scrutiny of regulatory authorities in this area of investigation, it is necessary to plan such interaction studies early in a development program.

17.4 GENERAL CONSIDERATIONS ON PATIENT STUDIES

17.4.1 Study Design

The initial studies in patients will usually be performed in the relatively young (under 65 years old) who are in all other respects healthy. The main purpose of these initial studies is to define the therapeutic range for investigation in later phase II and phase III studies. Hypnotics, in particular, are often prescribed to the elderly; therefore, at the time of registration, the database should contain a high percentage of elderly patients. The inclusion of healthy elderly subjects in early studies will facilitate their inclusion in late phase II studies. As the elderly often receive several other medications, it is also important to assess any possible drug interactions before commencing large multicenter trials. While most interaction studies can be performed in animals and *in vitro* systems and any potential interaction assessed in normal subjects, some interaction studies have to be performed in patients (e.g., potential interaction with digoxin).

Perhaps more than for any other treated conditions, the placebo response in the treatment of insomnia and anxiety is significant;[43] therefore, it is vital to include a matched placebo in all patient studies. A positive control, in the form of an established hypnotic or anxiolytic, will assist in the evaluation of relative efficacy and safety and help validate the trial. The design used in insomnia and anxiety clinical trials is generally parallel because a crossover design would result in a significant carryover effect between the two arms. It is therefore proposed that the optimal general trial design for hypnotics and anxiolytics is a parallel study of two (or more) doses of the new drug against placebo and a standard. Study duration is generally dictated by three kinds of considerations: (1) stage of development, (2) specifics of the condition (particularly for the different types of anxiety disorders), and (3) regulatory requirements with regard to collection of safety data and long-term efficacy data. The inclusion criteria and various study designs are reviewed extensively by Rickels et al.[44]

17.4.2 Tolerance

During periods of prolonged treatment, tolerance to the efficacy of a hypnotic or anxiolytic can develop, although the significance of this phenomenon has been questioned.[45] The reduction in efficacy can appear after just 2 weeks of treatment,[46,47] so careful monitoring of efficacy during repeat dose studies is important.

17.4.3 Withdrawal Reactions and Rebound Insomnia and Anxiety

Upon cessation of any drug treatment, rebound effects are not uncommon. For benzodiazepines, rebound insomnia is related to rebound anxiety and withdrawal syndromes.[48] Others have suggested that tolerance and dependence result from the same adaptive mechanisms.[49] Reynolds et al.,[50] however, have shown that administration of the benzodiazepine clobazam can result in a tolerance to its anticonvulsant property without producing dependence (e.g., withdrawal reactions). Tolerance and dependence, therefore, appear to be independent of each other.

Even the newer hypnotics such as quazepam, zolpidem, and zopiclone seem to cause rebound insomnia, although probably to a lesser extent than the classic hypnotics;[51] therefore, it is important that studies with new hypnotics and anxiolytics assess both tolerance and dependence. The most frequently reported effects upon withdrawal include anxiety, depression, somatic symptoms such as muscle trembling and muscle pain, malaise, weight loss, sweating, perceptual disturbance, sensory intolerance, hallucinations, psychosis, and seizures.[52,53]

The occurrence of any withdrawal reactions must be carefully monitored for any new hypnotic or anxiolytic. The U.S. Food and Drug Administration (FDA) recommends monitoring for three nights after cessation of treatment with hypnotics to assess any rebound insomnia,[54] but longer periods of monitoring (at least 2 weeks) are required to study all aspects of potential withdrawal problems. Spontaneous reporting of withdrawal symptoms may lead to great differences between investigators in frequency of occurrence; thus, a standardized method of assessment is advisable. Three examples of standard methods are (1) the Withdrawal Symptom Scale developed by Merz and Ballmer,[41] which is used in both normal populations and benzodiazepine-treated patients; (2) the Withdrawal Symptom Questionnaire,[55] which is used for benzodiazepine-treated patients;[52] and (3) a checklist of adverse events developed by Rickels et al.[42]

17.4.4 Pharmacokinetics and Metabolism Assessments

Hypnotics are widely used in the elderly, so it is likely that many patients will be suffering from some degree of impairment of renal or hepatic function. As a minimum, it is necessary to study the pharmacokinetics in the patients with well-characterized hepatic and renal impairment during phase II and phase III trials as part of a population pharmacokinetic approach. Alternatively, the pharmacokinetics may be studied in separate studies with hepatic and renally impaired patients. At the time a product license is applied for, it will certainly be important to have a sufficient number of elderly subjects within the database. As for anxiolytics, a major limitation to studies in the elderly is the difficulty in making a diagnosis of anxiety disorder in that population. Most clinical trials in anxiety exclude patients above the age of 65 or 70.

17.5 PRINCIPLES IN THE DEVELOPMENT OF HYPNOTICS

17.5.1 General Considerations on Measurements

Sleep studies in the laboratory are clearly an important part of the early patient studies of both hypnotics and anxiolytics; however, for longer term studies it is impractical to keep patients in a laboratory. In addition, it may be necessary to have a longer baseline period for patients than with volunteers to characterize the type and extent of any insomnia from which each patient suffers. It can be argued that laboratory studies are done in an artificial environment and studies with the patient at home better reflect the clinical situation, although the latter must rely on subjective assessments. One way to resolve this difficulty in obtaining objective sleep measures in clinical trials is to use ambulatory EEG recorders with either a standardized visual inspection or with automated analyzers. An even simpler, and perhaps equally valid, method is to monitor movement with wrist-worn sensors.[56] Hohagen and Berger[57] have produced detailed guidance on measurement and outcome variables in sleep studies. The emergence of new therapeutic targets[58] and subsequently of medications with novel modes of action (such as hypocretin or orexin antagonists or melatonin receptor agonists) is likely to have an impact on the choice of endpoints in future phase II or III clinical studies.

17.5.2 Measurements Used in Practice

Currently, polysomnography is the basic outcome for phase II trials, including all-night electrophysiological measurements of sleep with electroencephalograms (EEGs), electrooculograms (EOGs), and electromyograms (EMGs). Time to sleep onset is the primary endpoint, while the measurement of total sleep time (TST) and wake after sleep onset are secondary. A second set of outcomes consists of questionnaires completed in the morning that assess time to sleep onset, total sleep time, wake time, and quality of sleep. These questionnaires use either time estimates or visual analog scales. Finally, the next-day residual effects can be evaluated by ratings such as the digital symbol substitution test and a visual analog scale of sleepiness.

17.5.3 Target Profile

The target profile must consider the known pharmacological properties of the new hypnotic or anxiolytic and the intended marketing strategy. A potential clinical target profile for a new hypnotic could include the following:

- Greater than 50% reduction in sleep onset
- Plasma concentration half-life or mean residence time of less than 2 hours
- No active metabolites
- Psychomotor and cognitive performance equivalent to placebo if woken within 2 hours of sleep onset
- No rebound insomnia
- No amnestic properties
- Cardiopulmonary, ataxia, and other adverse effects less than with existing treatments
- Lack of tolerance over 6 weeks
- No physical dependence
- Production of physiological sleep
- No next-day impairment (hangover)
- Can be used in elderly patients

17.5.4 Main Steps in the Development of a Hypnotic

A simplified clinical development plan to evaluate a new drug with the above target profile could consist of the following:

1. Entry into humans, single dose in healthy volunteers:
   Establish pharmacokinetic profile.
   Establish effects on a limited range of tests of psychomotor function (EEG).
   Establish lack of major adverse events.
   Assess amnesic properties.
2a. Repeat-dose sleep laboratory study in patients (if a center is identified with the appropriate facilities and ability to rapidly conduct the study):
   Investigate efficacy dose range.
   Investigate hangover effect.
   Establish repeat-dose pharmacokinetics.
   Establish lack of major adverse events on repeat dosing.
2b. Perform mass balance study:
   Establish metabolic profile
3a. Study a range of doses in outpatients for 2 weeks of treatment (plus 2 weeks of follow-up) in a placebo-controlled study:
   Establish efficacy dose range.
   Establish lack of hangover effect.
   Establish lack of rebound.
   Investigate range of adverse events.
3b. Perform alcohol interaction study in healthy volunteers:
   Establish lack of interaction
4. Perform two separate phase III trials of one dosage of the new drug against the leading competitor hypnotics and against placebo, being allowed to continue with extended treatment for up to one year:
   Establish long-term safety profile.
   Establish market position.

Each of the proposed studies will provide information that could enable the making of go/no go development decisions. Such studies should also provide regulators with sufficient clinical information to consider a product license application or new drug application for a hypnotic, together with other studies generally required for any new drug.

17.6 DEVELOPMENT OF AN ANXIOLYTIC

17.6.1 Introduction

The development of drugs to treat anxiety has been transformed over the last 15 years by five trends:

- The finding that most antidepressants are anxiolytic and able to tackle panics, phobias, and generalized anxiety has made their development for anxiety indications a component in a wider strategy aimed at both depression and anxiety. In general, the study of depression has preceded the study of anxiety for serotonin-specific reuptake inhibitors (SSRIs) and serotonin–norepinephrine reuptake inhibitors (SNRIs), but a parallel development is conceivable for new molecular entities.
- Regulatory authorities have generally adopted clinical targets defined on the basis of widely accepted classificatory schemes, mainly DSM-IV and ICD-10. The validity and relevance of that approach have come under heavy criticism,[59] but it is unlikely to change in the near or medium term. Furthermore, the European authorities have issued detailed notes for guidance on clinical investigation[60] of therapeutics for anxiety based on the DSM-IV definition of clinical entities.

These guidelines should be taken into consideration for the development of any putative anxiolytic, as they cover in detail the selection of patients, design of studies, choice of efficacy outcome variables, requirements in the evaluation of safety, and duration of treatment. The FDA has not issued similar guidance documents in recent years.

- As is the case for depression, the field of anxiety trials is plagued by a very high percentage of placebo-controlled studies that are inconclusive ("failed") because the standard treatments do not differentiate from placebo.[61] Multicenter trials tend to be associated with high placebo responses, rater bias at baseline, enrollment of marginally ill patients, and the use of unrepresentative samples of symptomatic volunteers. Notwithstanding these hurdles, the use of a placebo control group is the only sure and acceptable way to evaluate the efficacy of an anxiolytic.[62,63] Placebo response rates tend to vary substantially within an indication and between indications; overall, the highest levels of placebo response have been observed in panic disorder (often close to or more than 50% of responders) and generalized anxiety disorder. More moderate response rates to placebo (close to 30%) occur in social anxiety disorder and obsessive–compulsive disorder.
- Regulatory authorities tend to prefer fixed-dose studies with as many as three or four arms for the tested drug in addition to the two controls, but evidence suggests that these are associated with a higher risk of "failure" (no difference between active control and placebo) than flexible-dose trials that are closer to clinical practice. Generally speaking, a higher number of arms increases the risk of inconclusive results.
- Academic clinicians and regulators are placing an increasing emphasis on evaluating efficacy beyond short-term improvement and assessing remission rates[64] as well as long-term efficacy.

17.6.2 Target Profile

A potential target profile for an anxiolytic could include some or all of the following:

- A predefined drug–placebo difference at endpoints on an itemized scale (e.g., at least four points on the Hamilton Anxiety Scales[65])
- Lack of any daytime psychomotor impairment
- Duration of action sufficient to permit once-daily dosing
- Onset of action on a par with that of benzodiazepines
- Absence of the development of tolerance or rebound anxiety
- Lesser withdrawal symptoms than existing standards (benzodiazepines or SSRIs)
- Lesser incidence of some specific adverse effects than with existing treatments: ataxia and daytime sedation for benzodiazepines, sexual and gastrointestinal dysfunctions for SSRIs

17.6.3 Main Steps in the Development of an Anxiolytic

A simplified clinical development plan to evaluate a new drug with the above target profile could consist of the following:

1. Entry into humans, single dose in healthy volunteers:
   Establish pharmacokinetic profile.
   Establish effects in a limited range of tests of psychomotor function (EEG).
   Establish lack of major adverse events.
   Assess amnestic properties.
2. Repeat-dose study with a range of doses in healthy volunteers, including the application of a model of anxiety at the beginning and end of treatment:
   Estimate efficacious dose range.
   Establish repeat dose pharmacokinetics.
3a. Study a range of doses in outpatients with treatment duration set as a function of indication (generally 6 to 12 weeks, plus 2 weeks of follow-up) against placebo:
   Establish acute efficacy dose range.
   Establish lack of psychomotor impairment.

           Establish lack of tolerance.

           Establish lack of rebound.

           Evaluate adverse events upon discontinuation.

  3b. Perform alcohol interaction study in healthy volunteers:

           Evaluate potential for interaction with most commonly used antidepressants (SSRIs or SNRIs) or with benzodiazepines.

    4. Perform at least two separate phase III trials of one dose (or of a dose range) of the new drug against the leading anxiolytic and placebo treatment, with treatment for 6 months with an optional extension for a further 6 months:

           Establish long-term safety.

           Establish market position.

17.6.4 Generalized Anxiety Disorder

Generalized anxiety disorder (GAD) is the most prevalent anxiety disorder in primary care. The current definition (DSM-IV) emphasizes its chronicity (6 months at least) and the significant distress and impairment it generates. Comorbidity with major depressive disorder or panic disorder is substantial. Patients present with a mix of somatic and psychological symptoms dominated by persistent, uncontrollable, and excessive chronic worries about everyday things. While GAD was traditionally treated with pure anxiolytics, primarily benzodiazepines, the use of SNRIs or SSRIs (in spite of their longer onset of action) is increasing due to the high rate of comorbid depression and to their absence of potential for addiction or abuse. Another trend is to treat for longer periods of time in order to protect patients from relapse and recurrence. The Hamilton Anxiety Scale (HAM-A)[65] is the most widely used rating instrument in GAD trials. It consists of 14 items (seven for somatic anxiety and seven for psychic anxiety); each item is scored from 0 (not present) to 4 (very severe). Disability is another important clinical outcome to assess. The Sheehan disability scale[66] is the most widely used for this purpose; it explores three domains: occupational, family, and social lives. It involves self-rating on a scale of 0 to 10 for each domain. Remission (see Table 17.1) is an important secondary endpoint.

    Most studies last 6 to 8 weeks, although study durations have ranged from 4 to 12 weeks. Placebo control and active control (SNRI or SSRI or benzodiazepine) ought to be used.

17.6.5 Panic Disorder with or without Agoraphobia

Clinically, panic disorder combines recurrent panic attacks and a fear of their recurrence. Often it is associated with agoraphobia, a fear and avoidance of the situations in which a panic attack might occur or has occurred. Patients with panic disorder are at risk for developing major depressive disorder. SSRIs have become the first-line therapy for panic disorder. High-potency benzodiazepines (alprazolam and clonazepam) are also often used, either alone or in combination with a SSRI, particularly at the beginning of treatment. Discontinuance of benzodiazepines requires a careful taper. Two main outcome variables should be used: (1) the number of panic attacks (with a breakdown between situational and spontaneous) or a panic attack factor (preferably), which multiplies the number of attacks by their intensity and by their duration; and (2) an itemized scale exploring the main clinical components (panics, anticipatory anxiety, phobic avoidance, and work or social impairment), either the seven-item Panic Disorder Severity Scale (PDSS)[67] or the 13-item Panic and Agoraphobia (P&A)[68] scale. Secondary efficacy parameters are the HAM-A[65] and level of disability; the Sheehan disability scale[66] is the most widely used for this purpose (see Section 17.6.4). Remission (see Table 17.1) is an important secondary endpoint.

    Most short-term studies last 8 weeks. Placebo control and active control (SSRI or high-potency benzodiazepine) ought to be used.

Table 17.1 Some Important Features of Clinical Trials in Anxiety Disorders

Feature	Generalized Anxiety Disorder	Panic Disorder	Social Anxiety Disorder	Obsessive–Compulsive Disorder	Posttraumatic Stress Disorder
Typical short-term study duration	6 weeks	8 weeks	12 weeks	12 weeks	12 weeks
Design	Parallel	Parallel	Parallel	Parallel	Parallel
Active control	SNRI (venlafaxine), or SSRI or benzodiazepine	SSRI, or high-potency benzodiazepine	SSRI or SNRI (venlafaxine)	—	—
Primary outcome	HAM-A	Number of panic attacks or panic attack index; itemized scale (PDSS or P&A)	LSAS	YBOCS	CAPS2; TOP-8
Secondary outcomes	Sheehan disability scale	HAM-A; Sheehan disability scale	SPIN; HAM-A; Sheehan disability scale	NIMH OCS scale	—
Remission criteria[64]	HAM-A score ≤7–10; Sheehan disability scale score ≤1 on each item	Free of panic attacks; no or mild agoraphobic avoidance; HAM-A score ≤7–10; Sheehan disability scale score ≤1 on each item	LSAS score ≤30; HAM-A score ≤7–10; Sheehan disability scale score ≤1 on each item	—	—

Note: CAPS2, Clinician-Administered PTSD Scale; HAM-A, Hamilton Anxiety Scale; LSAS, Liebowitz Social Anxiety Scale; NIMH OCS, National Institute of Mental Health Obsessive–Compulsive Scale; P&A, Panic and Agoraphobia; PDSS, Panic Disorder Severity Scale; SNRI, serotonin–norepinephrine reuptake inhibitor; SPIN, Social Phobia Inventory; SSRI, selective serotonin reuptake inhibitor; TOP-8, treatment-outcome PSD scale; YBOCS, Yale–Brown scale for obsessions and compulsions.

17.6.6 Social Anxiety Disorder (Social Phobia)

In its generalized form, social anxiety disorder is a chronic and disabling fear of negative evaluation by others and of embarrassment in a wide range of social situations (public speaking, dating, eating in restaurants, urinating in public bathrooms, talking with people in authority, etc.). The fears result in avoidance and anticipatory anxiety. Most areas of potential achievement (e.g., education, occupation) are affected. Comorbid depression, other anxiety disorders, and substance abuse are common. SSRIs are the first-line pharmacotherapy for this disorder. Clonazepam, a high-potency benzodiazepine, is also an efficacious treatment.

The primary rating instrument is the 24-item Liebowitz Social Anxiety Scale (LSAS).[69] Each item is rated on a 0 to 3 categorical subscale for fear and avoidance; thus, the total score can range from 0 to 144. Thirteen of the 24 items explore performance situations (e.g., eating in public or taking a test), while the remaining 11 items probe social interactions, such as making eye contact or talking to people in authority. The LSAS is used both as an outcome variable and as a selection tool (patients generally need to have a score of at least 70 in order to be included in a clinical trial). Secondary outcome measures include the HAM-A;[65] the Social Phobia Inventory (SPIN), a self-rating 17-item instrument that assesses physiological symptoms in addition to fear and avoidance;[70] and the Sheehan disability scale.[66]

Short-term trials are placebo controlled and last 12 weeks in general. Relapse prevention trials are being performed as well, similar to the relapse prevention of depression. They entail an initial 12-week, single-blind, acute-treatment phase with the test drug; responders are then randomized into a 24-week, double-blind, maintenance treatment phase[71] with two treatment groups (continuation of test drug or placebo). The main measurement is the proportion of patients relapsing during maintenance. In addition, time to relapse (using Kaplan–Meier survival curves) and efficacy at endpoint are assessed.

17.6.7 Obsessive–Compulsive Disorder

Two categories of chronic symptoms characterize obsessive–compulsive disorder (OCD): repeated intrusive thoughts or images (obsessions) and repetitive rituals (compulsions). The symptoms are experienced as senseless but are beyond the patient's control; the most frequent obsessions are fear of germs, fear of aggression, doubting, and need for symmetry, while most compulsions involve washing, counting, checking. The inclusion of OCD in the field of anxiety disorders has been challenged. SSRIs and clomipramine are the main pharmacotherapies for OCD.[72] The itemized Yale–Brown scale for obsessions and compulsions (YBOCS)[73] is generally used as primary outcome measure. It is a clinician-rated scale, consisting of five items for obsessions and five items for compulsions, resulting in two separate subtotals. Each item is rated from 0 to 4, on the basis of five parameters: (1) time spent experiencing the symptom, (2) interference with function, (3) distress induced, (4) ability to resist, and (5) ability to control. The NIMH obsessive–compulsive subscale[74] is frequently used as secondary outcome; it is a single-item, clinician-rated measure of severity with 15 levels ranging from minimal (1) to very severe (15). Most studies are placebo controlled and last 12 weeks

17.6.8 Posttraumatic Stress Disorder

The aftermath of an extremely frightening and dangerous event, posttraumatic stress disorder (PTSD) has three components: (1) reexperience in the form of flashbacks, dreams, and memories; (2) arousal with anxiety, irritability, insomnia, and hypervigilance; and (3) avoidance of trauma reminders. SSRIs are modestly effective pharmacotherapies for PTSD. The two main rating instruments are the Clinician-Administered PTSD Scale (CAPS2),[75] a reliable and sensitive (but time-consuming) instrument, and the TOP-8,[76] an eight-item anchored scale. Short-term clinical trials are placebo controlled and last 10 to 12 weeks.[77]

REFERENCES

1. Lader, M., Treatment of anxiety, *Br. Med. J.*, 309, 321–324, 1994.
2. APA, *Diagnostic and Statistical Manual of Mental Disorders*, 4th ed. (DSM-IV), American Psychiatric Association, Washington, D.C., 1994.
3. WHO, *International Classification of Diseases*, 10th rev. (ICD-10), World Health Organization, Geneva, 1992.
4. Harvey, S.C., Hypnotics and sedatives, in *The Pharmacological Basis of Therapeutics*, 7th ed., Gilman, A., Goodman, L.S., Rall, T.W., and Murad, F., Eds., Macmillan, New York, 1985.
5. Nicholson, A.N., Hypnotics and transient insomnia, in *Drugs and Driving*, O'Hanlon, J.F. and de Gier, J.J., Eds., Taylor & Francis, London, 1986.
6. Kunsman, G.W. et al., The use of microcomputer-based psychomotor tests for the evaluation of benzodiazepine effects on human performance: a review with emphasis on temazepam, *Br. J. Clin. Pharmacol.*, 34, 289–301, 1992.
7. Jochemsen, R., Clinical Pharmacokinetics of 5-Benzodiazepine Hypnotics, Ph.D. thesis, Pasmans, The Hague, 1983.
8. Jack, D.B., *Handbook of Clinical Pharmacokinetic Data*, Macmillan, Basingstoke, 1992.
9. Rosenbaum, J.F., Moroz, G., and Bowden, C.L., Clonazepam in the treatment of panic disorder with or without agoraphobia: a dose–response study of efficacy, safety and discontinuance, *J. Clin. Psychopharmacol.*, 17, 390–400, 1997.
10. Laties, V.G., Effects of meprobamate on fear and palmar sweating, *J. Abnorm. Soc. Psychol.*, 59, 155–161, 1959.
11. Uhr, L. and Miller, J.G., Experimental determined effects of envylcamate on performance, autonomic response, and subjective reactions under stress, *Ann. J. Med. Sci.*, 240, 204–211, 1959.
12. Pillard, R.C. and Fisher, S., Effects of chlordiazepoxide and secobarbitol on film induced anxiety, *Psychopharmacologia*, 12, 18–23, 1967.
13. Guimarães, F.S., Mbaya, P.S., and Deakin, J.F.W., Ritanserin facilitates anxiety in a simulated public speaking paradigm, *J. Psychopharmacol.*, 11, 225–231, 1997.
14. Grillon, C., Cordova, J., and Levine, L.R., Anxiolytic effects of a novel group II metabotropic glutamate receptor agonist (LY354740) in the fear-potentiated startle paradigm in humans, *Psychopharmacology*, 168, 446–454, 2003.
15. Traub, M., Lines, C., and Ambrose, J., CCK and anxiety in normal volunteers, *Br. J. Clin. Pharmacol.*, 36, 504P, 1993.
16. Hindmarch, I., Relevant psychometric tests for antidepressants and anxiolytics, *Int. Clin. Psychopharmacol.*, 9(Suppl. 1), 27–33, 1994.
17. Roehrs, T. et al., Sedative, memory and performance effects of hypnotics, *Psychopharmacologia*, 116, 130–134, 1994.
18. McClelland, G.R. and Jackson, D., Automated Testing of the Effects of Drugs on Cognitive Function, paper presented at XIth International Meeting of Pharmaceutical Physicians, Brighton, 1987.
19. Griffiths, A.N., Marshall, R.W., and Richens, A., Saccadic eye movement analysis as a measure of drug effects on human psychomotor performance, *Br. J. Clin. Pharmacol.*, 18, 735–825, 1984.
20. Tedeshi, G. et al., Rate of entrance of benzodiazepines into the brain determined by eye movement recording, *Br. J. Clin. Pharmacol.*, 15, 130–107, 1983.
21. Bond, A.J., and Lader, M.H., The residual effects of flurazepam, *Psychopharmacologia*, 32, 223–235, 1973.
22. McClelland, G.R. and Raptopoulos, P., Paroxetine and amylobarbitone, effects on psychomotor performance, *Br. J. Clin. Pharmacol.*, 22, 227P–228P, 1986.
23. Fink, M., EEG and human psychopharmacology, *Ann. Rev. Pharmacol.*, 9, 241–258, 1969.
24. Itil, T.M., Quantitative pharmacoelectroencephalography: use of computerised cerebral bipotentials in psychotropic drug research, in *Modern Problems of Pharmacopsychiatry*, Vol. 8, *Psychotropic Drugs and the Human EEG*, Itil, T.M., Ed., Karger, Basel, 1974.
25. Herrmann, W.M., Development and critical evaluation of an objective procedure for the electroencephalographic classification of psychotropic drugs, in *Electroencephalography in Drug Research*, Herrmann, W.M., Ed., Gustav Fischer, Stuttgart, 1982.
26. Fink, M., Quantitative pharmaco-EEG to establish dose–time relations in clinical pharmacology, in *Electroencephalography in Drug Research*, Herrmann, W.M., Ed., Gustav Fischer, Stuttgart, 1982.

27. Saletu, B. et al., Relation between pharmacodynamics and -kinetics: EEG and psychometric studies with cinolazepam and nomifensine, in *Electroencephalography in Drug Research*, Herrmann, W.M., Ed., Gustav Fischer, Stuttgart, 1982.

28. McClelland, G.R., Reaction Times and the Evoked Potential, paper presented at 29th Annual Meeting, European Society of Clinical Investigation, Cambridge, 1995.

29. Signorino, M. et al., Eliciting P300 in comatose patients, *Lancet*, 345, 255–256, 1995.

30. Engelhardt, M. et al., EEG and auditory evoked potential P300 compared with psychometric tests in assessing vigilance after benzodiazepines sedation and antagonism, *Br. J. Anaesth.*, 69, 75–80, 1992.

31. Parrott, A.C. and Hindmarch, I., Factor analysis of a sleep evaluation questionnaire, *Psych. Med.*, 8, 325–329, 1978.

32. Brogden, R.N. and Goa, K.L., Flumazenil: a preliminary review of its benzodiazepine antagonist properties, intrinsic activity and therapeutic use, *Drugs*, 35, 448–467, 1988.

33. Talbot, P.S. and Laruelle, M., The role of *in vivo* molecular imaging with PET and SPECT in the elucidation of psychiatric drug action and new drug development, *Eur. Neuropsychopharmacol.*, 12, 503–511, 2002.

34. Bixler, E.O. et al., Prevalence of sleep disorders in the Los Angeles metropolitan area, *Am. J. Psychiatry*, 136, 1257–1262, 1979.

35. Lader, M.H., The use of hypnotics and anxiolytics in the elderly, *Int. Clin. Psychopharmacol.*, 1, 273–283, 1986.

36. Swift, C.G., Postural instability as a measure of sedative drug response, *Br. J. Clin Pharmacol.*, 18, 875–905, 1984.

37. Ray, W.A. et al., Psychotropic drug use and the risk of hip fracture, *N. Engl. J. Med.*, 316, 363–369, 1987.

38. McClelland, G.R., Body sway and psychoactive drugs: a review, *Hum. Psychopharmacol.*, 4, 3–15, 1989.

39. Stanley, R.O., Tiller, J.W.G., and Adrian, J., The psychomotor effects of single and repeated doses of hypnotic benzodiazepines, *Int. Clin. Psychopharmacol.*, 2, 317–323, 1987.

40. Lee, A. and Lader, M., Tolerance and rebound during and after short-term administration of quazepam, triazolam and placebo to healthy human volunteers, *Int. Clin. Psychopharmacol.*, 3, 31–47, 1988.

41. Merz, W.A. and Ballmer, W., Symptoms of barbiturate/benzodiazepine withdrawal syndrome in healthy volunteers: standardised assessment by a newly developed self-rating scale, *J. Psychoactive Drugs*, 15, 71–84, 1983.

42. Rickels, K. et al., Long-term therapeutic use of benzodiazepines. 1. Effects of abrupt discontinuation, *Arch. Gen. Psychiatry*, 47, 899–907, 1990.

43. Spinweber, C.L. and Johnson, L.C., Effects of triazolam (0.5 mg) on sleep, performance, memory and arousal threshold, *Psychopharmacologia*, 76, 5–12, 1982.

44. Rickels, K. et al., Evaluating drug treatments of generalized anxiety disorder and adjustment disorders with anxious mood, in *Clinical Evaluation of Psychotropic Drugs: Principles and Guidelines*, Prien, R.F. and Robinson, D.S., Eds., Raven Press, New York, 1994.

45. Logan, K.E. and Lawrie, S.M., Long term use of hypnotics and anxiolytics may not result in increased tolerance, *Br. Med. J.*, 309, 742–743, 1994.

46. Kales, A. et al., Comparative effectiveness of nine hypnotic drugs: sleep laboratory studies, *J. Clin. Pharmacol.*, 17, 207–213, 1977.

47. Kales, A. et al., Rebound insomnia and rebound anxiety: a review, *Pharmacology*, 26, 121–137, 1983.

48. Lader, M.H. and Lawson, C., Sleep studies and rebound insomnia: methodological problems, laboratory findings and clinical implications, *Clin. Neuropharmacol.*, 10, 291–312, 1987.

49. Feely, M.P. and Haigh, J.R.M., Differences between benzodiazepines, *Lancet*, i, 1460, 1988.

50. Reynolds, E.H., Heller, A.J., and Ring, H.A., Clobazam for epilepsy, *Lancet*, ii, 565, 1988.

51. Lader, M., Rebound insomnia and newer hypnotics, *Psychopharmacologia*, 108, 248–255, 1992.

52. Schmauss, C., Apelt, S., and Emrich, H.M., Characterisation of benzodiazepine withdrawal in high and low dose dependent psychiatric in patients, *Brain Res. Bull.*, 19, 393–400, 1987.

53. Duncan, J., Neuropsychiatric aspects of sedative drug withdrawal, *Hum. Psychopharmacol.*, 3, 171–180, 1988.

54. FDA, *Guidelines for the Clinical Evaluation of Hypnotic Drugs*, U.S. Food and Drug Administration, Washington, D.C., 1977.

55. Tyrer, P. et al., Benzodiazepine withdrawal symptoms and propanolol, *Lancet*, i, 520–522, 1984.

56. Borbely, A.A., Ambulatory motor activity monitoring to study the time course of hypnotic action, *Br. J. Clin. Pharmacol.*, 17, 835–865, 1984.

57. Hohagen, F. and Berger, M., Testing the efficacy of new hypnotic drugs, in *Methodology of the Evaluation of Psychotropic Drugs*, Benkert, O., Maier, W., and Rickels, K., Eds., Springer-Verlag, Berlin, 1990.

58. Mignot, E., Taheri, S., and Nishino, S., Sleeping with the hypothalamus: emerging therapeutic targets for sleep disorders, *Nat. Neurosci.*, 5(Suppl.), 1071–1075, 2002.

59. Hyman, S.E. and Fenton, W.S., What are the right targets for psychopharmacology?, *Science*, 299, 350–351, 2003.

60. CPMP, *Notes for Guidance on Clinical Investigation of Medicinal Products for the Treatment of GAD, PD, SAD, OCD*, draft document, Committee on Proprietary Medical Products, European Agency for the Evaluation of Medicinal Products, London, 2003.

61. Robinson, D.S. and Rickels, K., Concerns about clinical trials, *J. Clin. Psychopharmacol.*, 20, 593–596, 2000.

62. Quitkin, F.M., Placebos, drug effects, and study design: a clinician's guide, *Am. J. Psychiatry*, 156, 829–836, 1999.

63. Leber, P., The use of placebo control groups in the assessment of psychiatric drugs: an historical context, *Biol. Psychiatry*, 47, 699–706, 2000.

64. Doyle, A.C. and Pollack, M.H., Establishment of remission criteria for anxiety disorders, *J. Clin. Psychiatry*, 64(Suppl. 15), 40–45, 2003.

65. Hamilton, M., The assessment of anxiety states by rating, *Br. J. Med. Psychol.*, 32, 50–55, 1959.

66. Sheehan, D.V., *The Anxiety Disease*, Scribner, New York, 1996.

67. Shear, M.K. et al., Multicenter collaborative panic disorder severity scale, *Am. J. Psychiatry*, 154, 1571–1575, 1997.

68. Bandelow, B., The assessment of efficacy of treatments for panic disorder and agoraphobia. II. The Panic and Agoraphobia Scale, *Int. Clin. Psychopharmacol.*, 10, 73–82, 1995.

69. Liebowitz, M.R., Social phobia, *Mod. Probl. Pharmacopsychiatry*, 22, 141–173, 1987.

70. Connor, K.M. et al., Psychometric properties of the Social Phobia Inventory (SPIN): new self-rating scale, *Br. J. Psychiatry*, 176, 379–386, 2000.

71. Stein, D.J. et al., Efficacy of paroxetine for relapse prevention in social anxiety disorder, *Arch. Gen. Psychiatry*, 59, 1111–1118, 2002.

72. Greist, J.H. et al. Efficacy and tolerability of serotonin transport inhibitors in obsessive–compulsive disorder, *Arch. Gen. Psychiatry*, 52, 53–60, 1995.

73. Goodman, W.K. et al., The Yale–Brown Obsessive Compulsive Scale. II. Validity, *Arch. Gen. Psychiatry*, 46, 1012–1016, 1989.

74. Goodman, W.K. and Price, L.H., Rating scales for obsessive compulsive disorder, in *Obsessive–Compulsive Disorders: Theory and Managment*, 2nd ed., Jenke, M.J., Baer, I., and Minichiello, W.E., Eds., PSG, Littleton, MA, 1990.

75. Blake, D. et al., A clinician rating scale for assessing current and lifetime PTSD: the CAPS-1, *Behav. Therap.*, 13, 187–188, 1990.

76. Davidson, J.R.T. and Colket, J.T., The eight-item treatment-outcome post-traumatic stress disorder scale: a brief measure to assess treatment outcome in post-traumatic stress disorder, *Int. Clin. Psychopharmacol.*, 12, 41–45, 1997.

77. Montgomery, S. and Bech, P., ECNP consensus meeting, March 5–6, 1999, Nice: posttraumatic stress disorder — guidelines for investigating efficacy of pharmacological intervention, *Eur. Neuropsychopharmacol.*, 10, 297–303, 2000.

78. Paulus, M.P. et al., Dose dependent decrease of activation in bilateral amygdala and insula by lorazepam during emotion processing, *Arch. Gen. Psychiatry*, 62, 282–288, 2005.

CHAPTER 18

Antidepressants

Lucia H. Lee, Christopher L. Wu, Benjamin R. Lee, and Chi-Jen Lee

CONTENTS

18.1 INTRODUCTION

Depression is a serious and common mood disorder. The lifetime prevalence of major depression is 17%, spread over the age group from 15 to 54 years; it is twice as common in women as in men.[1] Among elderly people living in the community, the prevalence of major depression is 3%, but it is 15 to 25% for those living in nursing homes, who have a 13% annual incidence of new episodes.[2] The exact etiology of the mood disorder is not clear. Various studies using computed tomography (CT), magnetic resonance imaging (MRI), positron emission tomography (PET), and single-photon emission computed tomography (SPECT) on patients with depression suggest that this disorder is associated with regional brain dysfunction, particularly changes in blood flow or metabolism in the frontal temporal cortex and caudate nucleus.[3] Many drugs have been reported to cause depression, but no drug has been shown to be causally related to depression with as high a frequency as depression that occurs naturally. These drugs include many antihypertensives (e.g., reserpine, propranolol, methyldopa, clonidine), hormones (e.g., estrogen, progesterone), corticosteroids, and antiparkinson drugs (e.g., levodopa and amantadine).[4]

The diagnostic criteria for major depression require that five or more of the following symptoms be present for 2 weeks:

- Depressed mood most of every day
- Marked decreased interest in most activities
- Appetite or weight change (more than 5% body weight in 1 month)
- Insomnia or hypersomnia
- Psychomotor agitation or retardation
- Fatigue or loss of energy
- Sense of worthlessness, excessive guilt
- Decreased ability to think or concentrate, indecisiveness
- Recurrent thoughts of death, suicidal attempt

Patients with major depression have experienced one episode of depression or have recurrent depressive episodes. Most patients with one major depressive episode will have more in the future. Among patients who recover from one depressive episode, 28% experience a recurrence within 1 year, 62% with 5 years, and 75% within 10 years.[5] The risk of completed suicide in patients with major depression is 15%, which is about 30% greater than the risk in the general population.

Two key concepts are important to the therapeutic plan for major depression:

- Continued therapy is necessary for all patients, and some patients may require lifelong maintenance therapy.
- Doses for continuation and maintenance therapy should be the same as the acute dose effective for eliminating depressive symptoms. When patients are given lower maintenance doses, their risk of relapse is much greater than when doses are maintained at acute dose levels.

18.2 PHARMACOTHERAPY FOR MAJOR DEPRESSION

The primary drugs used in the treatment of depression and the effective dose ranges in nonelderly adults are listed Table 18.1. Selection of an antidepressant drug or combination drug therapy is based on the mechanisms of action involved in the available antidepressants. Early antidepressants were the tricyclic antidepressants (TCAs), which blocked reuptake of norepinephrine and to some extent serotonin (5-HT) but also exhibited marked antagonistic effects on muscarinic, histaminic, and adrenergic receptors which caused many adverse effects. The toxicity of TCAs often resulted in frequent noncompliance with therapy. More recently, TCAs have been replaced by the more specific selective serotonin reuptake inhibitors (SSRIs), which selectively enhance serotonin. Thus, SSRIs have few to none of the cardiovascular, anticholinergic, and sedative side effects so common with TCAs. Most recently, the use of antidepressants has been based on multiple mechanisms, with a particular drug being selected to reduce unwanted effects while maintaining efficacy. For example, venlafaxine is a potent SSRI, but it also blocks reuptake of norepinephrine. Its adverse effects are similar to those of other SSRIs, but its dual neurotransmitter effect provides enhanced effectiveness. Nefazodone has selective serotonergic effects but has an added mechanism of blocking postsynaptic 5-HT_2 receptors, thus preventing the sexual dysfunction so common with SSRIs.[6–9]

18.2.1 Tricyclic Antidepressants

Tricyclic antidepressants are very effective antidepressants but with adverse reactions that limit their use in both acute and maintenance phases of treatment. All TCAs are well absorbed orally, extensively metabolized, highly protein bound in plasma and tissue, and eliminated slowly. Half-lives are prolonged in individuals over 55 years, thus the initial dose for older patients may require modification. One advantage TCAs have over newer antidepressants is that plasma levels can be

Table 18.1 Antidepressant Drugs and Their Effective Dose Ranges

Drug	Dose Range (mg)
Tricylic Antidepressants (TCAs)	
Amitriptyline (Elavil®)	150–300
Clomipramine (Anafranil®)	150–300
Desipramine (Norpramin®)	50–150
Doxepin (Sinequan®)	150–300
Imipramine (Tofranil®)	150–300
Nortriptyline (Pamelor®)	50–150
Protriptyline (Vivactil®)	20–60
Trimipramine (Surmontil®)	150–300
Selective Serotonin Reuptake Inhibitors (SSRIs)	
Fluoxetine (Prozac®)	10–60
Sertraline (Zoloft®)	50–200
Paaroxetine (Paxil®)	20–50
Fluvoxamine (Luvox®)	100–200
Citalopram (Celexa®)	20–60
Monoamine Oxidase Inhibitors (MAOIs)	
Phenelzine (Nardil®)	45–90
Tranylcypromine (Parnate®)	20–50
Others	
Venlafaxine (Effexor®)	225–375
Trazodone (Desyrel®)	200–600
Nefazodone (Serzone®)	300–600
Bupropion (Wellbutrin®)	300–450
Mirtazepine (Remeron®)	15–45

used to determine an effective TCA dose; for example, following are the plasma level ranges necessary for antidepressant efficacy for several TCAs:[10]

Nortriptylin	50–150 ng/mL
Desipramine	100–160 ng/mL
Amitriptyline	75–175 ng/mL
Imipramine	>200 ng/mL

Nortriptyline is unique in having a curvilinear response, in which clinical efficacy declines as the level exceeds 150 ng/mL. Plasma level monitoring indicates any lack of response at therapeutic doses, significant adverse effects at lower doses, suspected noncompliance, or changes in known enzyme inhibitors or inducers. With maintenance therapy, weight gain is the most common adverse effect and is often responsible for discontinuation of therapy. A major disadvantage of TCAs is the lethality of overdoses. Overdoses of more than 2000 mg of a TCA alone can be fatal.

18.2.2 Selective Serotonin Reuptake Inhibitors

Selective serotonin reuptake inhibitors (SSRIs) have been widely accepted as replacements for TCAs since the 1990s due to their lesser overdose lethality, lack of cardiovascular and anticholinergic effects, and convenience. An effective SSRI dose for depression is lower than the dose necessary to treat other disorders, such as obsessive–compulsive disorder and panic disorder. The initial dose of fluoxetine is 10 mg once daily; most patients require 20 mg daily. Sertraline is given initially at 50 mg, followed by dose titration in patients to an effective dose of 100 to 150 mg daily. Fluoxetine is well absorbed after oral administration, and peak plasma concentrations are attained 6 to 8 hours after a dose. Steady-state plasma concentrations are reached after 2 to 4 weeks. It is widely distributed throughout the body, and about 94% of a dose is bound to plasma protein. The drug is metabolized in the liver to norfluoxetine, which also selectively inhibits serotonin reuptake, and other metabolites. Fluoxetine is excreted in the urine, primarily as inactive metabolites. The elimination half-life is long: 1 to 4 days for fluoxetine and 7 to 10 days for norfluoxetine. Because of its long half-life, the drug can be administered once daily.

The SSRIs all produce similar adverse reactions, including some degree of activation and insomnia, gastrointestinal distress, and sexual dysfunction. More than 20 to 30% of patients taking venlafaxine or clomipramine experience sexual dysfunction, although some reports indicate 67 to 96%.[11] When SSRIs are discontinued, the dosage should be gradually reduced rather than abruptly stopped. A gradual taper allows monitoring for signs of relapse, with a prompt resumption of drug therapy if necessary. An SSRI discontinuation syndrome includes symptoms of dizziness, problems with balance, insomnia, fatigue, nausea, irritability, anxiety or agitation, flu-like chills, and headache.[12,13] Several SSRIs, such as fluvoxamine, proxetine, and nefazodone, are potent inhibitors of cytochrome P-450 isoenzymes, creating the potential for interactions with other drugs that rely on these isoenzymes for their metabolism.

18.2.3 Monoamine Oxidase Inhibitors

Monoamine oxidase inhibitors (MAOIs) are effective antidepressants indicated for atypical depression and treatment-resistant depression. Hypertensive reactions after ingestion of foods containing high concentrations of tyramine occur with drug use. Patients should avoid all aged cheeses and meats, concentrated yeast extracts, sauerkraut, and broad bean pods. Patients who cannot follow the dietary restrictions, those who drink excessive alcohol, and those with cardiovascular, hepatic, or renal diseases should not use MAOIs. Asthmatic patients and others who require pressor agents also should not take these drugs. Although food interactions have received much attention, several drug interactions are potentially more dangerous. These drugs include sympathomimetics (e.g., ephedrine, phenylpropanolamine), stimulants (e.g., amphetamines, cocaine), levodopa and meperidine, and SSRIs.[14]

18.2.4 Others

Venlafaxine causes potent serotonin and norepinephrine reuptake blockade. It requires dose titration and should be given in divided doses. In addition to adverse reactions similar to those of the SSRIs, venlafaxine has the unique effect of causing sustained increased diastolic pressure at higher doses, so regular blood pressure monitoring is necessary. It has no inhibitory effect on cytochrome P-450 isoenzymes. Nefazodone has SSRI activity with potent postsynaptic 5-HT$_{2a}$ antagonism. Its adverse reactions include initial sedation and orthostatic hypotension, thus initial doses should be lower and divided. It has established efficacy for severe depression. Nefazodone and bupropion exhibit the unique effect of increasing rapid eye movement (REM) sleep and normalizing sleep patterns, while TCAs and SSRIs decrease REM sleep and worsen sleep patterns.[15,16]

18.3 LABORATORY ASSESSMENTS OF ANTIDEPRESSANTS

An ideal antidepressant would effectively treat all forms of depression. The drug has a greater overall efficacy than currently used antidepressant drugs. It is effective in more than 70% of the patients treated and exhibits rapid speed of onset in therapeutic response. An antidepressant effect within one week after initiation of drug therapy constitutes a marked progress in treatment of depression. It can be used for long-term treatment with minimum adverse effects.

18.3.1 Pharmacodynamic Studies

Pharmacodynamic testing of antidepressants has focused on the biochemical characterization of the drug to confirm the mechanism of action. Because the brain is not accessible for direct measurement of neurotransmitters and their metabolites, indirect methods can be used. These methods are important for therapeutic studies to establish correlations with changes in severity of depression. Certain markers of depression are used to assess the response to antidepressant treatment. There are clinical and biological markers for evaluating treatment response. Among the clinical predictors, chronic depression, psychotic features, and morbidity are associated with a poor response, whereas severity of illness is an important predictor of the drug's short-term efficacy compared to placebo control.[17]

Biochemical markers focus on metabolites of central monoamines, such as 3-methoxy-4-hydroxy phenylglycol (MHPG) and 3-methoxy-4-hydroxy mandelic acid (VMA), their precursors, and the enzymatic processes. These are, however, poor markers. Serotonin is considered to be the major neurotransmitter involved in the etiology of depression. Several trace amines (e.g., phenylethylamine, tryptamine) play a role in the etiology of depression and in the mode of antidepressants. Some of these amines can be used as trait markers for depression. Platelets have been proposed as a model of central nervous system (CNS) neurons for studying neuronal β_2-adrenergic receptor regulation, and defective platelet L-tryptophan transport has been proposed as a marker of depression.[18] In addition, endocrine abnormalities found in depression and neuronal hormones may be useful markers in depression treatment. The dexamethasone suppression test and thyrotropin-releasing hormone stimulation test are widely used. The nocturnal hormone secretion is measured under the influence of antidepressant drugs. Elevated cortisol and testosterone secretion are used as state markers of acute depression.[19,20]

The noradrenaline-uptake-inhibiting effect of an antidepressant can be assessed in healthy volunteers by intravenous injection of sympathomimetic amines to assess its peripheral effects. Sensitivity to the directly acting noradrenaline is increased and to the indirectly acting tyramine is decreased.[21] The pressor tests are conducted by consecutive administration of increasing doses of amines until an increase in systolic blood pressure of 30 mmHg is reached. Plasma concentrations of TCAs correlate well with their effect on tyramine pressor tests. Effects of drugs on the autonomic nervous system can be studied by measuring papillary responses to adrenergic and cholinergic agents. Autonomic effects of antidepressants with a differentiation between muscarinic and adrenergic functions are also assessed. These studies are easily interpreted in healthy volunteers because the patients are associated with disturbances of autonomic function.

The effects of new drugs on cognitive and psychomotor performance such as vigilance, attention, and memory should be evaluated. Psychopharmacological studies examine the safety of the antidepressant with therapeutic doses and under conditions of real life. Laboratory tests can measure a spectrum of CNS function and evaluate real-life car handling ability. Quantitative pharmacoelectroencephalography is a promising technique for determining antidepressant drug effects because it directly focuses on the target human brain. Time– and dose–response relationships can be measured to establish the pharmacokinetic (PK)/pharmacodynamic (PD) relationships. In addition, *in vivo* nuclear magnetic resonance spectroscopy and positron emission tomography are potential useful in evaluating the drug effect on brain functions.

18.3.2 Pharmacokinetic Studies

Many aspects of the PK characteristics of a new antidepressant in humans are already established before beginning the clinical trial, such as protein binding and metabolism to human hepatocytes *in vitro*. Early elucidation of the metabolism of the drug in humans will indicate whether drug–drug interactions may occur. During PK studies of antidepressants, frequent monitoring of blood drug concentration is necessary because of the marked interindividual PK variability and proportional concentration–response relationships. Polymorphic hydroxylation reactions induce marked variability to the PK of TCAs, particularly with regard to excretion.[22] In general, patients who are poor metabolizers are more likely to experience adverse reactions on standard doses, whereas extensive metabolizers are at risk of efficacy failure. Phenotyping or genotyping tests are important in interpreting the PK of a new agent undergoing polymorphic drug oxidation.[23] Pharmacogenetic differences in the metabolism of SSRIs may not be related to the adverse reactions; however, they are important with regard to serious interactions with drugs metabolized by the same isozymes. It is important, therefore, to elucidate the metabolic pathways of new chemical entities and their interference with the metabolism of other drugs.[24]

Most antidepressant drugs form one or more active metabolites during metabolism in humans. Such metabolites contribute to both therapeutic and toxic effects. The mechanisms of action of the metabolites may be similar to or different from those of the parent compound. The biotransformation of TCAs is associated with a shift in the ratio of serotonin/noradrenalin reuptake inhibition. Differences between *in vivo* and *in vitro* studies indicate the formation of active metabolites *in vivo*. Determining the active metabolites of existing and new antidepressants will improve pharmacotherapy.[25] Also, PK–PD modeling to establish the relationships between concentration and pharmacological response is important to understanding the drug action in clinical psychopharmacology and providing information on appropriate dose selection and causal factors of variability in drug response.[26]

18.4 ASSESSMENTS OF ANTIDEPRESSANTS IN CLINICAL TRIALS

The primary objective of the phase I trials of new antidepressants is to determine their safety and tolerability. The trials are performed through single- and multiple-dose–response studies in healthy volunteers. Studies using elderly volunteers are appropriate, as the elderly form an important target population among depressed patients, and the age factor affects the variability of drug effectiveness. One approach is to conduct the single ascending dose study in young volunteers and the multiple ascending dose study in elderly volunteers. The PK–PD profiles are evaluated after the first dose to identify potential differences in the elderly before initiating the multiple dosing regimen. Phase I trials provide a unique opportunity to obtain information on PK and PD characteristics and their interrelationships over a wide dose range of the new drug.[27] The information obtained by integrated PK–PD studies in phase I is important in selecting the optimum dose for phase II trials and contributes to deciding whether or not the drug should be further developed.

Safety and tolerability are essential for new antidepressants intended for use in a broad population of depressed patients. These issues are studied in healthy volunteers using standard methods such as reporting adverse reactions, measuring vital signs, neurological examinations, and determining clinical laboratory parameters. The adverse reactions detected in the multiple-dose study are useful in judging a development of tolerance or an increase in intensity due to multiple-dose drug accumulation.

Phase II trials are designed to obtain information on safety and tolerability in depressed patients, explore dose–response relationships, and identify a therapeutic range to be used in phase III trials. Safety and tolerability remain critical issues in phase II trials. Even though information on a dose range is determined during phase I trials, special attention should be focused on adverse reactions in depressed patients. Physical examinations and clinical laboratory testing on patients should be conducted at regular intervals. Patients should be asked directly about adverse reactions, particularly sexual function.

For the diagnosis of depression and its subtypes, the following psychiatric systems are used:[28]

- *Diagnostic and Statistical Manual of Mental Disorders*, 4th ed. (DSM-IV)[29]
- International Classification of Diseases (ICD)-9/10
- Research Diagnostic Criteria (RDC)

Anxiety and personality disorders frequently complicate a differential diagnosis. The duration of depressive episode and psychiatric history should be recorded because these can influence the response rate. Phase II trials are preferably conducted with hospitalized patients. Diagnostic subgroups of patients are classified to allow assumptions on the generalization of results. Adequate inclusion and exclusion criteria of study patients should be established for the recruitment of depressive patients to participate in the trials. In addition, a drug history on over-the-counter drug use is necessary to rule out both drug and disease contributions to depression and to avoid drug interactions.

The common measures used to evaluate clinical status of depressed patients include:

- A relative reduction of baseline score on a rating scale
- A fixed endpoint cut-off score on a rating scale
- A combination of these two criteria

In short-term studies, a fixed, severity-independent cutoff score can lead to biases if treatment groups are not controlled for severity.[30,31] Before conducting large phase II trials, it is useful first to perform small-scale trials in depressed patients to establish the dose range to be used in phase II trials.

Placebo-controlled parallel group studies are used to assess the efficacy of a new antidepressant. Strong placebo responders can be detected within an initial 1- to 2-week period of placebo treatment before cross-treatment with trial medication. Usually a combination of fixed-dose and dose-titration designs is used.[32] A phase II trial is a dose-finding study that explores the full therapeutic range of a new compound. Fixed-dose designs are suitable to establish concentration vs. clinical response relationships, whereas titration designs within predefined dose ranges are more relevant to clinical settings.[33] In phase II trials of antidepressants, an effective dose escalation design is frequently used, in contrast to phase I trials where the selection of the next higher dose is based on tolerability. Testing on safety and tolerability must follow special evaluation techniques for dose titration.[34] Comparison of the new agent against active reference drugs is usually conducted during later phases of clinical trials. Reference drugs such as TCAs are frequently administered at a lower dosage in comparative studies with new antidepressants; however, sufficient doses should always be used.

For most antidepressant clinical trials, 4 weeks is adequate to determine whether a drug is effective in initially controlling acute symptoms but not sufficient to evaluate its effectiveness in treating the entire depressive episode. Many patients who do not show clear responses at 4 weeks exhibit improvement compared to placebo at 6 weeks. The chances of improving with drug therapy increase with time. In contrast, placebo does not improve effectiveness with time. Drug trials extended for 6 to 12 weeks can further increase the statistical differences between active drug and placebo.[35] For preventing relapse and recurrence, depressed patients after a first or second episode should be treated with full-dose antidepressants for at least 6 to 12 months. The prophylactic effects of antidepressants are usually studied in phase III trials and phase IV postmarketing surveys. Multicenter trials are frequently performed to recruit sufficient numbers of patients. These studies require the involvement of experienced investigators to ensure that the clinical protocol is followed and the results accurately analyzed by all centers.

Clinical trials for antidepressants are frequently conducted in subpopulations of female and elderly patients. Young women exhibit an enhanced response to nontricyclic antidepressants, and the administration of exogenous hormones and the menstrual cycle can interact with medications.[36] The U.S. Food and Drug Administration (FDA) guideline encourages early initiation of drug trials in females,[37] although pregnancy is usually an exclusion criterion for participating in clinical trials for antidepressants. Depression is common in the elderly and is associated with morbidity and mortality. The identification and treatment of depression are more difficult in the elderly than in young patients because of morbidity and concurrent drug use. Generally, initial therapy in the elderly uses lower doses than those recommended for younger adults. Excretion for many drugs is reduced in the elderly, and drug sensitivity is increased. The geriatric population is vulnerable to cardiovascular and anticholinergic side effects. Postural hypotension and the associated potential for falls and fractures should be avoided. The selection of an antidepressant drug in the elderly usually depends on side reactions and potential drug interactions rather than therapeutic effectiveness.

New mechanisms of action in the etiology and treatment of depression have been extensively studied. Serotonin receptors, such as 5-HTTA and 5-HT$_2$, may be involved in the major depression and the therapeutic effects of antidepressants.[38] Several agonists and antagonists for various serotonin receptor subtypes are currently involved in clinical trials for multiple psychiatric disorders. New antidepressants may be developed based on their ability to modify signal transducers (e.g., G proteins)[39] or to act at sites distal to receptors, such as second-messenger complexes.

REFERENCES

1. Blazzer, D.G., Kessler, R.C., McGonagle, K.A. et al., The prevalence and distribution of major depression in a national community sample: the national comorbidity survey, *Am. J. Psychiatry*, 151, 979–986, 1994.
2. Reynold, C.F., Treatment of depression in late life, *Am. J. Med.*, 97(Suppl. 6A), 39S–46S, 1994.
3. Cummings, J.L., The neuroanatomy of depression, *J. Clin. Psychiatry*, 54(Suppl. 9), 14–20, 1993.
4. Rush, D.R. and Stimmel, G.L., When drugs cause psychiatric symptoms, *Patient Care*, 23, 57–75, 1989.
5. Hirschfeld, R.M.A., Guidelines for the long-term treatment of depression, *J. Clin. Psychiatry*, 55(Suppl. 12), 61–69, 1994.
6. Stahl, S.M., Basic psychopharmacology of antidepressants. Part I. Antidepressants have distinct mechanisms of action, *J. Clin. Psychiatry*, 59(Suppl. 4), 5–14, 1998.
7. Frazer, A., Pharmacology of antidepressants, *J. Clin. Psychopharmacol.*, 17(Suppl. 1), 2S–18S, 1997.
8. APA, *Practice Guidelines for the Treatment of Psychiatric Disorders: Compendium*, American Psychiatric Association, Washington, D.C., 2000.
9. Richards, S. and Perri, M.G., Pharmacotherapy, in *Depression: A Primer for Practitioners*, Sage, Thousand Oaks, CA, 2002, pp. 180–199.
10. Perskorn, S.H., Pharmacokinetics of antidepressants, *J. Clin. Psychiatry*, 54(Suppl. 9), 14–34, 1993.
11. Segraves, R.T., Antidepressant-induced sexual dysfunction, *J. Clin. Psychiatry*, 59(Suppl. 4), 48–54, 1998.
12. Schatzberg, A.F., Haddad, P., and Kaplan, E.M., Serotonin reuptake inhibitor discontinuation syndrome: a hypothetical definition, *J. Clin. Psychiatry*, 58(Suppl. 7), 5–10, 1997.
13. Zajecka, J., Tracy, K.A., and Mitchell, S., Discontinuation symptoms after treatment with serotonin reuptake inhibitors: a literature review, *J. Clin. Psychiatry*, 58, 291–297, 1997.
14. Sweet, R.A., Brown, E.J., and Heimberg, R.G., Monoamine oxidase inhibitor dietary restrictions: what we asking patients to give up?, *J. Clin Psychiatry*, 56, 196–201, 1995.
15. Thase, M.E., Depression, sleep, and antidepressants, *J. Clin. Psychiatry*, 59(Suppl. 4), 55–65, 1998.
16. Dopheide, J.A., Stimmel, G.L., and Yi, D.D., Focus on nefaxodone, *Hosp. Formulary*, 30, 205–212, 1995.
17. Davidson, J.R.T., Giller, E.L., Zisook, S. et al., Predictors of response to monoamine oxidase inhibitors: do they exist?, *Eur. Arch. Psychiatry Clin. Neurosci.*, 241, 181–186, 1991.
18. Gronier, B., Azorin, J.M., Dassa, D. et al., Evidence for a defective platelet L-tryptophan transport in depressed patients, *Int. Clin. Psychopharmacol.*, 8, 87–93, 1993.
19. Mendlewicz, J., Sleep-related chronobiological markers of affective illness, *Int. J. Psychophysiol.*, 10, 245–252, 1991.

20. Dawkins, K. and Potter, W.Z., Gender differences in pharmacokinetics and pharmacodynamics of psychotropics: focus on women, *Psychopharmacol. Bull.*, 27, 417–426, 1991.

21. Ghose, K., Biochemical assessment of antidepressive drugs, *Br. J. Clin. Pharmacol.*, 10, 539–550, 1980.

22. Spina, E. and Caputi, A.P., Pharmacogenetic aspects in the metabolism of psychotropic drugs: pharmacokinetic and clinical implications, *Pharmacol. Res.*, 29, 121–137, 1994.

23. Alvan, G., Clinical consequences of polymorphic drug oxidation, *Fundam. Clin. Pharmacol.*, 5, 209–228, 1991.

24. van Harten, J., Clinical pharmacokinetics of selective serotonin reuptake inhibitors, *Clin. Pharmacokinet.*, 24, 203–220, 1993.

25. Bertilsson, L., Nordin, C., Otani, K. et al., Disposition of single oral doses of E-10-hydroxynortriptyline in healthy subjects, with some observations on pharmacodynamic effects, *Clin. Pharmacol. Ther.*, 40, 261–267, 1986.

26. Greenblatt, D.J. and Harmatz, J.S., Kinetic-dynamic modeling in clinical psychopharmacology, *J. Clin. Psychopharmacol.*, 13, 231–234, 1993.

27. Kroboth, P.D., Schmith, V.D., and Smith, R.B., Pharmacodynamic modeling: application to new drug development, *Clin. Pharmacokinetic.*, 20, 91–98, 1991.

28. Woggon, B., Methodology of measuring the efficacy of antidepressants: European viewpoint, *Psychopharmacology*, 106, S90–S92, 1992.

29. APA, *Diagnostic and Statistical Manual of Mental Disorders*, 4th ed., American Psychiatric Association, Washington, D.C., 1994.

30. Prien, R.F., Carpenter, L.L., and Kupfer, D.J., The definition and operational criteria for treatment outcome of major depressive disorder: a review of the current research literature, *Arch. Gen. Psychiatry*, 48, 796–800, 1991.

31. Angst, J., Delini-Stula, A., Stabl, M. et al., Is a cut-off score a suitable measure of treatment outcome in short-term trials in depression? A methodological meta-analysis, *Hum. Psychopharmacol.*, 8, 311–317, 1993.

32. D'Amico, M.F., Roberts, D.L., Robinson, D.S. et al., Placebo-controlled dose-ranging trial designs in phase II development of nefazodone, *Psychopharmacol. Bull.*, 26, 147–150, 1990.

33. Klimt, C.R., The conduct and principles of randomized clinical trials, *Controlled Clin. Trials*, 1, 283–293, 1981.

34. Hsu, P.H. and Laddu, A.R., Analysis of adverse events in a dose titration study, *J. Clin. Pharmacol.*, 34, 136–141, 1994.

35. Quitkin, F.M., Rabkin, J.G., Ross, D. et al., Duration of antidepressant drug treatment, *Arch. Gen. Psychiatry*, 41, 238–245, 1984.

36. Wilson, K., Sex-related differences in drug disposition in man, *Clin. Pharmacokinet.*, 9, 189–202, 1984.

37. FDA, Guideline for the study and evaluation of gender differences in the clinical evaluation of drugs, *Fed. Reg.*, 58(139), 1993.

38. Cowen, P.J., Serotonin receptor subtypes: implications for psychopharmacology, *Br. J. Psychiatry*, 159(Suppl. 12), 7–14, 1991.

39. Pataki, C.S., Feinberg, D.T., and McGough, J.J., New drugs for the treatment of attention-deficit/hyperactivity disorder, *Expert Opin. Emerg. Drug*, 9(2), 293–302, 2004.

CHAPTER 19

Drugs for Alzheimer's Disease and Other Dementias

Benjamin R. Lee, Lucia H. Lee, Christopher L. Wu, and Chi-Jen Lee

CONTENTS

19.1 INTRODUCTION

Dementia is a multifaceted cognitive impairment that involves memory, language, and reasoning. In many dementia patients, behavioral disturbances are also present. About one half to two thirds of all cases of dementia are due to Alzheimer's disease (AD). The prevalence of dementia increases drastically with advancing age; 3.5% of all persons over age 65 may be demented, whereas among those over age 85, the prevalence is 20 to 30% or even higher — up to 50% of those 85 years or older.[1-3] The other major type of dementia, vascular dementia (VaD), is less common in the West but is a major dementia in Japan and China.[4,5] The key clinical difference between AD and VaD lies in the gradual onset and progression of the former and the stepwise progression with focal neurological signs of the latter.

Dementia is associated with deterioration of both cortical and subcortical neurons. A marked loss of larger neurons in the neocortex, hippocampus, and locus coeruleus is characteristic of Alzheimer's disease, as well as the resulting decrease in brain concentrations of neurotransmitters, including norepinephrine, 5-hydroxytryptamine, glutamate, somatostatin, substance P, and especially acetylcholine (Ach). At autopsy, the brains of patients with Alzheimer's disease exhibit three major neuropathologic lesions:

- Neurofibrillary tangles that contain paired helical filaments consisting of hyperphosphorylated Tau protein
- Neuritic plaques consisting of dystrophic nerve endings, a core of β-amyloid peptide, plus micro-glia, astrocytes, and other components (β-amyloid is the proteolytic product of a larger precursor, amyloid precursor protein [APP], a glycoprotein expressed in most mammalian cells)
- β-Amyloid deposits in the walls of small pia blood vessels (angiopathy)

The deposition of β-amyloid triggers the pathogenic process in Alzheimer's disease. The gene for APP is located on chromosome 21. Many individuals with Down's syndrome develop diffuse plaques during adolescence, and these adults have symptoms characteristic of Alzheimer's disease in their brains by age 40. Mutations in the APP gene and in adjacent linkage sites on chromosome 21 have been identified in patients with early-onset Alzheimer's disease. A linkage site for these patients has been located on chromosome 14.

The β-amyloid fragment consists of parts of the transmembrane domain and a short portion of the extracellular domain of APP. It is produced in soluble form *in vitro* and *in vivo* during normal cellular metabolism. Aggregated β-amyloid is toxic to mature neuronal cell cultures and induces morphologic changes of apoptosis. Multi-infarct dementia associated with cerebrovascular athero-sclerosis and ischemia is more abrupt in onset than Alzheimer's disease. Alzheimer's disease is accurately diagnosed in 85 to 90% of patients based on criteria established in the *Diagnostic and Statistical Manual of Mental Disorders*:[6]

- Impairment in short- and long-term memory
- More than one of the following symptoms: (1) impairment in abstract thinking, (2) impaired judgment, (3) disturbances of higher cortical function (e.g., aphasia, constructional difficulty), or (4) personality change
- Impairment that significantly interferes with work, social activities, or interpersonal relationships
- Disturbance that does not occur exclusively during delirium
- Evidence from history, physical examination, or laboratory tests of a specific organic factor, or due to an etiologic organic factor

All patients suspected of having Alzheimer's disease receive a physical examination, including hearing and vision tests, to rule out other pathologies and may undergo various tests, including computed tomography (CT) or magnetic resonance imaging (MRI); blood count; serum chemistries; vitamin B_{12}, folic acid, and thyroid profiles; and a test for syphilis. Definitive diagnosis of Alzhe-imer's disease requires histopathologic confirmation.

19.2 AVAILABLE DRUG THERAPY

Drug therapy for dementia is limited because of insufficient understanding of its etiology and pathogenesis. Although progress has been made in understanding the neurodegenerative process of Alzheimer's disease, at present no cure or satisfactory restorative treatment is available. The objectives of investigational drug therapy include:

- Facilitating neural function that is involved in memory and other cognitive processes
- Inhibiting or reversing neuronal degeneration
- Increasing cerebral metabolism

Available drugs for treatment of Alzheimer's disease and other dementia are described in Table 19.1.

Table 19.1 Drugs for Treatment of Alzheimer's Disease and Other Dementia

Drug Category	Mechanism of Action
Ergoloid mesylates (Hydergine®)	Stimulate multiple neurotransmitter systems to act as metabolic enhancers
Cholinomemetic agents: tacrine (tetrahydroaminoacridine, THA; Cognex®); velnacrine	Enhance choline acetyltransferase and acetylcholinesterase activities
Nootropics: piracetam, oxiracetam, hydergine	Enhance cerebral metabolism
Others: nerve growth factor, neuroprotective agents (nimodipine, sabeluzole), cell membrane stabilizers (phosphatidylserine)	Enhance brain cell functions

19.2.1 Ergoloid Mesylates (Hydergine®)

Ergoloid mesylates are among the most widely used drugs for the treatment of Alzheimer's disease and other dementia. Hydergine® produces modest improvement in confusional states, depressed mood, dizziness, unsociability, and self-care.[7] The daily dose used in clinical trials for the treatment of dementia is 7.5 mg daily.

19.2.2 Cholinomimetic Agents

The use of cholinesterase inhibitors and other cholinomimetic agents in the treatment of AD is based on the observations that choline acetyltransferase and acetylcholinesterase activities are markedly reduced in the brains of these patients and the number of cholinergic (muscarinic) receptors is normal or slightly decreased. These enzymatic markers for cholinergic neurons parallel the severity of neuronal loss, density to neuritic plaques, and cognitive decline, especially in memory. Tacrine is a centrally active, noncompetitive, reversible cholinesterase inhibitor. Tacrine acts by inhibiting the hydrolysis of acetylcholine released from remaining cholinergic neurons in the cerebral cortex. In a clinical trial in which up to 150 mg of tacrine plus 10.8 g of lecithin was administered, 45% of the recipients improved by three or more points on the Mini-Mental State Examination, compared with 11% who received placebo.[8] In another study, patients exhibited significant improvement on the cognitive subscale of the Alzheimer's Disease Assessment Scale (ADAS COG) during a dose-finding (40 or 80 mg) phase before re-randomizing to a 6-week, double-blind phase with placebo.[9] Adverse reactions of tacrine involve elevation in aminotransferase, dyspepsia, nausea, vomiting, diarrhea, abdominal pain, and headache.

In clinical trials of a tacrine analog, velnacrine (Mentane), significant acute effects on the core symptoms of AD were demonstrated; 43% of patients improved by four points on the ADAS COG, and the drug (150 to 225 mg) was well tolerated. Similarly, patients with AD respond to physostigmine (Antilirium®). The use of metabolic enhancers such as acetyl-L-carnitine improves the function of surviving neuronal cells. Two randomized, placebo-controlled trials of acetyl-L-carnitine in patients with AD have been reported.[10,11] Patients who received the drug or placebo continued to worsen, but a modest reduction in the rate of deterioration on outcome measures was observed in those receiving the drug.

19.2.3 Nootropics

This class of drugs includes piracetam and its analogs, such as oxiracetam and pramiracetam. Nootropics are widely prescribed in Japan, Germany, and Italy. Deterioration of VaD was slowed using approaches to disease modification such as control of risk factors and antiplatelet therapy.

19.2.4 Others

Investigational approaches include the use of growth factors (e.g., nerve growth factor), neuroprotective agents (e.g., nimodipine, sabeluzole), and cell membrane stabilizers (e.g., phosphatidylserine). A 5-hydroxytryptamine receptor antagonist (ondansetron) and angiotensin-converting enzyme (ACE) inhibitors are also being investigated. Some drugs are available for both AD and VaD; however, all appear to be marginally effective and are symptomatic rather than disease-modifying agents. Thus, the development of a new drug is limited by the lack of a standard comparator, and clear-cut efficacy endpoints are difficult to determine.

19.3 LABORATORY ASSESSMENTS OF ANTIDEMENTIA DRUGS

Antidimentia drugs are intended to use for a prolonged period of time; therefore, oral administration is the route of choice. Specific pharmacokinetic issues include the problem of how readily the compound gets into the brain and how long it stays there. Theoretically, measuring drug concentrations in cerebrospinal fluid would answer this question; however, doing so is not always possible in early drug development. A more practical way is to measure brain concentrations by positron emission tomography (PET) scanning, which shows the kinetics of drugs in specific regions of the brain.[12] An alternative approach is to use the brain as a sort of bioassay of central drug levels; for example, changes in the EEG power spectrum and regional blood flow can show that the drug is distributed in the brain and reveal the duration of activity with different doses of the compound.[13] Several pharmacodynamic markers can be used for laboratory assessments:

- Direct measurements of cognition and memory
- Central pharmacological effects on brain physiology which may or may not be related to therapeutic effects
- Peripheral pharmacological effects of the compound as it interacts with receptors, enzymes, or their targets located on both sides of the blood–brain barrier
- Unanticipated peripheral pharmacological effects

Several test systems are available for direct measurement of cognition and memory. These include measurements on attention, speed, accuracy of information processing, short-term or working memory, long-term memory storage, and retrieval.[14] These functions act independently and can be affected by various stresses, such as trauma and drugs. A test should be specific to one function in order to facilitate interpretation of the test results from the behavior change. For measuring cognitive function, an adequate approach is to combine a variety of tests, each reflecting different aspects of mental function. Automated test systems, once properly developed and validated, can be more effective than oral examinations of patients.[15] Computerization allows assessments to be performed with greater sensitivity and to cover various functions. When selecting a test system, several requirements should be considered:

- The tests evaluate improvement or deterioration of the mental functions of subjects.
- The tests are easy to learn; after about four practice trials, subjects should be able to perform at their maximum level.
- Many alternative versions of the test are available so multiple trials within a subject are feasible.
- The tests are sensitive so active drugs can produce dose-related responses detectable with a statistical significance in 12 to 24 subjects.
- The tests are easy to administer and data generated are easy to analyze.
- The system are of short duration (15 to 45 minutes), thus allowing multiple daily tests to confirm the reliability and validity of the test procedure.

Clinical trials for evaluating improvement of cognitive function can be conducted in healthy young and elderly subjects; for example, trials in the elderly have been conducted to examine rising-dose safety and tolerability early in the development process. Two models in which impairment of various cognitive processes is induced and drugs are evaluated for their ability to prevent or counteract these effects are:

- The *hypoxia model*, which is based on one of two techniques: normobaric hypoxic hypoxidosis or hyperbaric hypoxia. Both have the same consequence of lowering the oxygen content of the blood, thus making less oxygen available for the central nervous system (CNS) and resulting in cognitive impairment. This model has been used to evaluate drugs in volunteer trials, and positive effects have been found with the nootropic piracetam under hypoxic hypoxidosis conditions.[16] This model has been used for the assessment of drugs aimed at the treatment of VaD symptoms.
- The *scopolamine model*, which is based on the cholinergic hypothesis of AD in that centrally active anticholinergic drugs can produce cognitive and memory impairments. The single-dose model is used to study procholinergic drugs such as nicotine, as well as anticholinesterases (e.g., physostigmine). The test should be well characterized to exhibit impairment in response to selected doses of scopolamine. The model is predictive for the anticholinesterase drug velnacrine; a confirmatory trial in AD patients showed similar improvements on the same measures as for the young, impaired volunteers.[17] Because the sensitivity of tacrine to anticholinesterases has been established in the scopolamine model, it provides an opportunity for future anticholinesterases to be modeled directly against physostigmine or tacrine so the dose–response relationships of candidate drugs can be determined. The scopolamine model is valuable for identifying potential efficacy and dose–response relationships.

Other techniques available to detect the effects of drugs in the brain include:

- *Pharmacoelectroencephalogram (EEG)* — EEG signals are monitored under two conditions (resting and alert) and via multiple leads. The combination of multiple leads, two conditions, many frequency bands, several doses of drugs, and various time points for assessment can lead to various statistical comparisons. The pattern and consistency of effects are as important as the presence or absence of the statistically significant differences. The pharmaco-EEG has been so effective in demonstrating drug activity that it was recommended as a technique for detecting drug-induced changes in vigilance.[18]
- *Neurophysiological tests* — Neurophysiological parameters that can be used to show drug-induced effects include sleep EEG and EEG brain mapping.[19,20]
- *Functional brain imaging studies* — The rapid development of new scanning techniques, such as PET, is providing new ways to study drug action. The oxygen consumption rate or glucose utilization rate can be measured using PET, which allows direct observation of drug-induced changes.[21] In addition, studies have been conducted with single photon-emission computed tomography (SPECT). Using this technique, it has been possible to image brain perfusion patterns before and after treatment to demonstrate effectiveness in clinical pharmacological studies of velnacrine[22] and physostigmine.[23] Similarly, magnetic resonance spectroscopy also allows direct measurement of local brain metabolism to demonstrate that the drug has entered into the brain and produces the desired functional effect.

Hormonal responses to a single dose of a drug are useful markers of central activity (e.g., cholinesterase inhibitors releasing growth hormone). Drugs that are active at serotogenic or dopaminergic receptors also have effects on prolactin, growth hormone, and adrenocorticotrophic hormone (ACTH) or cortisol. These neuroendocrine challenge studies are usually conducted as single-dose crossover studies using several doses and placebos. In addition, body temperature can be measured conveniently in neuroendocrine challenge studies for evaluation of centrally mediated drug action. Body temperature is decreased by some compounds acting on serotoninergic and dopaminergic receptors.[24]

Any pharmacologically active drug has effects peripherally as well as centrally unless the drug is specifically selective for central targets. Thus, cholinergic drugs exhibit various effects on the cardiovascular system, gastrointestinal secretion and motility, pupils, sweating, and salivation. All of these effects can be measured using standard techniques to help in defining pharmacologically active doses and setting limits in dosage for clinical trials.

19.4 ASSESSMENTS OF DRUG CANDIDATES IN CLINICAL TRIALS

Two objectives in the early development of an antidementia drugs are determining (1) the safety and kinetics of drugs, and (2) the dose-related pharmacodynamics. The target patients in efficacy studies are elderly, often frail and taking other medications. It is necessary to obtain appropriate drug interaction data, as well as to establish the tolerability and general safety of the drug in the elderly. In addition, an understanding of the dose–pharmacodynamic response relationship is critical to the choice of doses for clinical studies. Certain surrogate endpoints for cognitive enhancement, dose-related alerting effects in the EEG, or metabolic changes on PET scans can be used. Other specific aspects of the pharmacological activities of a drug can also be explored, such as blockade of 5-hydroxytryptamine (5-HT), induced skin wheal and flare by 5-HT_3 antagonist, or changes in urinary monoamine metabolites by selective monoamine oxidase inhibitors.

In the early stages of clinical trials, it is necessary to explore the fundamental biological characteristics of a drug in healthy subjects and then use this model to expedite patient studies. The selection criteria for volunteers and patients depend on the design and objectives of the study. Early tolerance studies in patients are important; for example, patients with Alzheimer's disease are more sensitive to the adverse effects of velnacrine than are healthy elderly volunteers.[25] Tolerance studies in young, healthy males are the usual way to begin; however, the target patient is generally elderly, female, and rather frail. Single- and multiple-dose studies should also be conducted in healthy elderly volunteers, including adequate numbers of individuals at least 75 years old and female.

Another key issue to explore is the potential for a drug to show pharmacokinetic (PK) or pharmacodynamic (PD) interactions with potential comedications. As the target patients will frequently be taking other medications, it is important to design a safe protocol for clinical studies that does not exclude too many patients. Drug interaction studies can be conducted in young, healthy volunteers; in fact, certain PD models are optimized in young, healthy, male subjects. Nicotine and caffeine have marked effects on the outcome of cognitive tests; thus, an adequate protocol would exclude smokers as well as heavy users of caffeine and restrict caffeine use during the study.

At present, for studies with antidementia drugs, it is not clear whether to select and use nondemented older individuals with self-reported cognitive and memory decline. One strategy is to regard these individuals as patients and to devise efficacy studies with the objective of treatment for their conditions. The other approach, however, is to regard these individuals as having a condition representing a model of dementia for testing an antidementia product. Both approaches have some advantages. Very few antidementia drugs have mechanisms of action that would limit their use only to dementia; thus, if a compound exhibits effectiveness in improving cognitive function in these trials, the information gained would be helpful in planning future phase II trials with demented patients.

Although most antidementia drugs should initially be studied in healthy volunteers, it is necessary to study the tolerance and bioavailability in patients to detect any differences between these two populations. Before entering a phase III program, the following information should be obtained:

- Evidence that the drug possesses the desired effect in humans
- Information on the effective dose range
- Dose–response relationship
- Time course of the effects with repeated dosing

Many efficacy trials of antidementia compounds have been conducted without sufficient evidence of efficacy from phase I and II. In some cases, the efficacy trials failed due to the wrong dose range, the dosing regimen used, or ineffectiveness of the drugs. In these cases, the compounds should not have progressed to efficacy trials. It is emphasized that the safety, tolerability, and pharmacokinetics of antidementia compounds should be measured in patients; in addition, the potential efficacy of the drug must be assessed in phase II.

Safety, tolerability, and PK trials must be conducted in demented patients regardless of whether or not they have been conducted in volunteers. The major question for efficacy testing in phase II trials is whether or not drug treatment can produce improvements in the symptoms of dementia. The issues here pertain to whether improvements in cognitive function can be identified in the short term (e.g., over days or weeks) and whether appropriate measurements for such improvement are available. The answer to the first question lies in the intended mechanism of action of the study compound. Drugs with direct effects on synaptic function (e.g., anticholinesterases) would produce rapid responses, whereas drugs acting through circuitous routes (e.g., desferrioxamine, which reduces brain aluminum levels) would show a slower onset of efficacy; however, as most cognition enhancers under development have direct actions on neurotransmitters or actions of calcium channel blockade, effects should be measured in the short term.

Because many patients are not properly cognizant of the risks involved in a trial, the issue of informed consent is difficult in dementia research. Caretakers are asked to give consent, but they are often the children of the patients, and the law does not hold children responsible for the actions of their parents. In addition, AD is a fatal disease without a known cure, which raises an ethical issue with regard to withholding a potentially effective treatment from a patient. Those individuals at risk or individuals concerned that they could develop the disease could give prospective consent, in case they do develop the disease, or they might nominate someone to give informed consent if necessary.

Patient selection in phase II efficacy studies is important — the more homogenous the population, the more likely that any positive effects of the drug will be detected in the trials. The diagnosis of the particular type of dementia should be accurate in order to improve the ability of the compound to ameliorate their symptoms. In addition, the severity of the illness should be identified. Many investigators recommend using mild or moderately demented patients in phase II trials. Severely demented patients should be avoided in phase II, because they are close to vegetative and thus unable to respond to the procedures required to identify change, and the neuronal damage is so extensive that manipulations of neurotransmitter functioning will have no detectable effect.

For AD, the diagnosis can be based on the criteria described in the *Diagnostic and Statistical Manual of Mental Disorders* (DSM-IV)[26] or the joint National Institute of Neurological and Communicative Disorders and Stroke and Alzheimer's Disease and Related Disorders Association (NINCDS–ADRDA).[27] Other confounding diseases should be ruled out, including pseudodementia, depression, hypothyroidism, pernicious anemia, and other forms of dementia, such as VaD, progressive supranuclear palsy, Creutzfeldt–Jakobs disease, Huntington's disease, and AIDS dementia.

Patients in phase II trials of antidementia products should receive adequate medical care to ensure their safety, similar to the care taken to protect healthy volunteers in phase I. It is necessary to evaluate each patient with comprehensive physical and neurological examinations, plasma and urine analyses, and electrocardiographs. During administration of a drug, the patient's physiological status should be monitored regularly. Such an approach in phase II produces a clear picture of what effects are attributable to the drug in patients that will be helpful when interpreting effects observed in phase III. In phase II trials, it is necessary to use placebo and positive internal (e.g., comparable effects to tacrine) controls. An alternative to using a placebo is to apply crossover designs where all patients receive active treatment for one period and placebo for another. If there is a carryover effect, this is in itself evidence of efficacy; also, the data can be analyzed using only the first period of treatment as if it were a parallel group design.

Phase II efficacy trials have two major stages:

- In the first stage, the maximum tolerated dose is established, safety and PK assessments are conducted, and evidence of efficacy is obtained.
- In the second stage, the most effective dose and one or two others are tested over a period of several months to confirm the effects and establish the stability of response profile over time.

A successful outcome leads to phase III trials; failure results in discontinuation of the project. A promising initial response is studied further with different dosing regimens.

Initially, a small study is conducted to establish the maximal tolerated dose in patients using the highest dose observed in phase I trials. When the highest tolerated dose has been identified, a range of doses is tested for the minimum dosing duration in which effects are expected to be identified. Adverse reactions are monitored throughout the trials, and regular assessments of plasma levels are performed. One or more post-drug cognitive testing assessments should be included on the first day of dosing. After the first dosing day, the cognitive tests are included as frequently as possible. This will identify the onset of any beneficial effects and permit an evaluation of the stability of any improvements. The number of subjects depends on the sensitivity of the cognitive test system used, but a minimum of 25 is necessary. At least three doses should be tested, although five or six would be better.

The next decision is to determine whether or not to proceed with further drug development. A demonstration in one or more studies of no effectiveness over a range of doses administered for a certain duration will be enough to stop development. If one or more doses show promising effects but fade afterwards, altering the dosing regimen can be considered. Such changes are based on the PK or considerations on receptor sensitivity. If one dose looks promising, a late phase II trial can be arranged. The purpose of a late phase II study is to confirm that the effects observed earlier persist over a longer dosing period (3 months or more). One or more doses can be used and run in parallel to a placebo group. Testing should be frequent to identify any tachyphylaxis. The number of subjects should be at least 50% greater than in the first stage.

Two critical keys to successful drug development are (1) fastest possible development time, and (2) effective use of resources on a potentially successful product. These strategies are as important for small companies with a single compound as for large companies with many compounds. Fund-limited companies require as much information as possible at each stage of development prior to committing further funding. Large companies may consider comparing various drug candidates and developing only those showing most promise. For any manufacturer, however, the decision to proceed to phase III should be made on the basis of supporting evidence of efficacy and low adverse effects. Rushing ahead into phase III trial without proper information presents a high risk of failure.

REFERENCES

1. Kokmen, E. et al., Prevalence of medically dementia in a defined U.S. population, *Neurology*, 39, 773–776, 1989.
2. Skoog, I. et al., A population-based study of dementia in 85-year-olds, *N. Engl. J. Med.*, 328, 153–158, 1993.
3. Evans, D.A. et al., Prevalence of Alzheimer's disease in a community population of older persons: higher than previously reported, *JAMA*, 262, 2551–2556, 1989.
4. Ueda, K., Kawano, H., Hasuo, Y. et al., Prevalence and etiology of dementia in a Japanese community, *Stroke*, 23, 798–803, 1992.
5. Shen, U.C., Li, G., Li, Y.T. et al., Epidemiology of age-related dementia in China, *Clin. Med. J. (Engl.)*, 107, 60–64, 1994.

6. APA, *Diagnostic and Statistical Manual of Mental Disorders*, 3rd ed. (rev.), American Psychiatric Association, Washington, D.C., 1987.

7. Hollister, L.E. and Yesavage, J., Ergloid mesylates for senile dementias: unanswered questions, *Ann. Intern. Med.*, 100, 894–898, 1984.

8. Eagger, S.A. et al., Tacrine in Alzheimer's disease, *Lancet*, 337, 989–992, 1991.

9. Davis, K.L. et al., A double-blind, placebo-controlled multicenter study of tacrine for Alzheimer's disease, *N. Engl. J. Med.*, 327, 1253–1259, 1992.

10. Spagnoli, A. et al., Long-term acetyl-L-carnitine treatment in Alzheimer's disease, *Neurology*, 41, 1726–1732, 1991.

11. Sano, M. et al., Double-blind parallel design pilot study of acetyl-levo-carnitine in patients with Alzheimer's disease, *Arch Neurol.*, 49, 1137–1141, 1992.

12. Kilbourn, M.R., DaSilva, J.N., Frey, K.A. et al., *In vivo* imaging of vesicular monoamine transporters in human brain using (^{11}C) tetrabenazine and positron emission tomography, *J. Neurochem.*, 60, 2315–2318, 1993.

13. Gustafson, K., Physostigmine and tetrahydroaminoacridine treatment of Alzheimer's disease, *Acta Neurol. Scand.*, 149, 39–41, 1993.

14. Hindmarch, I. and Stonier, P.D., Eds., *Human Psychopharmacology: Measures and Methods*, Vol. 1, Wiley, Chichester, 1987.

15. Cull, C. and Trimble, M., Automated testing in psychopharmacology, in *Human Psychopharmacology: Measures and Methods*, Vol. 1, Hindmarch, I. and Stonier, P.D., Eds., Wiley, Chichester, 1987, pp. 113–154.

16. Schaffler, K. and Kalausmitzer, W., Randomised placebo-controlled double-blind cross-over study on antihypoxidotic effects of piracetam using psychophysiological measures in healthy volunteers, *Arzneimittelforshung*, 38, 288–291, 1988.

17. Siegfried, K.P., Pharmacodynamic and early clinical studies with velnacrine, *Acta Neurol. Scand.*, 149, 26–28, 1993.

18. Amaduceei, L., Angst, J., Beech, P. et al., Consensus conference on the methodology of clinical trials of "nootropics," *Pharmacopsychiatry*, 23, 171–175, 1990.

19. Enz, A., Amstutz, R., Boddeke, H. et al., Brain selective inhibition of acetylcholinesterase: a novel approach to therapy for Alzheimer's disease, *Prog. Brain Res.*, 98, 431–438, 1993.

20. Saletu, B., Neurophysiological assessment of efficacy in drug trials with memory disorders, in *Guidelines for Drug Trials in Memory Disorders*, Canal, N. et al., Eds., Raven Press, New York, 1993.

21. Baron, J.C., Functional metabolic assessment using positron emission tomography, in *Guidelines for Drug Trials in Memory Disorders,* Canal, N. et al., Eds., Raven Press, New York, 1993.

22. Ebmeier, K.P., Hunter, R., Curran, S.M. et al., Effects of a single-dose of the acetylcholinesterase inhibitor velnacrine on recognition memory and regional cerebral blood flow in Alzheimer's disease, *Psychopharmacology*, 108, 103–109, 1992.

23. Gustafson, K., Physostigmine and tetrahydroaminoacridine treatment of Alzheimer's disease, *Acta Neurol. Scand.*, 149, 39–41, 1993.

24. Holland, R.L., Wsnes, K., and Dietrich, B., Single-dose human pharmacology of umespirone, *Eur. J. Clin. Pharmacol.*, 46, 461–469, 1994.

25. Cutler, N.R., Srameck, J.K., Murphy, M.F. et al., Implications of the study population in the early evaluation of anticholinesterase inhibitors for Alzheimer's disease, *Ann. Pharmacother.*, 26, 1118–1122, 1992.

26. APA, *Diagnostic and Statistical Manual of Mental Disorders*, 4th ed., American Psychiatric Association, Washington, D.C., 1995.

27. McKhann, G., Drachmann, D., Folstein, M. et al., Clinical diagnosis of Alzheimer's disease: report on the NINCDS–ADRDA work group under the auspices of the Department of Health and Human Services Task Force on Alzheimer's disease, *Neurology*, 34, 939–944, 1984.

PART VII

Assessment of Gastrointestinal and Liver Drugs

CHAPTER 20

Antiulcer Drugs

Benjamin R. Lee, Lucia H. Lee, Christopher L. Wu, and Chi-Jen Lee

CONTENTS

20.1 INTRODUCTION

Peptic ulcer is a chronic inflammatory condition characterized by ulceration in regions of the upper gastrointestinal (GI) tract where pepsin and hydrochloric acid are secreted. The most common sites are the duodenum and stomach. Peptic ulcer is caused by excessive digestive secretions, such as gastric acid, resulting from an imbalance between aggressive factors (e.g., hydrochloric acid, alcohol, nicotine, *Helicobacter pylori*, ulcerogenic drugs such as aspirin and nonsteroidal antiin-flammatory drugs [NSAIDs]) and protective factors (e.g., mucus and bicarbonate secretion, rapid epithelial cell turnover, mucosal blood flow). It is a common disease, with a prevalence of 3 to 5% and a lifetime incidence of 15 to 25%. Duodenal ulcers (DUs) are approximately four times more common than gastric ulcers (GUs) and occur more often in males than females; both types occur more frequently in the elderly population. DUs rarely become cancers, but approximately 5% of GUs are malignant.

Hydrochloric acid secretion by parietal cells is the result of the activation of a proton pump, hydrogen–potassium ion adenosine triphosphatase (H^+/K^+-ATPase). Three pathways stimulate gastric acid secretion: (1) the neurocrine pathway, which causes acetylcholine release from postganglionic vagal neurons in the stomach; (2) the endocrine pathway, which causes gastrin release from antral G cells; and (3) the paracrine pathway, which releases histamine from the mast cells. Gastrin is a key factor in acid secretion and is secreted in two forms: (1) G-34 (big gastrin), a 34-amino acid peptide, which is the predominant form in serum; and (2) G-17 (little gastrin), a 17-amino acid peptide, which is identical to the C-terminal half of G-34 and is the principal form in gastric antral mucosa.[1,2] Both forms of gastrin are equally potent in stimulating gastric acid secretion. Gastrin stimulates gastric acid and pepsinogen secretion, hepatic bile flow, insulin release from the pancreas, and pancreatic secretion. In addition, it also stimulates gastric and intestinal motility and increases lower esophageal sphincter pressure, which promotes closure of the sphincter. Gastrin may be assessed in the blood by radioimmunoassay; the normal level is less than 200 pg/mL. Peptic ulcer patients become more sensitive to the effects of gastrin. A gastrin assay is necessary for the diagnosis of gastrin-producing pancreatic adenoma, in which fasting blood gastrin levels increase greatly, between 200 and 1000 pg/mL. Histamine also plays an important role in gastric acid secretion. Gastric secretion can be divided into three phases: cephalic, gastric, and intestinal. The cephalic phase represents gastric acid secretion in response to the thought, sight, smell, or ingestion of food.

Vagal stimulation causes acetylcholine release, which triggers hydrochloric acid secretion and gastrin release. The gastric phase begins when food causes stomach distention and is mediated by both gastrin and cholinergic nerves. The intestinal phase begins when food enters the proximal portion of the small intestine. It has been shown that gastric secretion can be decreased through negative feedback. Several other substances are also secreted by the stomach, including vasoactive intestinal peptide, serotonin, growth factor, and prostaglandins.

The gastric mucosa is protected from ulceration by several mechanisms. Gastric epithelial cells secrete mucus and bicarbonate, which protects the mucosa from damage. Mucus and bicarbonate act as a barrier to hydrogen ion back-diffusion across the gastric mucosa. Rapid gastric mucosal blood flow allows removal of hydrogen ions. Prostaglandins stimulate mucus and bicarbonate secretion and maintain gastric mucosal blood flow. These protective mechanisms counteract aggressive factors on the gastric mucosa. Deficiencies in the protective mechanisms or excessive aggressive factors result in ulceration.

The presence of *Helicobacter pylori* is associated with antral gastritis and duodenal and gastric ulcers. *H. pylori* is a common gastric infectious agent, affecting more than 50% of the world's population, and is a major cause of gastritis and peptic ulcer disease.[3] Most patients with duodenal ulcer have *H. pylori* gastritis. *H. pylori* produces a urease enzyme that catalyzes urea to form ammonium and bicarbonate, thus allowing it to withstand the harsh gastric environment. Current detection methods rely on the reaction for positive results. Transmission of the organisms appears to occur through human-to-human contact, most likely through the fecal–oral route.

20.2 CLINICAL DIAGNOSIS

The diagnosis of peptic ulcer disease requires radiologic examination or endoscopic visualization of the ulcer. Radiologic examination with barium contrast is a common initial method of diagnosis for peptic ulcer. This method can detect 70 to 80% of ulcers found with endoscopy; detection rises to approximately 90% with double-contrast barium. Endoscopy is useful for detecting suspected ulcers that cannot be found radiographically; this technique is used to visualize and perform biopsies of gastric ulcers, to collect gastric biopsies for detection of *Helicobacter pylori*, and to identify sources of active GI bleeding. Because up to 10% of gastric ulcers are malignant, it is important to examine patients with follow-up endoscopy, which allows direct examination of the esophagus, stomach, and duodenum. Various lesions can be biopsied easily, and superficial erosions can be observed if not detected by radiological methods.

Bicarbonate produced in *Helicobacter pylori* by the urease reaction is excreted as carbon dioxide in lungs and forms the basis of measuring urease activity. Diagnostic tests for *H. pylori* can be divided into invasive and noninvasive measures. Invasive measures include endoscopy with gastric biopsy and histologic examination of organisms, biopsy with direct detection of urease activity in the tissue specimen, and biopsy with culture of the *H. pylori* organisms. Noninvasive measures include serologic tests for IgG antibodies to *H. pylori* and breath tests of urease activity, using orally administered urea labeled with ^{14}C or ^{13}C. Antibody levels may decrease slowly after eradication of *H. pylori* infection.

Table 20.1 Main Drugs Used for Treatment of Peptic Ulcers

Drug	Action Mechanism	Dosage and Duration	Adverse Effects and Precautions
Antisecretory Drugs			
H2-receptor antagonists			
Cimetidine	Inhibits gastric acid secretion (4–8 wk)	400 mg twice daily or 800 mg at night	Headache, dizziness, skin rash, nausea; interferes with hepatic metabolism of drugs (e.g., warfarin)
Ranitidine	Inhibits gastric acid secretion	150 mg twice daily or 300 mg at night (4–8 wk)	Headache, dizziness, nausea, diarrhea, skin rash
Others: famotidine, nizatidine, roxatidine			
Proton pump inhibitors (PPIs)			
Omeprazole	Inhibits gastric acid secretion; suppression of *Helicobacter pylori*	15–30 mg once daily (4–8 wk)	Diarrhea, headache, nausea, abdominal pain, dizziness
Lansoprazole	Inhibits gastric acid secretion	15–30 mg once daily (4–8 wk)	Diarrhea, headache, nausea, abdominal pain, dizziness
Others: pantoprazole			
Muscarinic M$_1$-receptor antagonist			
Pirenzepine	Inhibits gastric acid secretion; increases blood flow and mucus secretion	50 mg twice daily or 100 mg at night (4–6 wk)	Dry mouth, visual disturbances, skin rash
Cytoprotective Drugs			
Colloidal bismuth subcitrate	Binds to ulcer surface, providing barrier; inhibits *H. pylori*	120 mg 4 times daily or 240 mg twice daily (4–8 wk)	Renders stool black and discolors tongue and teeth; bleeding in long-term therapy
Sucralfate	Adheres to ulcer surface, providing barrier	1 g 4 times daily or 2 g twice daily (8 wk)	Constipation, nausea, headache, urticaria, dyspepsia; may interfere with drugs (e.g., warfarin)
Antisecretory and Cytoprotective Drugs			
Misoprostol	Inhibits acid secretion, increases blood flow and mucus secretion	400 mg twice daily	Diarrhea, nausea, dyspepsia, abdominal pain
Ranitidine bismuth citrate	Inhibits acid secretion, increases blood flow and mucus secretion; inhibits *H. pylori*	400 mg twice daily	Renders stool black and discolors tongue and teeth; headache, diarrhea, and pain
Antacids			
Aluminum hydroxide gel–magnesium hydroxide suspension	Decreases gastric acidity; binds pepsin	30 mL 1 hr before and 3 hr after meals and at bedtime	Constipation, phosphorus depletion; diarrhea, which interferes with the absorption of other drugs

20.3 CLINICAL PHARMACOLOGY OF ANTIULCER DRUGS

The mechanisms of action, dosage and duration of treatments, and adverse effects or precautions for antiulcer drugs are described in Table 20.1. H$_2$-receptor antagonists (cimetidine, ranitidine, famotidine, and nizatidine) competitively and reversibly bind to the H$_2$-receptor of the parietal cells, causing a dose-dependent inhibition of gastric acid secretion. They differ in potency, chemical structure, adverse effects, and ability to cause drug interactions. Famotidine is the most potent, followed by nizatidine, ranitidine, and cimetidine. Cimetidine is approved for acute and chronic treatment of DU, active benign GU, hypersecretory conditions, and gastroesophageal reflux disease. It has an oral bioavailability of 60 to 70%, with peak levels produced within 1 hour of administration. It is metabolized in the liver and has an elimination half-life of about 2 hours in patients with normal renal function. The half-life increases as the renal function diminishes, extending to approximately 5 hours in anephric patients.

Cimetidine, like the other H_2-receptor antagonists, has very few major side effects. Mild and transient diarrhea, dizziness, and headache have been reported in 1 to 7% of patients. Confusion, agitation, anxiety, or disorientation may occur, especially in severely ill patients and the elderly. It inhibits hepatic CYP1A2, CYP2C8-10, CYP2D6, and CYP3A3-5 enzymes in the liver, resulting in several drug interactions.

Proton pump inhibitors (PPIs), such as omeprazole and lansoprozole, are benzimidazole derivatives that irreversibly bind and inhibit the H^+/K^+-ATPase (acid pump). The maximum effect occurs within 2 hours of administration, reducing peak acid output by 80% or more. At 24 hours, 50% of maximum inhibition occurs, and effects may persist for up to 72 hours after a dose. The antisecretory activity of PPIs is greater than that of the H_2-receptor antagonists. Because these agents are acid unstable, they have been formulated using an enteric coating to delay the release of the drug. The bioavailability of omeprazole varies between 30 to 70%, whereas that of lansoprozole is between 80 and 90%. The PPIs play a primary role in eradicating *Helicobacter pylori*. In DUs, disease healing occurs with 2 to 4 weeks of single daily doses of PPIs, compared to 4 to 8 weeks with H_2-receptor antagonists. The PPIs are rapidly effective in treating GUs and are used extensively in the long-term treatment of GI hypersecretory conditions. PPIs inhibit cytochrome P-450 enzymes and may interact with drugs metabolized by this pathway.

Sucralfate (cytoprotective drug) is a unique therapeutic agent used for the acute and chronic treatments of DUs and GUs and the prevention of stress ulceration. It is an aluminum salt of a sulfated disaccharide that exerts its action locally on the GI mucosa. It binds to positively charged molecules and forms a gelatinous layer at the ulcer site, which protects the ulcer or involved mucosa from the aggressive action of acid, pepsin, and bile salts. It also absorbs pepsin and bile salts and may stimulate the secretion of endogenous cytoprotective prostaglandins. Sucralfate undergoes limited absorption from the GI tract (3 to 5%), although the aluminum ions released by its interaction with gastric acid may be absorbed significantly.[4] Because of its lack of systemic bioavailability, sucralfate is well tolerated. The small amount of aluminum absorbed from sucralfate is readily excreted by the kidney in patients with normal renal function; however, patients with chronic renal failure and patients who need dialysis may accumulate aluminum, leading to aluminum toxicity.

Because antacids can provide symptomatic relief and heal peptic ulcers, they are widely used. Common preparations include sodium bicarbonate, calcium carbonate, and salts of aluminum and magnesium. Antacids heal DUs by neutralizing gastric acid, which also inhibits the action of pepsin when the gastric pH increases above 4. Sodium bicarbonate and calcium carbonate have the greatest acid-neutralizing capacity but produce unacceptable side effects when administered chronically. Antacids may provide additional benefit by suppressing *Helicobacter pylori* growth.[5] Sodium bicarbonate and calcium carbonate are potent antacids but have side effects that preclude their use for peptic ulcer disease. Sodium bicarbonate produces gas from CO_2 formation in the stomach that may induce alkalosis and delivers a high sodium load when used chronically. Calcium stimulates gastrin release to produce acid rebound. Chronic administration of large dosages of calcium carbonate can be associated with the milk-alkali syndrome, producing hypercalcemia, hyperphosphatemia, increased blood urea nitrogen, and systemic alkalosis. Magnesium-containing antacids can cause diarrhea and are rarely used alone for peptic ulcer therapy. Aluminum hydroxide is a weaker antacid than magnesium hydroxide and can cause constipation.

Antacids can elicit drug interactions, usually by interfering with absorption or chelation of the drug (e.g., tetracycline). They reduce the serum concentrations of digoxin, ketoconazole, tetracycline, ferrous sulfate, isoniazid, and fluoroquinolones when administered concomitantly. Antacids can increase quinidine serum concentrations by enhancing renal tubular reabsorption of quinidine through an increase in urine pH.

Helicobacter pylori suppressive agents are used to eradicate *H. pylori* to reduce ulcer recurrence to less than 10% or eliminate recurrence.[6-8] The combination of an antisecretory agent with an antibiotic generally is necessary for ulcer healing and *H. pylori* eradication. Success rates are low with antibiotics alone for DU but may heal GUs. *H. pylori* eradication therapy depends on topical, local mucosal delivery of antibiotics. The oral route of antibiotic administration is preferred and produces high transient drug concentrations in the gastric mucosa. In addition, H_2-receptor antagonists are effective in increasing antibiotic concentrations in the gastric mucosa.

No suitable animal model exists to study therapy approaches; therefore, small trials in humans have been performed to obtain information on drug selection. Several antibiotics exhibit activity against *Helicobacter pylori*, including tetracycline, metronidazole, amoxicillin, clarithromycin, and azithromycin. The best combination of agents provides eradication rates of 80 to 90%. Such eradication rates have been reported for the combination of omeprazole (20 mg twice daily) and amoxicillin (1.5 to 2.0 g/day). Rates of 90% or higher have been achieved with three- and four-drug combinations. Single-antibiotic therapy should be avoided because of high rates of resistance.[9] Four-drug therapy involves the use of bismuth subsalicylate (two tablets four times daily), omeprazole (20 mg twice daily), tetracycline (500 mg four times daily), and metronidazole (500 mg three times daily) for 7 to 12 days. Eradication rates of greater than 95% have been achieved.[10,11]

In summary, H_2-receptor antagonists exhibit similar effectiveness in the treatment of DUs and GUs; however, the use of these products should be determined based on the potential adverse reactions and drug interactions. Sucralfate can be used as an alternative to H_2-receptor antagonists. Omeprazole has demonstrated better healing of DUs than conventional therapy. *Helicobacter pylori* eradication can reduce peptic ulcer recurrence and has become an important therapy.

20.4 DESIGN OF CLINICAL TRIALS AND PHARMACOKINETIC ISSUES

Healthy volunteers have been used for phase I and initial phase II clinical trials to determine the effectiveness of antisecretory agents. The observations in healthy volunteers usually show similar results in patients, although ulcer patients secrete more acid than do control groups.[12] Procedures used in the assessment of antisecretory drugs in patients involve invasive and inconvenient methods, whereas studies are usually completed faster when healthy volunteers are used. As an alternative, patients in remission from ulcer may be used. Clinical data obtained from volunteers or patients in remission are considered applicable to patients with active duodenal ulceration and gastric ulceration. In contrast, measurement of the reflux of gastric acid into the esophagus can only be performed in patients. Adequate methods for the assessment of cytoprotective agents are not currently available. Healthy volunteers and ulcer patients in remission have been used for studies of these agents.

Healthy volunteers may also be used to evaluate the effectiveness of drugs for treatment of *Helicobacter pylori*. The incidence rate of infection in healthy populations becomes high as age increases. In developed countries, approximately 50% of healthy individuals are infected at the age of 50 years. The incidence rate is much higher in the developing world, particularly in children, because of poor hygiene environment. The incidence in young healthy volunteers is low and screening would be required to identify individuals with asymptomatic infection. The benefit to patients in remission from duodenal ulceration is that eradication of *H. pylori* reduces the risk of recurrence.

Because of the potential adverse effects of the antibacterial agents used against *Helicobacter pylori* and the low incidence of infection in healthy people, it is convenient to use patients in remission for clinical studies. Healthy volunteers with high acid outputs such as males are the most appropriate group for study of antisecretory agents. It is necessary to measure the subjects' acid secretion the day before the study begins. It is also important to use volunteers who are familiar with the procedures involved in measuring gastric acid secretion. The passage of a nasogastric tube or electrode can cause anxiety in new volunteers. To avoid the disruption of safety monitoring, it is best to use experienced volunteers, particularly when measuring antisecretory effect in the first administration studies. New subjects can be used in later studies of antisecretory effects when it is no longer necessary to measure cardiovascular effects.

Most early studies of H_2-receptor antagonists tended to examine the activity of single doses, because they had relatively short elimination half-lives with no accumulation of drug levels on repeat dosing. Later, it was shown that the antisecretory effect of H_2 receptor antagonists diminishes on repeat dosing.[13] The presence of a short hypersecretory state has also been reported after stopping H_2 receptor antagonists. Because not all of the gastric parietal cell H^+/K^+-ATPase enzymes are active at the same time, repeat dosing with these rapidly eliminated drugs is required for at least one week before pharmacodynamic steady-state is attained. As a result, repeat doses are necessary to assess the pharmacodynamics of both H_2 receptor antagonists and H^+/K^+-ATPase inhibitors.

Studies involving 24-hour intragastric pH measurement usually use food to stimulate acid secretion. The presence or absence of a food interaction and its relevance must be assessed early in the project design. It is important to measure drug concentration in gastric secretion and urinary excretion. Two major methods for measuring antisecretory effect are (1) by aspiration of gastric contents, and (2) by continuous monitoring of intragastric pH using an intragastric electrode.

Regarding the technique of aspiration of gastric secretion, a nasogastric tube is positioned in the antrum of the stomach, either under fluoroscopic control or by using the water recovery test. Aspiration may be performed manually with a syringe or using continuous or intermittent aspiration with a low-pressure suction pump. Basal gastric acid secretory rate is variable and has an arrhythmic cycle in both healthy subjects and patients. Aspiration is technically difficult because of the relatively small volumes secreted; however, it is possible to show the pharmacological effect of low doses of drug on basal gastric acid secretion.[14] The variability in basal secretory rate can be overcome by using a stimulant of gastric acid secretion such as histamine, its analogs, and the H_2-receptor agonist impromidine. In addition, pentagastrin (Peptavlon®) is one of the most widely used and acceptable stimulants. An infusion rate of 0.6 µg/kg/hr is a near maximal stimulatory dose for the majority of healthy subjects; a higher dose level may be required in ulcer patients. Steady-state stimulation of secretion takes 30 minutes to attain. Maintaining the hydration of subjects with intravenous fluids during extended aspiration is necessary to replace the fluid loss from the stomach. Aspiration secretion is collected in 15-minute periods, and the pH and volume are recorded. The volume of secretion is multiplied by the hydrogen ion concentration to determine the total acid output during each period. When a drug is given orally, time must be allowed for the drug to leave the stomach before stimulation and aspiration begin. The effects of the drug are compared to those of a placebo, and the percentage inhibition of acid secretion is evaluated.

Other methods to assess gastric secretion include the "spit and chew" technique, which measures cephalic, vagally mediated stimulation of gastric secretion caused by the chewing and tasting of food. Aspiration methods also allow the measurement of other constituents of gastric secretion, such as pepsin and intrinsic factor.

The pH of gastric secretion may be monitored more conveniently by means of a nasogastric pH electrode. A small glass electrode is connected to a recording device by means of an insulted and protected wire. The electrode tip is positioned in the body of the stomach under fluoroscopic control or at the region of the gastroesophageal sphincter. Gastric pH data obtained by this technique are closer to physiological reality, because aspiration or instillation of alkali does not interfere with the intragastric contents. The antisecretory activity and duration on effect of two agents can be compared over a 24-hour period.

Several factors contribute to the resistance of the mucosa to aggressive agents. These include the properties of the mucus layer, the alkaline nonacid secretion of the mucosa, and rapid regeneration of mucosa. The functions of cytoprotective agents include the inhibition of aspirin-induced gastric bleeding, facilitating assessment of the endoscopic appearance of the mucosa, and inhibition of changes in potential mucosal difference. Several techniques have been applied for measuring the production of alkaline secretion in the stomach or duodenum;[15] for example, the defective secretion of bicarbonate was observed in the duodenum of ulcer patients. These methods can be used to evaluate the effectiveness of cytoprotective drugs.

Because of the marked individual differences in gastric secretion and antisecretory effect between different populations, it is important to use the placebo and comparator agent in studies of new antisecretory drugs. The desirable active comparator agents are either one of the H_2-receptor antagonists or omeprazole, because pharmacological data are available on these drugs.

Long-term studies of antisecretory agents are more appropriately performed in ulcer patients. In addition, studies of intraesophageal pH monitoring can only be performed in patients with acid reflux disease. In phase II trials, patients may be studied for up to 8 weeks and the response to therapy determined by endoscopy. The evaluation of drugs for treatment of *Helicobacter pylori* infection can be performed in patients with a history of chronic duodenal ulceration who are currently in remission and not on any medication. This population exhibits a near 100% incidence of infection.

20.5 EVALUATION METHODS

No clinically important differences exist in the pharmacokinetics of antisecretory agents in ulcer patients compared to healthy volunteers. The pharmacokinetics of drugs for treatment of *Helicobacter pylori* can be determined in early studies. Assessment of the local concentration of drug may be achieved by biopsy during endoscopic examinations of the patient. The total acid output measured over a given time is expressed as the volume of secretion multiplied by the H^+ ion concentration, which is determined by titration to pH 7 with alkali. This is greater than the H^+ activity in gastric secretion due to buffering of some H^+ ions by intragastric contents. In biological fluids, the pH is negatively related to the log of the H^+ ion activity, expressed as $pH = -\log (H^+ \text{ activity})$.

Low levels of antisecretory effect, if mediated through changes in volume of secretion, can be more easily detected by methods using aspiration to determine acid output. At higher doses, where near extinction of gastric secretion occurs, pH monitoring allows the clear separation of activity between two potent drugs. This implies that it is often easier to initially evaluate an antisecretory agent in a small number of subjects by measuring stimulated acid output before choosing a clinically relevant and relatively high antisecretory dose to evaluate further using pH monitoring.

The relationship between antisecretory effect and ulcer healing has been elaborated for duodenal ulceration using metaanalysis.[16] The duration of treatment and the time that the intragastric pH is maintained above pH 3 appear to be the critical factors. Maintaining intragastric pH above 3 for about 16 hours per day is associated with a healing rate of nearly 100% at 4 weeks. Adjusting to a higher pH threshold does not confer any additional benefit. Similar relationships have also been identified for gastric ulceration, where the duration of treatment appears to be a more critical factor related to ulcer healing. The relationship between the healing of reflux esophagitis and inhibition of acid secretion has also been observed; when intragastric pH is maintained above 4, the healing rate can be observed after 8 weeks of therapy. Intraesophageal pH monitoring may be performed in these patients using a method similar to that for intragastric monitoring. The results obtained from this technique are more variable than those for intragastric pH monitoring, because small differences in electrode placement can have considerable impact on the data. Also, marked day-to-day variations in the degree of acid reflux are observed. Despite this variability, healing rates can be inversely proportional to the degree of acid exposure on the esophagus.

The *in vitro* effects of drugs for the treatment of *H. pylori* infection do not correlate with *in vivo* activity; therefore, it is necessary to assess the activity of candidate agents for *in vivo* activity. Several methods are available, including the use of endoscopic biopsy.[17] Noninvasive methods are also available to detect the urea-splitting properties of the bacteria. These noninvasive tests involve drinking a solution of ^{13}C- or ^{14}C-labeled urea and measuring the amount of labeled carbon dioxide excreted by the subject. Although the eradication of *H. pylori* is associated with a reduced relapse rate of duodenal ulceration, confirmatory results are required in larger scale studies to assess effectiveness and safety. In studies on drugs for the treatment of *H. pylori* infection, the use of a placebo is not mandatory because the spontaneous rate of eradication of *H. pylori* is very low; however, the use of a placebo in a study provides more objective observations for assessment of effectiveness and safety. The use of an active comparator agent is necessary for more exhaustive studies. A triple-therapy approach using a bismuth salt, metronidazole, and erythromycin or amoxicillin is standard. A combination of antisecretory agents and antibiotics is also commonly used.

Studies of antisecretory agents can be performed with relatively few patients (e.g., 12 to 18) to demonstrate differences or similarities between two agents. Patients are usually treated for at least one week to assess antisecretory effect. Subsequent phase II trials to measure healing rates should be performed on a larger scale, with 100 patients or more per treatment arm. At least 2 weeks of treatment should be conducted to examine the effectiveness of drugs for treatment of *Helicobacter pylori* infection. These studies can be relatively small scale, using as few as 20 patients if detecting the presence or absence of activity is the primary objective. Large-scale studies are required if a dose–response or active comparator study is performed to assess anticipated response rates. Subsequent studies of the rate of recurrence of ulceration are performed in phase III trials.

When the relationship between antisecretory effects and upper gastrointestinal ulceration healing has been established, it is necessary to perform conventional dose-ranging studies in phase IIB trials. Antisecretory activity can be assessed from early studies in phase I and phase IIA trials, and a single-dose study can be designed for phase III trials. This approach should be discussed with the relevant regulatory agency in pre-investigational new drug (IND) meetings. Furthermore, in phase I and phase IIA trials, if a candidate agent is not capable of achieving antisecretory activity compared to currently available drugs, then there is no reason to develop that drug further. Clinical trials for cytoprotective agents are usually restricted to confirming tolerability and safety and elaborating possible mechanisms of action.

A dose–response relationship for drugs against *Helicobacter pylori* infection should be performed in early studies before progressing to large studies to confirm efficacy, safety, and rate of ulcer recurrence. For combination drug products, it is necessary to assess eradication of the bacteria and synergistic effect of each component using the eradication of *H. pylori* as an endpoint. The results on reduced recurrence rate of healing should be confirmed in large-scale phase III trials.

20.6 DEVELOPMENT AND EVALUATION OF
HELICOBACTER PYLORI VACCINE

The discovery of *Helicobacter pylori* led to the development of antibacterial therapies that, when properly applied, permanently cure the ulcer and eliminate the need for maintenance therapy; however, concerns about induction of antibiotic resistance and side effects of chemotherapy have generated interest in developing a *H. pylori* vaccine with both therapeutic and prophylactic effects for the treatment and prevention of peptic ulcer disease. Although the prevalence of *H. pylori* is decreasing in many areas of the world as living standards and health care improve, many millions still would benefit from immunization. In the United States, Europe, and Australia, 30% of the population are infected, and more than 60% of all Japanese are *H. pylori* positive. In developing countries, a million cases of ulcer, lymphoma, and adenocarcinoma could be prevented by a simple oral vaccine. Thus, vaccine development is an important and a cost-effective health priority.[18]

Helicobacter pylori produces many cellular products, such as vacuolating cytotoxin and phospholipases; however, most infected persons do not develop ulcers, so other factors must be involved. The only correlate of an ulcerogenic strain with an increased capacity to damage gastric tissue has been found in Cag-A-positive strains. The Cag-A gene codes for an immunogenic 120-kDa protein that is usually coexpressed with the vacuolating cytotoxin. The greater proportion of strains from gastric cancer patients are Cag-A positive; however, both ulcers and cancer can be caused by Cag-A-negative strains. These observations indicate that Cag-A-positive strains induce more vigorous inflammatory responses and make the tissue more susceptible to acid damage. In addition, high levels of serum IgG and vigorous humoral response to infection are observed with *H. pylori*.

In early studies on vaccine development, mice were administered *Helicobacter pylori* lysate alone or with the mucosal adjuvant cholera toxin (CT). A fivefold increase of IgA antibody in serum and a 16-fold increase in intestinal secretions were observed in immunized animals compared to the control group.[19] These results suggest that it is possible to develop an oral vaccine for the prevention of *H. pylori* infection and associated gastritis. Many investigators have subsequently shown that 90 to 100% protection could be achieved with *H. pylori* sonicate in the presence of CT adjuvant.[20,21] In addition, Agt11 was used to detect 66- and 31-kDa antigens in clones with antiserum raised against purified *H. pylori*. The DNA sequence of the cloned fragments corresponded to two polypeptides, UreA (26.7 kDa) and UreB (60.5 kDa).[22]

Immunization of cells derived from mice immunized with recombinant urease suggested the possibility that oral immunization could result in the accumulation and proliferation in gastric tissue of IgA antibody-secreting cells activated in mucosa-associated lymphoid tissue.[23,24] HspA and HspB proteins were shown to be immunogenic, as they were specifically recognized by sera from *Helicobacter pylori*-infected patients. Because of this and their apparent surface location, these proteins appeared likely to be vaccine candidates. Orogastric administration of 50 mg of HspA and HspB antigen with 5 µg CT protected 80 and 70% of mice, respectively, against *H. felis*. Combined vaccines of HspA and UreB showed better protection against *H. pylori* infection than either alone.[25]

Oral immunization of mice with disrupted *Helicobacter felis* or *H. pylori* plus CT exhibited therapeutic effect and cured the infection.[27] Furthermore, an oral vaccine of *H. pylori* urease and CT adjuvant immunized to ferrets, chronically colonized with infecting organism, showed that one third of the animals were cured of their natural infection, and, where cure was not achieved, inflammation was reduced. The discovery of a therapeutic effect of anti-*Helicobacter* immunization has had a catalyzing effect on research to develop a potentially therapeutic vaccine.

The protective immunity induced by vaccination in animal models of *Helicobacter* infection differs from the immunity induced by many other vaccines. The immune response induced by infection with *H. pylori* in human or *H. felis* in mouse models is inadequate to induce protective immunity. The bacteria continue to flourish. Animals cured of their infection with antibiotics can be reinfected with the same strains of *H. felis*.

In humans, the natural immunity induced by infection is also not effective enough to prevent further infection.[27] The presence of *Helicobacter pylori* in the mucous gel, the diffusion of bacterial products into the mucosal tissue, and damage to mucosal cells due to bacterial toxins or by-products (e.g., ammonia) all have the potential to act as signals to activate elements of both innate and adaptive immune responses.

The initial serum antibody response to gastric *Helicobacter* infection is production of IgM, followed by a significant serum IgG and, in 30 to 40% of cases, a detectable IgA response. IgG and IgA antibodies can also be detected in the gastric mucosa and on the surface of bacteria; however, these antibodies have little or no protective effect, and the *H. pylori* continue to thrive. Parenteral routes of immunization that induce high levels of serum antibodies do not protect animals from challenge. In addition, a cell-mediated response is also not responsible for protective immunity. If neither serum antibodies nor cell-mediated immune responses are protective, all that remains is an enhanced mucosal immune response mediated through the IgA antibody. It is shown that monoclonal IgA delivered at the time of infection can prevent the colonization of *H. felis*;[28] however, few differences in total IgA between infected and immunized animals can be detected. This is consistent with the demonstration of IgA antibody in the gastric mucosa of *H. pylori*-infected humans. Also, no differences exist between total levels of salivary IgA in mice immunized with *H. felis* sonicate alone or *H. felis* sonicate plus CT. Yet, cure has occurred only in the antigen plus CT group. In addition, oral immunization of mice with recombinant *H. pylori* urease plus *Escherichia coli* entero toxin (LT) induced a vigorous secretary IgA response against urease, and *Helicobacter*-infected mice showed no detectable IgA against urease. These results support the suggestion that IgA is the protective mechanism against *H. pylori* infection. The mechanism of action is explained by a process of immune exclusion, in which the antibody immobilizes the bacteria in a mucous gel, preventing them from moving against the mucous flow and moving down to the epithelial surface to attachment sites on the gastric mucosa. Thus, the bacteria are trapped in the mucous blanket that is flushed out of the stomach into the lower bowel together with infected epithelial cells. *H. pylori* cannot survive in the bile-rich small bowel, and the infection is destroyed. Surface exposure would be an essential feature of protective antigens if immune exclusion induces protective immunity. This feature of protective mechanism has been observed in mucosal immunization of three recombinant protein antigens including urease, heat-shock protein, and vacuolating cytotoxin in animal models.

Helicobacter pylori vaccine development is still in its early stage; however, we have passed the initial phase and have identified problems to be addressed. Extensive research and clinical trials are necessary to reveal future directions for the development of a safe and effective vaccine.

REFERENCES

1. Feldman, M., Peptic ulcer diseases, in *Scientific American Medicine*, Dale, D.C. and Federman, D.D., Eds., Scientific American, New York, 1997, pp. 1–15.
2. Friedman, L.S. and Peterson, W.L., Peptic ulcer and related disorders, in *Harrison's Principles of Internal Medicine*, 14th ed., Fauci, A.S., Braunwald, E., Isselbacher, K.J. et al., Eds., McGraw-Hill, New York, 1998, pp. 1566, 1616.
3. Del Valle, J., Cohen, H., Laine, L. et al., Acid–peptic disorders, in *Textbook of Gastroenterology*, 3rd ed., Yamada, T., Alpers, D.H., and Owyang, C., Eds., Lippincott, Philadelphia, 1999, pp. 1370–1444.
4. Lauritsen, K., Lauarsen, L.S., and Rask-Madsen, J., Clinical pharmacokinetics of drugs used in the treatment of gastrointestinal diseases, part II, *Clin. Pharmacokinet.*, 19, 94–125, 1990.
5. Berstad, A., Alexander, B., Weberg, R. et al., Antacids reduce *Campylobacter pylori* colonization without healing the gastritis in patients with nonulcer dyspepsia and erosive prepylonic changes, *Gastroenterology*, 95, 619–624, 1988.
6. Graham, D.Y., Lew, G.M., Klein, P.D. et al., Effect of treatment of *Helicobacter pylori* infection on the long-term recurrence of gastric or duodenal ulcer: a randomized, controlled study, *Ann. Intern. Med.*, 116, 705–708, 1992.
7. Adamek, R.J., Wegener, M., Labenz, J. et al., Medium-term results of oral and intravenous omeprazole/amoxicillin *Helicobacter pylori* eradication therapy, *Am. J. Gastroenterol.*, 89, 39–42, 1994.
8. Abu-Mahfouz, M.Z., Prasad, V.M., Sautograde, P. et al., *Helicobacter pylori* recurrence after successful eradication: 5 year follow-up in the United States, *Am. J. Gastroenterol.*, 92, 2025–2027, 1997.
9. Labenz, J., Ruhl, G.H., Bertrams, J. et al., Medium- or high-dose omeprazole plus amoxicillin eradicates *Helicobacter pylori* in gastric ulcer disease, *Am. J. Gastroenterol.*, 89, 726–730, 1994.
10. Howden, C.W. and Hunt, R.H., Guidelines for the management of *Helicobacter pylori* infection, *Am. J. Gastroenterol.*, 93, 2330–2338, 1998.
11. Salcedo, J.A. and Al-Kawas, F., Treatment of *Helicobacter pylori* infection, *Arch. Intern. Med.*, 158, 842–851, 1998.
12. Merki, H.S., Fimmel, C.J., Walt, R.P. et al., Pattern of 24-hour intragastric acidity in active duodenal ulcer disease and in healthy controls, *Gut*, 29, 1583–1587, 1988.
13. Broom, C., Eagle, S., Pue, M. et al., Comparison of the antisecretory activity of the reversible proton pump inhibitor SK&F 96067 and rantitidine, *Gastroenterology*, 104(4), A46, 1993.

14. Acton, G., Broom, C., Burnham, D. et al., Effects of low dose cimetidine on nocturnal acid secretion in healthy volunteers, *Aliment. Pharmacol. Ther.*, 5, 61, 1991.

15. Hogan, D.L., Ainsworth, M.A., and Isenberg, J.I., Gastro duodenal bicarbonate secretion, *Aliment. Pharmacol. Ther.*, 8, 5, 1994.

16. McIsaac, R.L., Dixon, J.S., Mills, J.G. et al., Ranitidine in the treatment of duodenal ulcer disease: relationship between antisecretory effect and ulcer healing rate, *Aliment. Pharmacol. Ther.*, 5, 227, 1991.

17. Marshall, B.J., Warren, R., Francis, G. et al., Rapid urease test in the management of *Campylobacter pyloridis*-associated gastritis, *Am. J. Gastroenterol.*, 82, 200–210, 1987.

18. Lee, A. and Doidge, C., Vaccines against *H. pylori*, in *New Generation Vaccines*, 2nd ed., Levine, M.M., Woodrow, G.C., Kaper, J.B., and Cobon, G.S., Eds., Marcel Dekker, New York, 1997, pp. 963–977.

19. Czinn, S.J. and Nedrud, J.G., Oral immunization against *Helicobacter pylori*, *Infect. Immun.*, 59, 2359–2363, 1992.

20. Lee, A. and Chen, M.H., Successful immunization against gastric infection with *Helicobacter* species: use of a cholera toxin B-subunit-whole-cell vaccine, *Infect. Immun.*, 62, 3594–3597, 1994.

21. Michetti, P., Corthesy-Theulaz, I., Davin, C. et al., Oral immunization with *H. pylori* urease A and/or B subunits protects against *H. felis* infection in the mouse, *Dig. Dis. Week*, 108, A577, 1994.

22. Clayton, C.L., Pallen, M.J., Kleanthous, H. et al., Nucleotide sequence of two genes from *Helicobacter pylori* encoding for urease subunits, *Nucleic Acids Res.*, 18, 362, 1990.

23. Pappo, J., Thomas, W.D., Kabok, Z. et al., Effect of oral immunization with recombinant urease on murine *helicobacter felis* gastritis, *Infect. Immun.*, 63, 1246–1252, 1995.

24. Ermak, T.H., Attardo, L., Ding, R. et al., Oral immunization of mice with *Helicobacter pylori* recombinant urease enhances the specific gastric IgA immune response, *Clin. Immunol. Immunopathol.*, 76(Pt. 2), S99, 1995.

25. Ferrero, R.L., Thiberge, J.M., Kansau, I. et al., The GroES homolog of *Helicobacter pylori* confers protective immunity against mucosal infection in mice, *Proc. Natl. Acad. Sci.*, 92, 6499–6503, 1995.

26. Doidge, C., Gust, I., Lee, A. et al., Therapeutic immunization against *Helicobacter* infection, *Lancet*, 343, 914–915, 1994.

27. Langenberg, W., Rauws, E.A., Oudbier, J.H. et al., Patient-to-patient transmission of *Campylobacter pylori* infection by fiberoptic gastroduodenoscopy and biopsy, *J. Infect. Dis.*, 161, 507–511, 1990.

28. Czinn, S.J., Cai, A., and Nedrud, J.G., Protection of germ-free mice from infection by *Helicobacter felis* after active oral or passive IgA immunization, *Vaccine*, 11, 637–642, 1993.

CHAPTER 21

Diuretics

Hitesh H. Shah, Pravin C. Singhal, and Joseph Mattana

CONTENTS

21.1 INTRODUCTION

The primary action of diuretics is to increase urinary sodium and water loss; hence, they are widely used in the treatment of edematous states. They are also indicated for the management of several nonedematous conditions, primarily hypertension, acute or chronic renal failure, calcium nephrolithiasis, and electrolyte disorders, including hyperkalemia, hyponatremia, and acute hypercalcemia. Most outcome trials have used thiazide-type diuretics as the basis of antihypertensive therapy.[1] Several of these trials, including the recently published Antihypertensive and Lipid-Lowering

Treatment To Prevent Heart Attack Trial (ALLHAT), have demonstrated that diuretic therapy can prevent cardiovascular complications of hypertension;[2] therefore, the Seventh Report of the Joint National Committee on Prevention, Detection, Evaluation, and Treatment of High Blood Pressure (JNC 7) recommends thiazide-type diuretics as initial therapy for most patients with uncomplicated stage 1 and 2 hypertension, either alone or in combination with other classes of antihypertensive agents.[3] A recent network metaanalysis also concluded that low-dose diuretics are the best first-line antihypertensive agents in preventing major cardiovascular disease endpoints in patients with hypertension.[4] The potassium-sparing diuretic spironolactone has been shown to reduce mortality in patients with advanced heart failure as a result of aldosterone antagonism.[5] Similarly, a recently approved potassium-sparing diuretic, eplerenone, has been shown to decrease death in patients who developed left ventricular dysfunction after acute myocardial infarction.[6]

21.2 RENAL CLEARANCE

Clearance is a theoretical concept that can be defined as the volume of plasma completely cleared of a given substance in unit time.[7] While studying diuretics, it is important to have a greater understanding of clearance.[8] Renal clearance of an endogenous or exogenous substance can be obtained by dividing the total urinary excretion of that substance by its plasma concentration during the collection period.[9] Different clearance techniques are used to determine glomerular filtration rate (e.g., inulin clearance, creatinine clearance), renal plasma flow (e.g., para-aminohippuric acid clearance), and renal tubular function; however, precautions should be taken to ensure the validity of these techniques, as several assumptions are made while calculating clearance.[8,9]

21.3 NORMAL KIDNEY WATER AND ELECTROLYTE HANDLING

Clinically used diuretic drugs act primarily on different renal tubular segments to inhibit sodium reabsorption, resulting in an increased fractional excretion of sodium and accompanying water loss; hence, to properly characterize a diuretic it is essential to have a basic understanding of renal (tubular) physiology. A normal individual may filter approximately 150 to 180 L of plasma water per day, of which 99% is reabsorbed by the renal tubules. Similarly, different tubular segments reabsorb 99% of the filtered sodium in order to maintain a normal fractional excretion of sodium of less than 1%. In the kidney, approximately two thirds of the filtered water and sodium chloride are reabsorbed passively in the proximal tubules. Fluid leaving the proximal tubule is isotonic with plasma. In the descending limb of the loop of Henle, solute is added, and an insignificant amount of water is removed. The ascending limb of the loop of Henle is impermeable to water; however, solute is reabsorbed in this segment, resulting in dilution of the tubular fluid and generation of solute-free water, measured as *free water clearance* (C_{H2O}). Tubular fluid then enters the cortical diluting segment, where a smaller amount of solute is reabsorbed. In the distal tubule, further dilution or concentration of urine will depend on the availability of antidiuretic hormone (ADH). In the absence of ADH, tubular fluid will be excreted without further reabsorption of water as dilute urine (low urine osmolality). While in the presence of ADH, further water will be reabsorbed from the distal tubular lumen into the hyperosmolar medullary interstitium leading to concentrated urine (high urine osmolality). This hypertonicity in the medullary interstitium is created primarily by the transport of solute from the loop of Henle and not from the cortical diluting segment. This extraction of water from the distal nephron in the presence of ADH results in *free water reabsorption* (denoted as TC_{H2O}).

21.4 CLASSIFICATION AND MECHANISM OF DIURETIC ACTION

Diuretics inhibit sodium chloride reabsorption at several sites along the nephron, leading to increased urinary electrolyte and water losses. Currently used diuretics are classified into three major groups depending on their site and mechanism of action along the nephron. Table 21.1 provides a summary of the various diuretic agents organized by site of action. The *loop diuretics* furosemide, bumetanide, and torsemide block the sodium–potassium–chloride cotransporter in the luminal membrane of the medullary and cortical aspects of the thick ascending loop of Henle. Although the exact mechanism by which ethacrynic acid (also a loop diuretic) inhibits sodium–chloride (NaCl) reabsorption is not known, its net effect on transport along the thick ascending limb of Henle is qualitatively similar to that of other loop diuretics.[10] In addition to promoting urinary loss of sodium and chloride, loop diuretics also increase potassium, magnesium, and calcium excretion. Increased urinary calcium excretion is clinically important in the management of patients with hypercalcemia.[11] The *distal convoluted tubule diuretics* include thiazide-type diuretics such as hydrochlorothiazide, chlorthalidone, and the quinazoline diuretic metolazone (all commonly prescribed drugs in this class of diuretics). Distal convoluted tubule diuretics inhibit the electroneutral sodium–chloride cotransporter in the luminal membrane of the distal tubule. Although distal convoluted tubule diuretics increase urinary magnesium excretion (like loop diuretics), they inhibit urinary calcium excretion; hence, distal convoluted tubule diuretics are commonly prescribed to hypercalciuric patients in order to prevent calcium nephrolithiasis.[10] *Collecting duct diuretics* include the two important groups of potassium-sparing diuretics. Amiloride and triamterene directly block the sodium channel activity, while spironolactone, and the recently approved eplerenone inhibit the action of aldosterone. These agents have weak natriuretic activity, so they are commonly used in combination with a thiazide or loop diuretic, either to decrease the degree of potassium loss or to increase the net diuresis. Other drugs such as *proximal tubule diuretics* (acetazolamide) and *osmotic diuretics* (mannitol) are less commonly used diuretic agents.

21.5 EXTRARENAL HEMODYNAMIC ACTIVITY

In addition to their diuretic action, loop diuretics have been known to have important renal and systemic hemodynamic effects. Intravenous furosemide induces a rapid and transient venodilation similar to morphine in patients with acute pulmonary edema. This in turn results in the fall of cardiac filling pressures and decreased pulmonary vascular congestion. This transient beneficial effect prior to the onset of diuresis is thought to be secondary to local prostaglandin production.[12,13] Furosemide in therapeutic concentrations has been shown to induce a dose-dependant direct venodilator effect on the dorsal hand vein of healthy individuals. This venodilator response was completely blocked by the prostaglandin inhibitor indomethacin. Local administration of nitric oxide synthesis inhibitor did not abolish furosemide-induced venodilation;[13] however, in certain conditions such as advanced chronic heart failure and cirrhosis, furosemide has an initial arteriolar vasoconstrictive effect. This deleterious response, which leads to acute elevation in systemic blood pressure and reduction in cardiac performance, is thought to be secondary to an acute rise in plasma renin levels.[14,15] This effect may be blocked by angiotensin-converting enzyme inhibitors and angiotensin receptor blockers. Similarly, certain thiazide diuretics have been shown to have direct vasodilator effect in addition to their diuretic effect; however, these effects are seen during chronic use and at higher doses.[16,17]

Table 21.1 Overview of Diuretics by Class

Class	Site of Action	Drug Names	Chemical Class	Mechanism	Adverse Reactions and Precautions
Carbonic anhydrase inhibitor	Proximal tubule	Acetazolamide (Diamox®)	Sulfonamide derivative	Inhibition of carbonic anhydrase	Allergic reactions, hyperchloremic metabolic acidosis, central nervous system effects, nephrolithiasis
Loop diuretic	Thick ascending limb	Furosemide (Lasix®), bumetanide (Bumex®), torsemide (Demadex®)	Sulfonamide derivative	Inhibition of Na–K–2Cl cotransporter	Allergic reactions, ototoxicity, hypokalemia, metabolic alkalosis, hypomagnesemia
Thiazide diuretic	Distal convoluted tubule	Hydrochlorothiazide (Hydrodiuril®, Microzide®), chlorothiazide (Diuril®), indapamide (Lozol®), metolazone (Zaroxolyn®)	Sulfonamide derivative	Inhibition of sodium chloride symport	Allergic reactions, hypokalemia, metabolic alkalosis, hyperuricemia, volume depletion, hypomagnesemia, hypercalcemia, hyponatremia, hyperglycemia, hyperlipidemia
Potassium-sparing diuretic	Cortical collecting duct	Amiloride (Midamor®), triamterene (Dyrenium®), spironolactone (Aldactone®)	Pyrazinoyl-guanidine, 17-spironolactone, and pteridine	Inhibition of luminal sodium entry (amiloride, triamterene); aldosterone antagonism (spironolactone)	Amiloride and triamterene: allergic reactions, hyperkalemia, nausea, vomiting, headache (triamterene may reduce glucose tolerance and increase risk of nephrolithiasis); spironolactone: allergic reactions, hyperkalemia, central nervous system effects, gynecomastia, impotence
Osmotic diuretic	Osmotic	Mannitol (Osmitrol®)	Sugar	Osmotic effect	Dehydration and hypernatremia or volume overload and hyponatremia

21.6 PHARMACOKINETICS

All diuretics (except osmotic diuretics) are secreted into the tubular fluid by the proximal tubular cells. As most diuretics (except spironolactone and eplerenone) act directly on the various luminal transport sites along the nephron, it is of greater pharmacodynamic importance to measure urinary drug levels of diuretics as compared to the measurement of plasma diuretic levels; however, the plasma concentration of diuretics may be required to assess certain pharmacokinetic features such as absorption and bioavailability. Important pharmacokinetic features of a diuretic include routes of metabolism, bioavailability, plasma half-life, and protein binding. Several of these features may play an important role in diuretic resistance. The following examples reinforce the importance of understanding the pharmacokinetics of diuretics. About half of the dose of furosemide is conjugated in the kidneys, while the remaining half is excreted unchanged in the urine; thus, the plasma half-life is prolonged in patients with renal dysfunction. Similarly the half-lives of the other two loop diuretics (bumetanide and torsemide) are increased in liver disease as the liver mainly metabolizes these drugs. Hence, clinically, one needs to avoid or change the dose of diuretics in certain diseases in order to avoid potential toxicities related to the drugs. The oral bioavailability of furosemide varies widely (ranges from 10 to 100%), thus making it difficult to predict how much of the drug will be absorbed in an individual patient. In comparison, the other two loop diuretics (bumetanide and torsemide) have a very high oral bioavailability. This pharmacokinetic feature may be clinically significant, as it has been reported that patients with heart failure required fewer hospitalizations when using a completely absorbed loop diuretic such as torsemide.[18] The frequency of administration of a diuretic depends upon its plasma half-life. Loop diuretics, for example, need to be administered several times in a day due to their shorter plasma half-lives as compared to distal diuretics, which have longer half-lives and can be administered once or twice a day. This feature may be important for improving the compliance of diuretic therapy. Diuretics are highly protein bound drugs (except osmotic diuretics). Binding of the diuretic to albumin in the urine is one of the most important mechanisms resulting in a decreased diuretic response in patients with severe nephrotic syndrome.[19]

21.7 PHARMACODYNAMIC ASSESSMENT

21.7.1 Dose-Ranging and Potency Determination

As part of the assessment of a new diuretic agent, the action of the drug must be determined. The potency and efficacy of the drug must be assessed, and for a diuretic it is important to establish the relationship between the amount of the diuretic and the natriuretic response. The response can be measured as urine sodium excretion by carrying out sodium balance studies or by measuring the fractional excretion of sodium. A diuretic acting at an efficacious dose would be expected to increase urinary sodium excretion and to increase the fractional excretion of sodium. Pharmacokinetic assessment of drugs examines many aspects of drug handling, including absorption, blood levels, bioavailability, metabolism, and routes of excretion. For many drugs, blood levels may serve as a useful variable to correlate with an outcome measure; however, to determine the pharmacodynamics for most diuretics, attempts to correlate blood levels of a diuretic with changes in sodium excretion may be unrewarding as most of these drugs work by being secreted into the lumen of the tubule, where they can interact with proteins on the luminal surface of the tubular epithelial cells.[19–22] For most diuretics, it is important to establish the relationships between urinary excretion of the drug and effect of the diuretic in terms of sodium excretion rate or fractional excretion of sodium. These drugs are characterized by a threshold effect such that a certain amount of the drug in the tubular lumen must be achieved for diuresis to occur. This is important in both dose-ranging and potency studies as well as in the clinical setting.[19] Typical relationships between urine sodium excretion and urinary excretion of the diuretic follow a sigmoid pattern.[19]

21.7.2 Measuring Glomerular Filtration Rate and Renal Plasma Flow

Another important aspect of diuretic pharmacodynamics is the potential effect on the glomerular filtration rate. Effects on renal function are important in drug development,[23] and for diuretics there are two important aspects in this regard. First, these drugs are often used in medical conditions characterized by a reduction in the glomerular filtration rate,[24] such as congestive heart failure, liver cirrhosis, and kidney diseases, so a further impairment in glomerular filtration rate must be seriously considered in the safe use of those drugs that may adversely impact upon renal function. Second, as these drugs are commonly used in these conditions, it is important to gain an understanding of how impairment of the glomerular filtration rate by the underlying disease process may impact upon the efficacy of the drug.[25] Several techniques are widely used for the measurement of the glomerular filtration rate and renal plasma flow. Measurement of serum creatinine levels along with urinary creatinine excretion rates are used clinically to estimate glomerular filtration rate through calculation of creatinine clearance, although this results in an overestimation and is more complex in the setting of chronic kidney disease.[26] Measuring the clearance of inulin has been widely used to accurately assess glomerular filtration and is described in detail elsewhere.[27–31] As part of the traditional protocol, a constant intravenous infusion of inulin must be administered, although some investigators have effectively carried out glomerular filtration determinations using bolus administration.[32] Clearance of [^{125}I]iothalamate has also been used for the determination of glomerular filtration rate, and comparisons have been made between the iothalamate, inulin, and other methodologies.[33] Recently, a method for the measurement of iothalamate has been described that utilizes liquid chromatography rather than radioisotopic methods.[34,35] Other methodologies are also currently under development.[36]

21.7.3 Segmental Tubular Function: Nephron Sites of Action

While animal studies may determine the precise site of action of a diuretic, it is helpful to make a determination of where the diuretic is acting in humans as well. Diuretics are typically classified by their site of action: (1) the proximal tubule, (2) the thick ascending limb of the loop of Henle, (3) the distal convoluted tubule, and (4) the cortical collecting tubule.[22] For a new diuretic, animal studies can directly demonstrate a site of action of the diuretic, while in humans, inferences can be made in phase I and phase II clinical trials regarding the site of action in the nephron based on the impact of some well-described maneuvers on water and solute handling as outlined below.

21.7.3.1 Proximal Tubule

The carbonic anhydrase inhibitors serve as a classical example of proximal tubule-acting diuretics. Acetazolamide inhibits carbonic anhydrase in the proximal tubule, thereby increasing urinary bicarbonate excretion.[37] Potassium excretion is also increased. These drugs are regarded as weak diuretics as the increase in sodium excretion is small. A decrease in serum bicarbonate levels as well as alkalinization of the urine is seen with these agents.[22] Lithium carbonate has been used for a number of years as a means of identifying the impact of various agents on proximal tubular function. A recent example of using fractional excretion of lithium as a marker of proximal tubular function is provided by Shirley et al.[38]

21.7.3.2 Thick Ascending Limb of the Loop of Henle

Furosemide and other loop diuretics serve as examples of agents that act at the thick ascending limb of the loop of Henle and have great clinical utility.[19,21,39] Inhibition of the Na–K–2Cl cotransporter results in a natriuresis, and drugs in this category have the greatest clinical efficacy of all the classes of diuretics. An effect on the thick ascending limb of the loop of Henle is suggested by the finding of a decrease in C_{H2O} and an increase in osmolar clearance.[22] This helps differentiate such agents from osmotic diuretics (discussed below), in which both C_{H2O} and solute clearance are increased.[40] A common consequence of administration of loop diuretics is enhanced urinary potassium excretion, which often requires supplementation. This appears, in part, to be a consequence of increased delivery of sodium chloride and water to the distal tubule, facilitating potassium secretion by increasing electrical and concentration gradients for potassium secretion, and by increased aldosterone levels due to the volume depletion with activation of the renin–angiotensin system.[41]

21.7.3.3   *Distal Convoluted Tubule*

Thiazide diuretics are examples of agents that act at the distal tubule although they have some effect on carbonic anhydrase as well. Diuretics acting on this site acutely increase excretion of sodium, chloride, potassium, bicarbonate, uric acid, and phosphate; however, chronically, these drugs are well known to potentially elevate uric acid and bicarbonate levels and can result in calcium retention. Inducing a water diuresis can help differentiate a drug acting at the loop of Henle vs. the distal tubule because an agent acting at the distal tubule under these conditions would be expected to decrease C_{H2O}. Inducing an antidiuresis, which will be discussed below, does significantly affect the reabsorption of solute-free water (TC_{H2O}) in the case of distal-tubule-acting agents, whereas agents that act on the loop of Henle will decrease TC_{H2O} under antidiuresis conditions.[22] Loss of medullary hypertonicity as a result of loop diuretic therapy in contrast to sparing of the medulla by distal-tubule-acting agents may contribute to this difference.

21.7.3.4   *Cortical Collecting Tubule*

Amiloride, triamterene, and spironolactone act at the level of the cortical collecting tubule. In contrast to loop diuretics and diuretics acting at the level of the distal convoluted tubule, these agents have a potassium-sparing effect as this site is responsible for the majority of potassium secretion and serves as the site where aldosterone is active. The hypokalemia induced by loop diuretics and thiazide diuretics is due in part to the delivery of sodium chloride and water to this site which facilitates potassium secretion. One mechanism, for example, is that sodium reabsorption at this site creates an electronegative charge on the luminal surface of the renal tubular epithelial cells given the relative impermeability of chloride. The negative charge enhances potassium secretion but amiloride, which blocks sodium channels here, decreases sodium reabsorption at this site, thus diminishing the electrochemical gradient for potassium secretion.[22] Spironolactone is an aldosterone antagonist that also has a potassium-sparing effect given the importance of aldosterone in sodium reabsorption and potassium secretion at this site. The potassium-sparing effect of these drugs makes them especially useful in combination with potassium-wasting agents. Other effects include a decrease in urinary acidification and a decrease in calcium excretion.[42]

21.7.3.5   *Osmotic Diuretics*

Some diuretic agents such as mannitol act by causing an osmotic diuresis. They are mentioned here for completion, although no anticipated tubular segmental issues should have to be addressed in a phase I or phase II clinical trial of a new osmotic diuretic. They act not by a specific effect on a transporter but by impairing water reabsorption from the tubular lumen and by increasing renal blood flow with a reduction in the hypertonicity of the renal medulla. The latter will decrease water reabsorption by further decreasing the osmotic gradient between the tubular lumen and the interstitium. Urinary excretion of sodium, potassium, chloride, bicarbonate, calcium, and magnesium increase.[22] Osmotic diuretics can cause volume contraction and hypernatremia secondary to urinary water losses.

21.7.4 Issues Regarding Diuretic Potency

Several issues must be considered when assessing diuretic potency. First, comparisons should be made only between diuretics that have the same known site of action;[43] therefore, the potency of a loop diuretic cannot be directly compared to that of a thiazide, for example. Second, clinical variables may confound the analysis.[44,45] For example, patients studied should all have a comparable volume status when the diuretic is given. Failure to take this into account may result in differences in diuretic response, with a volume-contracted individual experiencing less natriuresis than a volume-replete individual. Failure to replace urinary water and sodium losses during the study will likewise impact on the subsequent response to the diuretic. Third, the duration of action of the drug and compensatory responses are important.[19,45,46] A short-acting loop diuretic can pose a problem in assessing natriuresis given that, when the drug effect is gone, avid sodium absorption can occur such that a collection over a 24-hour period might lead to an underestimation of the natriuretic effect of the drug. This can be addressed by careful determination of appropriate urine collection times.

21.8 PROTOCOLS FOR DIURETIC EVALUATION

Diuretics require the same phase I and phase II testing that all drugs proposed for human usage must undergo. Phase I studies are done with small numbers of individuals and are intended to determine safe, tolerated doses. If no adverse effects occur after an initial dose, progressively higher doses are given up until a defined endpoint (natriuresis) is reached or toxicity develops. Drug pharmacokinetics may be assessed during this time, as well. If phase I studies indicate an acceptable level of safety, then phase II studies can be carried out. In addition to continued monitoring for adverse effects, these studies for diuretics should define optimal dose–response ranges for the drugs and a determination of the nephron segment on which they are active. More extensive data can be obtained in phase III trials based on the preliminary evidence provided in phase II trials. It is important at this time to identify any adverse effects of the drug that may have escaped detection in phase I or II studies. Additional information regarding the optimal use of the drug in different settings (for example, in different subpopulations of patients), as well as risks and adverse effects, is obtained during phase IV trials (postmarketing studies).

21.9 SEGMENTAL NEPHRON FUNCTION STUDIES

Detailed animal studies may reveal a precise segment of the nephron where the diuretic being tested is active. Given that such studies cannot be carried out in humans, other methods must be utilized in order to confirm the animal findings. Much information can be gained from some simple interventions designed to evaluate urinary excretion of water and electrolytes under conditions of water loading and dehydration as described thoroughly by McMurray and McEwen.[31] As an additional example, 72 hours before the start of the study, participants can be given a study diet (prepared by the general clinical research center where the study is being carried out) that consists of 200 mEq sodium, 1 g calcium, 2.4 to 3.8 g potassium (depending on the total caloric requirement), and 80 g protein daily.[35] Alcohol and caffeinated beverages should be avoided for at least 36 hours before the study, given their potential effects on urinary water and electrolyte handling.[38] Patients should fast beginning at midnight before the morning of the beginning of the study.[31] During the study, activity should be limited, with patients standing to void and otherwise remaining seated or lying down. Smoking is known to have renal effects, so it must be avoided as well.[47]

Several protocols of how to accomplish water loading or maximal hydration are available.[27,28,31,38] In one example, described by Miller et al.,[28] subjects voided at 8:00 a.m. and then ingested 800 mL of water over a 45-minute period. Each hour they drank an additional 200 mL. Intravenous lines were placed for blood sampling and for infusion of inulin and PAH for calculation of glomerular filtration rate and renal plasma flow. As described by McMurray and McEwen,[31] water loading can be accomplished by having subjects drink 20 mL/kg water over 20 minutes, followed by collection of urine samples at 15- to 20-minute intervals. Subjects then drink volumes of water to match their urine output plus an additional 1 mL/min to account for insensible losses. When a urine flow rate of 10 mL/min is achieved, urine osmolality is determined. Results of less than 80 mOsm/kg are considered to be consistent with adequate water loading and suppression of ADH such that the drug can then be given.[31] The volume of each voided urine is measured, and samples are saved for electrolyte and other analysis. Blood should be taken from the venous blood sampling catheter at the midpoint of each urine collection period.

The other maneuver carried out in segmental nephron function studies is the dehydration protocol.[31] At the beginning of the study, subjects can be given intravenous arginine vasopressin at a rate of 0.5 mU/kg/min along with hypertonic saline (3% sodium chloride). The 3% sodium chloride solution is given at a rate to achieve a urine volume of at least 4 mL/min. Given the lower urine volumes, it is suggested that the urine collection time be extended to at least 30 minutes. For both water diuresis and dehydration protocols, the glomerular filtration rate is determined using inulin or iothalamate, as described elsewhere,[27,30,31] and PAH is used to measure renal blood flow. Sodium, potassium, chloride, calcium, phosphate, magnesium, urate, and osmolality should be measured in blood and urine.[31]

21.10 INVESTIGATION OF POSSIBLE ADVERSE EFFECTS

Adverse effects must be determined when studying drugs, and diuretics are no exception. Several fluid, electrolyte, and acid–base disorders can develop during diuretic therapy. These disorders are unlikely to be found on single-dose studies; however, many of these complications will be seen during chronic diuretic use, especially when an appropriate active dose has been selected. These adverse effects could be a result of direct action of the diuretic agent on urinary fluid and electrolyte loss (e.g., hypokalemia) or secondary to the compensatory hemodynamic changes induced by these drugs (e.g., hyperuricemia). Therapy with loop or thiazide-type diuretics can commonly be associated with volume depletion, pre-renal azotemia, hypokalemia, hyponatremia (mainly thiazides), hypomagnesemia, hypocalcemia (mainly loop diuretics), hypercalcemia (mainly thiazides), and metabolic alkalosis. Potassium-sparing diuretics can induce hyperkalemia and metabolic acidosis. The hypokalemic potential of the study drug can be estimated from potency studies. A comparison of natriuretic vs. kaliuretic effect for the study drug with an established diuretic from the same class can give some estimation of the hypokalemic potency of the new drug.[48] Chronic use of thiazide-type diuretics and, less commonly, loop diuretics can also predispose to several metabolic disorders, including glucose intolerance, hyperlipidemia, and hyperuricemia. Hence, in addition to routine blood glucose measurement, an oral glucose tolerance test and lipid profile should be performed at baseline and after chronic dosing to evaluate the potential metabolic effects seen while studying a new diuretic. Uric acid excretion may be increased acutely by diuretic therapy; however, with chronic dosing most will decrease uric acid clearance. Assessment of urate handling by the body is complicated and is discussed in detail by Roberts and Daneshmend[49] and Mejia and Steele.[50] Hypersensitivity reactions secondary to the diuretic use can present with skin rash or, rarely, acute interstitial nephritis and acute renal failure. Ototoxicity with permanent deafness can be seen with high-dose and rapid infusion of loop diuretics in patients with renal failure.[51] High-tone audiometry should be considered when evaluating new loop diuretics. Endocrine side effects of potassium-sparing diuretic spironolactone, which results from nonselective binding to androgen and progesterone receptors, include gynecomastia, breast pain, menstrual irregularities, impotence, and decreased libido. Eplerenone, a more selective aldosterone antagonist has been shown to have a lower incidence of these side effects as compared to spironolactone.[6] Several adverse effects may not be seen until after a few months or years of new drug therapy; hence, careful evaluation of patients during the study period is recommended.

REFERENCES

1. Psaty, B.M. et al., Health outcomes associated with antihypertensive therapies used as first-line agents, *JAMA*, 277, 739, 1997.
2. The ALLHAT Officers and Coordinators for the ALLHAT Collaborative Research Group, Major outcomes in high-risk hypertensive patients randomized to angiotensin-converting enzyme inhibitor or calcium channel blocker vs. diuretic, *JAMA*, 288, 2981, 2002.
3. The Seventh Report of the Joint National Committee on Prevention, Detection, Evaluation, and Treatment of High Blood Pressure, The JNC 7 Report, *JAMA*, 289, 2560, 2003.
4. Psaty, B.M. et al., Health outcomes associated with various antihypertensive therapies used as first-line agents: a network analysis, *JAMA*, 289, 2534, 2003.
5. Pitt, B. et al., The effect of spironolactone on morbidity and mortality in patients with severe heart failure, *N. Engl. J. Med.*, 341, 709, 1999.
6. Pitt, B. et al., Eplerenone, a selective aldosterone blocker, in patients with left ventricular dysfunction after myocardial infarction, *N. Engl. J. Med.*, 348, 1309, 2003.
7. Smith, H., *Principles of Renal Physiology*, Oxford University Press, New York, 1956.
8. Levinsky, N.G. and Levy, M., Clearance techniques, in *Handbook of Physiology: Renal Physiology*, Orloff, J., Berliner, R.W., and Geiger, S.R., Eds., American Physiologic Society, Washington D.C., 1973, p. 103.
9. Maack, T., Renal clearance and isolated kidney perfusion techniques, *Kidney Int.*, 30, 142, 1986.
10. Ellison, D.H., Edema and the clinical use of diuretics, in *Primer on Kidney Diseases*, 3rd ed., Greenberg, A., Ed., Academic Press, San Diego, 2001, p. 116.
11. Bilezikian, J.P., Management of acute hypercalcemia, *N. Engl. J. Med.*, 326, 1196, 1992.
12. Dikshit, K. et al., Renal and extrarenal hemodynamic effects of furosemide in congestive heart failure after acute myocardial infarction, *N. Engl. J. Med.*, 288, 1087, 1973.
13. Pickkers, P. et al., Direct vascular effects of furosemide in humans, *Circulation*, 96, 1847, 1997.
14. Francis, G.S. et al., Acute vasoconstrictor response to intravenous furosemide in patients with chronic congestive heart failure: activation of the neurohumoral axis, *Ann. Intern. Med.*, 103, 1, 1985.
15. Daskalopoulos, G. et al., Immediate effects of furosemide on renal hemodynamics in chronic liver disease with ascites, *Gastroenterology*, 92, 1859, 1987.
16. Pickkers, P. et al., Thiazide-induced vasodilation in humans is mediated by potassium channel activation, *Hypertension*, 32, 1071, 1998.
17. Veld, A.J., and Schalekamp, M.A., Hemodynamic changes during long-term thiazide treatment of essential hypertension in responders and nonresponders, *Clin. Pharmacol. Ther.*, 27, 328, 1980.
18. Murray, M.D. et al., Open-label randomized trial of torsemide compared with furosemide therapy for patients with heart failure, *Am. J. Med.*, 111, 513, 2001.
19. Brater, D.C., Diuretic therapy, *N. Engl. J. Med.*, 339, 387, 1998.
20. Brater, D.C., Pharmacology of diuretics, *Am. J. Med. Sci.*, 319, 38, 2000.
21. Shankar, S.S. and Brater, D.C., Loop diuretics: from the Na–K–2Cl transporter to clinical use, *Am. J. Physiol.*, 284, F11, 2003.
22. Ellison, D.H., Okusa, M.D., and Schrier, R.W., Mechanisms of diuretic action, in *Renal and Electrolyte Disorders*, 6th ed., Schrier, R.W., Ed., Lippincott Williams & Wilkins, Philadelphia, 2003.
23. Brater, D.C., Measurement of renal function during drug development, *Br. J. Clin. Pharmacol.*, 54, 87, 2002.
24. McMurray, J. and Struthers, A.D., Role of neuroendocrine abnormalities in the enhanced sodium and water retention of chronic heart failure, *Pharmacol. Toxicol.*, 61, 209, 1987.
25. Wilcox, C.S., New insights into diuretic use in patients with chronic renal disease, *J. Am. Soc. Nephrol.*, 13, 798, 2002.

26. Levey, A.S. and Nephrology Forum, Measurement of renal function in chronic renal disease, *Kidney Int.*, 38, 167, 1990.

27. Levinsky, N.G. and Lieberthal, W., Clearance techniques, in *Handbook of Physiology*, Sec. 8, Vol. 1, Windhager, E.E., Ed., Oxford University Press, Oxford, 1992, p. 226.

28. Miller, J.A., Thai, K., and Scholey, J.W., Angiotensin II type 1 receptor gene polymorphism and the response to hyperglycemia in early type 1 diabetes, *Diabetes*, 49, 1585, 2000.

29. Uderman, H. et al., Omapatrilat: neurohormonal and pharmacodynamic profile when administered with furosemide, *J. Clin. Pharmacol.*, 41, 1291, 2001.

30. Lafayette, R.A., Perrone, R.D., and Levey, A.S., Laboratory evaluation of renal function, in *Renal and Electrolyte Disorders*, 6th ed., Schrier, R.W., Ed., Lippincott Williams & Wilkins, Philadelphia, 2003.

31. McMurray, J. and McEwen, J., Diuretics, in *Handbook of Phase I/II Clinical Drug Trials*, O'Grady, J. and Joubert, P.H., Eds., CRC Press, Boca Raton, FL, 1997, p. 415.

32. Orlando, R. et al., Determination of inulin clearance by bolus intravenous injection in healthy subjects and ascitic patients: equivalence of systemic and renal clearances as glomerular filtration markers, *Br. J. Pharmacol.*, 46, 605, 1998.

33. Perrone, R.D. et al., Utility of radioisotopic filtration markers in chronic renal insufficiency: simultaneous comparison of ^{125}I-iothalamate, ^{169}Yb-DTPA, ^{99m}Tc-DTPA, and inulin, *Am. J. Kidney Dis.*, 26, 224, 1990.

34. Agarwal, R., Vasavada, N., and Chase, S.D., Liquid chromatography for iothalamate in biological samples, *J. Chromatogr. B. Analyt. Technol. Biomed. Life. Sci.*, 785, 345, 2003.

35. Vasavada, N., Saha, C., and Agarwal, R., A double-blind randomized crossover trial of two loop diuretics in chronic kidney disease, *Kidney Int.*, 64, 632, 2003.

36. Gaspari, F., Perico, N., and Remuzzi, G., Application of newer clearance techniques for the determination of glomerular filtration rate, *Curr. Opin. Nephrol. Hypertens.*, 7, 675, 1998.

37. Dubose, T.D. and Lucci, M.S., Effect of carbonic anhydrase inhibition on superficial and deep nephron bicarbonate reabsorption in the rat, *J. Clin. Invest.*, 71, 55, 1983.

38. Shirley, D.G., Walter, S.J., and Noormohamed, F.H., Natriuretic effect of caffeine: assessment of segmental sodium reabsorption in humans, *Clin. Sci.*, 103, 461, 2002.

39. Lupinacci, L. and Puschett, J.B., An examination of the site and mechanism of action of torasemide in man, *J. Clin. Pharmacol.*, 28, 441, 1988

40. Suki, W.N. and Eknoyan, G., Physiology of diuretic action, in *The Kidney: Physiology and Pathophysiology*, Seldin, D.W. and Giebisch, G., Eds., Raven Press, New York, 1992.

41. Wilcox, C.S. et al., Factors affecting potassium balance during frusemide administration, *Clin. Sci.*, 67, 195, 1984.

42. Costanzo, L.S. and Weiner, I.M., Relationship between clearances of Ca and Na: effect of distal diuretics and PTH, *Am. J. Physiol.*, 230, 67, 1976.

43. Weiner, I.M., General pharmacological aspects of diuretics, in *Diuretics: Physiology, Pharmacology and Clinical Use*, Dirks, J.H. and Sutton, R.A.L., Eds., W.B. Saunders, Philadelphia, 1986, p. 183.

44. Wilcox, C.S., Roles of renin angiotensin aldosterone and autonomic nervous system in the response to diuretic drugs in man, in *Diuretics II: Chemistry, Pharmacology and Clinical Applications*, Puschett, J.B. and Greenberg, A., Eds., Elsevier, Amsterdam, 1987, p. 503.

45. McMurray, J. and Struthers, A.D., Frusemide pretreatment blunts the inhibition of renal tubular sodium reabsorption by ANF in man, *Eur. J. Clin. Pharmacol.*, 35, 333, 1988.

46. Ferguson, J.A. et al., Role of duration of diuretic effect in preventing sodium retention, *Clin. Pharmacol. Ther.*, 62, 203, 1997.

47. Halimi, J.M. and Mimran, A., Renal effects of smoking, *Nephrol. Dial. Transplant.*, 15, 938, 2000.

48. Puschett, J.B. and Rastegar, A., Comparative study of the effects of metolazone and other diuretics on potassium excretion, *Clin. Pharmacol. Ther.*, 15, 398, 1974.

49. Roberts, C.J. and Daneshmend, T.K., Assessment of natriuretic drugs, *Br. J. Clin. Pharmacol.*, 12, 465, 1981.

50. Mejia, G. and Steele, T.H., Uricosuric diuretics, in *Diuretics: Physiology, Pharmacology and Clinical Use*, Dirks, J.H. and Sutton, R.A.L., Eds., W.B. Saunders, Philadelphia, 1986, p. 135.

51. Rudy, D.W. et al., Loop diuretics for chronic renal insufficiency: a continuous infusion is more efficacious than bolus therapy, *Ann. Intern. Med.*, 115, 360, 1991.

CHAPTER 22

Medical Therapy of Benign Prostatic Hyperplasia

Benjamin R. Lee

CONTENTS

22.1 INTRODUCTION

Benign prostatic hyperplasia (BPH) is a condition in men that increases in prevalence and incidence as a direct correlation with age. Between the ages of 50 and 60, 50% of men are afflicted with this disease, and as many as 90% of men older than 80 years of age are affected.[1] Urinary frequency, urgency, nocturia (waking at night to void), decrease in force of urinary stream, post-void dribbling, intermittency, and hesitancy are some of the clinical manifestations. BPH is caused by cell proliferation in the transition zone of the prostate and increased tone in the smooth muscle of the prostate and bladder neck which can contribute to urethral obstruction.[2] Evidence also implicates the requirement of testicular androgens, the primary one being dihydrotestosterone, together with an aging prostate for growth and enlargement. The past decade has witnessed a dramatic change in the treatment paradigm, with a shift away from primary surgical management (transurethral resection of the prostate, or TURP) toward primary medical therapy with pharmacologic agents. The goal of this chapter is to discuss the contemporary medical treatment of BPH.

Table 22.1 Alpha-Adrenergic Blockers for Benign Prostatic Hyperplasia

Class	Drug Names	Mechanism of Action	Adverse Reactions
Alpha$_1$ blocker	Prazosin (Minipress®), terazosin (Hytrin®), doxazosin (Cardura®)	Selective inhibition of alpha$_1$ receptors	Dizziness, orthostatic hypotension, headache, drowsiness, lack of energy, weakness, palpitations, nausea, asthenia, nasal congestion
Alpha$_{1a}$ blocker	Tamsulosin (Flomax®)	Super-selective inhibition of alpha$_{1a}$ receptors	Decreased clearance with cimetidine, headache, dizziness, somnolence, asthenia, back pain
Five alpha reductase inhibitors	Finasteride (Proscar®), dutasteride (Avadart®)	Inhibition of both type I and type II 5-alpha reductase, blocking conversion of testosterone to dihydrotestosterone	CYP3A4 inhibitors: increased blood levels and impotence, decreased libido

22.2 ALPHA BLOCKERS

Histologically, the prostate is composed of smooth muscle, epithelium, and collagen. The disease is characterized by a gradual increase in both glandular and fibromuscular tissue in the periurethral and transition zones of the prostate. Stimulation of adrenergic receptors located within the smooth muscle element of the prostate by norepinephrine (an alpha$_1$ and alpha$_2$ agonist) and phenylephrine (an alpha$_1$ agonist) has produced an increase in muscle tone in *in vitro* prostate strip experiments.[3] This contraction of smooth muscle was inhibited by the addition of specific alpha$_1$ antagonists such as prazosin but was not suppressed by alpha$_2$-specific antagonists.[4] These findings suggest that the alpha-adrenoreceptors on prostate smooth muscle cells that mediate contraction are predominantly alpha$_1$-adrenoreceptors. Alpha$_1$ receptors for smooth muscle have been found to localize to the bladder neck and prostate, leading to the clinical development of alpha$_1$ antagonists to block these receptors with the ultimate goal of improved urinary voiding, flow rate, and quality of life. Table 22.1 summarizes the mechanism of action, adverse effects, and types of alpha$_1$ blockers.

22.3 PRAZOSIN

Studies have focused on developing agents for alpha$_1$-specific adrenoceptor blockers. Prazosin was the first alpha$_1$-specific adrenoceptor blocker studied for this application. Although initially introduced as an antihypertensive agent, it was found to increase bladder capacity and decrease the magnitude of hyperreflexic detrusor contractions in patients with detrusor–sphincter dyssynergia of neurogenic etiology.[5] Ultimately, selective alpha$_1$ blockers such as doxazosin, terazosin, and tamsulosin block alpha$_1$-adrenoreceptors in the prostate and bladder neck, inhibiting sympathetic stimulation of prostatic smooth muscle, reducing prostatic tone, and relieving urinary obstruction symptoms. These agents improve obstructive and irritative BPH symptoms and improve urinary flow, usually within 1 to 2 weeks of treatment.[6] Side effects from prazosin include first-dose syncope, postural hypotension, dizziness, and palpitations; therefore, dosing for this medication begins at 1 mg twice a day and is then increased according to the relief of symptoms to 5 mg twice a day.

22.4 TERAZOSIN

The mechanism by which terazosin and doxazosin suppress prostatic growth has recently been investigated by Kyprianou,[7] who reported that both doxazosin and terazosin induce apoptosis in prostate cancer cells both *in vitro* and *in vivo*. The apoptotic effect of doxazosin and terazosin is mediated by a mechanism independent of the alpha$_1$-adrenoceptor blockade, potentially under the direction of the quinazoline nucleus, since the nonquinazoline alpha$_1$-adrenoceptor antagonist tamsulosin does not elicit an apoptotic response. Furthermore, recent experimental evidence points to deregulation of signal transduction pathways involving transforming growth factor beta (TGF-beta) and disruption of cell attachment to the extracellular matrix as potential mechanisms underlying the apoptotic action of quinazoline-based alpha$_1$-adrenoceptor antagonists against prostate cells. Terazosin may also induce first-dose syncope, anaphylaxis, priapism, dizziness, and headache, and minor side effects may include asthenia, nasal congestion, somnolence, and peripheral edema; therefore, a test dose of 1 mg taken at night should be taken initially and gradually increased, according to the relief of symptoms, every 2 weeks to a maximum dose of 20 mg/day. Due to the clinical response, it may take 4 to 6 weeks to determine the effective dose.

22.5 DOXAZOSIN

Doxazosin is a selective inhibitor of the alpha$_1$ subtype of alpha-adrenergic receptors. Recently, a prospective, randomized, double-blind trial in 90 European study centers was conducted. This 52-week trial enrolled men 50 to 80 years old who had BPH; a total International Prostate Screening Score (IPSS) of 12 or greater, indicating moderate symptoms; a flow rate of 5 mL/sec or greater, but 15 mL/sec or less in a total voided volume of 150 mL or greater; and an enlarged prostate size based on digital rectal exam.[8] Men who received doxazosin showed a mean improvement in urinary flow rate of 8.3 ± 0.4 mL/sec. Maximal urinary flow rate was significantly improved from baseline to endpoint compared with placebo. Interestingly, when given in combination with finasteride, doxazosin was found to be more effective in improving urinary symptoms than finasteride alone or placebo. Doxazosin side effects include dizziness, headache, orthostatic hypotension, fatigue, somnolence, and dry mouth. To avoid first-dose hypotension, medications are started at 1 mg once a day and gradually increased to a maximum dose of 8 mg per day, according to the clinical relief of symptoms.

22.6 TAMSULOSIN

Tamsulosin is an antagonist of alpha$_{1A}$-adrenoceptors in the prostate. Absorption of tamsulosin is 90% complete following oral administration under fasting conditions. In two placebo-controlled, double-blind, 13-week, multicenter studies, 1486 men with signs and symptoms of BPH were enrolled. Patients were randomized to placebo or 0.4 mg or 0.8 mg tamsulosin. Primary efficacy assessments included the American Urological Association International Prostate Screen Score (AUA IPSS) symptom score questionnaire and peak urine flow rate. With 0.4-mg dosing, the AUA symptom scores decreased by 8.3 ± 6.5 from premedication values of 19.8 ± 5.0. Flow rates also improved by 1.75 ± 3.6 mL/sec. One factor that distinguishes tamsulosin from the other alpha blockers is its superselectivity for alpha$_{1A}$-adrenoceptors which has been reported to decrease the side effects of hypotension. Symptomatic hypotension was reported in 0.2% of patients, dizziness in 15%, and vertigo in 0.6%. Other side effects include headache, infection, asthenia, rhinitis, and abnormal ejaculation. Dosing of this medication begins at 0.4 mg by mouth once a day. Because of the superselectivity of alpha$_{1A}$-adrenoceptors, no significant degree of side effects due to hypotension has been observed.

22.7 5-ALPHA REDUCTASE INHIBITORS

Finasteride is a synthetic 4-aza steroid. It is a potent, reversible, type II 5-alpha reductase inhibitor.[9] The application of finasteride for the clinical treatment of symptomatic BPH is targeted at the key role that dihydrotestosterone has in the etiology of the disease. Finasteride is a competitive and specific inhibitor of type II 5-alpha reductase, with which a stable enzyme complex is slowly formed. Finasteride has no affinity for the steroid receptor. In clinical studies, finasteride has been shown to be potent at doses as low as 1.5 mg/day, even though current standard dosing is 5 mg/day. A multiple-dose safety and tolerability study that used 12.5 mg of the drug twice daily demonstrated an 80% decrease of serum dihydrotestosterone, from a baseline of 64 ± 16 ng/dL to 18 ± 17 ng/dL.[10] Daily dosing of finasteride at 5 mg/day for up to 4 years has been shown to reduce the serum dihydrotestosterone concentration by 70%. In patients with BPH treated with finasteride (1 to 100 mg) for 7 to 10 days prior to prostatectomy, an approximately 80% lower dihydrotestosterone content was measured in prostate tissue removed at surgery. Testosterone tissue concentration was increased up to ten times over pretreatment levels, relative to placebo. In terms of metabolism, finasteride is extensively metabolized in the liver, primarily via the cytochrome P-450 enzyme subfamily.

Finasteride was evaluated in the PROSCAR Long-Term Efficacy and Safety Study (PLESS), a double-blind, randomized, placebo-controlled, 4-year multicenter study. 3040 patients between the ages of 45 and 78 with moderate to severe symptoms of BPH and an enlarged prostate on digital rectal exam were randomized in the study. Patients who remained on therapy for 4 years had a mean decrease in symptom score of 3.3 ± 5.8 points compared to 1.3 ± 5.6 points in the placebo group. A statistically significant improvement in symptom scores was evident at 1 year and continued throughout treatment to year 4. In summary, finasteride has been shown to reduce prostate size by 29% and improve peak flow by 1.5 to 2 mL/sec. Data from several studies indicate that finasteride may be more effective than placebo in men with enlarged prostates[11] (greater than 40 cm^3) but may not be effective in men with smaller sized prostates. The use of finasteride has also been investigated as a chemopreventive agent for prostate cancer. A trial completed in 2004 randomized 18,882 men to finasteride or placebo treatment for 7 years. The goal of this study was to compare the prevalence of histologically confirmed prostate cancer. Side effects of this medication include a low incidence of retrograde ejaculation, dizziness, and ischemia. Furthermore, impotence (8%), decreased libido (6%), and decreased volume of ejaculate (3.7%) have been reported.

22.7.1 Effect on Urinary Retention and Need for Surgery

The results of 2- and 4-year studies of men with BPH demonstrate that finasteride decreases the risk of acute urinary retention[12] and surgical procedures on the prostate (namely, transurethral resection). The placebo-control arm had a urinary retention rate of 6.6%, whereas those patients on finasteride demonstrated a statistically significant decrease to 2.8%. Furthermore, compared to a placebo arm of 10.1% for surgical interventions for BPH, the finasteride arm decreased to 4.6%.

22.7.2 Treatment of Refractory Hematuria of Prostatic Origin

Puchner and Miller[13] were the first to describe the use of finasteride on patients with BPH and gross hematuria. A retrospective review was done of 18 patients who had been placed on finasteride (5 mg daily) for the treatment of gross hematuria associated with BPH. Using a grading system, improvement was observed in 11/12 patients with a follow-up of longer than 3 months. This work was corroborated by Delakas,[14] who demonstrated a 77% hematuria recurrence in untreated controls vs. 12% in patients who were on finasteride over a mean of 22 months. Further work has been performed by Pareek et al.[15] on the role of vascular endothelial-derived growth factor (VEGF), which is a potent promoter of angiogenesis. It is believed that VEGF increases endothelial cell permeability, thereby increasing prostatic blood flow. In this study, it was found that the expression of VEGF was reduced by finasteride, which inhibits angiogenesis. Furthermore, with decreased microvessel density in the prostatic suburethral tissue and resultant glandular shrinkage, this drug could help elucidate the pathway of reduced vascular inflow and promote the cessation of prostatic bleeding.

22.8 PROTOCOLS FOR BPH MEDICATION EVALUATION

New medical therapy for BPH requires the same phase I and phase II testing that all drugs proposed for human use must undergo. Phase I studies are done with small numbers of individuals and are intended to determine safe, tolerated doses. If no adverse effects occur after an initial dose, progressively higher doses are given until a defined endpoint (increase in flow rate, decrease in urinary symptoms) is reached or toxicity develops. Drug pharmacokinetics may be assessed during this time, as well. If phase I studies indicate an acceptable level of safety, then phase II studies can be carried out. In addition to continued monitoring for adverse effects, studies for BPH medication should define optimal dose–response ranges for the drug. More extensive data can be obtained in phase III trials based on the preliminary evidence provided in phase II trials. It is important to identify in phase III studies any adverse effects of the drug that may have escaped detection in phase I or phase II trials. Finally, phase IV trials should be performed to verify the safety of the drug postmarketing.

REFERENCES

1. Berry, S.J., Coffey, D.S., Walsh, P.C. et al., The development of human benign prostatic hyperplasia with age, *J. Urol.*, 132, 474–479, 1984.

2. Bartsch, G., Rittmaster, R.S., and Klocker, H., Dihydrotestosterone and the concept of 5-alpha-reductase inhibition in human benign prostatic hyperplasia, *Eur. Urol.*, 37, 367–380, 2000.

3. Lepor, H., Gup, D.I., Bauman, M., and Shapiro, E., Laboratory assessment of terazosin and alpha-1 blockade in prostatic hyperplasia, *Urology*, 32(Suppl.), 21–26, 1988.

4. Hedlund, H., Andersson, K.E., and Ek, A., Effect of prazosin in patients with benign prostatic obstruction, *J. Urol.*, 130, 275–278, 1983.

5. Jensen, D., Uninhibited neurogenic bladder treated with prazosin, *Scan. J. Urol. Nephrol.*, 15, 229–233, 1981.

6. Lepor, H., Williford, W.O., Barry, M.J. et al., for the Veteran Affairs Cooperative Studies Benign Prostatic Hyperplasia Study Group, The efficacy of terazosin, finasteride, or both in benign prostatic hyperplasia, *N. Engl. J. Med.*, 335, 533–539, 1996.

7. Kyprianou, N., Doxazosin and terazosin suppress prostate growth by inducing apoptosis: clinical significance, *J. Urol.*, 169(4), 1520–1525, 2003.

8. Kirby, R.S., Roehrborn, C., Boyle, P. et al., Efficacy and tolerability of doxazosin and finasteride, alone or in combination, in treatment of symptomatic benign prostatic hyperplasia: the prospective European doxazosin and combination therapy (PREDICT) trial, *Urology*, 61, 119–126, 2003.

9. Vermeulen, A., Giagulli, V.A., Schepper, P.D. et al., Hormonal effects of an orally active 4-azasteroid inhibitor or 5-alpha reductase in humans, *Prostate*, 14, 45–53, 1989.

10. Vermeulen, A., Giagulli, V.A., Scheppe, P., Buntinx, A., and Stoner, E., Hormonal effects of an orally active 4-azasteroid inhibitor of 5-alpha reductase in humans, *Prostate*, 14, 45–53, 1989.

11. Lepor, H., Williford, W.O., Barry, M.J. et al., for the Veterans Affairs Cooperative Studies Benign Prostatic Hyperplasia Study Group, The impact of medical therapy on BTH due to symptoms, quality of life, and global outcome and factors predicting response, *J. Urol.*, 160, 1358–1367, 1998.

12. McConnell, J.D., Bruskewitz, R., Walsh, P.C. et al., for the Finasteride Long-Term Efficacy and Safety Study Group, The effect of finasteride on the risk of acute urinary retention and the need for surgical treatment among men with benign prostatic hyperplasia, *N. Engl. J. Med.*, 338, 557–563, 1998.

13. Puchner, P.J. and Miller, M.I., The effects of finasteride on hematuria associated with benign prostatic hyperplasia: a preliminary report, *J. Urol.*, 154(5), 1779–182, 1995.

14. Delakas, D., Lianos, E., Karyotis, I., and Cranidis, A., Finasteride: a long-term follow-up in the treatment of recurrent hematuria associated with benign prostatic hyperplasia, *Urol. Int.*, 67(1), 69–72, 2001.

15. Pareek, G., Shevchuk, M., Armenakas, N.A., Vasjovic, L., Hochberg, D.A., Basillote, J.B., and Fracchia, J.A., The effect of finasteride on the expression of vascular endothelial growth factor and microvessel density: a possible mechanism for decreased prostatic bleeding in treated patients, *J. Urol.*, 169(1), 20–23, 2003.

PART IX

Assessment of Skin Drugs

CHAPTER 23

Drugs for the Treatment of Specific Skin Diseases

Muzlifah A. Haniffa, Anton B. Alexandroff Vrach,
Suzy N. Leech, and Clifford M. Lawrence

CONTENTS

23.1 INTRODUCTION

The skin is the largest organ in the human body. It is also anatomically varied in its structure and function. Both the underlying disease and the inherent site-specific differences influence the manifestations of skin disorders. This chapter begins by briefly outlining general concepts in the development, delivery and application, and efficacy and safety of drugs in skin disorders. This is followed by discussions on the use of existing drugs for the treatment of specific skin diseases. Several new advances in the treatment of skin disorders have been made in recent years. An important area of change has been the use of immunosuppressive agents and targeted immune-based therapies. Topical diclofenac, 5-fluorouracil, imidazoquinolines, and photodynamic therapy are the nonsurgical therapeutic armaments currently available for the treatment of premalignant and malignant skin disorders. In acne, therapy with antimicrobials, retinoids, and hormonal manipulation is currently used. Often, combination therapy is required for effective treatment. Psoriasis and two rare inflammatory dermatoses — pyoderma gangrenosum and toxic epidermal necrolysis — are also discussed, as these conditions illustrate the shift in dermatology treatment strategies toward targeted immune-based therapies. Psoriasis in the past has generally been managed with topical treatment, but more recently immunosuppressives such as methotrexate, cyclosporine, acitretin, and fumaric acid esters have been found to be highly effective. Targeted immune-based therapies such as the use of infliximab, etanercept, and other biologics are also highlighted. Intravenous immunoglobulin therapy is discussed in the treatment of toxic epidermal necrolysis.

23.2 DRUGS AND THE SKIN

The stratum corneum (the topmost layer of the epidermis) is the principal barrier to penetration of drugs into the skin. Drugs for skin application are presented in vehicles (e.g., cream and ointment). The entry of drugs into the skin is determined by the rate of diffusion of a drug from a particular type of vehicle to the surface of the skin, the individual physicochemical characteristic of a drug that allows it to partition between the vehicle and the stratum corneum, and the degree of hydration of the stratum corneum. Hydration improves diffusion of a drug through the skin, and vehicles vary in the extent of their ability to promote hydration. Absorption of a drug is also variable with anatomical site; absorption is higher on the face and scalp and lower where the skin is thicker, such as the palms and soles of the feet. Absorption is further increased in inflamed skin and when occlusion is applied. Following diffusion across the epidermis and dermis, a drug can then enter the microcirculation of the skin and the systemic circulation from thereon.

Topical cutaneous application is therefore ideal in skin disorders to target the drug to its site of action and limit systemic side effects. Topical applications can be lotions, which provide a cooling effect from evaporation; creams (oil-in-water or water-in-oil) for water-soluble drugs in a vehicle that is easy to spread and cosmetically appealing; or ointments, which are greasier and have varying degrees of water solubility but which allow hydration by preventing evaporation and heat loss. Water-based formulations contain preservatives, thus increasing the risk of allergic contact dermatitis. Where systemic effects are required for a drug to achieve its action, possible routes are oral, intravenous, subcutaneous, or transdermal (whereby a drug is released through a rate-controlling membrane into the skin and systemic circulation). Drug absorption through the epidermis can be enhanced by substances added to the preparation (e.g., squalene), liposomal delivery, or physical methods such as iontophoresis. The local duration of activity of a drug can also be enhanced by the administration of a vasoconstrictor — for example, adrenaline given with lidocaine for local anesthesia.

In skin disorders, important issues that should be addressed in drug design and development are the ability of a drug to remain active in its formulation, to remain confined to its site of action with minimal adverse local (irritant or allergic) and systemic effects, and to be clinically effective.

Table 23.1 Premalignant and Malignant Skin Lesions

	Nonmelanoma Skin Cancer	Nonmelanoma Skin Cancer	Melanoma Skin Cancer
Malignant	Squamous cell carcinoma	Basal cell carcinoma	Melanoma
Premalignant	Actinic keratosis; Bowen's disease	—	Lentigo maligna

Preclinical studies using organ culture or skin equivalents in conjunction with animal studies allow pharmacodynamic, pharmacokinetic, and toxicology studies to be performed. Human phase I trials normally follow on from these preclinical studies. In phase IV trials, surveillance for safety and efficacy and comparisons with other drugs are carried out.

Often in skin diseases, efficacy is judged clinically using visual scoring systems such as the Psoriasis Area and Severity Index (PASI) and the Leeds Acne Scale. Quality of life questionnaires, patient satisfaction, and tolerability scores are also important in evaluating a drug, as adherence to therapy is greatly influenced by these factors.

23.3 PREMALIGNANT SKIN LESIONS, MELANOMA, AND NONMELANOMA SKIN CANCER

Skin cancer can be categorized into melanoma and nonmelanoma skin cancer (NMSC). The most common NMSCs are basal cell carcinoma (BCC) and squamous cell carcinoma (SCC). Basal cell carcinoma, the most frequently occurring skin cancer, is found predominantly on the head and neck. It invades local structures but very rarely metastasizes. BCC does not appear to have a premalignant form. Squamous cell carcinoma, by contrast, has the potential to metastasize via the lymphatics and vascular system and is thus potentially life threatening. SCC has two types of premalignant forms: actinic keratosis (AK) and Bowen's disease. AKs, which occur on sun-exposed sites of 20 to 50% of white-skinned individuals over the age of 50, are made up of areas of dysplastic epidermis.[1] When the dysplasia involves the full thickness of the epidermis, the lesion is termed Bowen's disease, or squamous carcinoma *in situ*.

Fifty percent of melanomas arise from preexisting moles, and the remainder occur on normal skin. Melanoma incidence has doubled between 1971 and 1990.[1] Although melanomas account for approximately 10% of all skin cancers, it is the cause of 80% of the deaths from skin cancers.[1] Lentigo maligna (LM) is an *in situ* form of malignant melanoma. It has been estimated that the annual risk of an LM converting to malignant melanoma is a 2 to 5%.[1] LM presents as a flat brown mark in elderly patients at chronic sun-exposed sites.

The cause of these premalignant lesions, melanoma, and NMSC is multifactorial. Ultraviolet (UV) exposure leading to DNA damage is one of the strongest etiological factors for the pathogenesis of AKs, Bowen's disease, melanoma, and NMSC. UV-induced mutation of the p53 gene is a common finding in sun-damaged skin, and this may provide the oncogenic potential in a cell. The p53 mutation is present in 53% of AKs and in 69 to 90% of SCCs.[2,3] It has been suggested that 60 to 99% of all SCCs arise from AKs.[4] Other risk factors include genetic predisposition, immunosuppression, human papilloma virus infection, arsenic exposure, chronic injury, and x-irradiation damage to the skin. Table 23.1 summarizes the various premalignant and malignant skin lesions.

Both BCCs and SCCs are generally treated by surgical excision or radiotherapy. These lesions and premalignant lesions (AKs and Bowen's disease) are also treated by curettage and cryotherapy. Other treatment options include topical application of diclofenac, or 5-fluorouracil, and, more recently, the use of imidazoquinolines and photodynamic therapy. Malignant melanoma (MM) is treated by surgical excision with a 1- to 2-cm margin and LM with a 0.5-cm margin.[5] LM excision is complicated by the frequent occurrences of subclinical or amelanotic spread, the fact that more lesions are found on the face, and the frail conditions of the mostly elderly patients.

Recent developments with photodynamic therapy and topically applied immunomodulatory agents have shown promising results in the treatment of non-melanoma and melanoma skin cancer. This section will focus on the more recent agents that have become available including topical diclofenac, 5-fluorouracil, imidazoquinolines, and photodynamic therapy.

23.3.1 Topical Diclofenac

Diclofenac is a nonsteroidal antiinflammatory drug that inhibits cyclooxygenase enzymes and hence the downstream products of arachidonic acid metabolism, which are believed to have a role in inhibiting apoptosis and promoting carcinogenesis. Three studies have assessed topical diclofenac used twice daily for the treatment of AKs. Two placebo-controlled trials showed benefit with topical diclofenac 3% after treatment for 60 and 120 days.[6,7] Another study of 130 patients showed no benefit when topical diclofenac 3% was used twice daily for 180 days.[8] Topical diclofenac has no role in the treatment of Bowen's disease or malignant skin lesions. The most commonly reported side effects with this treatment include pruritus, xerosis, erythema, and skin reaction at the application site.

23.3.2 Topical 5-Fluorouracil

5-Fluorouracil (5-FU), acts as a nucleoside analog, inhibiting intracellular DNA synthesis. It selectively causes cell death in the precancerous lesions but not in normal skin. It is unclear if this is the result of enhanced vulnerability of the rapidly dividing cell population or different absorption levels of the drug between normal and precancerous cells.[9–11] It is the mainstay of treatment of AKs and is also used in the treatment of Bowen's disease and superficial basal cell carcinomas. Studies on its use in AKs have shown no difference in efficacy between the 5%, 1%, and 0.5% strengths of topical 5-FU preparations, although reduced adverse effects were noted with the low dose preparation.[12–15] The common side effects of treatment are mild to moderate facial erythema, dryness, and burning. Interestingly, one case of inflammatory colitis, neutropenia, and thrombocytopenia has been reported following topical 5-FU 5% application for basal cell carcinoma of the scalp in a patient with the very rare condition of dihydropyrimidine dehydrogenase (DPD) deficiency, which is the critical enzyme for 5-FU breakdown.[16]

23.3.3 Topical Imidazoquinolines

Imiquimod (1-[2-methylpropyl]-1H-imidazo[4,5-c]quinolin-4 amine) and its homolog resiquimod (4-amino-α, α-dimethyl-2-ethoxymethyl-1H-imidazo[4,5-c]-quinoline-1-ethanol) are immune-response modifiers. They act through the induction of innate and cell-mediated pathways by activating specific Toll-like receptors (TLRs) on dendritic cells. This leads to the synthesis and release of cytokines such as interferon-α (IFN-α), tumor necrosis factor α (TNF-α), and interleukin-12 (IL-12).[17] The locally generated cytokine milieu leads to a Th1-dominant response and cell-mediated immunity. In 1997, the U.S. Food and Drug Administration (FDA) approved imiquimod as a 5% cream for the treatment of genital and perianal warts caused by the human papilloma virus (HPV). Imiquimod has also been shown to exhibit antitumor effects in addition to its antiviral actions.[18]

Imiquimod has been used in the treatment of actinic keratosis. In a double-blind study, imiquimod was compared to a vehicle cream in different dosing groups to three target AKs for up to 16 weeks in 41 patients. The imiquimod group experienced clinical resolution of all target lesions.[17] In another study of 36 patients with AKs, resolution was observed in >80% of patients following 3 times/week application for 12 weeks or until resolution.[17] FDA approval for the use of imiquimod for the treatment of AKs on the face and scalp in immunocompetent adults was recently obtained.

Daily treatment for 16 weeks of biopsy-proven plaques of Bowen's disease with imiquimod in 16 patients in a phase II, open-label study showed no residual disease in 6-week post-treatment biopsies in 14/15 patients (six patients had to stop treatment early due to local skin inflammation during the study).[19] Imiquimod has been used successfully in combination with 5-FU for Bowen's disease following renal transplantation.[20] Case reports have also shown successful outcomes with imiquimod for the treatment of stucco keratosis[21] and porokeratosis of Mibelli.[22]

Several clinical trials and case reports regarding the effectiveness of imiquimod in treating superficial or nodular basal cell carcinomas on low-risk sites are available.[17,23–25] For superficial BCCs, cure rates range from 69.7 to 100%.[23,26] The cure rates for nodular BCCs are not as impressive.[25,27] No 5-year follow-up data are available at present to compare imiquimod with Mohs micrographic surgical treatment, which is associated with a 1 to 5% 5-year recurrence rate.[1]

The most effective imiquimod treatment regimen has yet to be established. Topical imiquimod produces a very brisk inflammatory reaction at the application site, and, unlike 5-FU, this occurs in normal and abnormal skin. When imiquimod was used in a patient with Gorlin's syndrome or nevoid basal cell carcinoma syndrome (NBCCS) and two patients with xeroderma pigmentosum (XP), it was found to reduce the rate of new tumor formation.[28–30] The results of a phase III trial comparing imiquimod to vehicle in patients with superficial BCCs and surgery for the treatment of nodular and superficial BCCs are currently awaited. The literature on imiquimod for AKs, BCCs, and Bowen's disease consists primarily of small studies and case reports. Additional studies over longer periods of time, with particular attention to recurrence rates and optimal dosing, are required.

The successful use of imiquimod in the management of LM has been reported, especially for patients for whom surgery is not a viable option.[31–33] A recent published study examined 12 patients with histologically proven LM who were treated with imiquimod three times a week for 6 weeks on the clinically affected areas and a 2-cm margin of normal surrounding skin. Histological resolution of the affected area was demonstrated one week after the end of treatment.[34] No clinical evidence indicated a recurrence at a median of 6 months follow-up.[34] It has also been used successfully in the management of cutaneous metastases of malignant melanoma.[35,36]

23.3.4 Topical Photodynamic Therapy

Topical photodynamic therapy (PDT) treatment involves activation of a photosensitizer in dysplastic or neoplastic cells by visible light in the presence of oxygen to produce reactive oxygen species that cause cell destruction. 5-Aminolevulinic acid (ALA) is the most widely used active agent for topical use. It is a precursor in the haem biosynthesis pathway. The photosensitizer protoporphyrin IX (PpIX) is formed following topical application of ALA. PpIX preferentially accumulates in dysplastic or neoplastic cells, probably because of increased penetration of ALA through the abnormal epidermis that overlies the tumor cells.[37] ALA is hydrophilic, and in most studies a 20% concentration in an oil-in-water emulsion is used.[38] Esterified derivatives of ALA such as methyl-5-aminolevulinate (methyl-ALA) are more lipophilic, allowing better intracellular penetration and hence enhanced efficacy. PpIX appears to be cleared from the body within 24 hours, and generalized photosensitization does not occur.[38,39]

Topical PDT has been used in the treatment of AKs, Bowen's disease, and BCCs. Both ALA–PDT and methyl-ALA–PDT are effective in clearing nonhyperkeratotic AKs on the face and scalp, with response rates comparable to topical 5-FU and cryotherapy.[38] The cosmetic response is felt to be superior to that with cryotherapy.[38] In Bowen's disease, ALA–PDT is similar in efficacy to cryotherapy and topical 5-FU. Topical photodynamic therapy may be advantageous for use over large or multiple lesions in areas of poor wound healing such as the lower leg and where existing treatments have recognized limitations.[38]

In a review of 12 studies treating 826 superficial and 208 nodular BCCs, the recurrence rates at 3 to 36 months' follow-up were 13 and 47% respectively.[40] Data are limited on the depth of response with this treatment. Morphoeic and pigmented lesions respond poorly to ALA–PDT.[40] At present, no 5-year follow-up data on the use of ALA–PDT in BCCs are available; therefore, no direct comparison can be made with conventional therapies.[41] Current evidence suggests that topical ALA–PDT may be as effective as cryotherapy for superficial or thin BCC but offers superior healing and cosmesis when used for large and multiple lesions.[38]

Photodynamic therapy is painful, although most patients can tolerate treatment without local anesthesia or analgesia. The face and scalp are more susceptible, and large or ulcerated lesions are more likely to be painful.[38] Topical or injected local anesthesia, premedication with benzodiazepine, the use of cooling fans, or spraying water on the lesions during therapy are strategies that have been employed to reduce pain.[38] Erythema and edema, with erosion, and crust formation can occur following photodynamic therapy.[38] Ulceration is a rare adverse event.[38] Hyper- and hypopigmentation can occur but usually resolve within 6 months; scarring is rare. Alopecia and a low risk of carcinogenicity are associated with ALA–PDT.[38]

23.4 ACNE

Acne affects almost 80% of those ages 11 to 30 years.[42,43] To understand the treatment options available for acne requires an understanding of the pathogenesis of acne. The pathophysiological factors involved in acne include the following:[44]

- Androgen-dependent sebaceous gland hyperplasia and increased sebum production
- Abnormal follicular differentiation and growth causing follicular blockage and sebum retention
- Colonization and overgrowth of the follicle with *Propionibacterium acnes*, which uses sebum as a metabolic substrate
- Release of inflammatory agents from the follicle due to *P. acnes* metabolism of sebum

Treatment options include topical and oral retinoids (isotretinoin), topical and oral antimicrobials such as benzoyl peroxide, hormonal manipulation, and mechanical or physical treatments involving cautery, laser, and chemical skin peeling. The following discussion focuses on retinoids, antimicrobials, and hormonal manipulation. Treatment is usually used as monotherapy or in combination. Table 23.2 shows the mechanisms of action of the available acne medications.

23.4.1 Topical Retinoids

Topical retinoids inhibit the formation of microcomedones, the precursor of acne lesions. Retinoids, by normalizing desquamation and reducing comedogenesis, enhance the penetration of other compounds such as topical antibiotics and benzoyl peroxide.[44] Several topical retinoids are currently available, including tretinoin, adapalene, tazarotene, isotretinoin, motretinide, retinaldehyde, and β-retinoyl glucoronide. They all act by targeting the microcomedo but differ somewhat in their antiinflammatory effects and tolerability.

Tretinoin, the first retinoid studied, is available in six strengths and three formulations: cream (0.025%, 0.05%, and 0.1%), gel (0.01% and 0.025%), and liquid (0.05%). Topical tretinoin has been found to be significantly more effective than vehicle in reducing both inflammatory and noninflammatory lesions in 12-week studies.[45,46] Once-daily tretinoin therapy (0.025% gel and 0.25% cream) reduced all types of acne lesions by 40 to 50%.[45,46] The early tretinoin formulations were associated with several side effects, including erythema, desquamation, burning, and pruritus. Two new formulations designed to reduce these tolerability problems include tretinoin microsphere (Retin-A MICRO 0.1% gel) and polymerized tretinoin (Avita 0.025% cream and 0.025% gel).[44] These formulations appear to improve tolerability by the slow release of tretinoin over time and improved localization to the follicles.[44]

Table 23.2 Types of Acne Treatment and Their Mode of Action

Acne Medication	Mechanism of Action
Topical retinoid	Normalize follicular desquamation; some reduce inflammatory response
Antibiotics	Reduce microorganisms; some reduce inflammatory response
Benzoyl peroxide	Reduce microorganisms
Hormonal therapy	Reduce sebum production; normalize follicular desquamation
Oral isotretinoin	Reduce sebum production; normalize follicular desquamation; reduce P. acnes indirectly; reduce inflammation

Adapalene is a third-generation retinoid. It is available in 0.1% concentration as cream, gel, solution, and pledgets.[44] Its efficacy has been demonstrated in numerous clinical trials.[47,48] A metaanalysis of five large controlled studies with more than 900 patients found that adapalene gel 0.1% was as effective as tretinoin gel 0.025%.[49] Adapalene was also found to be better tolerated than tretinoin in these studies.[49] Adapalene has been shown to have efficacy equivalent to that of tretinoin microsphere gel 0.1% and tretinoin cream 0.05% and greater tolerability than tretinoin cream 0.025%, although the tretinoin microsphere gel may have a faster onset of action than adapalene.[44] Isotretinoin in topical form does not reduce sebum secretion, unlike oral isotretinoin. It is similar to topical tretinoin but causes less skin irritation.[44]

23.4.2 Antimicrobial Therapy

Antimicrobial therapy can be prescribed topically or orally and has been used in acne treatment for more than 30 years. Topical agents are generally used for mild to moderate inflammatory acne, whereas oral antibiotics are used for moderate to severe inflammatory acne. Benzoyl peroxide acts as an antimicrobial agent in that it destroys both bacteria and yeasts.[44] By comparison with topical antibiotics, benzoyl peroxide has a greater and more rapid effect in suppressing *Propionibacterium acnes* without any evidence to date of resistance.[44] Antibiotics act by reducing the *P. acnes* and *Staphylococcal epidermidis* load in the skin.[44] They also have an antiinflammatory activity in that they inhibit macrophage functions, neutrophil chemotaxis, and cytokine production.[44,50,51] The oral antibiotic agents include tetracycline and its derivatives (e.g., minocycline, doxycycline, lymecycline), macrolides, cotrimoxazole, and trimethoprim. Topical antibiotics are less effective than oral antibiotics, and the most common side effects include erythema, peeling, itching, dryness, and burning. The most popular agents are clindamycin and erythromycin.[44] Topical tetracycline is no longer felt to be effective as acne therapy.[44]

Little or no significant difference exists in the therapeutic effects of these oral antibiotics.[44] The second generation of tetracyclines, such as minocycline, doxycycline, and lymecycline, induce a quicker clinical response than first-generation tetracyclines.[44] Oral treatment for 4 to 8 weeks is needed before any clinical effect is seen.[44] Side effects include gastrointestinal upset with the tetracyclines and macrolides, particularly erythromycin. Tetracyclines can also inhibit skeletal growth in the developing fetus and cause discoloration in the teeth of children under 10 years of age; it should not be prescribed to pregnant women and young children. Minocycline can cause drug-induced lupus erythematosus, pigmentation with long-term use, and benign intracranial hypertension.[44] Lymecycline in one study appears to have a better safety profile compared to minocycline.[52]

Various studies have been done to assess the efficacy of combination therapies in acne treatment. Combinations of topical antibiotics plus topical benzoyl peroxide, topical retinoids with topical or oral antibiotics, and topical retinoids with topical benzoyl peroxide have been shown to be more effective than monotherapy with the single agents alone.[53]

23.4.3 Hormonal Therapy

The aim of hormonal therapy is to oppose the effects of androgens on the sebaceous glands. For women, it can be a good option, especially if contraception is also desired. Estrogens suppress the ovarian production of androgens and stimulate the synthesis of sex-hormone-binding globulin (SHBG) by the liver.[44,54] The dose required to suppress sebum production is higher than the dose required to suppress ovulation.[44] Estrogens can be combined with a progestin in an oral contraceptive to avoid the risk of endometrial cancer with unopposed estrogens.[44] Some progestins may also have intrinsic androgenic activity, but the dose is believed to be insufficient to aggravate acne. The third-generation progestins (desogestrel, norgestimate, and gestodene) have the lowest intrinsic androgenic activity.[44] All combined oral contraceptives have a positive effect on acne; no single preparation has been shown to be superior to another.[44] Common side effects include gastrointestinal upset, breast tenderness, headache, menstrual irregularities, edema, and weight gain.[44] Flares of inflammatory acne can accompany the initiation of treatment with combined oral contraceptive.[44] Antiandrogens include cyproterone acetate (CPA), the diuretic spironolactone and its derivative drospirenone, and flutamide. CPA is unavailable in the United States. Both CPA and spironolactone can lead to feminization in men and should only be used in women. Spironolactone should be reserved for cases resistant to conventional therapy and where other antiandrogenic medication is unavailable.[44] Side effects of CPA include menstrual abnormalities, breast tenderness, nausea or vomiting, edema, headache, melasma, liver dysfunction, and blood-clotting disorders.[44] Spironolactone can cause hyperkalemia, menstrual irregularities, breast tenderness, headache, and fatigue. The use of flutamide in the treatment of acne is limited by its side-effect profile, which includes fatal hepatitis.[44] Pregnancy should be avoided with all antiandrogens due to the risk of feminization of the male fetus.[44] Glucocorticoids in low doses can suppress the adrenal production of androgens and are indicated in patients with the underlying endocrine abnormality, 11- or 21-hydroxylase deficiency.[44] It can also be used in acute flare of acne or in very severe acne for a few weeks.[44]

Hormonal therapy seems to work best in adult females with persistent papules and nodules involving the lower face and neck and who have flares before their menstrual periods.[44] In most cases, hormonal therapy should be combined with other antiacne therapies, including antibiotics and topical retinoids.

24.4.4 Oral Retinoids

Oral isotretinoin is indicated for severe nodular acne and moderate or severe acne unresponsive to conventional therapy.[55,56] It targets all of the pathophysiological factors in acne. Results are usually evident 1 to 2 months after the start of therapy. Generally, patients are started on a dose of no more than 0.5 mg/kg/day for the first month; if tolerated, it can be increased to 1 mg/kg/day over a 16- to 20-week course.[44] Most patients only require a single course of treatment but the recurrence of acne is not uncommon. In one study, 38% of patients were found to have no acne at 3-year follow-up after the first course of oral isotretinoin.[57] In the remainder of patients, acne was controlled with topical therapy in 17%, topical therapy plus oral antibiotics in 25%, or a second course of isotretinoin in 20%.[57] Relapse was more common in patients 16 years or younger and in women compared to men.[57] Maintenance therapy with topical retinoid therapy may reduce the relapse rate by controlling microcomedo formation.[44] Concomitant use of topical keratolytics and drying agents should be avoided because isotretinoin has a drying effect on mucocutaneous tissues.

Side effects are common and should be discussed before starting treatment. The common adverse effects of treatment include dry lips, skin, and eyes; myalgia and hypertriglyceridemia; epidermal fragility; nosebleeds; hair thinning; headaches; papilloedema; optic neuritis; and abnormal liver function. Regular monitoring of serum lipids and liver function is recommended.[44] Oral isotretinoin is a potent teratogen. Women of child-bearing age must not begin therapy until a negative pregnancy test result is obtained. Treatment should be initiated on the first 3 days of the menstrual period after the negative pregnancy test result is available, and adequate contraception is required during therapy and up to 6 weeks after therapy.[44] Some physicians believe that oral isotretinoin can occasionally cause mood changes, depression, and other significant psychiatric side effects leading to suicide. Long-term oral retinoid therapy has been known to cause skeletal hyperostosis and osteoporosis.[44,58]

24.5 PSORIASIS

Psoriasis is a common, chronic, relapsing, inflammatory inherited skin disease. It is characterized by an increased rate of epidermal turnover, hyperproliferation, and abnormal maturation of keratinocytes, accompanied by the dilatation of dermal blood vessels. The exact details of its molecular pathogenesis are unclear. It is generally believed that T-lymphocytes initiate and maintain the pathological process, although keratinocytes are also believed to play an important role.[59]

T-lymphocyte responses can be divided into T-helper 1 (Th1) or T-helper 2 (Th2) according to their cytokine secretion profile.[60] Psoriasis is characterized by a typical Th1 response involving but not limited to the production of interferon-gamma (IFN-γ), interleukin-2 (IL-2), tumor necrosis factor alpha (TNF-α), and tumor necrosis factor beta (TNF-β), as well as a largely cell-mediated immune response. In contrast, eczema, another common inflammatory dermatosis, produces a Th2 response with predominant antibody production and IL-4, IL-16, and IL-13 secretion. Antigen-presenting cells, especially dendritic cells, are important in directing the T-helper response by producing IL-12, IL-18, IL-23, and IL-27 in the Th1 and IL-10 in the Th2 response. Understanding the immunopathogenesis of psoriasis is essential for the design of new, targeted therapies.

Psoriasis can occur at any age and may affect any part of the skin. Various clinical patterns have been described: stable plaque psoriasis, localized palmoplantar psoriasis, guttate psoriasis, and generalized pustular psoriasis or erythrodermic psoriasis. It can also affect the scalp and nails, and in 10% of patients it is associated with arthritis. The treatment of psoriatic arthropathy has been reviewed elsewhere.[61] The existing treatments for psoriasis can be divided into topical therapy, phototherapy, and systemic therapy. A new group of drugs, referred to as biological response modifiers (BRMs), has recently been introduced.

The effectiveness of a new drug in psoriasis has been traditionally evaluated by the reduction of the psoriasis area and severity index (PASI), which is based on the proportion of erythema, scaling, and induration of the major body parts. A 75% reduction in PASI score may be necessary for the approval of a new drug by the FDA.[62]

24.5.1 Topical Treatments

Topical treatments are indicated for mild to moderate psoriasis. The commonly used topical agents are emollients, salicylic acid, corticosteroids, vitamin D analogs such as calcipotriol, anthralin (dithranol), and tar. Emollients and salicylic acid reduce scaling and improve penetration of other treatments, while mild- to moderate-strength topical steroids are used in the management of flexural and inflammatory psoriasis. Calcipotriol acts by skewing the T-cell response toward a Th2 type of response, as well as inhibition of IL-2, IFN-γ, and IL-12 secretion; T-cell proliferation; and maturation of dendritic cells.[63] A systematic review of 37 randomized controlled trials (RCTs) on calcipotriol found it to be more effective than coal tar and short-contact anthralin, with a 71% reduction in PASI score after 4 weeks when used in combination with topical steroids.[64,65] Drawbacks include irritation and hypercalcemia, if used in excess of more than 100 g a week.

Anthralin is an odorless, yellow substance with an as-yet unclear mechanism of action. Some evidence suggests that anthralin may affect keratinocyte proliferation and differentiation, T-lymphocyte activation, and neutrophil function. Anthralin has been used for over 100 years, and it remains an effective and safe treatment on its own or in combination with phototherapy.[66] It can be used as a short-contact topical application for 20 minutes and washed off, or it can be applied in Lassar's paste for 24 hours under bandages (Ingram's regime). Side effects of anthralin treatment include temporary skin burning and staining.

Coal tar is a by-product of coal distillation and has been used for the treatment of skin diseases for centuries.[67] Its mechanism of action is unclear but may involve the suppression of keratinocyte DNA synthesis. Coal tar consists of more than 10,000 compounds and is an inexpensive and effective treatment that can clear psoriasis but is malodorous and messy. Coal tar can be used alone or in combination with phototherapy and systemic agents. This treatment, however, has possible carcinogenic effects, but the data at present are conflicting. Epidemiological studies of industrial exposure, animal experiments, and one observational study in psoriasis patients suggest an increased risk of skin cancer, but a 25-year follow-up study of patients treated with coal tar did not confirm this finding.[67]

24.5.2 Phototherapy

Phototherapy plays an important role in the treatment of psoriasis on its own or in combination with tar or anthralin under occlusion as described above.[68] It possibly acts by reducing the number of T-lymphocytes in the skin as well as switching the immune response toward a Th2 response. The use of narrow-band or TLO-1 lamps (UVB spectrum with an emission peak between 310 and 313 nm) allows the delivery of a more precise and effective ultraviolet treatment; however, the most efficient phototherapy treatment, indicated for moderate to severe psoriasis, employs a combination of psoralen and ultraviolet A (PUVA). The psoralen can be applied topically or taken systemically and acts by sensitizing the skin to UVA, which cross-links DNA. This, unfortunately, also leads to an increased risk of skin cancer, especially squamous cell carcinoma, following prolonged use; therefore, it is recommended that the total treatment for one individual be restricted to a cumulative dose of 1500 J/cm². PUVA should not be combined with a potentially carcinogenic agent such as cyclosporine or azathioprine.[68] During the course of treatment, patients need to avoid sunlight exposure and, in the case of systemic PUVA treatment, wear protective sunglasses outside. Side effects of systemic PUVA include nausea, which can be severe; also, patients need to wear UV-absorbent glasses (e.g., Polaroid®) when outside for 24 hours.

24.5.3 Systemic Therapy

Systemic agents are indicated for the treatment of moderate to severe psoriasis. These include patients who have failed to respond to topical or light treatment, extensive plaque psoriasis with 10% to 20% body surface involvement, erythrodermic and pustular psoriasis, patients who are dysmorphophobic with regard to their psoriasis, or those who are unable to attend regularly for other treatment modalities (e.g., phototherapy).[69] Different systemic treatments are often used on a rotational basis and can be combined with topical therapy to increase its efficacy and reduce long-term adverse effects.

24.5.3.1 Methotrexate

Methotrexate was the first systemic drug used to treat psoriasis and still remains the most widely used systemic agent to date.[69] Methotrexate is a synthetic analog of folic acid, and through inhibition of dihydrofolate reductase it blocks thymidylate and DNA synthesis.[69] It has been shown to suppress lymphocyte and keratinocyte proliferation and secretion of IFN-γ and TNF-α. A recent study evaluated the effects of methotrexate in 88 patients who were randomized to receive either methotrexate or cyclosporine. In the group treated with methotrexate, up to 22.5 mg/week over 16 weeks, 40% achieved complete remission and the remaining 60% achieved a 75% reduction in PASI score.[70] Similar results were obtained in the cyclosporine group.

Frequent side effects of methotrexate include gastrointestinal upset, malaise, headache, and mouth ulcers. Bone marrow suppression, pulmonary fibrosis, and phototoxicity have all been reported. Hepatotoxicity is the most serious long-term adverse effect. Methotrexate is contraindicated in patients who use alcohol frequently; who have persistent renal and liver impairment, hepatitis, or myelosuppression; or who are pregnant. It is taken once weekly, has a slow onset of action, and requires regular monitoring of full blood count and renal and liver function.[69] With prolonged use, liver biopsies may be necessary, although measurement of serum levels of amino-terminal propeptide of type III collagen has been suggested as an alternative.[71]

24.5.3.2 Cyclosporine

Cyclosporine is an effective immunosuppressive agent widely used in solid organ transplantation. It inhibits calcineurin, which is required for IL-2 gene transcription, which prevents the activation of T-cells.[72] Cyclosporine has also been shown to inhibit the same pathway in keratinocytes.[59] Since its introduction in 1979, cyclosporine has become well established as a fast and efficient treatment of severe plaque, pustular, or erythrodermic psoriasis.[69,72,73] In patients with severe plaque psoriasis, a 50% and 90% reduction in PASI score can be achieved after 4 and 12 weeks of treatment, respectively.[73] More than 30% of patients were in remission for 6 months after a single 12-week course of treatment. Cyclosporine use, however, is limited by renal toxicity, hypertension, and the risk of malignancy, especially SCC of the skin in patients previously treated with PUVA. Short, intermittent courses of less than 12 weeks' duration are recommended for its use.[72] Regular monitoring of renal function, full blood count, and blood pressure is mandatory.

24.5.3.3 Retinoids

The retinoids affect proliferation and differentiation of keratinocytes. Acitretin and etretinate are teratogenic and persist in the liver for several years; therefore, acitretin must not be used in females who are pregnant or intend to become pregnant for up to 3 years after treatment cessation.[69] Acitretin is very effective for the treatment of pustular psoriasis, for which a response can be achieved within 10 days.[74] It has a slower onset of action in other forms of psoriasis and can be used in combination with phototherapy and oral hydroxyurea. In the management of erythrodermic psoriasis, methotrexate or cyclosporine can be used to gain a fast initial response before switching to acitretin. Acitretin side effects include dry skin and mucous membranes, hepatotoxicity, hyperlipidemia, gastrointestinal upset, alopecia, nail dystrophy, joint and muscle pains, and raised intracranial pressure. Regular monitoring of full blood count, renal and liver functions, and lipid profiles is necessary. In females of child-bearing age, pregnancy tests are also carried out.

24.5.3.4 Hydroxyurea

Hydroxyurea inhibits ribonucleotide reductase and DNA synthesis.[69] In psoriasis, it inhibits keratinocyte and vascular proliferation and reduces the number of dermal neutrophils. Hydroxyurea has been used in the management of psoriasis since the 1970s. In a recent prospective nonrandomized series, 75% of patients showed a 35% or greater reduction in PASI score after 8 weeks of treatment, with half of those achieving a 70% reduction in PASI score.[75] Its use is limited by the reversible bone marrow suppression commonly seen with the treatment.

24.5.3.5 Mycophenolate Mofetil

Mycophenolate mofetil (MMF) is an effective immunosuppressive drug used in transplantation and in the treatment of rheumatoid arthritis.[69] MMF is a morpholinoester of mycophenolic acid and acts as a noncompetitive inhibitor of inosine monophosphate dehydrogenase which leads to impaired purine synthesis and the proliferative responses of T- and B-cells.[76] MMF has been used alone or in combination with low doses of cyclosporine since the 1970s. A reduction of up to 47% in PASI score after 6 weeks of monotherapy with MMF can be expected.[76] Adverse effects with MMF include gastrointestinal symptoms, leucopenia, lymphoproliferative diseases, and increased incidence of herpes virus infections.

24.5.3.6 Fumaric Acid Esters

Fumaric acid esters (FAEs) have been used successfully in Germany, Switzerland, and The Netherlands since 1959. The mechanism of its action is not clear but is believed to involve switching the immune response toward a Th2 response by its actions on dendritic cells.[77] In addition, it may exert an antiproliferative effect on keratinocytes; suppress expression of chemokines, adhesion, and antigen-presenting molecules such as intercellular adhesion molecule 1 (ICAM-1) and human leukocyte antigen DR (HLA-DR); and cause apoptosis of T-lymphocytes. A prospective multicenter study demonstrated a mean reduction in PASI score of 80% after 4 months of treatment, and a randomized, double-blind, placebo-controlled trial showed an improvement in 70% of patients treated for 4 months.[78] The side effects are mild and consist of flushing, diarrhea, nausea, tiredness, relative lymphopenia, eosinophilia, and very rarely elevation of liver enzymes and renal failure. A study done on a group of 12 patients showed that treatment can be continued safely up to 14 years.[78] In a small number of patients, FAEs have been used in combination with cyclosporine, acitretin, or methotrexate.[79]

24.5.4 Biological Response Modifiers

Biological response modifiers (BRMs) is a generic term for hormones, neuroactive compounds, and immunoreactive compounds derived from living organisms that act at a cellular level and are used for the treatment, prevention, or cure of humans diseases.[62] To understand how such agents work in the setting of psoriasis, we need to outline the major points of the immune cascade involved in the disease process. In psoriasis, T-lymphocytes become activated. This happens when a T-cell receptor (TCR) recognizes a putative antigen associated with a major histocompatibility complex (MHC) molecule on an antigen-presenting cell such as a dendritic cell. This process is secured by the interaction of adhesion molecules such as ICAM-1/LFA-1, which hold the interacting cells together. In addition, a set of costimulatory signals is also required (IL-2/IL-2 receptor, LFA-3/CD2, CD28/CD80, CD40/CD40 ligand) for T-lymphocyte activation. Following successful activation and polarization toward a Th1 response, T-cells, directed by chemoattractants, home to the skin using adhesion molecules to migrate through blood vessels. The activated T-cells secrete a number of cytokines (e.g., TNF-α) which can act on keratinocytes and other immune cells. Based on this model, four basic strategies for the development of biological therapies in psoriasis have been developed. These strategies and the mode of action of current BRMs are summarized in Table 23.3.[80,81]

Tumor necrosis factor α plays an important role in the pathogenesis of psoriasis and may target T-lymphocytes, keratinocytes, Langerhans cells, and endothelial and natural killer (NK) cells.[82,83] It stimulates keratinocyte proliferation, the production of proinflammatory cytokines (e.g., IL-1, IL-6, IL-8), the expression of adhesion molecules on keratinocytes and endothelium, the maturation of dendritic cells, and the proliferation of blood vessels. Currently, two BRMs inhibit TNF-α: infliximab and etanercept. Infliximab is a chimeric, humanized mouse monoclonal antibody specific to TNF-α. It is given as an intravenous (i.v.) infusion every 4 to 8 weeks. It is approved for the treatment of rheumatoid arthritis and Crohn's disease and has been used in over 280,000 patients.[82] In a RCT involving 249 patients, infliximab achieved a 75% reduction in PASI score in 88% of patients at week 10.[84] In a small open-label follow-up study, half of the patients maintained a 75% reduction of PASI score for 6 months after the initial three infusions.[82] It should be used cautiously in patients with heart, renal, or liver impairment and demyelinating disorders.

Table 23.3 Mode of Action of the Biological Response Modifiers

Strategy or Mode of Action	Name and Function of the Drug	Mechanism of Action	Molecules Directly Involved
Decreases the number of effector T-cells	Alefacept (LFA-3 fusion protein)	Causes T-cell apoptosis	The LFA-3 fusion protein binds to CD2 on T-cells and causes their apoptosis by natural killer cells.
Inhibits T-cell contact and interactions with accessory cells and their subsequent activation	Efalizumab (monoclonal antibody to LFA-1)	Inhibits T-cell activation and migration	The monoclonal antibody binds to LFA-1 on T-cells and blocks the LFA-1/ICAM-1-dependent interaction of T-cells with antigen-presenting cells, endothelium, and keratinocytes.[a]
	Alefacept (LFA-3 fusion protein)	Inhibits T-cell activation and proliferation	The LFA-3 fusion protein blocks the CD2/LFA-3 interaction of T-cells and antigen-presenting cells.[a]
Switches Th1 to Th2 response	Human recombinant IL-10	Reduces secretion of Th1 cytokines (e.g., IFN-γ, IL-12) and inhibits cell-mediated immune response	Human recombinant IL-10.
Inhibits cytokines released by T-cells before they can exert their effect on target cells such as keratinocytes	Infliximab (monoclonal antibody to TNF-α)	Inhibits TNF-α	The monoclonal antibody binds to and neutralizes TNF-α.
	Etanercept (recombinant TNF-α receptor)	Inhibits TNF-α	The recombinant TNF-α receptor binds to and neutralizes TNF-α.

[a] Many other adhesion molecules, including LFA-1/ICAM-1 and LFA-3/CD2, also provide costimulatory signals.[87]

Etanercept is a recombinant human TNF-α receptor (fused with the constant region of an immunoglobulin molecule) and has a shorter half-life than infliximab. It is less immunogenic and is given subcutaneously (s.c.) every 2 weeks, thus allowing self-administration.[83] It has been approved by the FDA for the treatment of psoriatic arthritis. In a phase III trial, 49% of patients with plaque psoriasis achieved a 75% reduction in PASI score at 12 weeks and a 59% reduction at 24 weeks.[85] Adverse effects are mild and include local injection reactions and mild upper respiratory tract infections. No increase in the incidence of tuberculosis or lymphoma has been observed, but isolated cases of lupus erythematosus and heart failure have been described.

Efalizumab is a chimeric (human–mouse) monoclonal antibody directed against LFA-1 molecules expressed on memory T-lymphocytes.[86] Its ligands — ICAM-1, -2, and -3 — are expressed on antigen-presenting cells, endothelial cells, and keratinocytes.[87] The LFA-1/ICAM-1 interactions are important for T-cell activation, migration to skin, and interactions with keratinocytes.[86] It can be administered either intravenously or subcutaneously on a weekly basis. Two phase III clinical trials with over 1000 patients in total demonstrated a 75% reduction of PASI score in 30% of patients at week 12. The side effects are mild and transient and include upper respiratory tract infections, headache, nausea, chills, and fever. Abrupt discontinuation of therapy can lead to a rebound effect. The median time to relapse is 2 to 3 months. Trials to determine an optimal regime of withdrawal as well as the effect of continuous treatment are in progress.

Alefacept is a recombinant human LFA-3 molecule fused with the constant domain (Fc) of the immunoglobulin molecule (IgG$_1$), which binds to its ligand, CD2, on T-lymphocytes.[84,88] Normally, LFA-3 is expressed on antigen-presenting cells and delivers a costimulatory signal to T-cells. By blocking this interaction, alefacept suppresses T-lymphocyte activation and proliferation. It can also directly eliminate memory T-cells by inducing apoptosis. In a phase III RCT with 553 patients, alefacept given intravenously for 12 weeks resulted in a mean reduction of 47% in PASI after the first course and a 54% reduction after a second course.[89] Similar results were obtained in a trial with intramuscular injections. No rebound phenomena were observed, and maximum effects were achieved 8 weeks after the last administration. Mild and transient side effects of influenza-like symptoms were noted. Patients on alefacept maintained a normal immune response to novel and recall antigens as assessed in an open-labeled, randomized trial.[89] Regular monitoring of CD4/CD8 count is recommended.

Interleukin-10 (IL-10) and IL-4 are cytokines that can switch the immune response from a Th1 to a Th2 type. The mechanism of IL-10 action is complex, and it has been reported to induce or suppress the expression of up to 3000 different genes.[90] IL-10 promoter polymorphisms can also correlate with the severity of psoriasis and its response to therapy.[91] Data regarding its correlation with a family history of psoriasis are conflicting.[91,92] A number of small open-labeled trials previously reported improvement in patients treated with IL-10; however, a recent RCT of 28 patients failed to confirm these findings.[93] A small RCT of 17 patients demonstrated that IL-10 treatment can decrease the incidence of relapse and prolong remission in psoriasis.[94] IL-10 is well tolerated, but it can cause a reduction in platelet count, hemoglobin, and cholesterol levels. An increase in IgE levels was also observed. An encouraging phase I trial for IL-4 with 20 patients has been reported recently.[95] A large randomized, placebo-controlled trial is necessary to corroborate these results.

24.6 RARE INFLAMMATORY DERMATOSES

For numerous rare inflammatory dermatoses the use of immunosuppressive agents is beneficial, despite uncertainty about disease pathogenesis. The following section illustrates this point using two rare skin diseases: pyoderma gangrenosum and toxic epidermal necrolysis.

24.6.1 Pyoderma Gangrenosum

Pyoderma gangrenosum (PG) is a rare, ulcerative, potentially life-threatening, and frequently chronic inflammatory skin disease of uncertain etiology. PG affects individuals between the third and fifth decades of life.[96] It has a variety of forms and can be associated with other conditions such as rheumatoid arthritis, inflammatory bowel disease, and hematological malignancies.[97] Visceral involvement affecting the bone, liver, lung, and spleen has also been reported.[98] PG exhibits pathergy, whereby skin ulcers develop at the site of trauma such as a biopsy or needle puncture site.[96] The typical presentation of PG is of a rapidly developing painful ulcer with an undermined violaceous border predominantly affecting the lower extremities.

The treatment of PG is somewhat empirical and largely based on case reports. Local wound care must not be neglected, but surgical debridement is contraindicated due to the risk of pathergy. Topical nitrogen mustard[99] and tacrolimus[100] have been reported to be effective. The first-line systemic agents used are corticosteroids, alone or in combination with other agents. A high starting dose of prednisolone at 1 to 2 mg/kg/day is required to achieve control, and maintenance therapy at a lower dose is often needed to prevent relapse.[101] Often, one or more corticosteroid-sparing agents are required to achieve control during the acute stage and to prevent exacerbation as the corticosteroid dosage is adjusted.[101] Pulsed methylprednisolone has also been used, particularly in refractory PG. The benefits of long-term corticosteroids must be weighed against the potential harmful effects of hyperglycemia, osteoporosis, aseptic bone necrosis, infection, hypertension, and gastrointestinal bleeding. In patients receiving pulsed therapy, serious cardiovascular effects, including heart failure, hypotension, arrhythmias, and sudden death, have all been reported.[102]

More recently, cyclosporine and tacrolimus have been used successfully for the treatment of PG.[103,104] Tacrolimus shares the same mechanism of action as cyclosporine, which was discussed earlier in the chapter. Both agents appear effective at doses of 3 to 6 mg/kg/day for cyclosporine and 0.1 to 0.3 mg/kg for tacrolimus.[101] Topical tacrolimus 0.1% in combination with oral cyclosporine has been reported to be beneficial in PG.[100] Side effects include tremor, gingival hypertrophy, renal impairment, hypertension, and leucopenia for cyclosporine[105] and neurotoxicity, nephrotoxicity, infection, impaired glucose metabolism, and infection for tacrolimus.[106] Other agents that have been used in conjunction with corticosteroids include mycophenolate mofetil (MMF), azathioprine, methotrexate, and cyclophosphamide (pulsed and oral). MMF has been shown to be effective in PG with a good safety profile.[107]

Thalidomide has been used successfully in the treatment of recalcitrant PG in daily doses from 100 to 400 mg.[101] The adverse effects of thalidomide are peripheral neuropathy, sedation, and teratogenicity.[101] The use of human intravenous immunoglobulin (IVIG) for the treatment of recalcitrant PG has been reported;[108,109] improvement was seen one week after a 2-day course of IVIG at 1 g/kg, and complete healing after monthly treatment for 4 months.[108] IVIG used successfully as an adjunct to prednisolone and cyclosporine has also been reported.[109] Headache, myalgia, flushing, nausea, tachycardia, and labile blood pressure during the initial phase of infusion are some of the adverse reactions seen with IVIG.[109]

The most recent advance in the treatment of PG is the use of infliximab, a chimeric monoclonal antibody against tumor necrosis factor α (TNF-α). It has largely been used in patients with concomitant Crohn's disease.[110,111] A multicenter retrospective study of 13 patients with inflammatory bowel disease and refractory PG treated with infliximab showed that all patients responded well to the treatment.[112] Three patients had a complete response after one infusion, and 10 patients required multiple infusions.[112] Healing of ulcers is generally seen 1 to 4 months after therapy initiation.[101] Infusions at 4 weekly intervals may be required for acute control and 6- to 8-week intervals for maintenance therapy.[101]

24.6.2 Toxic Epidermal Necrolysis

Toxic epidermal necrolysis (TEN) is a severe drug reaction characterized by tenderness and erythema of the skin and mucosa, followed by destruction and extensive cutaneous and mucosal exfoliation and multisystem involvement. It can be fatal, with a mortality rate approaching 50%. When the disease predominantly involves the mucous membrane, it is referred to as Stevens–Johnson syndrome (SJS). The epithelial destruction is believed to be due to massive apoptosis. The exact mechanism leading to apoptosis is unclear, although the Fas/Fas ligand pathway has been implicated.[113]

Several studies have assessed the role of intravenous immunoglobulin in the treatment of TEN. IVIG contains antiidiotypic antibodies, antibodies against external antigens, and autoantibodies, all of which are exclusively of the IgG subtype. *In vitro* studies have shown both pro-apoptotic and anti-apoptotic effects of IVIG in different cell types. Clinical studies of IVIG use in adults with TEN have also shown conflicting outcomes. The first clinical study to be published (1998) assessed 10 consecutive patients with TEN or SJS (average skin detachment 28.5%, range 5 to 60%) treated with IVIG for 4 consecutive days. In this open study, the progression of skin disease was interrupted in all 10 patients 24 to 48 hours after IVIG infusions.[114] This was followed by rapid skin healing without significant adverse effects. A multicenter analysis of 48 TEN patients treated with IVIG over 4 days showed rapid cessation of skin and mucosal detachment following treatment. Six deaths were observed in this study.[115] Another open study on IVIG use in TEN looked at 16 patients with surface skin detachment ranging from 12 to 90% treated for 4 days with IVIG.[116] Cessation of disease and improvement in observed mortality compared to the predicted mortality using a validated prognosis score were found with IVIG use.[116] A prospective noncomparative study on IVIG in TEN and SJS that assessed 34 consecutive patients (9 with SJS, 5 with SJS-TEN, and 20 with TEN) treated for 2 days showed progression of epidermal detachment in 22 patients, regression in 4 patients, and no change in 7 patients following IVIG treatment.[117] No improvement in the observed mortality rate compared to the predicted mortality rate was found.[117] A nephrotoxic effect of high-dose IVIG with sucrose was also observed.[117] The reasons put forward in the literature to explain the conflicting results have been the use of different brands of IVIG, different doses and time of treatment initiation, referral bias leading to some centers having more severe cases, and variable prevalence of HIV infection in the patients with TEN treated with IVIG.[113] At the present time, no clear evidence supports the use of IVIG in TEN or SJS, and future randomized, double-blind, placebo-controlled clinical trials to address this issue are necessary. In clinical practice, however, severe cases of TEN are treated with IVIG.

24.7 CONCLUSION

In this chapter, we have illustrated the use of existing and several new agents that are available for the treatment of specific skin disorders. We have briefly described the role and mechanisms of action of commonly used drugs and described some of the newer drugs that have potential for further clinical application.

REFERENCES

1. Colver, G., *Skin Cancer: A Practical Guide to Management*, Martin Dunitz, London, 2002, pp. 25–82.
2. Ziegler, A., Jonason, A.S., Leffel, D.J. et al., Sunburn and p53 in the onset of skin cancer, *Nature*, 372, 773–776, 1994.
3. Nelson, M.A., Eiknspahr, J.G., Alberts, D.S. et al., Analysis of p53 gene in human precancerous actinic keratoses lesions and squamous cell cancers, *Cancer Lett.*, 85, 23–29, 1994.
4. Tutrone, W.D., Saini, R., Caglar, S. et al., Topical therapy for actinic keratoses. I. 5-Fluorouracil and imiquimod, *Cutis*, 71, 365–370, 2003.
5. Roberts, D.L.L., Anstey, A.V., Barlow, R.J. et al., U.K. guidelines for the management of cutaneous melanoma, *Br. J. Dermatol.*, 146, 7–17, 2003.
6. Wolf, Jr., J.E., Taylor, J.R. et al., Topical 3% diclofenac in 2.5% hyaluronan gel in the treatment of actinic keratoses, *Int. J. Dermatol.*, 40, 709–713, 2001.
7. Rivers, J.K., Arlette, J., Shear, N. et al., Topical treatment of actinic keratoses with 3% diclofenac in 2.5% hyaluronan gel, *Br. J. Dermatol.*, 146, 94–100, 2002.
8. McEwan, L.E. and Smith, J.G., Topical diclofenac/hyaluronic acid gel in the treatment of actinic keratoses, *Dermatology*, 38, 187–189, 1997.
9. Chabner, B.A., Allergra, C.J., Curth, G.A. et al., Antineoplastic agents: pyrimidine analogs, in *Goodman and Gilman's The Pharmacological Basis of Therapeutics*, 9th ed., Hardman, J.G. and Limberd, L., Eds., McGraw-Hill, New York, 1996, pp. 1247–1251.
10. Dineheart, S.M., The treatment of actinic keratoses, *J. Am. Acad. Dermatol.*, 42, 525–528, 2000.
11. Jansen, G.T., Topical therapy with 5-fluorouracil, *J. Surg. Oncol.*, 3, 317–323, 1971.
12. Levy, S., Furst, K., and Chern, W., A comparison of the skin permeation of three topical 0.5% fluorouracil formulations with that of a 5% formulation, *Clin. Ther.*, 23, 901–907, 2001.
13. Levy, S., Furst, K., and Chern, W., A pharmacokinetic evaluation of 0.5% and 5% fluorouracil topical cream in patients with actinic keratoses, *Clin. Ther.*, 23, 908–919, 2001.
14. Loven, K., Stein, L., Furst, K. et al., Evaluation of the efficacy and tolerability of 0.5% fluorouracil cream and 5% fluorouracil cream applied to each side of the face in patients with actinic keratoses, *Clin. Ther.*, 24, 990–1000, 2002.
15. Weiss, J., Menter, A., Heria, O. et al., Effective treatment of actinic keratoses with 0.5% fluorouracil cream for 1, 2, or 4 weeks, *Cutis*, 70(2, Suppl.), 22–29, 2002.
16. Johnson, M.R., Hageboutos, A., Wang, K. et al., Life-threatening toxicity in a dihydropyrimidine dehydrogenase-deficient patient after treatment with topical 5-fluorouracil, *Clin. Cancer Res.*, 5, 2006–2011, 1999.
17. Berman, B., Poochareon, V.N., and Villa, A.M., Novel dermatologic uses of the immune response modifier imiquimod 5% cream, *Skin Ther. Lett.*, 7, 1–6, 2002.

18. Gupta, A.K., Browne, M., and Bluhm, R., Imiquimod: a review, *J. Cutan. Med. Surg.*, 6, 554–560, 2002.

19. Mackenzie-Wood, A., Kossard, S., de Laurey, J. et al., Imiquimod 5% cream in the treatment of Bowen's disease, *J. Am. Acad. Dermatol.*, 44, 462–470, 2001.

20. Smith, K.J., German, M., and Skelton, H., Squamous cell carcinoma *in situ* (Bowen's disease) in renal transplant patient treated with 5% imiquimod and 5% 5-fluorouracil therapy, *Dermatol. Surg.*, 27, 561–564, 2001.

21. Stockfleth, E., Rowert, J., Arndt, R. et al., Detection of human papillomavirus and response to 5% imiquimod in a case of stucco keratosis, *Br. J. Dermatol.*, 143, 846–850, 2000.

22. Agarwal, S. and Berth-Jones, J., Porokeratosis of Mibelli: successful treatment with 5% imiquimod cream, *Br. J. Dermatol.*, 146, 338–339, 2002.

23. Marks, R., Gebauer, K., Shumack, S. et al., Imiquimod 5% cream in the treatment of superficial basal cell carcinoma: results of a multicentre 6-week dose-response trial, *J. Am. Acad. Dermatol.*, 44, 807–813, 2001.

24. Bentner, K.R., Geisse, J.K., Helman, D. et al., Therapeutic response of basal cell carcinoma to the immune response modifier imiquimod 5% cream, *J. Am. Acad. Dermatol.*, 41, 1002–1007, 1999.

25. Salasche, S., Imiquimod 5% cream: a new treatment option for basal cell carcinoma, *Int. J. Dermatol.*, 41(Suppl. 1), 16–20, 2002.

26. Drehs, M.M., Cook-Bolden, F., Tanzi, E.L. et al., Successful treatment of multiple superficial basal cell carcinomas with topical imiquimod: case report and review of the literature, *Dermatol. Surg.*, 28, 427–429, 2002.

27. Shumack, S., Robinson, J., Kossard, S. et al., Efficacy of topical 5% imiquimod cream for the treatment of nodular basal cell carcinoma: comparison of dosing regimens, *Arch. Dermatol.*, 138, 1165–1171, 2002.

28. Kagy, M.K. and Amorette, R., The use of imiquimod 5% cream for the treatment of superficial basal cell carcinomas in a basal cell naevus syndrome patient, *Dermatol. Surg.*, 26, 577–579, 2000.

29. Geisse, J.K., Commentary: the use of imiquimod 5% cream for the treatment of superficial basal cell carcinoma in a basal cell naevus patient, *Dermatol. Surg.*, 26, 579–580, 2000.

30. Weisberg, N.K. and Varghese, M., Therapeutic response of a brother and sister with xeroderma pigmentosum to imiquimod 5% cream, *Dermatol. Surg.*, 28, 518–523, 2002.

31. Ahmed, I. and Berth-Jones, J., Imiquimod: a novel treatment for lentigo maligna, *Br. J. Dermatol.*, 143, 843–845, 2000.

32. Chapman, M.S., Spencer, K.D., Brenwick, J.B., Histological resolution of melanoma *in situ* (lentigo maligna) with 5% imiquimod cream, *Arch. Dermatol.*, 139, 943–944, 2003.

33. Epstein, E., Extensive lentigo maligna clearing with topical imiquimod, *Arch. Dermatol.*, 139, 944–945, 2003.

34. Powell, A.M., Russel-Jones, R., and Barlow, R.J., Topical imiquimod: immunotherapy in the management of lentigo maligna, *Clin. Exp. Dermatol.*, 29, 15–21, 2004.

35. Steinmann, A., Funk, J.O., Schuler, G. et al., Topical imiquimod treatment of cutaneous melanoma metastasis, *J. Am. Acad. Dermatol.*, 43, 555–556, 2000.

36. Ugurel, S., Wagner, A., Pionier, C. et al., Topical imiquimod eradicates skin metastases of malignant melanoma, *Dermatology*, 205, 135–138, 2002.

37. Svanberg, K., Anderson, T., Killander, D. et al., Photodynamic therapy of non-melanoma malignant tumours of the skin using topical 5-aminolevulinic acid sensitisation and laser irradiation, *Br. J. Dermatol.*, 130, 743–751, 1994.

38. Morton, C.A., Brown, S.B., Collins, S. et al., Guidelines for topical photodynamic therapy: a report of a workshop of the British Photodermatology Group, *Br. J. Dermatol.*, 146, 552–567, 2002.

39. Rhodes, L.E., Tsoukas, M.M., Anderson, R.R. et al., Iontophoretic delivery of ALA provides a quantitative model for ALA pharmacokinetics and PpIX phototoxicity in human skin, *J. Invest. Dermatol.*, 108, 87–91, 1997.

40. Peng, Q., Warloe, T., Berg, K. et al., 5–ALA based photodynamic therapy, *Cancer*, 79, 2282–2308, 1997.

41. Fink-Puches, R., Soyer, H.P., Hofer, A. et al., Long term follow-up and histological changes of superficial nonmelanoma skin cancers treated with topical delta-aminolevulinic acid photodynamic therapy, *Arch. Dermatol.*, 134, 821–826, 1998.

42. Leyden, J.J., New understandings of the pathogenesis of acne, *J. Am. Acad. Dermatol.*, 32(Suppl.), S15–S25, 1995.

43. Cunliffe, W.J. and Gould, D.J., Prevalence of facial acne vulgaris in late adolescence and in adults, *Br. Med. J.*, 1, 1109–1110, 1979.

44. Gollnick, H., Cunliffe, W., Berson, D. et al., Management of acne: a report from a global alliance to improve outcomes in acne, *J. Am. Acad. Dermatol.*, 49(Suppl.), S1–S38, 2003.

45. Lucky, A., Cullen, S., Funicella, T. et al., Double-blind, vehicle-controlled multicentre comparison of two 0.025% tretinoin creams in patients with acne vulgaris, *J. Am. Acad. Dermatol.*, 38(Suppl.), S24–S30, 1998.

46. Lucky, A., Cullen, S., Jarrat, M. et al., Comparative efficacy and safety of two 0.025% tretinoin gels with results from a multicentre, double-blind, parallel study, *J. Am. Acad. Dermatol.*, 38(Suppl.), S17–S23, 1998.

47. Shalita, A.R., Weiss, J.S., Chalker, D.K. et al., A comparison of the efficacy and safety of adapalene gel 0.1% and tretinoin gel 0.025% in the treatment of acne vulgaris: a multi-centre trial, *J. Am. Acad. Dermatol.*, 34, 482–485, 1996.

48. Dunlap, F.E., Mills, O.H., Turley, M.R. et al., Adapalene 0.1% gel for the treatment of acne vulgaris: its superiority compared to tretinoin 0.025% cream in skin tolerance and patient preference, *Br. J. Dermatol.*, 139(2, Suppl.), 17–22, 1998.

49. Cunliffe, W.J., Pncet, M., Loesche, C. et al., A comparison of the efficacy and tolerability of adapalene 0.1% gel versus tretinoin 0.025% gel in patients with acne vulgaris: a meta-analysis of five randomised controlled trials, *Br. J. Dermatol.*, 139(Suppl. 52), 48–56, 1998.

50. Eady, E.A., Core, J.H., Holland, K.T. et al., Superior antibacterial action and reduced incidence of bacterial resistance in minocycline compared to tetracycline treated acne patients, *Br. J. Dermatol.*, 122, 233–244, 1990.

51. Esterly, N.B., Koransky, J.S., Furey, N.L. et al., Neutrophil chemotaxis in patients with acne receiving oral tetracycline therapy, *Arch. Dermatol.*, 120, 1308–1313, 1984.

52. Grosshans, E., Belaich, S., Meynadier, J. et al., A comparison of the efficacy and safety of lymecycline and minocycline in patients with moderately severe acne vulgaris, *Eur. J. Dermatol.*, 8, 161–166, 1998.

53. Leyden, J.J., A review of the use of combination therapies for the treatment of acne vulgaris, *J. Am. Acad. Dermatol.*, 49(Suppl.), S200–S210, 2003.

54. Lucky, A., Henderson, T., Olson, W. et al., Effectiveness of norgestimate and ethinyl oestradiol in treating moderate acne vulgaris, *J. Am. Acad. Dermatol.*, 37, 746–754, 1997.

55. Cunliffe, W., van de Kerkhof, P., Caputo, R. et al., Roaccutane treatment guidelines: results of an international survey, *Dermatology*, 194, 351–357, 1997.

56. Ortonne, J.P., Oral isotretinoin treatment policy: do we all agree?, *Dermatology*, 195(Suppl. 1), 34–40, 1997.

57. White, G.M., Yao, J., and Wolde-Tsadik, G., Recurrence rates after one course of isotretinoin, *Arch. Dermatol.*, 134, 376–378, 1998.

58. Margolis, D., Attie, M., Leyden, J. et al., Effects of isotretinoin on bone mineralisation during routine therapy with isotretinoin for acne vulgaris, *Arch. Dermatol.*, 132, 769–774, 1996.

59. Al-Daraji, W.I., Grant, K.R., Ryan, K. et al., Localization of calcineurin/NFAT in human skin and psoriasis and inhibition of calcineurin/NFAT activation in human keratinocytes by cyclosporin A, *J. Invest. Dermatol.*, 118, 779–788, 2002.

60. Murphy, K.M., Ouyang, W., Farrar, J.D. et al., Signaling and transcription in T helper development, *Annu. Rev. Immunol.*, 18, 451–494, 2000.

61. Ruderman, E.M., Evaluation and management of psoriatic arthritis: the role of biologic therapy, *J. Am. Acad. Dermatol.*, 49(2, Suppl.), S125–S132, 2003.

62. Enter, M.A., Krueger, G.C., Feldman, S.R. et al., Psoriasis treatment 2003 at the new millennium: position paper on behalf of the authors, *J. Am. Acad. Dermatol.*, 49(2, Suppl.), S39–S43, 2003.

63. Mathieu, C. and Adorini, L., The coming of age of 1,25–dihydroxyvitamin D(3) analogs as immuno-modulatory agents, *Trends Molec. Med.*, 8(4), 174–179, 2002.

64. Ashcroft, D.M., Po, A.L., Williams, H.C. et al., Systematic review of comparative efficacy and tolerability of calcipotriol in treating chronic plaque psoriasis, *Br. Med. J.*, 320(7240), 963–967, 2000.

65. Kaufmann, R., Bibby, A.J., Bissonnette, R. et al., A new calcipotriol/betamethasone dipropionate formulation (Dovobet) is an effective once-daily treatment for psoriasis vulgaris, *Dermatology*, 205(4), 389–393, 2002.

66. Mahrle, G., Dithranol, *Clin. Dermatol.*, 15(5), 723–737, 1997.

67. Thami, G.P. and Sarkar, R., Coal tar: past, present and future, *Clin. Exp. Dermatol.*, 27(2), 99–103, 2002.

68. Zanolli, M., Phototherapy treatment of psoriasis today, *J. Am. Acad. Dermatol.*, 49(2, Suppl.), S78–S86, 2003.

69. Yamauchi, P.S., Rizk, D., Kormeili, T. et al., Current systemic therapies for psoriasis: where are we now?, *J. Am. Acad. Dermatol.*, 49(2, Suppl.), S66–S77, 2003.

70. Heydendael, V.M., Spuls, P.I., Opmeer, B.C. et al., Methotrexate versus cyclosporine in moderate-to-severe chronic plaque psoriasis, *N. Engl. J. Med.*, 349(7), 658–665, 2003.

71. Zachariae, H., Heickendorff, L., and Sogaard, H., The value of amino-terminal propeptide of type III procollagen in routine screening for methotrexate-induced liver fibrosis: a 10-year follow-up, *Br. J. Dermatol.*, 144(1), 100–103, 2001.

72. Griffiths, C.E., Dubertret, L., Ellis, C.N. et al., Ciclosporin in psoriasis clinical practice: an international consensus statement, *Br. J. Dermatol.*, 150(Suppl. 67), 11–23, 2004.

73. Ho, V.C., The use of ciclosporin in psoriasis: a clinical review, *Br. J. Dermatol.*, 150(Suppl. 67), 1–10, 2004.

74. Ling, M.R., Acitretin: optimal dosing strategies, *J. Am. Acad. Dermatol.*, 41(3, Pt. 2), S13–S17, 1999.

75. Kumar, B., Saraswat, A. and Kaur, I., Rediscovering hydroxyurea: its role in recalcitrant psoriasis, *Int. J. Dermatol.*, 40, 530–534, 2001.

76. Geilen, C.C., Arnold, M., and Orfanos, C.E., Mycophenolate mofetil as a systemic antipsoriatic agent: positive experience in 11 patients, *Br. J. Dermatol.*, 144, 583–586, 2001.

77. Litjens, N.H., Rademaker, M., Ravensbergen, B. et al., Monomethylfumarate affects polarization of monocyte-derived dendritic cells resulting in down-regulated Th1 lymphocyte responses, *Eur. J. Immunol.*, 34, 565–575, 2004.

78. Hoefnagel, J.J., Thio, H.B., Willemze, R. et al., Long-term safety aspects of systemic therapy with fumaric acid esters in severe psoriasis, *Br. J. Dermatol.*, 149, 363–369, 2003.

79. Balasubramaniam, P., Stevenson, O., and Berth-Jones, J., Fumaric acid esters in severe psoriasis, including experience of use in combination with other systemic modalities, *Br. J. Dermatol.*, 150, 741–746, 2004.

80. Mehlis, S.L. and Gordon, K.B., The immunology of psoriasis and biologic immunotherapy, *J. Am. Acad. Dermatol.*, 49(2, Suppl.), S44–S50, 2003.

81. Singri, P., West, D.P., and Gordon, K.B., Biologic therapy for psoriasis: the new therapeutic frontier, *Arch. Dermatol.*, 138, 657–663, 2002.

82. Gottlieb, A.B., Infliximab for psoriasis, *J. Am. Acad. Dermatol.*, 49(2, Suppl.), S112–S117, 2003.

83. Goffe, B. and Cather, J.C., Etanercept: an overview, *J. Am. Acad. Dermatol.*, 49(2, Suppl.), S105–S111, 2003.

84. Weinberg, J.M., An overview of infliximab, etanercept, efalizumab, and alefacept as biologic therapy for psoriasis, *Clin. Ther.*, 25, 2487–2505, 2003.

85. Leonardi, C.L., Powers, J.L., Matheson, R.T. et al. and Etanercept Psoriasis Study Group, Etanercept as monotherapy in patients with psoriasis, *N. Engl. J. Med.*, 349, 2014–2022, 2003.

86. Leonardi, C.L., Efalizumab: an overview, *J. Am. Acad. Dermatol.*, 49(2, Suppl.), S98–S104, 2003.

87. Alexandrov, A.V., Jackson, A.M., and Rumyantsev, A.G., Mechanism of modulation of intercellular adhesion molecules ICAM, *Immunologia*, 1, 4–13, 1997.

88. Krueger, G.G. and Callis, K.P., Development and use of alefacept to treat psoriasis, *J. Am. Acad. Dermatol.*, 49(2, Suppl.), S87–S97, 2003.

89. Gottlieb, A.B., Casale, T.B., Frankel, E. et al., CD4+ T-cell-directed antibody responses are maintained in patients with psoriasis receiving alefacept: results of a randomized study, *J. Am. Acad. Dermatol.*, 49, 816–25, 2003.

90. Jung, M., Sabat, R., Kratzschmar, J. et al., Expression profiling of IL-10-regulated genes in human monocytes and peripheral blood mononuclear cells from psoriatic patients during IL-10 therapy, *Eur. J. Immunol.*, 34, 481–493, 2004.

91. Kingo, K., Koks, S., Silm, H. et al., IL-10 promoter polymorphisms influence disease severity and course in psoriasis, *Gen. Immun.*, 4, 455–457, 2003.

92. Asadullah, K., Eskdale, J., and Wiese, A. et al., Interleukin-10 promoter polymorphism in psoriasis, *J. Invest. Dermatol.*, 116, 975–978, 2001.

93. Kimball, A.B., Kawamura, T., Tejura, K. et al., Clinical and immunologic assessment of patients with psoriasis in a randomized, double-blind, placebo-controlled trial using recombinant human interleukin 10, *Arch. Dermatol.*, 138, 1341–1346, 2002.

94. Friedrich, M., Docke, W.D., Klein, A. et al., Immunomodulation by interleukin-10 therapy decreases the incidence of relapse and prolongs the relapse-free interval in psoriasis, *J. Invest. Dermatol.*, 118, 672–677, 2002.

95. Ghoreschi, K., Thomas, P., Breit, S. et al., Interleukin-4 therapy of psoriasis induces Th2 responses and improves human autoimmune disease, *Nat. Med.*, 9, 40–46, 2003.

96. Blitz, N.M., Rudikoff, D. et al., Pyoderma gangrenosum, *Mt. Sinai J. Med.*, 68, 287–297, 2001.

97. Callen, J.P., Pyoderma gangrenosum, *Lancet*, 351, 581–585, 1998.

98. Vadillo, M., Jucgla, A., Podzamezer, D. et al., Pyoderma gangrenosum with liver, spleen, and bone involvement in a patient with chronic myelomonocytic leukaemia, *Br. J. Dermatol.*, 141, 541–543, 1999.

99. Tsele, E., Yu, R.C.H., and Chu, A.C., Pyoderma gangrenosum: response to topical nitrogen mustard, *Clin. Exp. Dermatol.*, 192, 252–254, 1992.

100. Reich, K., Vente, C., and Neumann, C., Topical tacrolimus for pyoderma gangrenosum, *Br. J. Dermatol.*, 139, 738–759, 1998.

101. Gettler, S.L., Rothe, M.J., Grin, C. et al., Optimal treatment of pyoderma gangrenosum, *Am. J. Clin. Dermatol.*, 4, 597–608, 2003.

102. White, K.P., Driscoll, M.S., Rothe, M.J. et al., Severe adverse cardiovascular effects of pulse steroid therapy: is continuous cardiac monitoring necessary?, *J. Am. Acad. Dermatol.*, 30, 768–773, 1994.

103. Chow, R.K.P. and Ho, V.C., Treatment of pyoderma gangrenosum, *J. Am. Acad. Dermatol.*, 34, 1047–1060, 1996.

104. Curley, R.K., Macfarlane, A.W., and Vickers, C.F.H., Pyoderma gangrenosum treated with ciclosporin A, *Br. J. Dermatol.*, 113, 601–604, 1985.

105. Lebwohl, M., Ellis, C., Gottlieb, A. et al., Cyclosporine consensus conference: with emphasis on the treatment of psoriasis, *J. Am. Acad. Dermatol.*, 39, 464–475, 1998.

106. Weichert, G. and Sauder, D.N., Efficacy of tacrolimus (FK 506) in idiopathic treatment resistant pyoderma gangrenosum, *J. Am. Acad. Dermatol.*, 39, 648–650, 1998.

107. Hohenleutner, U., Mohr, V.D., Michael, S. et al., Mycophenolate mofetil and ciclosporin treatment for recalcitrant pyoderma gangrenosum, *Lancet*, 350, 1748, 1997.

108. Dirschka, T., Kastner, U., Behrens, S. et al., Successful treatment of pyoderma gangrenosum with intravenous human immunoglobulin, *J. Am. Acad. Dermatol.*, 39, 789–790, 1998.

109. Gupta, A.K., Shear, N.H., and Sauder, D.N., Efficacy of human intravenous immunoglobulin in pyoderma gangrenosum, *J. Am. Acad. Dermatol.*, 32, 140–142, 1995.

110. Tan, M.H., Gordon, M., Lebwohl, O. et al., Improvement of pyoderma gangrenosum and psoriasis associated with Crohn's disease with anti-tumour necrosis factor α monoclonal antibody, *Arch. Dermatol.*, 137, 930–933, 2001.

111. Mimouni, D., Anhalt, G.J., Kouba, D.J. et al., Infliximab for peristomal pyoderma gangrenosum, *Br. J. Dermatol.*, 148, 813–816, 2003.

112. Regueiro, M., Valentine, J., Plevy, S. et al., Infliximab for the treatment of pyoderma gangrenosum associated with inflammatory bowel disease, *Am. J. Gastroenterol.*, 98, 1821–1826, 2003.

113. Bachot, N. and Rojeau, J.-C., Intravenous immunoglobulins in the treatment of severe drug eruptions, *Curr. Opin. Allergy Clin. Immunol.*, 3, 269–274, 2003.

114. Viard, I., Wehrli, P., Bullani, R. et al., Inhibition of toxic epidermal necrolysis by blockade of CD35 with human intravenous immunoglobulin, *Science*, 282, 490–493, 1998.

115. Prins, C., Kerdel, F.A., Padilla, S. et al., Treatment of toxic epidermal necrolysis with high-dose intravenous immunoglobulins: multicentre retrospective analysis of 48 consecutive cases, *Arch. Dermatol.*, 139, 26–32, 2003.

116. Trent, J.T., Kirsner, R.S., Romanelli, P. et al., Analysis of intravenous immunoglobulin for the treatment of toxic epidermal necrolysis using SCORTEN; the University of Miami experience, *Arch. Dermatol.*, 139, 39–43, 2003.

117. Bachot, N., Revuz, J., and Roujeau, J.C., Intravenous immunoglobulin treatment for Steven–Johnson syndrome and toxic epidermal necrolysis: a prospective noncomparative study showing no benefit on mortality or progression, *Arch. Dermatol.*, 139, 33–36, 2003.

CHAPTER 24

Drugs for the Treatment of Atopic Eczema

Christopher L. Wu, Lucia H. Lee, Benjamin R. Lee, and Chi-Jen Lee

CONTENTS

24.1 INTRODUCTION

Atopic eczema, frequently referred to as atopic dermatitis, is a chronic inflammatory skin disorder characterized by an itchy red rash that most commonly occurs in persons with a family history of allergic diseases, such as rhinitis, asthma, or conjunctivitis. The disorder occurs in infants, children, and adults, with an onset usually before 5 years of age. The prevalence is high in children (10% or greater in the 1990s). The cumulative incidence is 10 to 15% in children up to 14 years of age, and the incidence is increasing. Heredity plays a role, with a possible genetic defect in some bone-marrow-derived cells.[1–3] The word *atopic* is an indicator of the frequent association with atopy and the need to separate this clinical phenotype from the other forms of eczema such as irritant, allergic contact, discoid, venous, and photosensitive eczemas, which have other causes and distinct patterns.

    The exact cause of atopic eczema is unknown. Abnormalities in both immunologic and physiologic characteristics are observed in certain areas: (1) frequent association of atopic eczema with other allergic disorders; (2) elevations of serum IgE; (3) positive wheal and flare reactions to a wide variety of scratch tests; (4) increased susceptibility to bacterial, viral, and fungal infections; and (5) association with immunodeficiency diseases. Patients exhibit abnormal humoral and cell-mediated immunity, such as an impaired delayed hypersensitivity response and increased production of IgE. The identification of cytokines, such as interferons (IFNs) and interleukins (ILs), has allowed further delineation of mechanisms and the development of new treatment strategies; for example, the mononuclear leukocytes in atopic eczema patients produce lower levels of IFN-γ and higher levels of IL-4. IFN-γ mediates delayed hypersensitivity reactions, and IL-4 stimulates IgE synthesis.[4] The presence of decreased numbers of T-lymphocytes indicates a lack of sufficient T-cells to control B-cell production of immunoglobulin, resulting in high IgE levels. In addition, high numbers of *S. aureus* bacteria are observed on both the diseased and normal skin of eczema patients.

Eczema occurs in acute, subacute, and chronic stages, each with a wide range of severity, with corresponding clinical and histological features. In addition, eczema exhibits several distinct clinical subtypes, each associated with various predisposing and triggering factors. In general, a given background predisposes to the mixed factors of immunological, pharmacological, and physiological features that respond to triggering factors leading to the inflammatory response and clinical symptoms of eczema.

The objectives of this chapter are (1) to provide a background and overall plan for the drug development process in eczema, and (2) to facilitate further research and development of a new generation of agents with benefits for treatment of disease.

24.2 CLINICAL PRESENTATION AND DIAGNOSIS

The diagnostic marker is itching, frequently accompanied by erythema and dry skin. Major environmental factors that induce or exacerbate atopic eczema include dry skin, sweating, exercise, scratching, prickly clothes, temperature change, and allergies to foods. Laboratory test and histologic examination of biopsy may not provide confirmatory evidence, although an estimated 85% of patients have elevated IgE levels and positive immediate skin test to foods and inhalant allergens.

A close relationship exists between food allergy and atopic disease, primarily in children. The types of foods most commonly involved include eggs, peanuts, milk, soy, wheat, and fish. Inhalant allergens, such as dust mites, are more involved in causing the disease for adults. In infants, atopic eczema is most likely to occur at 3 months of age. Intense itching is observed as the infant scratches constantly and rubs against garments and bedding. Some infant cases continue to childhood or recur years after resolution of disorder. In children, the flexor surfaces as well as neck, wrists, and ankles are usually involved rather than exterior areas. In adults, papules tend to become confluent, forming large lichenified areas. Crusts result from scratching due to the intense itching.

The course of atopic eczema is variable and generally marked by remissions and exacerbations. Most cases begin in infancy but onset may not occur until childhood or after puberty. The reported frequency of persistence varies widely from 10 to 83%. Such variance may be due to the inaccurate diagnostic criteria used. Atopic eczema in childhood is often associated with a family history of atopic disease, the presence of allergic rhinitis and/or asthma, female sex, and early age of onset (less than 1 year old).

24.3 DRUGS FOR THE TREATMENT OF ATOPIC ECZEMA

Therapeutic strategies involve drug treatment and environmental change. The most common measures include the use of topical and occasionally systemic corticosteroids, systemic antihistamines, topical or systemic antibiotics, orally administered immunosuppressants such as azathioprine and cyclosporine, skin maintenance care, and environmental change. The therapeutic goals are to decrease skin inflammation, eliminate exacerbating factors, and relieve the itching and dry skin. It is necessary to avoid extremes of temperature and humidity; strenuous exercise; rough, scratchy clothing; bathing with harsh soaps and hot water; irritant chemicals; and allergens. These factors can perpetuate the itch–scratch cycle. Stress, anger, or anxiety may contribute to exacerbations of atopic eczema. The ideal drug is one that can be used safely, effectively, and conveniently to intervene, at the earliest possible stage, in the disease process. When more than 10 to 20% of the surface area of skin is involved, oral therapy may be the preferred mode of administration.

24.3.1 Corticosteroids

Patients with mild or localized atopic eczema require only treatment with a topical corticosteroid ointment or cream. For patients with extensive disease, a combination of topical measures may be necessary. In the acute phase, high-potency topical steroids can be used for 7 to 10 days. Therapy is then switched to less potent products for up to several more weeks. Patients with severe conditions may require long-term use of nonfluorinated (hydrocortisone 1% or desonide 0.05%) or low-potency fluorinated preparations (triamcinolone 0.025%). Long-term use of fluorinated corticosteroids, particularly high-potency agents, causes thinning of the skin and can lead to atrophy on the face and skinfold areas. Systemic corticosteroids may be useful under certain conditions.

24.3.2 Antimicrobial Agents

Secondary infection frequently due to *Staphylococcus aureus* can be treated with topical antibiotics. Preparations containing erythromycin or bacitracin are preferred because of less sensitization compared to agents such as neomycin. Mupirocin is also effective. Systemic antibiotic therapy may be indicated to treat secondary bacterial infections such as folliculitis. Therapy is directed toward Gram-positive cocci, particularly *S. aureus*. A 7-day course of an antistaphylococcal agent (e.g., dicloxacillin, erythromycin, cephalexin) is often used.

24.3.3 Antihistamines

Systemic antihistamines may be useful under certain circumstances. Benefits of oral administration of antihistamines include relief of pruritus and sedation. If sedation is the desired goal, then patients should benefit more from the traditional H_1-blockers.[5] After intense therapy to break the cycle of scratching, the major challenge is to keep the skin clear by eliminating the urge to scratch. If the worst scratching occurs during sleep, a higher dose of a sedating antihistamine may be adequate. For example, if diphenhydramine 25 mg is not adequate, then 50 mg should be administered; if hydroxyzine 25 mg is not adequate, then 50 mg or higher dose should be administered.

24.3.4 Agents Affecting the Immune System

Cyclosporine inhibits T-lymphocyte-dependent immune responses and downregulates cytokine production. Oral cyclosporine in doses of 2.5 to 6.0 mg/kg/day (5.0 mg/kg/day most common) has provided benefit to patients with atopic eczema. Improvement usually occurs within 1 to 2 weeks with some continuing improvement over a 6- to 8-week period. Discontinuation results in relapse in a high percentage of patients (50 to 75%). Reduced maintenance doses, ranging from 0.5 to 2 mg/kg/day or 5 mg/kg given every 5 days, have been used in maintaining response.[6] Hypertension, nephrotoxicity, and serious drug interactions are concerns with long-term therapy.[6,7] Tacrolimus, an inhibitor of T-lymphocyte proliferation, has been used systematically and topically. Most data concern the topical form. A 0.01% tacrolimus ointment results in diminished pruritus within 3 days.

Other approaches involve immunomodulation with cytokines, including IFNs and ILs. Daily subcutaneous injections of IFN-γ (50 to 100 μg) for 12 weeks resulted in more than 50% improvement in 45 to 66% of patients studied. Relief of pruritus occurred in some patients within 2 to 4 days. Relapse within 4 to 7 days has occurred in some patients after discontinuation of therapy. Side effects with this therapy include flu-like symptoms, such as fever, chills, headache, and myalgia, which respond well to acetaminophen. Leukopenia and thrombocytopenia have been reported but are uncommon. Eosinophil counts are reduced, although no significant changes occur in serum IgE levels. IL-2 showed benefit in one group of six patients with severe disease; relapse occurred 4 to 6 weeks after discontinuation of therapy, and serum IgE levels were unaffected.

Thymopentin, a synthetic pentapeptide derived from thymic hormone thymopoietin, enhances production of cytokines such as IL-2 and IFN-γ. This agent was used to treat several groups of patients with atopic eczema. Doses (50 mg) administered intramuscularly or subcutaneously result in clinical improvement but relapse occurs.[7] Current first-line treatments in the United Kingdom include emollients, topical corticosteroids, and sedative antihistamines. Second-line treatments include allergen avoidance and ultraviolet light. Third-line treatments include systemic immuno-modulatory treatments such as cyclosporine A and azathioprine.[8]

24.4 EVALUATION OF DRUGS FOR ECZEMA

Some techniques for evaluating eczema subtypes and the effects of all potentially useful drugs will be more suitable than others in any given situation. When applying a drug topically or systemically for the treatment of skin diseases, it is important to gather information on all aspects of its effects in humans. For a topical corticosteroid, key questions will relate to its speed and degree of efficacy vs. the risk of well-known adverse reactions, such as skin thinning. When developing a new drug, it is important to investigate the mechanism of action. The following issues should be emphasized in the early phases of clinical trials to evaluate both topical and systemic agents:

- Determine the effectiveness of the testing agent in the treatment of eczema.
- Define the optimal dosage.
- Define the pharmacokinetic and pharmacodynamic patterns of the drug in human skin, as well as systemically.
- Compare the effectiveness of the agent with standard therapies, allowing further decisions to be made on subsequent studies.
- Estimate the risk–benefit profile of the agent.

In topical therapy, the vehicle and concentration of active agent in the formulation must be optimized. In the early stages of clinical trials for topical corticosteroid, inadequate conditions were observed in the dosing regimens, as well as a failure to determine with precision the necessary adjustments in corticosteroid concentration in a given vehicle to improve clinical efficacy.[9,10] The exact timing of critical activities in clinical development plans for topical and systemic drugs may vary from project to project. Clinical changes are readily visible and usually occur quickly, and, in case of topical therapy, the safety margin is generally good. In addition, the skin represents the ideal organ for exploring human tissue pharmacology in a relatively less invasive manner.[11]

For topical applications, it is necessary to collect data on its use in normal human skin before proceeding to patients, because of the inflammatory nature of the eczema process and its exacerbation following irritation. This can be done in healthy volunteers using an occlusive technique involving double-blind assessment to evaluate epidermal and dermal changes, such as erythema, papules, vesiculation, infiltration, and ulceration, similar to methods used for allergic contact dermatitis.[12,13] Alternatively, repeated application techniques with or without occlusion, can be used. For systemic drugs, standard phase I studies are used to evaluate safety and general human pharmacology.

During early clinical trials, it is important to establish the efficacy of the drug for the treatment of patients with eczema; however, well-defined experimental volunteer models can be valuable. Important issues in the early phases of clinical trials for eczema drugs include:

- Population to use (patients or healthy volunteers?)
- Model of eczema subtype to study and the experimental design
- Endpoints and surrogate markers to be measured (clinical symptoms and signs; pharmacological, immunological, anatomical, or structural parameters?)
- Methods and procedures to perform measurements

The study design should be double-blind, controlled, and randomized and should follow statistical considerations. Whenever possible, bilateral, symmetrical, paired comparison methods should be used to reduce variability. The study should utilize the valuable resource of the study population efficiently, with subjects acting as their own controls.[14,15] The concern that drug administration to one site may affect another is unlikely to be of practical significance if small amounts of drug are applied to limited areas of diseased skin.

The ideal model of experimental design would be ethical, simple to use, reliable in responses to both the challenge modality and test therapies, noninvasive and nonscarring, reproducible, and clinically relevant.[16–19] In patient or healthy volunteer models, croton oil, tetrahydrofurfuryl nicotinate, or sodium lauryl sulfate can be used to induce inflammation; wheal and flare reactions occur following histamine administration and antigen challenge. These models appear to represent potentially useful methods. Rapid screening with small numbers of volunteers should be conducted to examine any given agent. The inflammation models using different agents are useful for inducing various types of inflammatory changes in the skin which may respond to particular antiinflammatory drugs. These models can be considered when evaluating a novel agent with a suitable antiinflammatory profile.

Adhesive tape stripping may be used to produce epidermal derangement accompanied by hyperemia as an adjunct to the human vasoconstriction assay for corticosteroid assessment and as a method for ensuring greater penetration of drug into skin challenged by various modalities.[20,21] Wheal and flare reactions are useful in the evaluation of both systemic and topical agents with antihistamine effects, as well as those that can modify mast cells and basophil cell activity. This model can be extended to assess drug effects on various other vasoactive agents.[22,23] The human vasoconstriction assay has been used successfully to screen topical corticosteroids for clinical activity, for determining the bioavailability of corticosteroids from their vehicles, and for predicting the relative clinical potencies of topical corticosteroid preparations.[24]

Volunteer models for the assessment of itching utilize intracutaneous injections of histamine and various proteases (e.g., trypsin, papain) or the epicutaneous application of cowhage extract. Parameters measured include itch threshold, duration, and intensity. The sensation induced by pruritogenic agents varies qualitatively depending on the depth to which the injection is given.[25,26] Measurement of itching in patients may be performed by subjective evaluation using data loggers or by limb meters, which evaluate scratching as a direct correlate of itching.[27,28] For studies in patients, preference should be given in the early stages to evaluate subtypes of eczema that lend themselves to assessment by the bilateral paired comparison method. Atopic eczema, venous stasis eczema, and contact dermatitis would be appropriately selected in circumstances where a broad-spectrum, antiinflammatory effect is anticipated.

Methods for evaluating drug effects on eczema and experimentally challenged skin are described in Table 24.1. In all clinical and volunteer studies, characteristic symptoms (e.g., itching, stinging, burning, pain, erythema, blanching, papules, vesicles, pustules, infiltration, and scaling) produced by challenge modality and modification of these by the test agent can be evaluated by utilizing scoring systems under blinded conditions.[14] Scoring systems for individual symptoms should include the full range of possibilities (e.g., no response to intense response) using a 5- to 10-point scale with clinically meaningful and evenly separated spacing between descriptive terms. An overall severity score incorporating grouped symptoms should also be included. Progress in the condition, to complete clearing of symptoms, should be scored using a similarly constructed scale. Despite the subjective nature of these assessments, they are of central importance in dermatological studies and are accurate and reproducible when performed by trained and experienced researchers.

Measurement of the area of wheals and flares produced by various intradermally injected challenge substances (e.g., histamine) is a simple, reliable, and reproducible method of evaluating drug effects that has been used extensively to determine the time of onset, intensity, and duration of drug activity in clinical trials. Laser Doppler velocimetry and flowmetry are useful objective measures of cutaneous blood flow that have been utilized to study the pharmacodynamic response

Table 24.1 Methods for Evaluating Drug Effects on Eczema

Methods	Applications
Blind-arranged subjective scoring system based on clinical symptoms[22,35]	Patient studies and healthy volunteer models
Measurement of area or volume[36]	Wheal and flare studies
Laser Doppler velocimetry or flowmetry[24,37–39]	Volunteer models with a sufficient inflammatory component to increase skin blood flow, including wheal and flare studies; specially adapted forms of human vasoconstriction assays
Measurement of transepidermal water loss (TEWL) by evaporimetry[28,31,40]	Patient studies and healthy volunteer models that involve functional disturbances of the epidermis
Skin thickness determination, using calipers, ultrasound, or radiography[41]	Healthy volunteer studies to determine skin-thinning potential of topical agents
Skin absorption of radiolabeled drug[42,43]	Studies to determine drug pharmacokinetics where the use of pharmacodynamic endpoints is not feasible
Suction blisters and skin windows[38,40]	Patient studies and healthy volunteer models of eczema or inflammation to determine skin drug levels and effects at a molecular and cellular level

following application of topical vasodilators. They can be used to provide objective data to augment subjective evaluations when assessing drug effects in skin inflammatory models where the drug being tested has an effect on cutaneous blood flow.[29,30]

The measurement of transepidermal water loss (TEWL) by evaporimetry provides a practical and objective method for assessing the effect of treatment on the return to full functional integrity of the epidermis, particularly the stratum corneum. Normal function of the stratum corneum, as determined by TEWL, may occur several days after the skin has returned to normal.[31,32] Suction blister and skin window methods permit the sampling of biological fluids from deeper into the epidermis and allow the determination of skin drug concentrations at the target site following systemic administration, as well as the study of the effects of topical and systemic drugs on mediators of inflammation and other parameters at a molecular or cellular level. For example, these methods can be used to verify whether an agent (e.g., lipoxygenase blockade) actually performs its suggested role in the skin *in vivo*.[33,34]

The skin is an ideal organ for the study of human tissue pharmacology. Continual efforts to validate and standardize evaluation methods complement the advancement of new drugs for eczema, all of which are important goals of scientific efforts in this field.

REFERENCES

1. Rothe, M.J. and Grant-Kels, J.M., Atopic dermatitis: an update, *J. Am. Acad. Dermatol.*, 35, 1–13, 1996.
2. Leung, D.Y., Diaz, L.A., Deleo, V. et al., Allergic and immunologic skin disorders, *JAMA*, 278, 1914–1923, 1997.
3. Sampson, H.A., Pathogenesis of eczema, *Clin. Exp. Allergy*, 20, 459–467, 1990.
4. Chan, S.C. and Hanifin, J.M., Immunologic aspects of atopic dermatitis, *Clin. Rev. Allergy*, 11, 523–541, 1993.
5. Advenier, C. and Queille-Roussed, C., Rational use of antihistamines in allergic dermatological conditions, *Drugs*, 38, 634–644, 1984.
6. Brehler, R., Hildebrand, A., and Luger, T.A., Recent developments in the treatment of atopic eczema, *J. Am. Acad. Dermatol.*, 36, 983–994, 1997.
7. Lim, K.K., Daniel, W.P., Schroeter, A.L. et al., Cyclosporine in the treatment of dermatologic disease: an update, *Mayo Clin. Proc.*, 71, 1182–1191, 1996.

8. Hoare, C., Li Wan Po, A., and Williams, H., Systematic review of treatments for atopic eczema, *Health Technol. Assess.*, 4(37), 1–140, 2000.

9. Gibson, J.R., Kirsch, J.M., Darley, C.R. et al., An assessment of the relationship between vasoconstrictor assay findings, clinical efficacy and skin thinning effects of a variety of undiluted and diluted corticosteroid preparations, *Br. J. Dermatol.*, 111(Suppl. 27), 204–212, 1984.

10. Gibson, J.R., Hough, J.E., Marks, P. et al., Effect of concentration on the clinical potency of corticosteroid ointment formulations, in *Pharmacology and the Skin*, Vol. I, Shroot, B. and Schaefer, H., Eds., S. Karger AG, Basel, 1987, p. 214.

11. Camp, R.D.R. and Greaves, M.V., Inflammatory mediators in the skin, *Br. Med. Bull.*, 43, 401–414, 1987.

12. Wilkinson, J.D. and Rycroft, R.J.G., Contact dermatitis, in *Textbook of Dermatology*, 4th ed., Vol. I, Rook, A., Wilkinson, D.S., Ebling, F.I.G., Champion, R.H., and Burton, J.L., Eds., Blackwell Scientific, Oxford, 1992, pp. 611–715.

13. Marks, J.G. and DeLeo, V.A., *Contact and Occupational Dermatology*, 2nd ed., Mosby-Yearbook, St. Louis, MO, 1997.

14. Allen, A.M., Design methodology in trials of topical drugs, in *Safety and Efficacy of Topical Drugs and Cosmetics*, Kligman, A.M. and Leyden, J.I., Eds., Grune & Stratton, New York, 1982, p. 25.

15. Hanifin, J.M., Cooper, K.D., and Roth, H.L., Atopy and atopic dermatitis, *J. Am. Acad. Dermatol.*, 15, 703–706, 1986.

16. Meurer, M., Fartasch, M., Albrecht, G. et al., Long-term efficacy and safety of pimecrolimus cream 1% in adults with moderate atopic dermatitis, *Dermatology*, 208(4), 362–372, 2004.

17. Furue, M., Terao, H., Morai, Y. et al., Dosage and adverse effects of topical tacrolimus and steroids in daily management of atopic dermatitis, *J. Dermatol.*, 31(4), 277–283, 2004.

18. Hanifin, J.M., Atopic dermatitis: broadening the perspective, *J. Am. Acad. Dermatol.*, 51(1, Suppl.), S23–S24, 2004.

19. Grundmann-Kollmann, M. et al., Mycophenolate mofetil is effective in the treatment of atopic dermatitis, *Arch. Dermatol.*, 137(7), 870–873, 2001.

20. Frodin, T. and Skogh, M., Measurement of transepidermal water loss using an evaporimeter to follow the restitution of the barrier layer of human epidermis after stripping the stratum corneum, *Acta Derm. Venereol.*, 64, 537–540, 1984.

21. Wells, G.C., The effect of hydrocortisone on standardized skin-surface trauma, *Br. J. Dermatol.*, 69, 11, 1957.

22. Cornell, R.C. and Stoughton, R.B., Correlation of the vasoconstriction assay and clinical activity in psoriasis, *Arch. Dermatol.*, 121, 63–67, 1985.

23. Ruzicka, T., Bieber, T., Schopf, E. et al., A short-term trial of tacrolimus ointment for atopic dermatitis, *N. Engl. J. Med.*, 337, 816–821, 1997.

24. Barry, B.W., Dermatological formulations: percutaneous absorption, in *Drugs and the Pharmaceutical Sciences*, Vol. 18, Swarbrick, J., Ed., Marcel Dekker, New York, 1983, p. 164.

25. Spilker, B., Clinical evaluation of topical antipruritics and antihistamines, in *Models in Dermatology*, Vol. 3, Maibach, H.I. and Lowe, N.J., Eds., S. Karger AG, Basel, 1987, p. 55.

26. Woodward, D.F., Conway, J.L., and Wheeler, L.A., Cutaneous itching models, in *Models in Dermatology*, Vol. 1, Maibach, H.I. and Lowe, N.J., Eds., S. Karger, Basel, 1985, p. 187.

27. Doherty, V., Sylvester, D.G.H., Kennedy, C.T.C. et al., Treatment of itching in atopic eczema with antihistamines with a low sedative profile, *Br. Med. J.*, 298, 96, 1989.

28. Savin, J.A., Dow, R., Harlow, B.J. et al., The effect of a new non-sedative H_1-receptor antagonist (LN2974) on the itching and scratching of patients with atopic eczema, *Clin. Exper. Dermatol.*, 11, 600, 1986.

29. Guy, R.H., Tur, E., and Maibach, H.I., Optical techniques for monitoring cutaneous microcirculation: recent applications, *Int. J. Dermatol.*, 24, 88–94, 1985.

30. Bisgaad, H., Kristensen, J.K., and Sondergaard, J., A new technique for ranking vascular corticosteroid effects in humans using laser Doppler velocimetry, *J. Invest. Dermatol.*, 86, 275–278, 1986.

31. Blichmann, C.W. and Serup, J., Reproducibility and variability of transepidermal water loss measurement: studies on the Servo Med evaporimeterer, *Acta Derm. Venereol.*, 67, 206–210, 1987.

32. Grice, K.A., Transepidermal water loss in pathological skin, in *Pathophysiology of the Skin*, Vol. 6, Jarret, A., Ed., Academic Press, London, 1980, p. 2147.

33. Kobza Black, A., Greaves, M.W., Hensby, C.N. et al., A new method for recovery of exudates from normal and inflamed human skin, *Clin. Exp. Dermatol.*, 2, 209–216, 1977.

34. Cunningham, F.M. and Camp, R.D.R., New assays for inflammatory mediators in skin diseases, in *Models in Dermatology*, Vol. 3, Maibach, H.I. and Lowe, N.J., Eds., S. Karger AG, Basel, 1987, p. 39.

35. Wendt, H. and Frosch, P.J., *Clinico-Pharmacological Models for the Assay of Topical Corticoids*, S. Karger AG, Basel, 1982.

36. Fowle, A.S.E., Hughes, D.T.D., and Knight, G.J., The evaluation of histamine antagonists in man, *Eur. J. Clin. Pharmacol.*, 3, 215, 1971.

37. Drouard, V., Wilson, D.R., Maibach, H.I. et al., Quantitative assessment of UV-induced changes in microcirculatory flow by laser Doppler velocimetry, *J. Investig. Dermatol.*, 83, 188–192, 1984.

38. Michel, L. and Dubertret, L., A simple method for studying chemotaxis, vascular permeability and histological modifications induced by mediators of inflammation *in vivo* in man, *Br. J. Dermatol.*, 113(Suppl. 28), 61–66, 1985.

39. Stevenson, J.M., Maibach, H.I., and Guy, R.H., Laser Doppler and photoplethysmographic assessment of cutaneous microvasculature, in *Models in Dermatology*, Vol. 3, Maibach, H.I. and Lowe, N.J., Eds., S. Karger AG, Basel, 1987, p. 121.

40. Cunningham, F.M. and Camp, R.D.R., New assays for inflammatory mediators in skin diseases, in *Models in Dermatology*, Vol. 3, Maibach, H.I. and Lowe, N.J., Eds., S. Karger AG, Basel, 1987, p. 39.

41. Tan, C.Y., Statham, B., Marks, R. et al., Skin thickness measurement by pulsed ultrasound: its reproducibility, validation and variability, *Br. J. Dermatol.*, 106, 657–667, 1982.

42. Guy, R.H., Bucks, D.A.W., McMaster, J.R. et al., Kinetics of drug absorption across human skin *in vivo*, in *Pharmacology and the Skin*, Vol. I, Shroot, B. and Schaefer, H., Eds., S. Karger AG, Basel, 1987, p. 70.

43. Rougier, A. and Lotte, C., Correlations between horny layer concentration and percutaneous absorption, in *Pharmacology and the Skin*, Vol. I, Shroot, B. and Schaefer, H., Eds., S. Karger AG, Basel, 1987, p. 81.

PART **X**

Assessment of Metabolism Drugs

CHAPTER 25

Drugs for Treatment of Disorders of Lipid Metabolism

Christopher L. Wu, Lucia H. Lee, Benjamin R. Lee, and Chi-Jen Lee

CONTENTS

25.1 INTRODUCTION

Disorders of lipid metabolism and transport induce the risk of developing atherosclerotic plaque with subsequent myocardial infarction. Impaired lipid metabolism or ingestion of a high cholesterogenic diet can result in increased risk of coronary heart disease (CHD) due to elevated serum concentrations of total cholesterol, low-density lipoprotein (LDL) cholesterol, very-low-density lipoprotein (VLDL) cholesterol, lipoprotein (a), and triglyceride-rich chylomicrons and low serum concentrations of high-density lipoprotein (HDL) cholesterol. Factors that further increase the risk of CHD include hypertension, cigarette smoking, sedentary habits, diabetes mellitus, obesity, chronic renal failure, and a family history of CHD.[1,2] Intervention, such as coronary artery bypass surgery and angioplasty, can reduce the incidence of CHD in hypercholesterolemia patients.

In general, a 1% serum reduction of total cholesterol or 1.5% reduction of LDL cholesterol or a 1-mg/dL increase in HDL cholesterol concentration reduces the risk of myocardial infarction in high-risk hypercholesterolemic patients by approximately 2 to 3%.[3,4] In addition, reducing serum total cholesterol concentration from 300 to 200 mg/dL increases life expectancy by up to 3 years and delays symptomatic CHD by up to 5 years.[5]

Dietary and endogenous fatty acids and cholesterol are transported after incorporation into lipoprotein molecules. The lipoproteins involved in lipid transport are metabolically interrelated. They are separated by density and electrophoretic migration into five classes:

- Chylomycrons, the largest lipoproteins, consist of 90% triglycerides and about 5% cholesterol by weight.
- Very-low-density lipoprotein (VLDL) consists of 60% triglycerides and 10 to 15% cholesterol.
- Intermediate-density lipoprotein (IDL) consists of approximately equal proportions of cholesterol and triglycerides.
- Low-density lipoprotein (LDL) consists of almost 50% cholesterol and <10% triglycerides; it carries 60 to 70% of total circulating cholesterol.
- High-density lipoprotein (HDL) consists of about 20 to 30% cholesterol and <5% triglyceride.

The endogenous lipid transport pathway originates in the liver, where triglycerides and cholesterol are either synthesized or recycled through VLDL, IDL, and LDL. LDL particles can become highly atherogenic after oxidation in the peripheral vasculature. This process is accelerated by the presence of prooxidants. Oxidized LDL is toxic to endothelial cells and triggers secretion of platelet activation factors, which stimulate smooth-muscle cell proliferation, tissue hyperplasia, and progression of atherosclerotic lesions. HDL particles are synthesized in the liver and intestine. HDL may inhibit atherogenesis. It facilitates lipoprotein metabolism, inhibits LDL oxidation, stimulates prostacyclin secretion, and promotes fibrinolysis. It also inhibits platelet activation, oxidized LDL aggregation, and binding to scavenger receptors.[6]

The major lipoprotein disorders (dyslipidemias) are classified based on the lipid abnormality and clinical manifestations. Primary dyslipidemias are genetically determined, whereas secondary dyslipidemias are associated with certain diseases, diets, and drug therapy. Dyslipidemia results from malfunction of the metabolic steps involved in the synthesis, transport, interconversion, or catabolism of lipoproteins.

Definitions of desirable (<200 mg/dL), borderline (200 to 239 mg/dL), and high (240 mg/dL) serum total cholesterol concentrations reflect the ranges associated with, respectively, baseline, increasing, and more than double risk of death from cardiovascular disease.[7] Because LDL cholesterol is the principal atherogenic component of circulating lipids, ranges of serum LDL cholesterol concentrations have been classified as desirable (<130 mg/dL), borderline high risk (130 to 159 mg/dL), and high risk (160 mg/dL). Hypercholesterolemia is redefined in the presence of multiple risk factors. Patients with CHD or atherosclerotic diseases are at substantially increased risk for adverse events when serum LDL cholesterol concentrations exceed 130 mg/dL; in these patients, serum LDL cholesterol concentrations that are <100 or <70 mg/dL and serum HDL cholesterol concentrations up to >35 (or 45) mg/dL are now considered desirable. In addition, fasting plasma triglyceride concentrations are now classified as normal (<200 mg/dL), borderline high (200 to 400 mg/dL), high (400 to 1000 mg/dL), and very high (>1000 mg/dL).[7] Evaluations should be conducted at 5-year intervals in adults not at risk and more often in those at risk and during therapeutic intervention.

25.2 AVAILABLE DRUGS AND THEIR MECHANISMS OF ACTION

No single drug is effective in the treatment of all types of lipoprotein disorders, and the long-term safety of some agents has not been established. The drugs used to treat lipoprotein disorders can be grouped on the basis of common mechanisms of action or on common effects on plasma lipids (see Table 25.1).[8–11]

Table 25.1 Available Drugs for Treatment of Disorders of Lipid Metabolism

Drug Category	Mechanism of Action
Bile acid sequestering resins:	
Cholestyramine resin Colestipol	Reversibly bind bile acids in the small intestine
Fibric acid derivatives:	
Clofibrate Fenofibrate Bezafibrate	Reduce serum very-low-density lipoprotein (VLDL) and plasma triglyceride concentrations
Hydroxy-3-methylglutaryl coenzyme A (HMG-CoA) reductase inhibitors:	
Fluvastatin Lovastatin Prabastatin Simvastatin	Inhibit cholesterol synthesis
Others:	
Niacin (nicotinic acid)	Decreases hepatic VLDL synthesis and secretion
Probucol	Decreases serum LDL cholesterol concentrations

25.2.1 Bile-Acid-Sequestering Resins

Cholestyramine and colestipol interfere with the absorption of cholesterol-derived bile acids from the gut, resulting in a reduction in hepatic cholesterol content and an increase in hepatic uptake of circulating LDL. The resins are interchangeable, used both for their hypocholesterolemic effect and in the treatment of lipoprotein disorders in which LDL cholesterol concentration cannot be decreased by diet alone. They are the drugs of choice for familial and polygenic hypercholesterolemia to reduce the risks of atherosclerotic coronary artery disease and myocardial infarction. When used as adjuncts to dietary control, they reduce serum LDL cholesterol concentration an average of an additional 20 to 30% in a dose-dependent manner.

The combination of niacin and cholestyramine has reduced LDL-cholesterol concentrations more than maximal doses of either agent alone (e.g., 40 to 60%). Similar decreases have followed a combination of a resin and a hydroxy-3-methylglutaryl coenzyme A (HMG-CoA) reductase inhibitor. Colestipol (15 g/day) lowered serum cholesterol concentrations, significantly reduced the incidence of cardiovascular disease-related death, and stabilized atherosclerotic lesions in similar populations of patients.[12] Patients with hypercholesterolemia and a history of coronary artery disease who were given either cholestyramine (16 or 24 g/day) or colestipol (15 g/day) in addition to dietary therapy for up to 7 years had decreased progression of coronary artery narrowing, increased frequency of lesion regression, and decreased frequency of fatal and nonfatal myocardial infarction, stroke, angina, coronary artery bypass surgery, and angioplasty.[13] Cholestyramine and colestipol are among the safest drugs currently available to treat hypercholesterolemia; cholestyramine has been no more toxic than placebo during up to 13 years of use.[14]

25.2.2 Fibric Derivatives

The fibric acid derivatives (clofibrate, gemfibrozil, fenofibrate, benzafibrate) produce variable decreases in serum total or LDL cholesterol concentrations but are effective in controlling hypertriglyceridemia. They are useful in disorders characterized by hypertriglyceridemia and in familial dysbetalipoproteinemia.[15] When combined with bile-acid-sequestering resins or niacin, fenofibrate or benzafibrate have additive effects in decreasing serum LDL cholesterol and plasma triglyceride concentrations and in increasing serum HDL cholesterol concentrations. They are frequently combined with cholestyramine or colestipol because their actions on serum LDL cholesterol concentration are complementary. In double-blind trials, fenofibrate (100 mg three times daily) or benzafibrate (400 to 600 mg daily) combined with modified-fat diets for 1 to 6 months reduced serum LDL cholesterol concentrations by an additional 5 to 37% and plasma triglyceride concentrations by 13 to 67% and increased serum HDL cholesterol concentrations by 10 to 34% in hypercholesterolemic patients with mild hypertriglyceridemia when compared with the effects achieved by diet therapy or placebo.[16]

25.2.3 HMG-CoA Reductase Inhibitors

The 3-hydroxy-3-methylglutaryl coenzyme A reductase inhibitors (fluvastatin, lovastatin, provastatin, and simvastatin) directly inhibit cholesterogenesis and accelerate LDL clearance. They are more potent in reducing serum total and LDL cholesterol concentrations than other available drugs and are well tolerated.[17] Combining HMG-CoA reductase inhibitors with bile-acid-sequestering resins or niacin enhances the effects on cholesterol metabolism. Inhibition of cholesterol synthesis stimulates upregulation of high-affinity cell surface receptors for LDL; as hepatic uptake of LDL increases, serum total and LDL cholesterol concentrations decrease. In addition, hepatic synthesis of apolipoprotein B and VLDL is inhibited by HMG-CoA reductase inhibitors, especially fluvastatin.[18] HMG-CoA reductase inhibitors inhibit the absorption of dietary cholesterol by reducing acyl coenzyme A:cholesterol acyltransferase activity in intestinal cells. They also decrease the susceptibility of LDL to peroxidation.[19] HMG-CoA reductase inhibitors are well tolerated for at least 5 years and cause fewer adverse reactions than bile-sequestering resins.[20,21] Rhabdomyolysis with myalgia, with or without acute renal failure secondary to myoglobinuria, has occurred in fewer than 0.2% of patients receiving HMG-CoA reductase inhibitor monotherapy.[22]

25.2.4 Others

Niacin decreases hepatic VLDL synthesis and secretion. As a result, plasma triglyceride and serum VLDL and LDL cholesterol concentrations decrease. Niacin also stimulates the synthesis and secretion of HDL and apo A-1, which increase serum HDL_3 concentrations, as well as serum HDL_2 concentrations. In familial dysbetalipoproteinemia, serum lipid concentrations are reduced to normal. Probucol decreases serum LDL cholesterol concentrations by enhancing hepatic LDL uptake through a receptor-independent pathway and by increasing fecal bile acid excretion. It does not reduce serum triglyceride concentrations in most patients. It inhibits oxidative modification of LDL particles, reducing their atherogenicity. The antioxidant actions of probucol are more important than its lipid-lowering effects in preventing cardiovascular disease.

25.3 LABORATORY ASSESSMENTS OF LIPID-ACTING DRUGS

Most lipid-acting drugs are designed to lower blood levels of low-density lipoprotein cholesterol or triglycerides, to raise levels of high-density lipoprotein cholesterol, or to provide a combination of these effects. It is ideal to test experimental drugs in the absence of other medications to ensure that the effects on the therapeutic endpoints and side effects are due to the new drug candidate. In early studies, it is necessary to exclude patients taking other medications, but late phase II studies may include such patients as they are likely to be eligible for later trials. Patients with any illness that affects lipid levels or lipoprotein regulation mechanisms, such as diabetes, hypothyroidism, renal, pancreatic, or liver disease, or who are severely obese should not participate in the trials. Routine biochemical tests on liver and renal function should be normal except for minor elevations in some patients with dyslipidemia; for example, results might include:

- Borderline low thyroid function tests
- Mild elevations of serum creatine phosphokinase (SCPK) levels
- Mild elevations in serum bilirubins
- Mild elevations of serum creatinine due to some degree of renal atherosclerosis

Abnormal liver function tests are frequently seen in dyslipidemias with fatty infiltration of the liver. Monitoring levels for abnormalities in these tests are important to rule out hepatotoxic effects of drugs; therefore, in the early clinical trials, liver function tests, such as alanine aminotransferase (ALT) levels, must be normal before drug administration. Minor elevation in serum aspartate aminotransferase (AST) can be tolerated only if ALT levels are normal. Patients with fasting hyperbilirubinemia are acceptable in trials if they have no other abnormalities in liver function or bilirubin metabolism. Alkaline phosphatase levels are to be normal or not larger than twice the upper limit of normal at baseline. Fasting blood glucose levels should be normal, but levels up to 140 mg/dL are usually accepted in the absence of any other symptom of diabetes.

One of the following levels of laboratory assessments of lipoprotein can be used, depending on the specific study requirements:

- Level 1 — Basic serum concentrations of lipid content including total cholesterol, triglycerides, HDL, and an estimated LDL
- Level 2 — Above, plus directly measured LDL for studies allowing serum triglyceride levels above 400 gm/dL
- Level 3 — Above, plus apolipoproteins A-1 and B-100, lipoprotein (a), and LDL/HDL cholesterol subfraction analyses
- Level 4 — Above, plus apolipoprotein E genotype and LDLC oxidation susceptibility, as well as measurement of lipoprotein (a), a newly discovered proatherogenic and prothrombotic risk factor, and intestinal cholesterol or fat absorption to determine drug actions on these parameters

Total serum cholesterol and triglycerides are measured enzymatically.[23] The total cholesterol value is the sum of all cholesterol in the blood including LDL, HDL, and VLDL. About 70% of the cholesterol is esterified, and 30% is free. When triglyceride levels are the primary target for therapy, glycerol blanking (removal of background serum glycerol levels) is necessary. Free glycerol present in the serum is measured before the addition of lipase and then subtracted from the total triglyceride measured after incubation with lipase.

For determination of LDL cholesterol, three approaches are available:

- Measure the total cholesterol, HDL cholesterol, and triglyceride concentrations, then estimate the LDLC concentration using the Friedwald equation:[24] LDLC = Total cholesterol – HDL cholesterol – (triglycerides/5). This method is adequate for estimation of LDL cholesterol in routine patient care, but in trials of new drugs it is more appropriate to measure LDL cholesterol directly.
- In the beta-quantification method,[25] the plasma is ultracentrifuged to float the VLDL fraction, which is then removed. The cholesterol content is determined enzymatically, and the HDL cholesterol value is subtracted to obtain the LDL cholesterol content.
- A newer method for direct measurement is performed using immunoseparation.[26] In this method, whole serum is mixed with a reagent containing microbeads to which all non-LDL binds. After centrifugation, the remaining LDL cholesterol fraction is determined. The VLDL cholesterol value is estimated using the Friedwald equation or the beta-quantification procedure.

High-density lipoprotein is measured directly in serum or plasma after precipitation of all apolipoprotein B-containing lipoproteins with a divalent cation and a polyanion.[27] Apolipoprotein A-1 (apo A-1) and apo B-100 are the major proteins of HDL and LDL/VLDL, respectively. Apo-A measurement can be used as a surrogate of HDL, whereas apo B-100 estimates the total number of LDL and VLDL fractions. In addition, because oxidized LDL is atherogenic, its content has been tested in lipid-acting drugs and antioxidative vitamins for their effectiveness to reduce the susceptibility of LDL to *in vitro* oxidation. In this procedure, the lag time is measured after incubation of isolated LDL with copper ions.[28] Laboratories for conducting tests in clinical trials with dyslipidemic drugs should be standardized. The Centers for Disease Control and Prevention (CDC) lipid standardization program was designed for lipid research laboratories to evaluate total cholesterol, triglycerides, HDL, and other lipid contents.

25.4 ASSESSMENTS OF LIPID-ACTING DRUGS IN CLINICAL TRIALS

Early clinical trials, which are strategically important in the development of drugs for the treatment of disorders of lipid metabolism, are designed to estimate short-term safety and efficacy as well as dosage of a new compound. Potential interactions with commonly used drugs (e.g., analgesics, hormones) or other drugs frequently administered to dyslipidemic patients are also examined in these trials. Patients who are healthy except for dyslipidemia symptoms can substitute for healthy volunteers in late phase I or early phase II clinical trials. This approach has several advantages:

- Evidence can be obtained earlier regarding the efficacy of the lipid-acting compound on treatment of abnormal serum lipids.
- Dose–efficacy response can be measured.
- Evaluation in subjects with elevated serum lipoprotein indicates whether or not the new drug has pharmacokinetic parameters that differ in these patients compared to healthy subjects.

Parallel, controlled, double-blind, placebo vs. drug studies are ideal; however, the use of placebo controls becomes more difficult in trials longer than 3 to 6 months. Ethical considerations make it necessary to use positive controls with a dose of a drug for which short-term side effects are similar to placebo and the therapeutic potency is established (e.g., 10 to 20 mg/day of lovastatin). Crossover designs are not as desirable as parallel designs; however, crossover designs are useful in studying effects on parameters that have a wide range of individual abnormality, such as serum triglyceride concentrations.

It is important to establish efficacy endpoints for clinical trials.[29] Any new hypolipidemic drug must lower cholesterol levels by a mean of at least 15% in dyslipidemic patients. It is now desirable for treatments of lipid metabolism disorders to reduce serum LDL cholesterol concentrations to 100 or even 70 mg/dL, reduce triglycerides to below 200 mg/dL, and raise HDL cholesterol to over 45 mg/dL.

Early clinical trials should be aware of the following possible adverse reactions:

- Eyes — Cataract formation or other ocular dysfunction; because of the role of lipids in the metabolism of the lens tissue, these side effects are potentially irreversible.
- Liver — Hepatotoxicity; the liver plays important roles in lipoprotein regulation mechanisms, as well as first-pass effects and biliary excretion of many drugs.
- Muscle — Myopathies and associated myotoxicity; dyslipidemia is related to muscle-associated disorders with or without drug treatment.
- Neuropsychiatric system — Insomnia and behavioral changes; lipid components are contained in the nervous system, and many drugs induce differences in the lipid/water partition coefficient.

Phase II trials are ideal for conducting in-depth pharmacodynamic and pharmacokinetic studies of the new compound. Pharmacokinetic data obtained from phase II studies facilitate the planning of large-scale clinical trials by demonstrating the following:

- Important kinetic changes among populations of different age, sex, and ethnic characteristics
- Potential kinetic changes in different lipoprotein abnormality patterns

- Pharmacokinetic characteristics that establish the best time of drug administration for optimum efficacy and safety
- Inappropriate dosages and administration
- Drug interactions that might arise during future drug therapy

Careful planning of phase II trials provides the data required to perform subsequent large-scale, scientifically valid phase III trials.

Phase III trials are designed to demonstrate and confirm the efficacy of a new drug in the actual target population based on statistically and clinically significant evidence. A phase III trial is a randomized, double-blind, controlled study that balances potential variables affecting disease risk and avoids possible bias in the assessment of the clinical endpoints. The design maximizes the chance that a difference in clinical symptoms between two equivalent groups is due to the effect of the drug compound being evaluated. The sample size of a phase III trial (often several hundred to several thousand subjects from the high-risk population) must be adequate to support rigorous hypothesis testing. Trial conclusions supported by statistically valid comparisons provide convincing evidence for effectiveness and safety.

Following licensure of the drug product, a postmarketing survey is conducted to address concerns arising during review of prelicensure data. The postmarketing survey monitors drug efficacy and safety in a large population or in certain subpopulations, such as the elderly. When a drug is used in a large population, very rare adverse reactions, unrecognized drug interactions that may occur with commonly administered medications, and the incidence of nonresponders can be determined.

REFERENCES

1. Ross, R., The pathogenesis of atherosclerosis: a perspective for the 1990s, *Nature*, 362, 801–809, 1993.
2. Neaton, J.D. and Wentworth, D., Serum cholesterol, blood pressure, cigarette smoking, and death from coronary heart disease: overall findings and differences by age for 316,099 white men, *Arch. Intern. Med.*, 152, 56–64, 1992.
3. Manson, J.E. et al., The primary prevention of myocardial infarction, *N. Engl. J. Med.*, 326, 1406–1416, 1992.
4. Stampfer, M.J. et al., A prospective study of cholesterol, apolipoproteins, and the risk of myocardial infarction, *N. Engl. J. Med.*, 325, 373–381, 1991.
5. Grover, S.A. et al., The benefits of treating hyperlipidemia to prevent coronary heart disease: estimating changes in life expectancy and morbidity, *JAMA*, 267, 816–822, 1992.
6. Badimon, J.J. et al., Role of high density lipoproteins in the regression of atherosclerosis, *Circulation*, 86(Suppl. III), III-86–III-94, 1992.
7. Expert Panel, *Second Report of the Expert Panel on Detection, Evaluation, and Treatment of High Blood Cholesterol in Adults (Adult Treatment Panel II)*, National Cholesterol Education Program, National Heart, Blood, and Lung Institute, Washington, D.C., 1993.
8. Dujovne, C.A., New lipid lowering drugs and new effects of old drugs, *Curr. Opin. Lipidol.*, 8(6), 362–368, 1997.
9. Dujovne, C.A., Drug intervention trials in dyslipidemia: the past and the future, *Clin. Cardiol.*, 14(2, Suppl. 1), 148–152, 1991.
10. Wierzbicki, A.S., New lipid-lowering agents, *Expert Opin. Emerg. Drugs*, 8(2), 365–376, 2003.
11. McKenney, J.M., Pharmacotherapy of dyslipidemia, *Cardiovasc. Drugs Ther.*, 15(5), 413–422, 2001.
12. Kuo, P.T. et al., Use of combined diet and colestipol in long-term (7–7.5 years) treatment of patients with type II hyperlipoproteinemia, *Circulation*, 59, 199–211, 1979.
13. Brensike, J.F. et al., Effects of therapy with cholestyramine on progression of coronary atheriosclerosis: results of the NHLBI type II coronary intervention study, *Circulation*, 69, 313–324, 1984.
14. Lipid Research Clinics Investigators, The Lipid Research Clinics Coronary Primary Prevention Trial: results of 6 years of post-trial follow-up, *Arch. Intern, Med.*, 152, 1399–1410, 1992.

15. Frick, M.H. et al., Helsinki Heart Study: primary-prevention trial with gemfibrozil in middle-aged men with dyslipidemia — safety of treatment, changes in risk factors, and incidence of coronary heart disease, *N. Engl. J. Med.*, 317, 1237–1245, 1987.

16. Balfour, J.A. et al., Fenofibrate: a review of its pharmacodynamic and pharmacokinetic properties and therapeutic use in dyslipidaemia, *Drugs*, 40, 260–290, 1990.

17. Mantell, G., Lipid lowering drugs in atherosclerosis: the HMG-CoA reductase inhibitors, *Clin. Exp. Hypertens. A*, 11(5–6), 927–941, 1989.

18. Levy, R.I. et al., A quarter century of drug treatment of dyslipoproteinemias, with a focus on the new HMG-CoA reductase inhibitor fluvastatin, *Circulation*, 87(Suppl. 4), III45–III53, 1993.

19. Hoffman, R. et al., Hypolipidemic drugs reduce lipoprotein susceptibility to undergo lipid peroxidation: *in vitro* and *ex vivo* studies, *Atherosclerosis*, 93, 105–113, 1992.

20. Boccuzi, S.J. et al., Long term experience with simvastatin, *Drug Invest.*, 5, 135–140, 1993.

21. McGovern, M.E. and Mellies, M.J., Long-term experience with provastatin in clinical research trials, *Clin. Ther.*, 15, 57–64, 1993.

22. Bradford, R.H. et al., Expanded clinical evaluation of lovastatin (EXCEL) study results. I. Efficacy in modifying plasma lipoproteins and adverse event profile in 8245 patients with moderate hypercholesterolemia, *Arch. Intern. Med.*, 151, 43–49, 1991.

23. Warnick, G.R., Enzymatic methods for quantitation of lipoprotein lipid, *Methods Enzymol.*, 129, 101–123, 1986.

24. Friedewald, W.T., Levy, R.I., and Fredrickson, D.S., Estimation of the concentration of LDL cholesterol in plasma without the use of the ultracentrifuge, *Clin. Chem.*, 18, 499–502, 1972.

25. Belcher, J.D., McNamara, J.R., Grinstead, G.F. et al., Measurement of low-density lipoprotein cholesterol concentration, in *Laboratory Measurement of Lipids, Lipoproteins and Apolipoproteins*, Rifai, N. and Warnick, G.R., Eds., American Association for Clinical Chemistry Press, Washington, D.C., 1994, pp. 107–124.

26. Singh, J., Kulig, K., and Lucco, L., Determination of direct LDL cholesterol in human serum triglycerides 400 mg/dl by Genzyme Immunoseparation reagent (Gen-LDL) kit, *Clin. Chem.*, 40, 1099–1100, 1994.

27. Wiebe, D.A. and Warnick, G.R., Measurement of high density lipoprotein cholesterol concentration, in *Laboratory Measurement of Lipids, Lipoproteins and Apolipoproteins*, Rifai, N. and Warnick, G.R., Eds., American Association for Clinical Chemistry Press, Washington, D.C., 1994, pp. 91–106.

28. Jialal, I. and Scaccini, C., Laboratory assessment of lipoprotein oxidation, in *Laboratory Measurement of Lipids, Lipoproteins and Apolipoproteins*, Rifai, N. and Warnick, G.R., Eds., American Association for Clinical Chemistry Press, Washington, D.C., 1994, pp. 307–321.

29. Steiner, G., Clinical trial assessment of lipid-acting drugs in diabetic patients, *Am. J. Cardiol.*, 81(8A), 58F–59F, 1998.

CHAPTER 26

Antidiabetic Drugs

Christopher L. Wu, Lucia H. Lee, Benjamin R. Lee, and Chi-Jen Lee

CONTENTS

26.1 INTRODUCTION

The term "diabetes mellitus" is derived from the Greek word *diabetes* for "siphon" and *mellitus* for "sweet," based on the original diagnosis of polyurea and sweet-tasting urine. The disease is comprised of a spectrum of conditions, with hyperglycemia being the common medical finding. It is a prevalent biochemical abnormality where insulin-sensitive cells are deficient for glucose metabolism, despite a paradoxical abundance of glucose in the plasma. The two main forms are type 1 diabetes (insulin-dependent diabetes mellitus, or IDDM) and type 2 diabetes (non-insulin-dependent diabetes mellitus, or NIDDM). Diabetes is a chronic disease characterized by disorders in carbohydrate, fat, and protein metabolism caused by a deficiency in the action of insulin and possibly abnormally high amounts of glucagons and other counter-regulatory hormones such as growth hormone, sympathomimetic amines, and corticosteroids. Insulin secretion in patients with type 1 diabetes is normally deficient to nonexistent, whereas those with type 2 diabetes may have normal, high, or low insulin secretion.

Type 1 diabetes results from immune-mediated destruction of the β-cells of the pancreas, resulting in insulin deficiency. Patients with type 1 disease are more likely to develop ketoacidosis than patients with type 2. Genetic susceptibility to type 1 diabetes is linked to two genes on chromosome 6. These genes control production of human lymphocyte antigens (HLAs) DR3 and

DR4. Of patients with type 1 diabetes, 95% have one or both of these antigens. In addition, most patients have circulating antibodies, islet cell antibodies (ICAs), and insulin autoantibodies (IAAs) before overt type 1 disease develops. On the other hand, patients with type 2 diabetes usually have insulin resistance with variable insulin secretion and are obese. Their blood sugars remain elevated because of tissue resistance to the action of insulin. Many patients have hypertension, dyslipidemia, and impaired fibrinolysis, a collection of conditions referred to as syndrome X. These patients are more likely to experience cardiovascular disease and develop long-term complications of diabetes. They exhibit two major metabolic defects: (1) decreased sensitivity of target tissues, primarily the liver and skeletal muscle, to the actions of insulin, and (2) relatively deficient endogenous insulin secretion. Impaired insulin secretion and increased glucagons contribute to continued hepatic glucose output, resulting in elevated fasting glucose levels.

26.2 CLINICAL SYMPTOMS AND DIAGNOSIS

Type 1 diabetes usually occurs rapidly, with excessive thirst, quantity of urine, and desire to eat; weakness; weight loss; dry skin; and ketoacidosis. On the other hand, type 2 diabetes is slow and insidious in onset and frequently unaccompanied by symptoms. Type 2 disease often is discovered when glucose is found in the urine or when elevated blood sugar is observed during a routine health examination. The patients usually are over 40 years old and obese. Examination of these patients often reveals glucosuria, proteinuria, hyperglycemia after eating, microaneurysms, and retinal exudates. Other symptoms of hyperglycemia associated with diabetes include blurred vision, numbness of the extremities, slow-healing skin infections, itching, drowsiness, and irritability. Patients with these symptoms and who have a family history of diabetes should be examined closely for hyperglycemia. Generally, type 1 diabetes is easy to diagnose because patients exhibit all of the classic symptoms of diabetes and high concentrations of glucose in the urine and blood. Type 2 diabetes is more difficult to diagnose because patients do not present with the classic symptoms. Diabetes can be diagnosed in three ways:

- *Fasting plasma glucose concentration* is the preferred testing method, because it is fast, inexpensive, and easy to perform. Blood is drawn from the patient after an overnight fast. Normal values are in the range of 65 to 110 mg/dL. The diagnosis of diabetes is confirmed in patients with two or more fasting plasma glucose levels above 126 mg/dL (7 mmol/L).
- The *oral glucose tolerance test (OGTT)* is a less commonly used and more cumbersome test. This test measures the patient's ability to utilize a glucose load over a period of time. After an overnight fast, a morning fasting blood sugar is drawn and the patient ingests a 75-g glucose load. Blood samples are then drawn at half-hour intervals for 2 hours and then at 3 hours. In normal subjects, the blood glucose level returns to normal in less than 2 hours. In patients with diabetes, the glucose peak is higher and occurs much later than in healthy subjects, and the glucose level declines at a slower rate. A normal OGTT occurs when the fasting plasma glucose is less than 115 mg/dL, the 2-hour plasma glucose is less than 140 mg/dL, and the glucose peak values are below 200 mg/dL.
- *Urine tests* are performed for evaluating glucose, ketones, and protein levels. Glycosuria is observed under many conditions. It occurs when the renal threshold of glucose level exceeds 180 mg/dL or higher; however, older patients may have obvious diabetes that may not be detected by urine analysis. Urine ketone testing should be performed for the patient with diabetes during acute illness or stress or when blood glucose levels are not well controlled. Patients with type 1 disease should test for urine ketones when blood sugar readings are greater than 240 mg/dL. Urine protein tests are used as a screening tool for the presence of diabetic nephropathy. Patients who test negative with standard dipstick methods may be further evaluated with a microalbumin test or by 24-hour urine collections.

Hemoglobin glycosylation occurs when hemoglobin is exposed to ambient glucose concentrations in the blood. When higher concentrations of blood glucose are present, the percentage of glycosylated hemoglobin (HbAlc) increases. The HbAlc reflects glycemic control for that time period and most precisely reflects the average blood sugar from the previous 2 to 3 months. Generally, a person without diabetes has a HbAlc in the range of 4 to 6%, and a patient with diabetes may have values as high as 20%. Usually for each 1% rise in HbAlc value, the average serum blood sugar increases by 30 mg/dL. Thus, a patient with an HbAlc value of 6% would correlate with an average blood sugar of 120 mg/dL. The clinical endpoint for glycosylated hemoglobin is less than 7%.

Proteins in the blood can become glycated, similar to hemoglobin. The half-life of serum abumin ranges from 14 to 20 days, and it acts as a marker of glycemic control over a shorter time frame than HbAlc. Serum fructosamine assay is a common method of measuring glycated abumin in the body and is highly correlated with HbAlc values.

26.3 DRUGS USED FOR TREATMENT OF DIABETES

The number of drugs available in the United States for the treatment of diabetes has expanded greatly in the past few years. Currently, six main categories of drugs are available for treating diabetes (see Table 26.1).[1-3]

26.3.1 Insulin

Insulins may be categorized into groups on the basis of their time–activity profiles: ultrashort-acting (2- to 4-hr duration), short-acting (6- to 8-hr duration), intermediate-acting (16- to 24-hr duration), and long-acting (24- to 36-hr duration) (see Table 26.1). Human insulin analogs have a structure and function similar to human insulin but are developed with DNA recombinant technology. By altering the amino acid sequence in human insulin, various alterations in the actions of insulin can be prepared. In insulin lispro, the normal sequence of proline and lysine is reversed at the amino acid 28 and 29 positions. The change in amino acid sequence results in rapid absorption from the subcutaneous tissues, resulting in a faster pharmacologic action than human regular insulin.[4]

Semilente, a short-acting insulin, is an amorphous precipitate of insulin and zinc in the form of a suspension; it has a slightly delayed onset and peak and a greater duration of action than regular insulin. Intermediate-acting insulin (hagedorn [NPH] insulin preparation) contains a suspension of zinc–insulin crystals and protamine. Certain patients taking these preparations can become allergic to protamine. Lente® insulin is composed of a 30:70 mixture of semilente and Ultralente®. The Lente® insulins are produced from various forms of the zinc–insulin complex and are useful in patients sensitive to protamine. The only available long-acting insulin is Ultralente®. Human insulin is the least antigenic of the available insulins and tends to be more soluble than animal insulins, resulting in more rapid absorption and shorter duration. Biosynthetic insulin formed by recombinant DNA using *Escherichia coli* (Eli Lilly), baker's yeast (Novo Nordisk), and semi-synthetic (Novo Nordisk) insulin are therapeutically similar.

26.3.2 Sulfonylureas

Sulfonylureas are one of the main therapeutic options for patients with type 2 diabetes. These products increase insulin secretion directly and decrease glucagon release. They may affect glucose levels by increasing insulin receptor binding affinity, increasing insulin effect by post-receptor action, and decreasing hepatic insulin extraction. Chlorpropamide has the longest half-life of the first-generation agents and is associated with the highest incidence of adverse reactions. Drug interactions with the first-generation agents include alcohol, anabolic steroids, beta-blockers, dicumarol, monoamine oxidase inhibitors, salicylates, and sulfonamides. Second-generation sulfonylureas are more potent and tend to have fewer drug interactions, because they bind nonionically

Table 26.1 Drugs for the Treatment of Diabetes

Product	Brand Name	Mechanism of Action	Side Effects
Insulin			
Insulin lispro	Humalog®	Stimulates the release of insulin from pancreatic β-cells	Hypoglycemia, lipohypertrophy, lipoatrophy
Insulin (systemic)	Humulin® R, Novolin® R, Velosulin® Human R	Stimulates the release of insulin from pancreatic β-cells (short-acting)	
	Lente®, NPH Iletin® II, Novolin® L, Novolin® N	Stimulates the release of insulin from pancreatic β-cells (intermediate-acting)	
	Humulin® 50/50, Humulin® 70/30, Humulin® U, Novolin® 70/30, Ultralente®	Stimulates the release of insulin from pancreatic β-cells (long-acting)	
Sulfonylureas (First Generation)			
Acetohexamide	Dymelor®	Stimulate the release of insulin	Hypoglycemia, weight gain, syndrome of inappropriate antidiuretic hormone (SIADH), disulfiram reaction
Tolazamide	Tolinase®		
Tolbutamide	Orinase®		
Sulfonylreas (Second Generation)			
Glimepiride	Amaryl®	Stimulate the release of insulin	Hypoglycemia, weight gain, syndrome of inappropriate antidiuretic hormone (SIADH), disulfiram reaction
Glipizide	Glucotrol® and Glucotrol® XL		
Glyburide	Diabeta®, Micronase®, and Glynase®		
α-Glucosidase Inhibitors			
Arabose	Precose®	Competitive and reversible inhibition of intestinal α-glucoside hydrolast and pancreatic α-amylase, resulting in delayed carbohydrate metabolism and absorption	Diarrhea, abdominal pain, increase in liver function test values
Miglitol	Glyset®	Competitive and reversible inhibition of intestinal α-glucoside hydrolast and pancreatic α-amylase, resulting in delayed carbohydrate metabolism and absorption	Diarrhea, abdominal pain

Biguanide			
Metformin	Glucophage®	Decreases hepatic glucose production and increases peripheral insulin sensitivity	Diarrhea, abdominal pain, megaloblastic anemia, lactic acidosis, and alterations in taste
Thiazolidinediones			
Troglitazone	Rezulin®	Increases skeletal muscle cell sensitivity and decreases hepatic glucose production	Liver failure, risk of pregnancy in anovulatory women, and hypoglycemia
Rosiglitazone	Avandia®	Increases skeletal muscle cell sensitivity and decreases hepatic glucose production	Mild to moderate edema, anemia, increase in blood cholesterol
Pioglitazone	Actos®	Increases skeletal muscle cell sensitivity and decreases hepatic glucose production	Mild to moderate edema, anemia, increase in blood cholesterol
Meglitinides			
Repaglinide	Prandin®	Increases insulin secretion by the pancreas	Hypoglycemia, weight gain

and are present at much lower concentrations than the first-generation agents. Tolbutamide, tolazamide, and glipizide are metabolized to inactive metabolites and are favored in patients with renal failure. The newest sulfonylurea, glimepiride, has effects similar to those of the other agents and can be given once daily. In addition, it has a lower incidence of hypoglycemia than other sulfonylureas.[5] The primary side effects of sulfonylureas include hypoglycemia and weight gain. Conditions in which the sulfonylureas are contraindicated include acidosis, severe infections, major surgery, sulfa sensitivity, and pregnancy. Approximately 40% of patients with type 2 diabetes do not achieve satisfactory control with the sulfonylureas.

26.3.3 α-Glucosidase Inhibitors

The α-glucosidase inhibitors, such as acarbose and miglitol, reduce the small intestinal absorption of starch, dextran, and disaccharides by competitively inhibiting the action of the intestinal brush border enzyme, α-glucosidase, which is responsible for the generation of monosaccharides. Inhibition of α-glucosidase, which is the final step in carbohydrate transfer across the small intestine, slows down the absorption of carbohydrates. These drugs are used for the treatment of patients with type 2 diabetes who are inadequately controlled by diet or other oral antidiabetic drugs. Clinical trials of α-glucosidase inhibitors show decreases in postprandial glucose levels and glycosylated hemoglobin (HbA1c) levels of 0.5 to 1%. Miglitol reduces HbA1c less effectively than glyburide and causes more gastrointestinal side effects. Miglitol, which must be taken with each meal, has little effect on fasting blood glucose concentrations but decreases postprandial glucose levels at lower insulin concentrations than those observed with sulfonylureas. It is not associated with hypoglycemia, hyperinsulinism, or weight gain. Significant hepatic injury has been observed with chronic acarbose therapy, which was not detected in clinical trials. The incidence appears to be low and unpredictable. Transaminase levels should be checked regularly in patients taking acarbose.

26.3.4 Biguanides

Three biguanides — metformin, phenformin, and buformin — have historically been used for the treatment of type 2 diabetes, but only metformin remains in use today. Phenformin was removed from the market in 1976 because of a high incidence of lactic acidosis. Metformin lowers blood glucose by reducing hepatic glucose production and glycogen metabolism in the liver and enhancing insulin-mediated glucose uptake by skeletal muscle. Abdominal bloating, nausea, intestinal cramping, and diarrhea are common adverse effects of metformin. Metoformin is not metabolized and is secreted by the renal tubules, so it is contraindicated in patients with renal dysfunction, hepatic dysfunction, lactic acidosis, alcoholism, or congestive heart failure. Administration of metformin reduces fasting plasma glucose levels an average of 58 mg/dL and HbA1c an average of 1.8%. In addition, it is associated with a reduction in triglyceride concentration (16%), low-density lipoprotein (LDL) cholesterol (8%), and total cholesterol (5%), as well as a slight increase in high-density lipoprotein (HDL) cholesterol (2%).[6] Many patients lose a small amount of body weight.

26.3.5 Thiazolidinediones

Troglitazone, a thiazolidinedione product, is an insulin sensitizer that lowers blood glucose by enhancing the action of insulin and reducing insulin resistance. Its main action is on muscle tissue and the liver. Two other agents, rosiglitazone and pioglitazone, act similarly to troglitazone. Troglitazone is well tolerated; however, it is associated with rare hepatocellular injury that has resulted in liver transplant or death. Routine liver function testing should be performed. It is hepatically metabolized and is an inducer of cytochrome P-450 (CYP) 3A4, which can interact with other drugs metabolized by the same enzyme system. Troglitazone causes in increases of LDL (up to 13%), HDL (up to 16%), and total cholesterol levels (5%), but the ratios of these are not altered.

Postprandial and fasting triglyceride levels are reduced by up to 26%. Reductions in HbA1c of 0.5% are observed when it is given as single dose, with drops of 1.4 and 1.8% when it is used in combination with insulin or sulfonylureas, respectively. Modest weight gain is observed when troglitazone is used in combination with other oral agents or insulin; however, troglitazone was withdrawn from the U.S. market in 2000 due to serious adverse reactions and drug interactions. Pioglitazone has been substituted for troglitazone in patients with type 2 diabetes.[7]

26.3.6 Meglitinides

Meglitinides are derived from the unrelated sulfonylurea part of the glyburide molecule. Sulfonylureas and meglitinides have similar clinical effects; both classes cause an increase in insulin secretion from the pancreas and thus require functioning β-cells for their action. Repaglinide binds competitively to the sulfonylurea receptor of the pancreatic β-cell and stimulates insulin release by inhibiting K_{ATP} channels in the β-cells. Repaglinide is rapidly absorbed and eliminated ($t_{1/2}$ less than 1 hour) and is most effective when given within 30 minutes after meal. Adverse events common with repaglinide administration include weight gain and hypoglycemia. Antifungal agents such as ketoconazole and miconazole and the antibiotic erythromycin may inhibit the metabolism of repaglinide. Also, hepatic inducers of the CYP 3A4 enzyme can increase the metabolism of repaglinide. Because it is hepatically metabolized and excreted through the feces, it should be used in patients with caution. Its clinical effect is most obvious in the first couple weeks of administration, and HbA1c reductions of 1.7 to 2.1% are observed.[8]

26.4 CLINICAL TRIALS AND ANTIDIABETIC DRUG DEVELOPMENT

The goals of antidiabetic drug development include:

- Earlier diagnosis (through random screening or screening of first-degree relatives of diabetes)
- Prevention of diabetes and treatment of obesity
- Control of glucose metabolism through insulin-releasing and -sensitizing activities, delaying postprandial absorption of carbohydrate, reducing hepatic glucose output, or increasing energy expenditure
- Control of lipid metabolism by reducing the concentration of plasma free fatty acids or inhibiting hepatic fatty acid oxidation
- Prevention of complications, such as neuropathy (aldose reductase inhibitors have been developed on the basis that the nerve damage is caused by formation of sorbitol from glucose, catalyzed by the enzyme aldose reductase)

One clinically relevant change for a glucose-lowering agent is a reduction of HbA1c 1 to 10% relative to placebo. The relationship between the rate of progression of retinopathy and glycated hemoglobin level is considered to be a continuum, and the use of drug combinations is important to bringing glycerated hemoglobin as close to normal. Because the primary endpoint for a glucose-lowering drug is HbA1c, dose-ranging studies should be conducted for a minimum of 2 to 3 months, and efficacy trials are expected to be at least 6 months long.

The landmark Diabetes Control and Complication Trial (DCCT) conclusively determined that glycemic control affects the appearance and progression of chronic diabetic complications.[9] This study evaluated patients with type 1 disease, randomized to receive either conventional therapy (one to two insulin injections per day) or intensive therapy (three or more injections per day). The results overwhelmingly support intensive therapy, which demonstrated a 60% reduction in clinical neuropathy development, 56% reduction in macroalbuminemia, and 45% reduction in progression to severe retinopathy. The clinical trial was stopped 1 year earlier than initially planned. A renewed emphasis has been placed on strict but reasonable glycemic control to prevent the severe and debilitating chronic complications of diabetes. Strict glycemic control is particularly important before and during pregnancy for reducing the incidence of perinatal complications and mortality in mothers with diabetes.

The U.K. Prospective Diabetes Study (UKPDS) was a 20-year study involving more than 4000 patients with type 2 diabetes.[10–13] Four separate trials were conducted to determine the effects of:

- Intensive blood glucose control with sulfonylureas or insulins
- Intensive blood glucose control with metformin in overweight patients
- Tight blood pressure control in hypertensive diabetic patients
- Atenolol and captopril on blood pressure control

In these studies, intensive control was defined as achieving a fasting plasma glucose of less than 6 mmol/L (108 mg/dL), and conventional treatment was defined as achieving a fasting plasma glucose of less than 15 mmol/L (270 mg/dL). Patients treated with conventional therapy were treated with diet and weight maintenance and with sulfonylureas, metformin, or insulin if severe hyperglycemia occurred. Blood sugars were controlled with chlorpropamide, glyburide, glipizide, or insulin in the intensively treated group. The following endpoints were evaluated:

- Any diabetes-related endpoint (sudden death, death from hyperglycemia or hypoglycemia, myocardial infarction)
- Other cardiovascular events, amputation, or ophthalmic events
- Death-related diabetes, including sudden death, stroke, peripheral vascular disease, renal disease, and glycemic derangements

Results of the clinical trials showed that HbA1c values over a 10-year period were 7.0% in the intensive group and 7.9% in the conventional group, with all agents having similar efficacy in the intensively treated patients. Patients in the intensively treated group had a 12% lower risk of any diabetes-related endpoint and a 25% lower risk of microvascular complications than those in the conventionally treated group.

The objective of a phase I clinical trial is to provide preliminary tolerability, metabolism, and kinetic data in order to set safe parameters for phase II studies. Estimations of dose range, regimen, food interactions, and drug interactions can be made for use later in more extensive and costly trials. Phase I trials are conducted in healthy volunteers, but complications arise when developing biosynthetic agents or in the case of immunosuppressive agents for which an adequate toxicological examination is required. An ascending-dose, crossover design in two alternating parallel groups has the advantage of speed and limited individual drug exposure. The use of a randomized placebo and double-blinding is recommended.

The upper dose can be set on a case-by-case basis, taking into account the animal pharmacology and threshold levels determined from the toxicity tests. The design can incorporate an oral glucose tolerance test 2 to 3 hours after dosing, when an effect from a single dose is evident and blood samples can be analyzed for glucose and hormone levels. When the drug produces a glucose-lowering activity in healthy subjects, a dose–response curve should be examined to identify appropriate doses for future studies. Preliminary kinetic profiles will help in selecting the regimen and design of subsequent kinetic studies.

Subjects are fasted overnight for a further 8 or 10 hours after dosing. Proportional doses to cover the dose range and placebo are administered and clinical tests performed. Dynamic kinetic modeling[14] should confirm the optimal dose range within which the presence of active metabolites can be used to interpret any unusual kinetic observations. To assess the effects of food on a drug product, a two-way study or a three-way crossover study with a placebo can be used to examine postprandial glucose levels. A kinetic study on drug–food interactions has indicated that it is necessary to determine blood glucose levels of diabetic patients at different times after drug administration, as their testing results will be affected by their eating before administration of the drug.

It is necessary to establish repeat-dose tolerability in healthy subjects or patients as early as possible. The upper doses may be curtailed in healthy subjects due to hypoglycemia, a limited degree being acceptable; further treatment-related changes in glucose and insulin may imply and detect insulin resistance. The use of diabetic patients in such study requires a longer time period but allows preliminary dose findings. Patients may be exposed to several 5-day or 7-day periods of different treatments based on previous toxicology studies. Two or more parallel groups afford a good range of doses or regimens. This type of study may include oral glucose tolerance tests with ten subjects and two placebos to evaluate drug tolerability.

Possible drug interactions can be identified during studies on the pharmacology and metabolism of the drug. Protein displacement occurs when protein binding is high and the volume of distribution low and usually is not clinically important if the drug is a base. High renal clearance indicates the possibility of drug competition for one of the renal excretion systems; interactions at the hepatic level can be determined by *in vitro* cytochrome P-450 enzyme, identification of the P-450 subtype involved, and information on other substrates or inhibitors.

For phase II trials, a parallel group study is best as a baseline run-in and requires 2 to 3 months of treatment to estimate HbA1c. The placebo-controlled dose-range study can be applied. When an estimate of likely dose and regimen is available, a 24-hour profile study can be conducted in patients randomized to drug or placebo in a crossover design. Useful data will be obtained, such as hormone data and postprandial effects. Formal dose-range studies ideally require HbA1c measurements.

Based on metabolic route, appropriate investigations in kidney- or liver-impaired subjects should be undertaken. Diabetics have a high prevalence of renal impairment, and it will be useful to know the dosing schedule in kidney-impaired subjects before phase III. In addition, as type 2 diabetes is prevalent in the elderly, the International Conference on Harmonisation (ICH) guidelines for geriatrics can be applied.[15] These guidelines also comment on the scope and nature of interaction studies and usefulness of kinetic data from young and elderly subjects.

For new drug development and determining its market potential, mode of action studies should be performed in phase I or phase II with the objective of confirming animal pharmacology and developing optimal conditions for phase III studies:

- Insulin sensitivity — The hyperglycemic clamp technique[16] is useful for estimating changes in insulin sensitivity following treatment with a drug product. An insulin releaser may induce the endogenous release of insulin, which will flaw the study. This is detected by measurement of C-peptide and overcome by the addition of a somatostatin infusion. Assessment for an insulin releaser should be done in C-peptide-negative, type 2 diabetes patients. Other methods of assessing insulin sensibility can also be used.[17]
- Pancreatic response to glucose — The hyperglycemic clamp technique demonstrates first- and second-phase insulin response to glucose *in vivo*. First- and second-phase responses are diminished in type 2 diabetes patients but may be restored by drugs or an improvement in the levels of glucose.[18]
- Liver metabolism — The study design should consider the suppression of hepatic glucose production due to a lack of tracer steady state and implications of the position of the label on tracer recycling.[19] Gluconeogenesis is followed by using labeled precursors, such as alanine or glycerol. Adequate time (e.g., 10 hours) should be allowed to achieve a steady state.
- Muscle metabolism — Muscle biopsy or nuclear magnetic resonance may be used to examine glycogen synthesis. Cannulation of the forearm artery and vein allows estimation of metabolite flux and extraction through forearm skeletal muscle.[20]
- Fat metabolism — Metabolite flux across human subcutaneous adipose tissue may be examined by cannulation of a superficial vein on the anterior abdominal wall and venous sampling during exercise or periprandially.[21,22]

Phase III trials are expanded controlled studies to establish the safety and effectiveness of a product in an expanded patient population. They are used to evaluate the overall risk–benefit ratio of the product and to supply necessary data for product licensure. These studies also provide the labeling information that enables physicians to utilize the product effectively. The optimum dosage should also be established at this time. Trials usually include several hundred to several thousand target patients.

Following licensure of a new drug, further studies are undertaken to monitor and confirm the efficacy and safety of the drug in a large population. Phase IV studies are designed to observe long-term drug efficacy; adverse reactions that occur with long-term use or in particular patient subpopulations, such as children and the elderly; drug interactions that may occur with concomitantly given drugs; and the incidence of nonresponders.

REFERENCES

1. Rosak, C., The pathophysiologic basis of efficacy and clinical experience with the new oral antidiabetic agents, *J. Diabetes Complicat.*, 16(1), 123–132, 2002.
2. Harrigan, R.A., Nathan, M.S., and Beattie, P., Oral agents for the treatment of type 2 diabetes mellitus: pharmacology, toxicity, and treatment, *Ann. Emerg. Med.*, 38(1), 68–78, 2001.
3. Setter, S.M., White, J.R., and Campbell, R.K., Diabetes, in *Textbook of Therapeutics: Drug and Disease Management*, Herfindal, E.T. and D.R. Gourley, D.R., Eds., Lippincott Williams & Wilkins, Baltimore, MD, 2000, pp. 377–406.
4. Campbell, R.K. and Campbell, L.K., Insulin lispro: its role in the treatment of diabetes mellitus, *Ann. Pharmacother.*, 30, 1263–1271, 1996.
5. Campbell, R.K., Glimepiride: role of a new sulfonylurea in the treatment of type 2 diabetes mellitus, *Ann. Pharmacol.*, 32, 1044–1052, 1998.
6. DeFronzo, R.A., Goodman, A.M., and the Multicenter Metformin Study Group, Efficacy of metformin in patients with NIDDM, *N. Engl. J. Med.*, 333, 541–549, 1995.
7. Kane, M.P., Busch, R.S., Bakst, G., and Hamilton, R.A., Substitution of pioglitazone for troglitazone in patients with type 2 diabetes, *Endocr. Pract.*, 10(1), 18–23, 2004.
8. Cheatham, W.W., Repaglinide: a new oral blood glucose lowering agent, *Clin. Diabetes*, 16, 70–72, 1998.
9. DCCT Research Group, The effect of intensive treatment of diabetes on the development and progression of long-term complications in insulin-dependent diabetes mellitus, *N. Engl. J. Med.*, 329, 977–986, 1993.
10. U.K. Prospective Diabetes Study (UKPDS) Group, Intensive blood-glucose with sulfonylurea or insulin compared with conventional treatment and risks of complications in patients with type 2 diabetes (UKPDS 33), *Lancet*, 353, 837–853, 1998.
11. U.K. Prospective Diabetes Study (UKPDS) Group, Intensive blood-glucose with metformin on complications in overweight patients with type 2 diabetes (UKPDS 34), *Lancet*, 352, 854–865, 1988.
12. U.K. Prospective Diabetes Study (UKPDS) Group, Tight blood pressure control and risk of macrovascular and microvascular complications in type 2 diabetes (UKPDS 38), *Br. Med. J.*, 317, 703–713, 1998.
13. U.K. Prospective Diabetes Study (UKPDS) Group, Efficacy of atenolol and captopril in reducing risk of macrovascular and microvascular complications in type 2 diabetes (UKPDS 39), *Br. Med. J.*, 317, 13–20, 1998.
14. Byron, W.D., Rotherham, N.E., and Bratty, J.R., Relationship between hypoglycemia response and plasma concentration of BTS 67 582 in healthy volunteers, *Br. J. Clin. Pharmacol.*, 38, 433–439, 1994.
15. ICH, *Studies in Support of Special Populations: Geriatrics*, Guideline III/3388/93, International Conference on Harmonisation of Technical Requirements for Registration of Pharmaceuticals for Human Use, Geneva, 1995.
16. De Fronzo, R.A., Tobin, J.D., and Andres, R., Glucose clamp technique, a method for quantifying insulin secretion and resistance, *Am. J. Physiol.*, 237, E214–E223, 1979.
17. Fulcher, G.R., Walker, M., and Alberti, K.G.M.M., The assessment of insulin action *in vivo*, in *International Textbook of Diabetes Mellitus*, Alberti, K.G., De Fronzo, M.M., Keen, H., and Zimmimet, P., Eds., John Wiley & Sons, New York, 1992.
18. Fermer, R.E., Rawlins, M.D., and Alberti, K.G., Impaired beta-cell responses improve when fasting blood glucose concentration is reduced in noninsulin-dependent diabetes, *Q. J. Med.*, 66, 137–146, 1988.
19. Wolfe, R.R., *Radioactive and Stable Isotope Tracers in Biomedicine: Principles and Practice of Kinetic Analysis*, Wiley-Liss, New York, 1992.
20. Walker, M., Fulcher, G.R., Catalano, C. et al., Physiological levels of plasma non-esterified fatty acids impair forearm glucose uptake in normal man, *Clin. Sci.*, 79, 167–174, 1990.
21. Hodgetts, V., Coppack, S.W., Frayn, K.N. et al., Factors controlling fat metabolisation from human subcutaneous adipose tissue during exercise, *J. Appl. Physiol.*, 71, 445–451, 1991.
22. Frayn, K.N., Coppack, S.W., Humphreys, S.M. et al., Periprandial regulations of lipid metabolism in insulin treated diabetes mellitus, *Metabolism*, 42, 504–510, 1993.

Assessment of Chemotherapeutic Drugs

CHAPTER **27**

Antibiotics

Lucia H. Lee, Christopher L. Wu, Benjamin R. Lee, and Chi-Jen Lee

CONTENTS

27.1 INTRODUCTION

Antibiotics are chemical compounds produced by living cells that inhibit the growth of microorganisms and are used for treatment of bacterial infections. Drug development made a great leap forward with the discovery of antibiotics. In 1928, the Scottish scientist Sir Alexander Fleming found a zone in a culture of bacteria that was caused by the invasion of a mold. Penicillin, the extract from that mold, was shown to cure bacterial infections. The golden age of antimicrobial therapy began in 1941 when a brilliant group of investigators, led by Howard W. Florey and Ernst Chain, purified penicillin and produced quantities sufficient to permit clinical trials; subsequently, many other antibiotics have been developed. Antibiotics have almost entirely replaced sulfonamides in the treatment of bacterial infection. Dozens of biosynthetic penicillins have been prepared in an attempt to obtain compounds better than penicillin G with respect to physical, chemical, and pharmacological properties. In 1958, methods were devised for preparing the penicillin nucleus, thus making it possible to biosynthesize penicillins that could not be formed in a normal medium. The resulting compounds were usually more acid stable and penicillinase resistant and had a wider antibacterial spectrum.

The wide use of antibiotics in animal nutrition and treatment of disease has resulted in the sensitization of a large number of susceptible individuals, many of whom have serious reactions upon contact with these drugs. Such agricultural use also contributes to the pool of antibiotic-resistant strains in a community. Because bacteria mutate easily, drug-resistant strains of bacteria develop quickly. As a result, researchers are forced to continually develop new antibiotics to stay ahead of the steady emergence of drug-resistant strains.[1]

The detection of antibiotic-producing organisms is based on the ability of cultures of the candidate organism to inhibit certain test bacteria *in vitro*. Several test organisms such as *Staphylococcus aureus* and *Escherichia coli* are used because no one organism is representative of all antibiotic susceptibilities. The screening method involves plating out in serial dilution an aqueous extract of soil or other natural substance into an agar medium. The forming antibiotic substances are distinguished by a clear zone around the colony, indicative of inhibition of the test organism, which grows abundantly in the form of a marked turbidity throughout the agar.

Many modifications of this method are employed; thus, the use of various media, pH, temperatures, and substrates can be used for screening different types of soil organisms. The best condition for detecting the largest number of antagonists is preincubation of agar cultures containing the soil dilutions but not the test bacteria. The preincubation is followed by a secondary incubation after the test organism has been applied to the plate by homogeneous streaking. In this way, slow-growing organisms are given a chance to develop and manifest their antibiotic-producing ability.

When detected, the antagonist is isolated in pure culture and identified, and the optimal conditions for producing antibiotic substance are examined. When an optimum medium is established, other strains of the antagonist are compared for the properties and amount of the antibiotic produced. The highest yielding strain is selected for further investigation. The antibacterial spectrum obtained includes the minimum inhibitory concentration (MIC) necessary to inhibit the growth of a large variety of Gram-positive and Gram-negative bacteria, as well as other pathogenic microorganisms. Such data suggest the infections against which certain antibiotics may be useful.

Furthermore, toxicity and pharmacological studies are conducted in animals and, if the results are favorable, in clinical trials on high-risk populations. When the clinical trials show the antibiotic to be a promising therapeutic agent, the process for large-scale manufacture should be established. Chemical studies of the structure of the pure compound will indicate the feasibility of chemical synthesis. Generally, antibiotics are complex substances for which synthesis may be extremely difficult compared with microbiologic production.

27.2 ANTIBIOTICS USED IN CHEMOTHERAPY
AND THEIR MECHANISMS OF ACTION

Antibiotics are classified by various categories, the two most important being the mechanisms of action and their chemical structures and relationships. The primary antibiotics used in chemotherapy are listed in Table 27.1.

27.2.1 Beta-Lactam Antibiotics

All penicillins are bacteriostatic at low concentrations and bactericidal at high concentrations. Their antimicrobial spectra differ according to the pattern of beta-lactamase resistance, the ability to penetrate the outer membrane of Gram-negative bacteria, and their selectivities for the various bacterial transpeptidases. Although penicillin G is destroyed by gastric acid, its low oral bioavailability can be compensated by increased dosage. Penicillin V is the only marketed acid-stable compound. The spectrum is narrow and primarily limited to Gram-positive bacteria, such as *Streptococcus pyogenes*, pneumococci, *Bacillus anthracis*, and Gram-negative cocci. The penicillin resistance is due to their reaction to penicillin-destroying enzymes known as beta-lactamase which convert penicillin into inactive penicilloid acid. In addition, non-penicillinase-mediated resistance, referred to as methicillin resistance, is caused by an alteration in the target transpeptidase (penicillin-binding protein I).

Penicillin is known to interfere with the synthesis of peptidoglycans that are part of the cell wall. As a result, the growing protoplast cannot form a protective cell wall. Several wall enzymes are reversibly inhibited, the most important being a D,D-carboxypeptidase that also functions as a transpeptidase. The potency of penicillin is expressed in units per milligram. One International Unit (IU) is equivalent to the activity of 0.6 µg of pure sodium penicillin G. Because of the large doses used, it is usually expressed in megaunits (i.e., 1 megaunit equals 10^6 units).

Penicillin is practically nontoxic; however, hypersensitivity reactions occur in certain patients. The most common symptom of this allergic response is a skin rash. Nondermatological manifestations of allergy include serum sickness, angioedema, nephropathy, rare hemolytic anemia, Arthus reaction, and anaphylaxis. Side effects of oral administration of penicillins include nausea, vomiting, and diarrhea. Like other antibiotics, penicillin can markedly alter the normal bacterial flora.

The cephalosporins are a group of antibiotics closely related to the penicillins. The cephalosporanic acid moiety characteristic of cephalosporins is an analog of the penicillanic acid moiety. Both compounds have a beta-lactam ring. The cephalosporins have a mechanism of action similar to that of the penicillins. They bind to one or more penicillin-binding proteins (PBPs) that are transpeptidases and inhibit the cross-linking of the peptidoglycan units in the bacterial cell wall. The intrinsic activity of a cephalosporin depends on resistance to beta-lactamases, affinity to PBPs, and their ability to reach these targets in Gram-positive and Gram-negative bacteria.[2] As with the penicillins, one common mechanism of resistance is their reaction to a beta-lactamase. Other resistance mechanisms include failure to bind to PBPs, as occurs with methicillin-resistant strains of staphylococci.

Hypersensitivity occurs in 5 to 10% of recipients of cephalosporins, causing symptoms of eosinophilia, drug fever, rash, urticaria, serum sickness, edema, anaphylaxis, rare hemolytic anemia, and transient hepatic abnormalities. Other adverse effects of cephalosporins include pain, induration, sterile abscess and sloughing at the site of injection, nausea, vomiting, diarrhea, abdominal pain, and heartburn. Cephalosporins should not be used in combination with other antibiotics or diuretics that cause nephrotoxicity.

27.2.2 Aminoglycosides

The aminoglycosides each contain one or more aminosugars; for example, glucosamine is linked by glycosidic linkages to a basic amino or guanidine six-carbon ring. The major spectrum of activity of aminoglycosides includes aerobic Gram-negative bacilli and *Staphylococcus aureus*. The aminoglycosides combine with bacterial ribosomes to inhibit protein synthesis. The initiation complex can be formed but cannot pass into subsequent stages of protein synthesis. The drugs also interfere with the binding of aminoacetyl-tRNA, which prevents chain elongation. Further, they cause misreading of some RNA codons such that inappropriate proteins are formed. Aminoglycosides have

Table 27.1 Primary Antibiotics Used in Chemotherapy[21,22]

Category	Administration Route, Spectrum, and Remarks
Beta-Lactam Antibiotics	
Penicillins	
Natural penicillins:	
Penicillin G	Intravenous, intramuscular; best narrow spectrum (streptococci)
Penicillin V	Oral only; same spectrum as penicillin G
Penicillinase-resistant penicillin (antistaphylococcal):	
Cloxacillin	Oral
Dicloxacillin	Oral
Methicillin	Intravenous; interstitial nephritis may occur
Nafcillin	Intravenous
Oxacillin	Oral
Aminopenicillins (improved Gram-negative; *Haemophilus influenzae*, *Shigella*, *Salmonella*):	
Amoxacillin	Oral
Ampicillin	Intravenous; incomplete oral absorption, diarrhea, rash
Bacampicillin	Oral prodrug converted to ampicillin
Extended-spectrum penicillins (antipseudomonal):	
Carbenicillin	Intravenous; high sodium
Ticarcillin	Intravenous; similar to carbenicillin but less sodium
Piperacillin	Intravenous; best negative spectrum
Mezlocillin	Intravenous; similar to piperacillin
Beta-lactamase combinations (expand spectrum to *Staphylococcus*, beta-lactamase producers):	
Clavulanalate–amoxacillin	Oral; more diarrhea than amoxacillin
Sulbactam–ampicillin	Intravenous; beta-lactamase producing *Haemophilus influenzae* and *Streptococcus pneumoniae*
Clavulanate–ticarcillin	Intravenous; more active against Gram-negative bacilli
Tazobactam–piperacillin	Intravenous; more active against Gram-negative bacilli
Cephalosporins	
First-generation (*Staphylococcus*, enteric Gram-negative bacilli):	
Cefadroxil	Oral; intermediate acting
Cefazolin	Intramuscular, intravenous; intermediate duration, less painful
Cephalexin	Oral; short acting
Cephalothin	Intramuscular, intravenous; narrow spectrum; short acting
Cephapirin	Intramuscular, intravenous; short acting
Cephradine	Intramuscular, intravenous, oral; short acting
Second-generation (more active against Gram-negative; active against *Haemophilus influenzae* and anaerobes):	
Cefaclor	Oral, short acting
Cefamandole	Intramuscular, intravenous; short acting
Cefmetazole	Intravenous; short acting
Cefonicid	Intramuscular, intravenous; intermediate to long acting
Ceforanid	Intramuscular, intravenous; intermediate acting
Cefotetan	Intramuscular, intravenous; intermediate to long acting
Cefoxitin	Intramuscular, intravenous; short acting
Cefprozil	Oral; short acting
Cefuroxime	Intramuscular, intravenous, oral; beta-lactamase resistance
Loracarbef	Oral; short acting
Third-generation (best Gram-negative spectrum, beta-lactamase resistant, poor against *Staphylococcus*):	
Cefixime	Oral; intermediate to long acting
Cefpodoxime	Oral; intermediate acting, similar to cefixime
Cefoperazone	Intramuscular, intravenous; intermediate acting, good against *Pseudomonas*
Cefotaxime	Intramuscular, intravenous; shortest acting
Ceftazidime	Intramuscular, intravenous; short acting, good against *Pseudomonas*
Ceftizoxime	Intramuscular, intravenous; short acting

Table 27.1 Primary Antibiotics Used in Chemotherapy (cont.)

Category	Administration Route, Spectrum, and Remarks
Ceftriaxone	Intramuscular, intravenous; long acting, good against *Gonococci*
Ceftibuten	Oral; similar to cefixime
Cefdinir	Oral; similar to cefixime
Fourth-generation:	
Cefepime	Intravenous; better against *Staphylococcus* and *Streptococcus* than third-generation
Aminoglycosides	
Amikacin	More resistant to bacterial enzymes, active against gentamicin resistance strains
Gentamicin	Least expensive
Netilmicin	Similar to gentamicin spectrum
Tobramycin	Similar to gentamicin spectrum
Streptomycin	Used primarily for tuberculosis
Macrolides	
Azithromycin	Expanded spectrum, less GI effects, does not affect liver enzymes, long-half-life
Clarithromycin	Improved spectrum over erythromycin, less GI effects, inhibits liver enzymes
Erythromycin	Frequent GI effects, inhibits liver enzymes
Tetracyclines	
Chlortetracycline	Short acting, incomplete oral absorption
Demeclocycline	Intermediate acting, more phototoxicity
Doxycycline	Long acting, good oral absorption, biliary excretion
Minocycline	Long acting, good oral absorption, dizziness
Methacycline	Intermediate acting
Oxytetracycline	Short acting, incomplete oral absorption
Tetracycline	Short acting, incomplete oral absorption
Fluoroquinolones	
Classical fluoroquinolones	
Ciprofloxacin	Intermediate spectrum
Norfloxacin	Incomplete oral absorption, limited spectrum
Ofloxacin	Intermediate spectrum
Levofloxacin	More active than ofloxacin, long acting
Enoxacin	Limited spectrum
Lomefloxacin	Intermediate spectrum, phototoxicity
Pefloxacin	Intermediate spectrum, long acting, phototoxicity
New fluoroquinolones	
Sparfloxacin	Expanded spectrum, long acting, phototoxicity
Grepafloxacin	Expanded spectrum, long acting
Trovafloxacin	Expanded spectrum
Polypeptides	
Bacitracin	Topical use; systemic toxicity
Polymyxin B	Topical use; systemic toxicity

been very important antibiotics for the treatment of infections caused by Gram-negative bacilli. Toxicity in humans results from blockade of N-type calcium channels and inhibition of lysosomal phospholipase and sphingomyelinase. Resistance to aminoglycosides develops very rapidly with some bacteria (e.g., meningococcus, *Haemophilus*). Most of the toxic actions of antibiotics are common among all aminoglycosides. Hypersensitivity, rashes, and drug fever occur in 5 to 10% of recipients; eosinophilia is common. A history of sensitization contraindicates use, and cross-sensitization can occur.

27.2.3 Macrolides

The macrolides are hydroxylated macrocyclic lactones containing 12 to 20 carbon atoms in the primary ring. This class has 37 known compounds, but only erythromycin and its derivatives have been used widely. Two new macrolides, clarithromycin and azithromycin, were approved in 1991. These are chemically similar to the 14-membered-ring macrolide, erythromycin. The macrolides are active against Gram-positive bacteria, mycoplasmas, and *Legionella*. Erythromycin is used less frequently because of the emergence of resistant strains of streptococci and staphylococci plus problems with gastrointestinal intolerance. The new macrolides are better tolerated and offer a broader spectrum against *Haemophilus influenzae* and *Mycobacterium avium*. Macrolides bind to the 50s subunit of the bacterial ribosome. Their main activity involves inhibition of the translocation step in protein synthesis. These drugs are primarily bacteriostatic in therapeutic concentrations. They bind equally to ribosomes from Gram-positive and Gram-negative bacteria.

27.2.4 Tetracyclines

The tetracyclines are all very much alike with respect to their antimicrobial spectra and the side effects they elicit. They differ mainly in their absorption, duration of action, and suitability for parenteral administration. The tetracyclines are broad-spectrum antibiotics and are primarily bacteriostatic. They bind to the bacterial 30s ribosomes and prevent tRNA from combining with mRNA; thus, protein synthesis is inhibited. The drugs have activities against both Gram-positive and Gram-negative bacteria, mycobacteria, *Mycoplasma*, rickettsia, actinomyces, *Chlamydia*, and plasmodia.[3] Resistance to the tetracyclines is not acquired as rapidly as to penicillin, but it nevertheless occurs readily. Among the Gram-positive bacteria, up to 44% of *Streptococcus pyogenes* are resistant and 74% of *Enterococcus fecalis*. The incidence of resistance among hospital strains of *Staphylococcus aureus* may run from 30 to 50% but may increase to as high as 75% after several days of treatment. Highly resistant gonococci have become prevalent. Various streptococci and pneumococci have also become resistant. The incidence of resistance among various Gram-negative bacteria is also very high, especially among the Enterobacteriaceae. Resistance to one tetracycline usually confers resistance to all others.

The tetracyclines have several adverse effects. Gastrointestinal toxicity is common with oral use, causing local irritation and alteration of the intestinal flora. Symptoms include heartburn, epigastric distress, nausea, vomiting, diarrhea, and rare esophageal ulceration in persons with esophageal obstruction or spastic disease. The broad-spectrum antibacterial activity of the tetracyclines causes marked alterations in the floral ecology, so microorganisms formerly held in check overgrow to cause superinfections. The most common superinfection is candidiasis, but overgrowth from staphylococci, enterococci, *Proteus*, and *Pseudomonas* occurs. Staphylococcal enteric superinfections are frequently fatal. Various hypersensitivity reactions, especially urticaria, asthma, facial edema, and phototoxicity, occur. Tetracyclines can discolor developing teeth and reversibly impair bone growth through complexation with the bone salts and fixation to matrix proteins.

27.2.5 Fluoroquinolones

The fluoroquinolones are bacteriostatic at low doses and bactericidal at high doses. They are highly active against most Gram-negative pathogens, including *Pseudomonas aeruginosa*. The Enterobacteriaceae, *Staphylococcus aureus* and *S. epidermidis*, *Legionella*, mycobacteria, mycoplasma, and chlamydia have intermediate sensitivities. The newly approved levofloxacin, sparfloxacin, grepafloxaxin, and trovafloxacin have improved activity against *Streptococcus pneumoniae* and some Gram-negative bacteria resistant to older fluoroquinolones. The drugs inhibit DNA gyrase (topoisomerase II), which results in abnormal linkage between opened DNA and the gyrase. Negative supercoiling is impaired, so efficient transcription of DNA into RNA and subsequent protein synthesis is inhibited. Resistance to one fluoroquinolone usually confers resistance to all other quinolones but not to other classes of antibiotics.[4] Adverse effects are usually mild and transient. They include gastrointestinal disturbances, such as nausea, vomiting, diarrhea, constipation, heartburn, and abdominal discomfort (2 to 8%); central nervous system symptoms, such as headache, restlessness, malaise, dizziness, tremor, insomnia, nightmares, depression, visual disturbances, rare hallucinations, phobias, manic excitement, and convulsions (0.5 to 6%); and hematologic perturbations, including eosinophilia, anemia, elevated erythrocyte sedimentation rate (1.5 to 5%), mild or moderate rash and pruritus (1%), dry mouth, and photosensitivity.

27.2.6 Polypeptides

The polypeptide antibiotics, including bacitracin and polymyxin B, are restricted to topical use because of their systemic toxicity. They differ from each other in their mechanism of action and antibacterial spectrum; for example, bacitracin is primarily effective against Gram-negative bacteria and inhibits cell wall synthesis by interfering with the transfer of peptidoglycan subunits to the cell wall, while polymyxin B is active against Gram-negative bacteria due to its cationic detergent-like disruption of bacterial cytoplasmic membranes. The high incidence of nephrotoxicity that follows the injection of bacitracin precludes systemic use except in life-endangering staphylococcal infections in infants for which other antibiotics are ineffective or in the treatment of antibiotic-associated enterocolitis. Other toxic effects of injection route include pain, induration, skin rash, malaise, anorexia, nausea, and vomiting. Topical application is not irritating and rarely induces allergic reactions. Development of bacterial resistance is much less frequent and slower for bacitracin than for penicillin. The *in vitro* and *in vivo* antimicrobial spectra of polymyxin B activity are restricted to Gram-negative bacteria. All Gram-positive bacteria are resistant. It is used topically for the treatment or prevention of external ocular infections caused by susceptible microorganisms, especially *Pseudomonas aeruginosa*.[5] In topical therapy, it is often combined with neomycin, gramicidin, or bacitracin. When administered by injection, it causes toxicity in the central nervous system and kidney.

27.3 LABORATORY ASSESSMENTS OF ANTIBIOTICS

The development of antibacterial agents involves preselection of a series of compounds screened from natural products or synthesized by chemists. When a promising compound is found or synthesized, its *in vitro* activity on several strains of selected bacteria is determined. The selection of testing bacteria depends on the design requirements of the new research project and systemic analyses of the activity of all new antibacterial agents against various pathogens. For example, the objective of research on new macrolides is to increase antibacterial activity for naturally susceptible species but also to counter cross-resistance to erythromycin and to extend the activity to strains resistant to erythromycin (e.g., *Streptococcus pneumoniae*).[6]

27.3.1 Preselection and Laboratory Assessments

Choosing strains with various antibiotic phenotypes and comparative compounds is important in the early stages of developing a new compound. Activity *in vivo* determines the next step, which consists of testing the efficacy of preselected compounds in nonspecific models of infection when administered by the injection or oral route. Data gathered during the preselection phase will lead to the selection of candidates for clinical trials. The selection is based on *in vitro* and *in vivo* activity, as well as on the toxicity of the different compounds. Even though some preselected compounds may be more active than the final selected candidate, they may not be chosen because of their toxicity. The screening process is aimed at selecting the compound with the most effective and well-balanced antibacterial spectrum and the most promising safety profile in animal studies. After the selection phase, the next step involves chemical characterization and microbiological studies, a prerequisite for clinical trials. The following physical and chemical properties should be characterized:

- Solubility of the compound in water and the various solvents used in microbiological studies
- Chemical content, structure, and molecular weight
- Quantitative analysis
- Interactions with calcium, zinc, magnesium, and other metal ions
- Need for particular growth factors in the culture medium
- Stability of the compound in culture medium with time and at different temperatures and pH

The factors influencing bacterial growth should be determined. The effect of different media on the MIC value should also be tested. Certain compounds become less bactericidal as the inoculum increases. For example, the bactericidal activity of the fluoroquinolones decreases at bacterial inoculum above 10^8 cfu/mL. Several bacteria require an atmosphere enriched in CO_2 for growth, but CO_2 influences antibacterial activity (e.g., that of macrolides) by modifying the pH of the culture medium.[7] The pH of the medium can also modify the activity of a compound. Fluoroquinolones that possess a piperazine ring in position 7 are less active in acid media than in alkaline media. In contrast, compounds that do not have substitutes in position 7 are more active in acid than alkaline media.[8]

Adding horse serum to the culture medium is often necessary for bacterial growth, but it is necessary to check that the MIC values do not change as a result. The enriched media can be used to determine the MICs of the different cephalosporins, regardless of the strain of *Streptococcus pneumoniae*. The effect of human serum on the activity of a new agent could be evaluated using pooled normal human serum combined with Mueller–Hinton medium to yield a 50% final concentration. It is essential to test the antibiotic against reference strains for quality control. The inhibition zone diameters and MIC values for reference strains should be measured.

The microbiological data are important in the license application for the new antibacterial agent. It involves determination of the antibacterial spectrum and activity of the compound, including bacteriostatic (MIC) and bactericidal (MBC) activities. The compound should be tested on a sufficient number of strains of pathogens (about 100) to determine the MIC_{50} and MIC_{90} values. In addition, three types of strain should be tested: (1) reference strains to identify possible resistance mechanisms, (2) collection strains from a laboratory that has participated in other studies and can serve as a reference, and (3) freshly isolated clinical strains.

The MIC_{50} value can be calculated in two different ways: (1) assemble all data into an orderly array and select the median value as the MIC_{50}, and (2) accumulate data and then determine the MIC_{50} by interpolating from a graph of accumulated strains inhibited (%) vs. the MIC.[9] The MIC_{50} reflects the intrinsic activity of the compound and establishes the spectrum and activity of the compound, whereas the MIC_{90} reflects the various resistance mechanisms and depends on the particular study center and the way in which the strains are collected. To determine the intrinsic value of a compound, it is necessary to conduct tests on the various bacterial species comprising a genus and also on the isolates with resistance strains. It is also necessary to determine the antibacterial activity of the potential metabolites of the antibacterial agent. When a metabolite is active and accounts for an important part of the drug kinetics, the parent compound and its metabolite should be tested together to ensure that no antagonism exists.

The choice of culture medium, pH, and test strain is critical for the assessment of a compound. The method should be sufficiently sensitive, exhibiting large inhibition zone relative to the standard curves, and should be reproducible. A chemical assay method such as high-performance liquid chromatography (HPLC) should be utilized and a correlation obtained between microbiological and chemical methods. Regression lines are evaluated by comparing the inhibition zones between the edge of the paper disk and the edge of the growth zone of a reference strain and the clinical isolate on the same plate. The radius of difference between these two zones is used to determine whether an antibiotic is active, moderately active, or inactive.

Table 27.2 Pathogenic Bacteria Used To Evaluate Antibiotic Activity

Bacterial Species	Microorganisms
Gram-positive cocci	Coagulase-negative staphylococci *Enterococcus* spp. *Streptococcus* spp. (e.g., *Streptococcus pneumoniae*) Others: *Gemella* spp., *Stomatococcus* spp., *Micrococcus* spp., *Aerococcus* spp.
Gram-positive bacilli	*Bacillus anthracis* *Corynebacterium diphtheriae* *Corynebacterium* spp. (e.g., *C. jeikeium, C. urealyticum*) *Lactobacillus* spp. *Listeria monocytogenes*
Gram-negative cocci	*Neisseria meningitides, N. gonorrhoeae*
Gram-negative bacilli	*Citrobacter diversus, C. freundii* *Enterobacter cloacae, E. aerogenes* Enterobacteriaceae *Escherichia coli* *Klebsiella pneumoniae* *Pseudomonas aeruginosa* *Salmonella* spp. *Shigella* spp. *Yersinia enterocolitica* Others: *Acinetobacter* spp., *Vibrio cholerae, Haemophilus* spp., *Moraxella* spp. (e.g., *M. catarrhalis*)
Anaerobes	*Bacteroides* spp. *Clostridium difficille* *Peptococcus* spp. *Peptospreptococcus* spp. *Porphyromonas* spp. *Veillonella* spp.
Other microorganisms	*Borrelia* spp. *Campylobacter* spp. *Helicobacter pylori* *Mycoplasma* spp. Intracellular pathogens: *Mycobacterium tuberculosis, M. avium complex, M. leprae, Chlamydia* spp. (e.g., *C. trachomatis*)

27.3.2 Common Pathogens for Evaluation of Antibiotics

The pathogenic bacterial species used for assessment of antibiotic activity are shown in Table 27.2.

27.3.2.1 Gram-Positive Cocci

A distinction can be made between *Staphylococcus aureus* strains that produce penicillinases and those that are resistant to methicillin. Strains that produce penicillinases account for more than 80% of isolates in some areas. When testing a new antibacterial agent, it is necessary to use strains possessing the four enzymes A, B, C, and D. Cephalosporin is more stable to penicillinase A hydrolysis than cefazolin. Other antistaphylococcal agents should be tested in comparison. The emergence of strains resistant to penicillin G and multiresistant strains requires determining the antipneumococcal profile of a new compound. A simple method is to determine the comparative *in vitro* activity of the compound on strains that are susceptible (MIC < 0.12 mg/L), intermediately susceptible (0.12 MIC < 1 mg/L), or resistant (MIC 1 mg/L) to penicillin G. It is necessary to add strains resistant to cefotaxime (MIC 2 mg/L) and those with diminished susceptibility (0.5 < MIC < 1 mg/L), as well as multiresistant strains to erythromycin (MIC 1 mg/L), tetracycline, chloramphenicol, and cotrimoxazole. It is preferable to determine the MIC in agar rather than broth media, which show more variable results. Bactericidal activity should be tested on strains with different resistance phenotypes to beta-lactams with different inocula. Antibacterial activity on streptococcal groups A, B, C, G, and F should be tested. The pathogens should include strains resistant to erythromycin, particularly *Streptococcus pyogenes*.

27.3.2.2 Gram-Positive Bacilli

Activity against *Corynebacterium diphtheriae* and *C. jeikeium* should be tested, as few active drugs are available.

27.3.2.3 Gram-Negative Cocci

A decrease in the penicillin G activity to *Neisseria meningitides* has been observed, and the resistance mechanism is similar to that of *Streptococcus pneumoniae*. The intensive use of rifampicin prophylaxis accounts for the emergence of resistant strains to this antibiotic. The testing should include susceptible strains to antibacterial agents, strains with diminished susceptibility to penicillin G, and strains resistant to rifampicin and macrolides. The emergence of strains of *N. gonorrhoeae* resistant to penicillin G, tetracyclines, and fluoroquinolones makes it necessary to test the compound on strains with different resistance phenotypes.

27.3.2.4 Gram-Negative Bacilli

Enterobacteriaceae produce enzymes that hydrolyze beta-lactams and inactivate aminoglycosides to a varying degree or become resistant to the fluoroquinolones by chromosomal mechanisms.[10–12] The new compound should be tested on:

* Isogenic strains, such as *Escherichia coli* 600, which possesses different enzymes capable of hydrolyzing beta-lactams or inactivating aminoglycosides
* Strains resistant to fluoroquinolones by known mechanisms
* Reference strains that produce the different beta-lactamases or enzymes that inactivate aminoglysocides

Initially, studies are limited to species frequently involved in infectious diseases. Activity on less frequent species has to be tested as a second step. *Salmonella* and *Shigella* are important among the Enterobacteriaceae. Any new antibacterial agent should be tested on strains resistant to antibiotics recommended in the chemotherapy, such as ampicillin, chloramphenicol, and cotrimoxazole for *Salmonella* and tetracyclines and nalidixic acid for *Shigella*. New antibacterial agents should be tested for their activity on clinical isolates and collection strains of *Pseudomonas aeruginosa*, strains with known resistance (e.g., beta lactamase producers), and strains resistant to fluoroquinolones and aminoglycosides. Bactericidal activity should be determined alone and in combination with other antibacterial agents. A sufficient number of strains of species other than *P. aeruginosa* should be included when determining antibacterial activity. The susceptibility of *Haemophilus influenzae* should be examined on strains comprising beta-lactamases producers and nonproducers, as well as strains resistant to ampicillin through nonenzymatic mechanisms. Cephalosporins have decreased activity on these strains, and oral and parenteral cephalosporins should be included in the comparators.

27.3.2.5 Anaerobes

Antibacterial activity against anaerobes should be tested in a special laboratory. Gram-negative bacilli that are tested include strains resistant to clindamycin and cephamycins. Activity should be tested on two different culture media. Combination activities with metronidazole and clindamycin must be tested with the new antibacterials against pathogens involved in intraabdominal sepsis or in dental infections.

27.3.2.6 Other Microorganisms

Helicobacter pyrori has been found to be involved in duodenal ulcers and chronic gastritis type B. Antibacterial activity *in vitro* is tested at gastric pH if the compounds are acid stable. It is necessary to examine antibacterial activity in combination with Hep-2 cells. Because antiulcer drugs such as H_2-blockers and proton pump inhibitors are often used in therapy, the activity of an antibacterial agent should be tested in their presence. A few antibiotics are able to penetrate into phagocytic cells (e.g., macrolides, fluoroquinolones, and tetracyclines). The first step in the testing of intracellular bioactivity is to determine the kinetics of penetration and efflux, as well as the precise subcellular site of accumulation. This testing should be compared in the same class of antibacterials. As methods vary in different laboratories, it is necessary to obtain results from at least two different groups. The next step involves testing the intracellular activity of the antibacterial agent on intracellular pathogens, such as *Mycobacterium tuberculosis* and *M. avium complex*.[13]

27.3.3 Animal Models

Two types of animal models can be used: nondiscriminatory models or specific models of experimental infections.[14] Nondiscriminatory models are used in the preselection phase. *In vitro* activity may not correlate with *in vivo* activity (e.g., absorption, metabolism, toxicity). Systemic infections in these models are used to test activity on Gram-positive cocci (*Staphylococcus aureus*, *Streptococcus pyogenes*, *Streptococcus pneumoniae*, and *Enterococcus faecalis*), Enterobacteriaceae, and *Pseudomonas aeruginosa* using comparators in the same chemical group. The procedure includes strains with different antibiophenotypes, such as *P. aeruginosa* strains with different susceptibility to imipenem and ceftazidime.

In discriminatory models, two types of experimental infections can be used. Target infections include lower respiratory tract infection (e.g., *Klebsiella pneumoniae*), experimental pyelonephritis, endocarditis, experimental abscesses due to *Bacteroides fragilis*, experimental osteomyelitis due to *Staphylococcus aureus* or *Pseudomonas aeruginosa*, and experimental diarrhea in the piglet. Mice immunosuppressed with steroids or cyclophosphamide, or neutropenic mice, are used to predict activity in the target patients. Activity in otitis media due to *Haemophilus influenzae* is tested in the gerbil or in the chinchilla.

The second type of infection is more specific for the microorganism. These models are prerequisites for clinical testing in respiratory tract infections by *Legionella pneumophila* (guinea pig) and genital tract infections by *Chlamydia trachomatis* (mice).

Pharmacologic studies should be conducted to determine clinical indications. For activity against pneumococcal infection, microbiological validation is necessary, assessing effectiveness on the emergence of strains with decreased susceptibility (resistant to penicillin G or multiresistant). The first step is to test *in vitro* activity (MIC and MBC) on strains with variable susceptibility to penicillin G and cefotaxime. Multiresistant strains to erythromycin, tetracyclines, and kanamycin are also tested. If the activity of a fluoroquinolone is to be examined, it is also necessary to test strains of variable susceptibilities, such as to ofloxacin (MICs of 2 mg/L and >2 mg/L). The second step involves determining bactericidal activity using the killing curves method with different inocula (10^5 and 10^7 cfu/mL). An additional study involves determining the selective potential of the compound and the frequency and rate of mutations. These experiments are carried out *in vitro* and *in vivo*.[15] Comparative experimental models of systemic infection are used to determine potential therapeutic activity and will guide the choice of doses for phase II trials. The same approach is used for other pathogens, such as *Staphylococcus aureus* and *Pseudomonas aeruginosa*.

27.4 CLINICAL TRIALS TO EVALUATE EFFICACY AND SAFETY

The dosage and route of administration are important in the development of a new antibacterial agent. Studies conducted *in vitro* and *in vivo* examine the proposed dose and route of administration to be used during phase II studies. The antibacterial activity of roxithromycin is similar to that of erythromycin A, but it is three to ten times more active *in vivo* in nondiscriminative models of experimental infections due to its favorable pharmacokinetics.[16] The roxithromycin phase II trials were conducted with one third of the erythromycin A recommended dose (i.e., 600 mg/day), but later, the optimal daily dose was found to be 300 mg.[17] In the second phase, a certain number of models can be used to validate the chosen dosage. For meningitis, cerebrospinal fluid (CSF) levels of the agent should be at least ten times the MIC for the pathogen, depending on the stage of meningitis. After a cefotaxime dose of 200 mg/kg/day by intravenous injection, concentrations were found to be higher during the acute phase of the infection (1.7 to 7 mg/L), and they fell slightly during the attenuation phase (1.2 to 4 mg/L). During the resolution phase, the concentrations were 0.7 to 1.3 mg/L. When antibacterial activity falls, as seen with penicillin G in *Streptococcus pneumoniae*, the dosage should be increased to maintain the minimum ratio of CSF/MIC values of 10:1 and CSF bactericidal activity titer of 1:8.[18]

27.4.1 Pharmacokinetic Assessments

The following pharmacokinetic parameters are examined: area under the curve (AUC) above the MIC, the peak serum concentration/MIC ratio, the time during which serum concentrations are above the MIC (T > MIC), and AUIC (the AUC/MIC ratio). The concentration of the drug in the fluid surrounding the microorganism is related to what drives it into the bacterial cell and delivers it to the binding site. Because the majority of microorganisms live in the interstitial fluid, drug concentrations and kinetics should be examined in the extravascular fluid. The pharmacokinetics and pharmacodynamic properties of a drug must be evaluated with regard to patient responses to treatment. The AUIC is the best predictor of clinical response. It has been applied to the evaluation of cephalosporins, fluoroquinolones, aminoglycosides, metronidazole, and daptomycin but could be used for other antibiotics. The AUIC should be at least 125.

The killing rate of beta-lactams is time dependent and concentration independent. The time during which serum concentrations are above the MIC is the best predictor of therapeutic activity for beta-lactams. The bactericidal activity of beta-lactams can be saturated and reaches optimal when the serum concentration is four to eight times higher than the relevant MBC. Above this concentration, bactericidal activity no longer increases and may decrease. Efficacy is optimum if the T > MIC values are 100% and 50%, respectively, for Gram-negative bacteria and Gram-positive cocci; that is, serum concentrations should be above the MIC between two drug intakes for Gram-negative bacteria but only for 50% of the time for Gram-positive cocci, given the absence of a post-antibiotic effect.[19]

In conventional *in vitro* tests, bacteria are exposed to a constant concentration of antibiotic throughout the test period. This does not reflect the situation in humans, where the concentration of antibiotic in the serum and tissue is constantly changing, depending on the absorption, metabolism, and elimination rates of the compounds. *In vitro* kinetic models can be used to simulate the concentrations of antibiotics measured in the serum and extravascular fluid of individuals following conventional dosage and to assess their antibacterial activities.[20] This model may be used to study direct comparative activity, the effect of different dosage regimens (to predict breakpoints values more accurately), and the potential for any synergistic or antagonistic interactions at concentrations in humans.

27.4.2 Microbiological Assessments

Microbiological assessments involve several aspects:

- Collection and transport of pathological specimens
- Isolation and identification of pathogens
- Determination of the antibacterial activity of the test compound and comparators
- Phenotyping and genetic analysis of the strain
- Correlation of *in vitro* activity with clinical efficacy for the determination of breakpoints

During clinical trials, the MIC values and zone diameter inhibition should be determined for each clinical isolate. Reference strains must also be used and their MIC values and zone diameter determined. The sampling conditions and the way in which specimens are transported to the clinical laboratory should be established and standardized. Pathological specimens include blood, urine, stool, bronchial secretions, bronchoalveolar lavage fluid, CSF, pleural fluid, pericardial fluid, ascites, joint fluid, pharyngotonsillar samples, and various pus. Cytological and microscopic examinations after staining are conducted for bacterial isolation and identification.

Quantitative analyses are necessary for certain pathological samples such as urine and bronchial brushing specimens. Cytobacteriological and biochemical examinations are conducted in certain infections such as purulent meningitis. Bacterial species must be identified. Streptococci are identified by their group, and pneumococcal serotypes are determined. In the case of *Haemophilus influenzae*, not only must the serotype be analyzed (e.g., type b and non-type b) but also the biotype, which is useful if eradication is not achieved. Identification of the strains is conducted at the beginning of the infection and during the treatment.

When the same bacterial species is isolated after completion of or during the treatment, it is necessary to check that it is the same as the strain present at the outset of infection. Certain bacterial species, such as the Enterobacteriaceae, can be analyzed by gel-electrophoresis. The antibiotic susceptibility of the clinical isolate responsible for the infection should be tested in the clinical microbiology laboratory. The MIC and inhibition zone diameter for the sample and reference strains are measured.

Certain tests are conducted routinely; for example, testing with *Streptococcus pneumoniae* using disks loaded with 1 μg of oxacillin can be used to predict if the strain is resistant to penicillin G. It is necessary to add a cefizoxime disk when the diameter is 15 mm, because it is possible that the strain is resistant to cefotaxime and ceftriaxone (MIC 2 mg/L). These data can be confirmed by determining the MIC value. In addition, the activity of a new beta-lactam on Enterobacteriaceae must be determined. Cefotaxime, cefazidime, and aztreonam should be tested in association with coamoxyclav to detect extended spectrum beta-lactamase. For aminoglycosides, it is necessary to determine the enzymatic profile of a bacterial strain for different enzymes and abnormality of membrane permeability in the inhibition zone diameters.[11]

All isolates should be stored under adequate conditions. A centralized laboratory tests all strains isolated during the clinical trials. All strains should be reidentified and confirmed, including serotypes, beta-lactamase, and enzymes inactivating aminoglycosides. The MIC is routinely redetermined. For bacterial species for which growth is variable (e.g., *Streptococcus pneumoniae*, *Streptococcus pyogenes*, *Moraxella catarrhalis*, and *Haemophilus influenzae*), it is necessary to run antibacterial susceptibility tests and to examine the MIC values of antibiotics tested in parallel. Other tests, such as killing curves, can be conducted on a given strain when the microbiological response occurs slower than expected in comparison with the majority of isolates for a given bacterial species.

Certain bacterial species are tested for tolerance using MIC and MBC methods, such as benzylpenicillin and viridans streptococci or 2-amino-5-thiazolyl cephalosporins and *H. influenzae*. Correlations between the disk method and MIC technique should be established, which involves multicenter studies using fresh clinical isolates collected over a given period that include the major bacterial species growing aerobically or in anaerobic conditions (e.g., Enterobacteriaceae and bacteria commonly responsible for clinical infections).

Most phase II clinical trials are conducted as preliminary studies to establish a basis for phase III trials by identifying the optimal dosage and administration route for large-scale evaluation. Phase III trials are expanded controlled trials to establish the efficacy and safety of the drug, information that is necessary to evaluate the overall risk–benefit relationship of the product and provide necessary data for product license application.

Following licensure of the product, further studies are undertaken to monitor and confirm its efficacy and safety in a large population. These studies are usually required as a condition of license approval. Phase IV studies are designed to observe long-term product efficacy, to detect any adverse reactions that occur with long-term administration in patient subpopulations (e.g., children and the elderly), and to determine the incidence of nonresponders. Studies of rare adverse reactions attributable to drug therapy are of particular importance.

REFERENCES

1. Levin, B.R., Noninherited resistance to antibiotics, *Science*, 305(5690), 1578–1579, 2004.
2. Kim, G.T., Ryu, E.J., Jang, Y.J. et al., Cephalosporins with the dichlorophenyl group at C-7 position and pyrimidine at C-3 position exhibiting potent activity against Gram-positive strains, *J. Antibiol. (Tokyo)*, 57 (7): 468–472, 2004.
3. Del Rosso, J.Q., A status report on the use of subantimicrobial-dose dexyclcline: a review of biologic and antimicrobial effects of the tetracyclines, *Cutis*, 74(2), 118–122, 2004.
4. Mohapatra, P.R., Fluoroquinolones in multidrug-resistant tuberculosis, *Am. J. Respir. Crit. Care Med.*, 170(8), 920–921, 2004.
5. Spann, C.T., Taylor, S.C., and Weinberg, J.M., Topical antimicrobial agents in dermatology, *Dis. Mon.*, 50(7), 407–421, 2004.
6. Agouridas, C., Bonnefoy, A., Chantot, J.F. et al., A New Distinct Semi-Synthetic Class of Macrolides: *In Vitro* and *In Vivo* Antibacterial Activity, paper presented at the 34th Interscience Conference on Antimicrobial Agents and Chemotherapeutics, Orlando, FL, 1994.
7. Siebor, E. and Kazmierczak, A., Factors influencing the activity of macrolide antibiotics *in vitro*, in *Macrolides: Chemistry, Pharmacology and Clinical Use*, Bryskier, A.J., Butzler, J.P., Neu, HC., and Tulkens, P.M., Eds., Blackwell-Arnette, Paris, 1993, pp. 197–203.
8. Bryskier, A., Veyssier, P., and Kazmierczak, A., Fluoroquinolones: proprietes physicochimiques et microbiologiques, *Encyclopédie Médico: Chirurgicales-Maladies Infectieuses*, Elsevier, Amsterdam, 1994.
9. Hamilton-Miller, J.M.T., Towards greater uniformity in sensitivity testing, *J. Antimicrob. Chemother.*, 3, 385–392, 1997.
10. Philipon, A., Arlet, G., and Lagrange, P.H., Origin and impact of plasmid-mediated extended-spectrum beta-lactamases, *Eur. J. Clin. Microbiol. Infect. Dis.*, 13(Suppl. 1), 17–29, 1994.
11. Miller, G.H. and Aminoglycoside Resistance Study Group, Resistance to aminoglycosides in *Pseudomonas*, *Trends Microbiol.*, 2, 347–352, 1994.
12. Bryskier, A., Fluoroquinolones: mechanisms of action and resistance, *Int. Antimicrob. Agents*, 2, 151–184, 1993.
13. Rastogi, N., Labrousse, V., and Bryskier, A., Intracellular activities of roxithromycin used alone and in association with other drugs against *Mycobacterium avium* complex in human macrophages, *Antimicrob. Agents Chemother.*, 39(4), 976–978, 1995.
14. Zak, O. and O'Reilly, T., Animal models as predictors of the safety and efficacy of antibiotics, *Eur. J. Clin. Microbiol. Infect. Dis.*, 9, 472–478, 1990.

15. Barry, A.L. and Sabath, L.D., Special tests: bactericidal activity and activity of antimicrobics in combination, in *Manual of Clinical Microbiology*, 2nd ed., Lennette, E.H., Spaulding, E.H., and Truant, J.P., Eds., American Society for Microbiology, Washington, D.C., 1974.
16. Chantot, J.F., Bryskier, A., and Gasc, J.C., Antibacterial activity of roxithromycin: a laboratory evaluation. *J. Antibiotics*, 39, 660–668, 1986.
17. Akoun, G., Bertrand, A., and Cambarrere, I., Clinical evaluation of rexithromcin (RU 28965) in the treatment of hospitalized patients with lower respiratory tract infections, in *Macrolides: A Review with an Outlook on Future Development*, Butzler, J.P. and Kobayashi, H., Eds., Excerpta Medica, Amsterdam, 1986, pp. 95–99.
18. Tauber, M.G., Kunz, S., Zak, O. et al., Influence of antibiotic dose, dosing interval, and duration of therapy on outcome in experimental pneumococcal meningitis in rabbits, *Antimicrob. Agents Chemother.*, 33, 418–423, 1989.
19. Vogelman, B.S. and Craig, W.A., Postantibiotic effects., *J. Antimicrob. Chemother.*, 15(Suppl. A), 37–46, 1985.
20. Grasso, S., Meinardi, G., De Carneci, I. et al., New *in vitro* model to study the effect of antibiotic concentration and rate of elimination on antibacterial activity, *Antimicrob. Agents Chemother.*, 13, 570–576, 1978.
21. Division of Drugs and Toxicity, Cephalosporins and related agents, in *Drug Evaluations*, American Medical Association, Washington, D.C., 1995, pp. 1413–1480.
22. Nichols, W.K., Anti-infectives, in *Remington: The Science and Practice of Pharmacy*, Gennaro, A.R., Ed., 20th ed., Lippincott Williams & Wilkins, Baltimore, MD, 2000, pp. 1507–1561.

CHAPTER 28

Antiviral Drugs

Lucia H. Lee, Christopher L. Wu, Benjamin R. Lee, and Chi-Jen Lee

CONTENTS

28.1 INTRODUCTION

Viruses cause extensive morbidity and mortality worldwide, but advances in the chemotherapy of viral diseases are limited. Only a few antiviral agents of proven clinical effectiveness are available for a limited number of indications. Antiviral drug development has become a very active area during the past 20 years, especially with the challenges presented by the acquired immunodeficiency syndrome (AIDS), hepatitis, and severe acute respiratory syndrome (SARS) epidemics. The need to develop more selective inhibitors of viral function has resulted in many antiviral drug clinical trials for human immunodeficiency virus (HIV) as well as other viral diseases and should lead to important progress in the future.

Viruses are obligate intracellular parasites that utilize many biochemical pathways of the infected host cells. Viruses cannot replicate independently because they use the energy-generating DNA or RNA and protein-synthesizing pathways of the host cells to replicate; thus, the development of virus-specific inhibitors has received considerable attention recently. With nonselective inhibitors of viral replication, it is difficult to achieve a useful antiviral therapy without also affecting some aspect of normal host cell metabolism and inducing potentially toxic effects in the host cells. Searching for selective inhibitors of viral replication is an important goal for drug development.

Viral replication can be targeted at several processes:

- Adsorption to host-cell surface receptors and penetration into cells
- Uncoating of viral nucleic acid
- Synthesis of early regulatory enzymes, such as nucleic acid polymerase, thymidine kinase, and reverse transcriptase
- Synthesis of RNA or DNA
- Synthesis of late structural proteins
- Assembly of viral particles
- Release of infectious virions from the cell

Replication of the virus peaks after acute illness or before the clinical symptoms appear; thus, early initiation of therapy and prevention of infection are important for optimal clinical treatment, such as using acyclovir to treat varicella-zoster infection and amantadine prophylaxis against influenza A. The development of pyrimidine and purine nucleoside analogs has led to new drugs that selectively inhibit viral DNA synthesis. Several reverse transcriptase inhibitors have been selected as drugs for the HIV retrovirus to block transcription of the HIV RNA genome into DNA and protein synthesis. More recently, protease inhibitors have been developed to prevent the synthesis of late protein and packaging of the virion.

In contrast to acute illnesses, infections by hepatitis B and C, papillomavirus, and cytomegalovirus cause chronic diseases leading to serious clinical sequelae. Antiviral drugs for these chronic viral infections, therefore, should interrupt the progression of the disease and reduce the chance of late adverse consequences. Because drugs for chronic viral diseases will be used for long periods of time, tolerability becomes a critical element in the risk–benefit assessment for drug development.

Immunization should be the primary approach for the prevention of viral infections. When effective vaccines are not available or in a particular high-risk population (e.g., immunodeficient individuals and those with hypersensitivity to existing vaccines), chemoprophylaxis should be considered. For diseases such as influenza, drug therapy should be initiated as soon as an outbreak is recognized. For other prophylactic use, the duration and the timing for initiating prophylaxis will depend on conditions of the natural history of the disease.

28.2 ANTIVIRAL DRUGS AND THEIR MECHANISMS OF ACTION

The major antiviral drugs are categorized as inhibitors of viral uncoating, inhibitors of viral nucleic acid synthesis, reverse transcriptase inhibitors, protease inhibitors, and immunostimulants; the main antiviral drugs are shown in Table 28.1. Most antiviral drugs, such as zidovudine, idoxuridine, and didanosine, are nucleoside analogs that interfere with viral nucleic acid synthesis by inhibiting viral DNA polymerases.[1] This inhibition of viral enzyme, however, is not selective, and all these drugs cause toxicities due to their inhibitory actions on host enzymes. Other drugs, such as amantadine and rimatadine, interfere with entry of the influenza virus. Recently, HIV protease has been recognized as a new target of virus-specific functions.[2] Several potent inhibitors of HIV replication have exhibited promising results in early-phase clinical trials. Other target sites include virus-specific integrase and regulatory enzymes responsible for amplification of viral replication.[3] Rational drug design based on structure analysis and simple screening procedures suitable for high-flux random screening can now be used to identify drug candidates that inhibit these target sites.

Table 28.1 Antiviral Drugs

Drug Category	Treatment and Remarks
Nucleic Acid Synthesis Inhibitors	
Purine analogs	
Acyclovir	Antiherpes; central nervous system (CNS) effects
Cidofovir	For cytomegalovirus (CMV); nephrotoxicity
Famciclovir	Prodrug of penciclovir
Ganciclovir	For CMV, bone marrow suppression
Penciclovir	Antiherpes; similar to acyclovir
Ribovarin	For respiratory syncytial virus (RSV); potential embryo toxicity
Valacyclovir	Prodrug of acyclovir; better oral absorption
Pyrimidin analogs	
Fluorouracil	For warts
Idoxuridine	For herpes simplex
Trifluridine	For herpes simplex
Nonnucleosides	
Foscarnet	For CMV, acyclovir-resistant herpes; nephrotoxicity
HIV Reverse Transcriptase Inhibitors	
Pyrimidine nucleosides	
Lamivudine	Well tolerated
Stavudine	Peripheral neuropathy
Zalcitabine	Peripheral neuropathy
Zidovudine	Anemia, neutropenia, gastrointestinal (GI) effects, CNS effects
Purine nucleosides	
Didanosine	Peripheral neuropathy, pancreatitis, GI effects
Nonnucleosides	
Nevirapine	Rash, fever, nausea, headache
HIV Protease Inhibitors	
Indinavir	For kidney stones; good bioavailability, inhibits CYP3A4
Nelfinavir	Fewer side effects, some diarrhea
Ritonavir	Good bioavailability, more side effects and drug interactions
Saquinavir	Low bioavailability, fewer side effects, inhibits CYP3A4
Inhibitors of Influenza Viral Penetration or Uncoating	
Amantadine	Renal excretion, greater CNS toxicity
Rimantadine	Metabolized, similar toxicity as amantadine
Interferons and Immunoglobulins	
Interferon-alpha, -beta, -gamma	Inhibit viral protein synthesis or assembly or stimulate the immune system
Immunoglobulins	Prevent viral infections by specific binding to viruses

In addition, immunomodulators have been used in antiviral therapy to enhance the cytotoxic killing of infected cells that serve as reservoirs for further spread of the virus. For example, alpha-interferon, which has been studied extensively, has independent immunomodulatory and antiviral effects against viral hepatitis and papilloma viral infection.[4] Other immunomodulators such as gamma-interferon, interleukin (IL)-2, and IL-12 have also been examined for their potential use against various viral diseases. These immunomodulators do not exhibit a direct antiviral effect.[5,6]

28.2.1 Nucleic Acid Synthesis Inhibitors

28.2.1.1 Purine Analogs

Acyclovir and other guanosine analogs (e.g., ganciclovir, valacyclovir, famciclovir) are the most important group of antiherpes drugs that act by inhibition of viral nucleic acid synthesis. They inhibit virus growth in three ways: (1) the drug (e.g., acyclovir triphosphate) can act as a competitive inhibitor of DNA polymerases, while the human enzyme is much less susceptible than the viral enzyme; (2) the drug can be a chain terminator; or (3) the drug can produce irreversible binding between DNA polymerase and the interrupted chain, causing permanent inactivation.[7,8] Ribovaran is a synthetic purine nucleoside analog that is phosphorylated by host cell adenosine kinase, resulting in a monophosphate that inhibits cellular inosine monophosphate formation. The result is depletion of guanosine triphosphate and inhibition of viral protein synthesis, plus suppression of initiation or elongation of viral mRNA.

28.2.1.2 Pyrimidine Analogs

Idoxuridine and trifluridine are pyrimidine analogs that are incorporated into viral DNA, resulting in inhibition of DNA synthesis. They are only used topically for herpes simplex infections of the cornea because of their toxicity. Fluorouracil acts by blocking production of thymidine and interrupts normal cellular RNA and DNA synthesis. It is also restricted to topical therapy of warts.

28.2.1.3 Nonnucleosides

Foscarnet, a phosphonoformic acid, inhibits DNA polymerases, RNA polymerases, and reverse transcriptases. It is used primarily for AIDS patients with cytomegalovirus (CMV) retinitis but can be used against CMV herpes viruses resistant to acyclovir.[9]

28.2.2 HIV Reverse Transcriptase Inhibitors

Zidovudine and several dideoxynucleosides (e.g., zalcibine, lamuvidine, stavudine) are competitive inhibitors of the HIV enzyme that converts viral RNA into DNA and act as DNA chain terminators upon phosphorylation to the triphosphate nucleotide derivatives. These nucleoside antivirals also inhibit mammalian DNA polymerases but require higher concentrations than those effective on HIV reverse transcriptase. Two reverse transcriptase inhibitors are usually combined with a protease inhibitor to decrease the development of resistance. Nevirapine is a non-nucleoside inhibitor of reverse transcriptase that also disrupts the catalytic site of this enzyme.

28.2.3 HIV Protease Inhibitors

Indinavir, nelfinavir, ritonavir, and saquinavir are peptide analogs that inhibit the HIV-1-specific protein-cleaving enzyme necessary for the production of infectious HIV virions and act synergistically with reverse transcriptase inhibitors. It is important to use them in combination for HIV therapy because resistance occurs if they are used alone. Two reverse transcriptase inhibitors may be used in combination with one protease inhibitor. Combination therapy can decrease viral replication, improve the immunologic status, delay complications, and prolong life.

28.2.4 Inhibitors of Influenza

Amantadine and rimantadine are effective for prophylaxis of influenzae A. These antiviral drugs are tricyclic amines that differ only in their pharmacokinetics. Renal excretion predominates for amantadine while rimantadine is extensively metabolized.

28.2.5 Interferons and Immunoglobulins

Interferons and immunoglobulins are endogenous compounds that stimulate immune responses to virus infections. Interferon-alpha, -beta, and -gamma are glycoproteins produced by lymphocytes, macrophages, fibroblasts, and other cells. They act by inhibiting viral protein synthesis or assembly or by stimulating the immune system. Interferons have specific intracellular actions that produce several effects, including inhibition of viral penetration, uncoating, translation of viral proteins, and assembly and release of virus.[10] Immunoglobulins can be used to prevent some viral infections through the use of antibody preparations with high titers of those that bind to specific viruses, especially hepatitis B and rabies.

28.3 LABORATORY ASSESSMENTS OF ANTIVIRAL DRUGS IN ACUTE AND CHRONIC INFECTIONS

The goal of chemoprophylaxis is to prevent the infection and clinical manifestation of disease caused by a pathogenic virus. For viral infections leading to chronic diseases, prevention of infection is important. For viral infections causing only acute diseases, prevention of clinical manifestation should be adequate. The development of an immune response to subclinical infection is a desirable approach of prophylaxis, as immunity can be established against reinfection. Evaluating the efficacy of chemoprophylaxis usually requires a large number of patients because of low natural infection rates. This problem can be approached in early-phase clinical studies by the selection of a subpopulation with higher infection rates such as nursing home residents, other institutionalized populations, and less immunocompetent individuals. Because of the unpredictability of the outbreak and the variability of the immune status of each individual against a particular viral infection, efficacy data from uncontrolled, open studies are not reliable. Phase II efficacy studies should be double blinded and controlled; phase I single- and multiple-dose–response pharmacokinetic and tolerance studies can remain open and uncontrolled.

Efficacy trials of chemoprophylaxis in the prevention of chronic viral infections, such as HIV, are difficult due to the low incidence rate. A very large sample size will be required for drugs with high efficacy. Early-phase studies can be used primarily to establish drug safety. Because of the high rate of perinatal transmission of HIV, the efficacy of chemoprophylaxis can be evaluated with a large number of patients. Extensive controlled trials can be planned based on efficacy and safety data from early studies in pregnant women.[10–13]

Many laboratory methods are now available to confirm viral infection. Antibody determinations can be used for the detection of seroconversion or increases in antibody titers.[14] Other tests, such as antigen-capture assays, detect the presence of the virus or its components in the infected patients. Viral culture, when positive, is a useful indication for the infectivity of the patients. Negative culture, however, may not indicate the absence of the virus and could be due to the difficulty in reaching optimum conditions of the culture method. Diagnostic tests based on polymerase chain reaction (PCR) and branched-DNA assays will facilitate the confirmation of viral infection.[15–17]

For acute viral infection, viral culture data provide key assessments of any antiviral effect. The presence of viruses in herpetic lesions or the nasal washes of patients with influenza disease can be identified by culture. The sensitivity of a culture method depends on the particular viral infection. For influenza virus, quantitative analysis for viral isolation has been well established, and data on viral shedding are reliable. These culture assays were used to demonstrate that fewer patients with influenza disease were shedding virus after 2-day therapy with rimantadine compared to those who received placebo. In addition, those who continued to shed virus despite rimantadine therapy had significantly lower viral titers compared to placebo recipients.[18] On the other hand, viral culture data from studies with herpes simplex were not clear. Positive culture could not be obtained from herpetic lesions in up to 50% of recurrent episodes.[19] PCR assays will greatly increase the sensitivity in the identification of viral diseases.[20]

Commercial assays are available for quantitative determinations of components associated with various viruses, such as hepatitis B virus (HBV), hepatitis C virus (HCV), and HIV. In HBV infection, the plasma levels of both HBV DNA and HBV DNA polymerase correlate well with the amount of viral particles. A decrease in these parameters with therapy should therefore reflect antiviral activity of the drug. Moreover, continuous suppression of these HBV viral markers has been associated with reversion of serological status of patients and improvement in liver histology.[21] Hepatitis B surface antigen is an accepted marker for HBV; however, no such antigen has been observed for HCV. It has been suggested that HCV RNA levels parallel the course of alanine transaminase (ALT) values, indicating the possible utility of using the viral marker as a surrogate. In HIV infection, the reduction of viral counts as measured by amplification strategy (e.g., RNA-PCR) correlates better with clinical outcome.

Viral cultures have not been reliable efficacy parameters for chronic viral infection due to problems with reproducibility. The recently developed method of microculture titering of plasma HIV viral load has helped to establish another valid viral load measurement. Antibodies to specific viral antigens represent another important marker for laboratory assessments. The presence of specific antibodies is correlated with a less active phase of viral replication. The appearance of these antibodies during drug therapy, therefore, indicates that the activity of the disease has been slowed down or arrested. Improvement of immune function can be used as key evidence for the efficacy of a drug for HIV infection. In other viral infections, improvements in immune function can also be used as evidence for efficacy.

Several immunologic tests have been used for the evaluation of immune functions. Cell counts of total subtypes of white blood cells provide a quick analysis of overall status of the immune system. Measurements of subsets of T-lymphocytes, such as helper (CD4) and suppressor (CD8) populations, are useful as surrogate markers for evaluating the efficacy of HIV therapy but are not generally useful for other viral infection. *In vitro* assay of lymphocyte response to mitogenic and antigenic stimulation is the most commonly used method to assess the overall function of cellular immunity.[22] More specific assays such as antibody-dependent, cell-mediated cytotoxicity should be used when infected cells can serve directly as target cells for cytotoxic killing in the *in vitro* assay. Cutaneous delayed-type hypersensitivity tests have been used to evaluate T-cell functionality *in vivo*.

When to initiate therapy and how frequently efficacy measurements should be made are two issues critical to a successful treatment study of acute viral infection. The earlier a drug treatment begins, the more likely it is that the drug will offer noticeable benefits. Studies on influenza A and herpes simplex showed that, to be effective in treatment against these acute infections, drugs must be given within 48 to 72 hours after the first clinical symptom of the diseases. In general, drug therapy should not be initiated until a laboratory diagnosis has been made; however, when a rapid diagnostic test cannot be performed, treatment may be started without laboratory diagnosis — for example, if the disease is serious or the experimental drug has fewer adverse effects. Under these conditions, a retrospective laboratory diagnosis should be conducted. Earlier drug therapy may also be needed for the effective treatment of acute viral infection in children.

Many patients recover from acute infections within several days without therapy; therefore, a drug must exhibit efficacy within a narrow time frame. Demonstration of effectiveness with therapy requires frequent monitoring of patients and making several observations each day. This close monitoring may require housing patients with diseases; otherwise, hospitalization generally is not necessary because it can increase the cost of a study and require additional management.

Because of the variation in the process of acute disease among infected patients, drug efficacy for symptomatic relief should be evaluated in double-blind, controlled studies. A randomized trial of vidarabine vs. foscarnet in patients with acyclovir-resistant herpes simplex virus (HSV) was terminated early due to clear evidence of the superiority of foscarnet in terms of time to healing, resolution of pain, and cessation of viral shedding.[23,24] When the trial was terminated, only 14 of projected 26 patients had been enrolled, indicating the potential power of a controlled trial to rapidly detect large differences in efficacy between treatments. Although early phase tolerance studies can be open and uncontrolled, the toxicities of a drug can be confused with the clinical symptoms of the disease being treated. In this case, further clarification of drug toxicity should be obtained from a controlled trial.

28.4 CLINICAL TRIALS FOR EFFICACY AND SAFETY

The primary efficacy endpoint is prevention of laboratory-confirmed viral infection during chemo-prophylaxis. Laboratory analyses are critical in respiratory viral infection because many different respiratory viruses cause diseases with similar clinical symptoms; however, laboratory analyses may not be required for evaluating suppression of recurrence because in this case patients are usually familiar with the specific clinical symptoms associated with the disease, and an accurate diagnosis can be made. The severity of a viral disease that develops during chemoprophylaxis should be monitored. Disease that develops during chemoprophylaxis can be less severe or have fewer complications, thus further supporting the activity of the drug.

In acute viral infections, the most important efficacy parameters in early-phase trials are clinical symptoms. One approach to simplifying and facilitating the assessment of symptoms is to establish a scoring system, such as the one used in studies with rimantadine for the treatment of influenza A.[25] A second approach is to select key symptoms as the primary parameters for analysis. For example, only pain and itching were evaluated in most studies with acyclovir and interferons for the treatment of herpes simplex, but both acute pain and postherpetic neuralgia have been used as key efficacy parameters for herpes zoster.[19,26] A third approach uses transformed parameters that provide general measurements of the rate of recovery from disease, such as time to 50% improve-ment and time to last fever, which were used to analyze data from the rimatadine studies.[27] These parameters help to eliminate conducting an analysis at each time point.

Improving the quality of life of patients with acute viral infection can provide evidence for the efficacy of a drug. Evaluations of productivity (e.g., return to work, class attendance) can provide useful evidence regarding the benefits of a drug. More accurate methods can be used to evaluate changes in overall behavior or perceptions such as psychosocial functioning and general well-being.

The clinical assessment of acute infection is primarily restricted to herpetic lesions. Resolution of viral lesions is measured by time to healing, time to crusting, and duration of vesicle or ulcer. Some of these parameters are more appropriate than others for a particular type of herpetic lesion, depending on the natural course of the disease. It is necessary to conduct consistent observations of lesions by the same investigator because the assessment of lesions can be subjective.

The main objectives of therapy for chronic viral infection are to arrest disease progression and reduce possible late adverse reactions. The ultimate goal is to completely eliminate viral infection. This goal is probably not realistic because of viral–gene integration and the development of latency. Active viral replication does not take place in many infected cells; phenotypically and functionally, these cells closely resemble the noninfected cells, thus leaving only a few selective targets for drug activity.

The evaluation of antiviral drugs for chronic infection follows a two-step process. Virological or immunologic surrogate markers are usually used as endpoints for drug activity during early-phase studies. When drug activity and the therapeutic index have been determined, long-term trials to determine the efficacy and safety of the drug can be conducted based on the clinical endpoints established. It is necessary to discuss with the regulatory agency the use of surrogate markers to evaluate drug activity in early-phase trials. Responses in CD4 cell counts have been used as the basis for the approval of didanosine, zalcitabine, and stavudine for the treatment of advanced HIV disease. CD4 cell counts, however, have partially satisfied the criteria as a valid surrogate marker defined by the Institute of Medicine.[28] Other endpoints, including β_2-microglobulin, HIV p24 antigen, and neopterin, have been used as surrogate markers in early trials. In addition, viral load measurement based on the amplification method may be used to evaluate the effectiveness of a drug against HIV disease, as well as drug therapy against hepatitis C.[29]

In the early phases of clinical trials, when control group are not used, the toxicities of a drug may be exaggerated because it can be difficult to separate toxicities associated with the drug from clinical symptoms of diseases. For example, the gastrointestinal toxicities observed in patients receiving rimantadine or amantadine for acute influenza infection could be due to either drug or the disease.[25] When no control group is included in a trial for comparison, it is important to state the relationship of the observed toxicity and drug therapy, as well as the reversibility of side effects after termination of therapy. If possible, readministration of the drug should be considered to provide direct evidence for the causal relationship.

Most phase II clinical trials are conducted as preliminary studies to lay the basis for phase III trials and are designed to identify the dosages and schedules for large-scale evaluation. Phase III studies, expanded controlled trials to establish the drug's efficacy and safety in an expanded patient population, are necessary to evaluate the overall risk–benefit relationship of the product and provide necessary data for product license application. The optimum dosage should be established at this time.

Sometimes, the evidence of safety and effectiveness obtained from phase II studies are so convincing that phase III trials are not necessary. For example, in studies on the anti-AIDS drug zidovudine, one AIDS patient died while being treated with zidovudine, compared to 10 AIDS patients given placebo. In this study, 1338 asymptomatic patients with T4 lymphocyte counts <500/mm³ received either zidovudine 100 or 300 mg or placebo, each given five times daily. Participants were monitored for the development of the signs and symptoms of HIV disease and tolerance to the regimens employed. The study was terminated early because a statistically significant difference in progression to AIDS was observed between the group receiving 500 mg/day and the placebo group.[30] Because the results were dramatically better with zidovudine, as compared with the placebo, the FDA was able to approve the drug for marketing in March 1987, only 4 months after receiving an application from Burroughs Wellcome.

Following licensure of the product, further studies are undertaken to monitor and confirm its efficacy and safety in a large population. These studies are usually required as a condition of license approval. Phase IV studies are designed to observe long-term product efficacy and adverse reactions that occur with long-term administration in patient subpopulations (e.g., children, the elderly) and the incidence of nonresponders. Studies of rare adverse reactions attributable to drug therapy are of particular importance. These rare reactions cannot be observed during phase II or phase III clinical trials, even with sample sizes of tens of thousands.

REFERENCES

1. Herdewijin, P.A., Novel nucleoside strategies for anti-HIV and anti-HSV therapy, *Antiviral Res.*, 19, 1–14, 1992.
2. Vacca, J.P., Dorsey, B.D., Schleif, W.A. et al., L-735,524: an orally bioavailable human immunodeficiency virus type 1 protease inhibitor, *Proc. Natl. Acad. Sci. USA*, 91, 4096–4100, 1994.
3. Mitsuya, H. and Broder, S., Strategies for antiviral therapy in AIDS, *Nature*, 325, 773–778, 1987.
4. Clements, M.J. and McNurlan, M.A., Regulation of cell proliferation and differentiation by interferons, *Biochem. J.*, 226, 345–360, 1985.
5. Scott, P., IL-12: initiation cytokine for cell-mediated immunity, *Science*, 260, 496–497, 1993.
6. Sneller, M., Cytokine Therapy of HIV Infection, paper presented at the Fourth Triennial Symposium, New Directions in Antiviral Chemotherapy, San Francisco, CA, November 10–12, 1994.
7. Bacon, T.H., Levin, M.J., Leary, J.J. et al., Herpes simplex virus resistance to acyclovir and penciclovir after two decades of antiviral therapy, *Clin. Microbiol. Rev.*, 16, 114–128, 2003.

8. Tyring, S.K., Baker, D., and Snowden, W., Valacyclovir for herpes simplex virus infection: long-term safety and sustained efficacy after 20 years' experience with acyclovir, *J. Infect. Dis.*, 186(Suppl. 1), S40–S46, 2002.

9. Morfin, F. and Thouvenot, D., Herpes simplex virus resistance to antiviral drugs, *J. Clin. Virol.*, 26, 29–37, 2003.

10. Sen, G.C., Viruses and interferons, *Ann. Rev. Microviol.*, 55, 255–281, 2001.

11. Connor, E.M., Sperling, R.S., Gelber, R. et al., Reduction of maternal–infant transmission of human immundeficiency virus type I with zidovudine treatment, *N. Engl. J. Med.*, 331(18), 1173–1180, 1994.

12. O'Sullivan, M.J., Boyer, P.J., Scott, G.B. et al., The pharmacokinetics and safety of zidovudine in the third trimester of pregnancy for women infected with human immunodeficiency virus and their infants: phase I acquired immunodeficiency syndrome clinical trial group study (Protocol 082), *Am. J. Obstet. Gynecol.*, 168(5), 1510–1516, 1993.

13. Sperling, R.S., Roboz, J., Dische, R. et al., Zidovudine pharmacokinetics during pregnancy, *Am. J. Perinatol.*, 9(4), 247–249, 1992.

14. Sninsky, J.J., Application of the polymerase chain reaction to the detection of viruses, in *Viral Hepatitis and Liver Disease*, Hollinger, F.B., Lemon, S.M., and Margolis, H.F., Eds., Lippincott Williams & Wilkins, Baltimore, MD, 1991, p. 799.

15. Mulder, J., McKinney, N., Christopherson, C. et al., Rapid and simple PCR assay for quantitation of human immunodeficiency virus type I RNA in plasma: application to acute retroviral infection, *J. Clin. Microbiol.*, 32(2), 292–300, 1994.

16. Martinot-Peignoux, M., Marcellin, P., Gournay, J. et al., Detection and quantitation of serum HCV-RNA by branched DNA amplification in anti-HCV positive blood donors, *J. Hepatol.*, 20(5), 676–678, 1994.

17. Urdea, M.S., Horn, T., Fultz, T.J. et al., Branched DNA amplification multimers for the sensitive, direct detection of human hepatitis viruses, *Nucleic Acids Symp. Ser.*, 24, 197–200, 1991.

18. Van Voris, L.P., Betts, R.F., Hayden, F.G. et al., Successful treatment of naturally occurring influenza A/USSR/77 H1N1, *J. Am. Med. Assoc.*, 245, 1128–1131, 1981.

19. Sacks, S.L., Treatment of genital herpes, in *Clinical Use of Antiviral Drugs*, DeClercq, E., Ed., Martinus Nijhoff, Boston, 1988, p. 87.

20. Cone, R.W., Hobson, A.C., Brown, Z. et al., Frequent detection of genital herpes simplex virus DNA by polymerase chain reaction among pregnant women, *JAMA*, 272(10), 792–796, 1994.

21. Alexander, G.J.M., Brahm, J., Fagan, E.A. et al., Loss of HBsAg with interferon therapy in chronic hepatitis B virus infection, *Lancet*, ii, 66, 1987.

22. Yarchoan, R. and Nelson, D.L., A study of the functional capabilities of human neonatal lymphocytes for *in vitro* specific antibody production, *J. Immunol.*, 131, 1222–1228, 1983.

23. Safrin, S., Crumpacker, C., Chatis, P. et al., A controlled trial comparing foscarnet with vidarbine for acyclovir-resistant mucocutaneous herpes simplex in the acquired immunodeficiency syndrome, *N. Engl. J. Med.*, 325, 551–555, 1991.

24. Brady, R.C. and Bernstein, D.I., Treatment of herpes simplex virus infection, *Antivir. Res.*, 61, 73–81, 2004.

25. Hall, C.B., Dolin, R., Gala, C.L. et al., Children with influenza a infection: treatment with rimantadine, *Pediatrics*, 80, 275–282, 1987.

26. Gilden, D.H., Herpes zoster with postherpetic neuralgia: persisting pain and frustration, *N. Engl. J. Med.*, 330(13), 932–934, 1994.

27. Wingfield, W.L., Pollack, D., and Grunert, R.R., Therapeutic efficacy of amantadine HCl and rimantadine HCl in naturally occurring influenza A2 respiratory illness in man, *N. Engl. J. Med.*, 281, 579–584, 1969.

28. Weiss, R. and Mazade, L., Eds., *Surrogate Endpoints in Evaluating the Effectiveness of Drugs Against HIV Infection and AIDS*, National Academy Press, Washington, D.C., 1990.

29. Osada, T., Iwabuchi, S., Takatori, M. et al., Serum levels of HCV–RNA determined by branched DNA (bDNA) probe assay in chronic hepatitis C: method and clinical significance on interferon (IFN) therapy, *Nippon Rinsho*, 52(7), 1747–1753, 1994.

30. Volberding, P.A. et al., Zidovudine in asymptomatic human immunodeficiency virus infection: a controlled trial in persons with fewer than 500 CD4-positive cells per cubic millimeter, *N. Engl. J. Med.*, 322, 941–944, 1990.

CHAPTER 29

Anticancer Drugs

Robert E. Martell, Christiane Langer, and Renzo Canetta

CONTENTS

29.1 INTRODUCTION

The unique nature of cancer biology impacts therapeutic strategy. The tissue of origin (often referred to as the "primary site") of a cancer can usually be determined by the pattern of growth or spread and then confirmed by pathologic or molecular evaluation. Attention to the primary site of cancer is important because it often correlates with disease course and treatment sensitivity. Clinical staging of cancer takes into consideration clinical characteristics of the tumor (T), the involvement of lymph nodes (N) by the tumor, and the presence of metastasis (M) to other locations within the body. A compilation of these parameters (TNM) forms the basis of the most commonly used staging system by the American Joint Committee on Cancer (AJCC).[1]

The development of cancer involves alterations in cellular functions as diverse as proliferation and apoptosis. Typically, multiple alterations exist that affect a variety of signaling pathways or cellular functions. Because these alterations can be redundant, targeting a single molecule or cellular mechanism may be successful only for a short period or not successful at all. Furthermore, many tumors evolve over time, developing resistance to a previously active therapy or developing other phenotypic characteristics that increase morbidity or mortality. One of the most successful anticancer paradigms involves clonal elimination (elimination of every cancer cell in the body). Often the best way to accomplish clonal elimination of a cancer is by using multiple modalities that might include surgery, radiotherapy, or chemotherapy. Unfortunately, when malignant cancer has progressed to a metastatic state, localized therapies such as radiotherapy and surgery cannot be practically employed to eradicate the disease. Currently available systemic therapies rarely achieve clonal elimination of metastatic solid tumors (primary from body tissues other than blood, bone marrow, or the lymphatic system). Certain hematologic malignancies (primary from blood, bone marrow, or the lymphatic system) can be successfully treated systemically; however, a large number of patients still succumb to their disease. Metastatic cancer is therefore a life-threatening disease for which a substantial medical need exists. Because of this dire situation, toxic therapy has been accepted.

Agents with a wide variety of classes and mechanisms of action have been employed to treat cancer (see Table 29.1).[2,3] These include agents that directly destroy proliferating cells (such as inhibitors of DNA replication or transcription, antimetabolic agents, tubulin-binding agents, membrane-active agents, or inhibitors of reparases). Other agents indirectly affect neoplastic cells (such as cytokines or immune-stimulating agents). Certain agents target genes or proteins known to be involved in the development or maintenance of cancer (e.g., hormonal agents, tyrosine kinase inhibitors, monoclonal antibodies, gene therapy). Through the increased use of pharmacogenomic approaches, new targets in cancer are being discovered, identified, and moved into the early stages of drug development more rapidly. These include targets outside of cells, such as receptor ligands and cell surface proteins (e.g., receptors), as well as various proteins or enzymes within the cell plasma, mitochondria, or nucleus. Finally, other modalities are employed to treat cancer, the most frequent example being ionizing radiation, which acts by damaging DNA. The term "cytotoxic" is often used loosely to indicate an agent that has specific or nonspecific cell-killing activity, while "cytostatic" has been used to refer to an agent that causes disruption of cell growth but not necessarily sudden cell death. Many of the new molecularly targeted agents are considered to have cytostatic activity, which could result in prolonged, chronic treatment with less toxicity. This trend may result in evolution of the field of oncology drug development away from traditional toxic cytotoxic therapies toward treatment paradigms more similar to those of other therapeutic areas.

The development of oncology drugs involves general steps similar to those of other therapeutic areas, including nonclinical studies; investigational new drug (IND) or equivalent application; phases I, II, and III; marketing approval; and phase IV. The average drug development time (from first-in-human to approval), however, can require as long as 8 years for an oncology agent, while 4 to 6 years are required for most drugs in other therapeutic areas. Phase I development for oncology drugs tends to be slower in patients, considering the narrow therapeutic index of many agents and the incremental process required to safely identify a maximum tolerated dose (MTD). Given the significant medical need in oncology, development of a drug is less likely to be discontinued in phase I based on a less-than-ideal pharmacokinetic or adverse event (AE) profile. The failure of a drug to exhibit evidence of activity in the phase II setting is a more common situation for discontinuing development.

Special initiatives have been implemented in the United States to facilitate development of anticancer drugs, including the Accelerated Approval mechanism for marketing approval (also known as subpart H of Federal Regulations, Title 21, Part 314), facilitating patient access to unapproved anticancer agents, giving membership and voting rights to patients and patient representatives on advisory committees, and reducing the need for IND applications for investigator-initiated studies for marketed agents in nonlabeled cancer indications.[4]

Table 29.1 Agents Used To Treat Cancer

Class	Mechanism	Examples (Not Exhaustive)
Alkylating agents	Alkylation of DNA	Cyclophosphamide, chlorambucil, melphalan, ifosfamide, temozolomide
Platinum agents	Covalent binding to DNA	Cisplatin, carboplatin, oxaliplatin
Antimetabolites	Incorporation of abnormal nucleotide analog into RNA or DNA	Gemcitabine, 5-fluorouracil, cytosine arabinoside, 5-azacytidine, 6-mercaptopurine, tegafur/uracil, fludarabine, 2-chlorodeoxyadenosine
Antifolates	Inhibition of dihydrofolate reductase	Methotrexate, pemetrexed
Topoisomerase agents	Inhibition of DNA topoisomerase I and II	Topotecan, irinotecan, etoposide, mitoxantrone
Antimicrotubule agents	Inhibit or enhance microtubule formation	Vincristine, vinorelbine, paclitaxel, docetaxel
Anthracyclines	Inhibition of DNA topoisomerase II; reactive oxygen intermediates	Doxorubicin, epirubicin
Tyrosine kinase inhibitors	Inhibit receptor tyrosine kinases	Gefitinib, erlotinib, imatinib
Hormonal therapies	Various; perturbation of hormone-dependent cell signaling, proliferation, and apoptosis	Adrenal steroids and antagonists (dexamethasone), androgens and antiandrogens (flutamide, bicalutamide), estrogens and antiestrogens (tamoxifen, fulvestrant), progestins (medroxyprogesterone), aromatase inhibitors (letrozole, anastrozole, exemestane) gonadotropin-releasing hormone analogs (leuprolide, goserelin), somatostatin analog (octreotide)
Cytokines	Direct effects on cell signaling, growth, and differentiation; indirect enhancement of host immune function	Interferons, interleukins
Differentiation agents	Induce cell differentiation	All-*trans* retinoic acid
Antibodies (unconjugated and conjugated)	Antibody-dependent cellular cytotoxicity; delivery of cytotoxin to cells	Rituximab, alemtuzumab, cetuximab, trastuzumab, ibritumomab, tositumomab
Angiogenesis agents	Inhibition of tumor angiogenesis	Bevacizumab, thalidomide
Immune system agents	Immune system augmentation or stimulation	Lentinan, schizophyllus, vaccines (in development)
Proteasome agents	Inhibition of ubiquitin proteasome pathway, stabilization of IkB	Bortezomib
Enzyme therapy	Depletion of an essential amino acid	L-Asparaginase
Miscellaneous	Apoptosis by incompletely understood mechanism	Arsenic trioxide
	Inhibition of ribonucleotide reductase	Hydroxyurea
	DNA cleavage (respectively)	Bleomycin

29.2 KEY ISSUES FOR PHASE I AND II ONCOLOGY STUDIES

29.2.1 Impact of Nonclinical Studies

The requirements for nonclinical studies of cancer agents vary from region to region. In Europe, detailed toxicology studies are required in mice and rats;[5] in the United States, the two essential studies required to begin phase I clinical trials in cancer patients are (1) a rodent study to identify doses that produce life-threatening and non-life-threatening toxicity, and (2) a nonrodent study to better characterize the tolerability of the drug in that species.[6] Additional studies may be necessary for development in Japan.[7]

Nonclinical studies may include safety pharmacology, toxicokinetic, pharmacokinetic, single-/ multiple-dose toxicity, local tolerance, genotoxicity, carcinogenicity, reproduction toxicity, and pharmacodynamic studies. The main achievement of animal toxicology studies in the oncology field is that they offer a safe starting dose for phase I trials in humans. Guidelines for some of these studies in oncology drug development may differ from those in other therapeutic areas due to the patient population and the nature of the agent being studied. For example, the top dose evaluated in nonclinical studies limits treatment of subjects who do not have a life-threatening condition; however, it may not necessarily limit the top dose in a carefully escalated clinical study of patients with metastatic cancer and no available therapeutic options. Likewise, carcinogenicity studies are not usually required prior to oncology clinical studies. For certain serious disease indications, carcinogenicity studies may be performed after marketing approval and may not even be required at all (e.g., a cytotoxic drug for treatment of advanced systemic disease). However, carcinogenicity evaluation is important for drugs intended for chronic use, chemoprevention, or adjuvant therapy of patients expected to be disease free for an extended period. Finally, nonclinical studies are valuable for determining potential drug toxicities.[8–10]

An important goal of nonclinical studies of anticancer agents is prediction of clinical activity. Substantial efforts have been undertaken by the National Cancer Institute's (NCI) Developmental Therapeutics Program since the mid-1950s to establish preclinical efficacy models for anticancer agents.[11] A broad understanding of antiproliferative activity of an agent can be evaluated by using a panel of human cancer cell lines.[12,13] These studies have evolved from primarily evaluating antiproliferative effects to characterizing the molecular signature of an agent.[14] The ability of *in vitro* cell line activity to predict clinical activity is variable.[15] Alternatively, animal allograft (relatively unreliable) and xenograft models offer the opportunity to evaluate anticancer activity *in vivo*.[16–18] Even in this more realistic setting, such experiments fail to precisely predict the clinical activity of oncology agents. Well-designed pharmacodynamic studies evaluating biologic activity (including biomarkers; see below) and efficacy can assist in estimating effective doses, dosing schedules, and target plasma concentrations.

Given the frequent need to combine anticancer agents in the clinical setting, nonclinical studies offer the opportunity to evaluate the effect of dose, schedule, and sequencing on efficacy and toxicity of drug combinations; for example, the clinical development of taxol/platinum combinations was facilitated by this approach.[19,20] The results of combining agents in preclinical models, however, are not always predictive of the clinical outcome as illustrated by the example of gefitinib, which preclinically was more efficacious when combined with chemotherapy compared to each component alone. Unfortunately, large phase III studies failed to show meaningful clinical benefit from adding gefitinib to chemotherapy given to patients with non-small-cell lung cancer.[21]

29.2.2 Nature of Oncology Studies

Key objectives of clinical studies evaluating new oncology agents include safety and efficacy. While most studies have components of both of these endpoints, phase I development tends to focus on safety considerations, while later phase development tends to focus on efficacy. Historically, efficacious doses for oncology agents (especially cytotoxic agents) have had significant levels of toxicity, including life-threatening adverse events. Cancer treatment is also often time sensitive and has improved outcomes when therapy is administered in a timely fashion. For these reasons, first-in-patient studies with an unproven agent are usually performed in patients with advanced systemic disease who have exhausted available therapies or who have no available treatment options. Certain agents may achieve biologically active exposure well below a toxic dose. In such cases, it may be possible to pursue early clinical development in less extreme medical situations, such as an earlier line of treatment (first or second line rather than last line), an earlier stage disease (localized disease at stages 1, 2, and 3 rather than metastatic at stage 4), adjuvant therapy (following localized therapy, such as surgery), neoadjuvant therapy (prior to localized therapy), or concomitantly (with another agent or modality). All studies should be guided by prudent consideration of the risks and benefits to which the subjects will be exposed. For example, if a patient population has a window of opportunity for a clinically significant outcome with an existing therapy, this opportunity should be considered in the clinical study design for a new agent.

Several types of special phase I or II studies have relevance to development of oncology agents. A study can be dedicated to characterizing the pharmacodynamic impact of a drug or evaluating the dose/exposure effect of a drug on specific or exploratory biomarkers (described below in Section 29.2.4). For solid tumors, evaluation of pharmacodynamic endpoints poses a challenging problem because access to the relevant tumor tissue is often difficult to achieve. Tumor biopsies are usually acquired only in a minority of patients when the biopsies are an optional secondary endpoint of the study. In contrast, neoadjuvant studies, or studies that require tumor tissue as part of the primary endpoint, can more consistently evaluate tumor pharmacodynamic endpoints. Additionally, tumor tissue may be more readily available in patients with hematologic malignancies (such as leukemias or lymphomas) or easily accessible solid tumors (such as skin cancer or malignant ascites). Other non-cancer tissues can be evaluated, such as skin, buccal mucosa, or peripheral blood cells; however, these may be limited by lack of reflection of the drug effect on the target tissue.

Monotherapy can provide proof of principle for a drug and a clear toxicity profile, a strategy that allows optimization of therapy from the beginning and gives important feedback to preclinical drug developers. Many of the most effective therapies for cancer involve combinations of anticancer agents or modalities. Combinations can be with other anticancer drugs; sensitizing agents; agents intended to attenuate toxicity of the drug, radio-, or phototherapy; or any of a variety of other modalities. Promising combinations often involve agents with disparate mechanisms of action or nonoverlapping toxicity profiles. As described above, nonclinical interaction studies can provide evidence of synergism with respect to toxicity or efficacy; however, such studies are not necessarily required prior to human evaluation.[6] Based on preclinical data on additive or synergistic effects, the novel agent is usually paired with a standard drug or combination. Combinations with one or more other investigational agents are also possible; however, the regulatory implications should be taken into account. Phase I studies are required to understand how combined agents interact. Untoward interactions involving metabolism, activity, or toxicity must be detected and character-ized. Other types of phase I studies that are important for oncology drug development include equivalence studies (compare pharmacokinetics between two populations of patients or two for-mulations of drug), special populations (pediatric, elderly, hepatic failure, renal insufficiency, metabolic polymorphism), drug metabolism, and drug interaction studies.

29.2.3 Nature of Oncology Patients

The overall population of patients with cancer is heterogeneous in numerous ways, including factors that significantly affect conduct of oncology clinical trials. Enrollment onto oncology clinical trials varies depending on the objective of the study. Considerations for enrollment criteria (depending on study objectives) for oncology clinical trials are shown in Table 29.2. Defining tumor histology and other characteristics (such as molecular phenotype/genotype) are very important because many

Table 29.2 Considerations for Inclusion and Exclusion Criteria in Oncology Studies

Define life expectancy (e.g., 3 months). Short life expectancy may not allow sufficient time to characterize safety or efficacy of an agent.

Define performance status. This is an important oncology prognostic factor.

Diagnose malignancy (histologically or cytologically). Documentation is usually required prior to initiating most anticancer interventions.

Define primary malignancy, stage, molecular characteristics, radiographic characteristics, and recent progression. The range of each of these may be broad or focused depending on the study. Clarify whether brain metastases are allowed (poorer prognosis; sheltered from many anticancer agents)

Identify prior anticancer chemo-, radio-, hormonal, or immunotherapy, along with period since therapy. These variables may impact safety or efficacy of the study drug. A minimum of 4 weeks from prior cytotoxic chemotherapy is usually required.

Identify organ function parameters, concurrent disease status, and medical history to ensure safe administration of the agent in light of expected toxicities.

Define genomic population of interest to allow possible enrichment of treatment population.

of these factors are associated with disease course or responsiveness to a particular therapy. In general, patients with cancer must have histologically or cytologically documented disease. Characterization of other phenotypes (molecular or histologic) or genotypes may be required. Documentation of disease from a sample obtained immediately prior to the initiation of a clinical study is usually not required; however, if documentation comes from a sample obtained in the past, there should be sound clinical or radiographic evidence that the patient continues to harbor the disease. Additionally, consideration should be given to the fact that a cancer will likely evolve over time, possibly resulting in significant changes over extended periods. Phase I studies often allow a heterogeneous patient population, including different tumor primaries, whereas later phase studies require a more strict definition of patient or tumor characteristics.

Exposure of patients to prior anticancer therapy is important because it often leads to the development of drug resistance by their tumors that reduces the anticancer activity of subsequent agents. This resistance is most significant when subsequent treatment is with a similar agent; however, induction of multidrug resistance mechanisms can affect the efficacy of other types of anticancer agents. Agents with significantly disparate mechanisms (e.g., cytotoxic and hormonal agents) are less likely to be affected by cross-resistance. A second important consideration is the potential for cumulative toxicity. For example, in a patient who had received prior doxorubicin, caution would be required if another anthracycline were being evaluated due to the elevated potential for the development of cardiomyopathy. Neuropathy is another toxicity of certain anticancer agents that can be cumulative.

Performance status is often correlated with the outcome of cancer patients and should therefore be considered when enrolling patients into a clinical study.[22] In phase I, performance status may affect the ability of patients to tolerate therapy, thus affecting the MTD or the ability of patients to stay on therapy through multiple courses. In later phases, poor performance status may result in the inability of patients to tolerate effective doses of therapy. Oncology studies often use the Eastern Cooperative Oncology Group (ECOG) performance status guidelines (Table 29.3).[23]

Cancer incidence increases exponentially with age. Elderly cancer patients with good performance status have been shown to benefit from active therapeutic intervention, in some cases as much as a younger cohort.[24–27] However, many physiologic and pathophysiologic changes occur with aging that may affect drug efficacy and toxicity, including significant changes in drug pharmacokinetics, drug metabolism, renal function, vessel elasticity and distensibility (increased risk for hypotension), cardiac functional reserve, and susceptibility to confusion, ataxia, and incontinence.[28–30] In addition, polypharmacy is a significant issue in the elderly that increases the potential for untoward drug–drug interactions;[31] therefore, it is important to thoroughly characterize oncology agents in this population.

Table 29.3 ECOG Performance Status

Grade	Description
0	Fully active, able to carry on all predisease performance without restriction
1	Restricted in physically strenuous activity but ambulatory and able to carry out work of a light or sedentary nature (e.g., light housework, office work)
2	Ambulatory and capable of all self care but unable to carry out any work activities; up and about more than 50% of waking hours
3	Capable of only limited self care; confined to bed or chair more than 50% of waking hours
4	Completely disabled; cannot carry on any self care; totally confined to bed or chair
5	Dead

The pediatric population continues to have a significant need for more effective, less toxic anticancer agents. Challenges compared to adult oncology development include a relatively smaller patient population (may require multiple-institution studies), drug metabolism differences, tumor biology differences (different patterns of efficacy), and differences in toxicity susceptibility.[32,33] Important ethical considerations have led to the desire to treat patients as close as possible to therapeutic doses; therefore, phase I studies are often initiated at relatively high starting doses (e.g., 80% of the adult MTD). This assumes that pediatric studies can only begin after characterization of a drug in adults.

29.2.4 Endpoints

Endpoints for oncology studies have several unique aspects. The important endpoint of safety is monitored using one of a number of AE grading systems, some of which are specifically designed for oncology. The World Health Organization (WHO) guidelines have been widely used in the past.[34] Oncology cooperative groups, including the ECOG and the South West Oncology Group (SWOG), have developed AE scales.[23,35] The NCI has developed a widely used standard called the Common Terminology Criteria for Adverse Events (CTCAE; earlier versions of this scale were termed the Common Toxicity Criteria).[36] This standard provides oncology-friendly terminology and an objective severity grading scale for most events. The possibility of delayed effects and cumulative toxicity exists with anticancer therapies; therefore, monitoring for AEs should occur throughout the study and for an appropriate period after the study. The frequency of monitoring depends on the level of understanding of toxicity of an agent and on the timing and nature of expected adverse events. Early human studies may require weekly, or even daily monitoring because toxicities are unknown. Hematologic evaluation often occurs 1 to 2 weeks after a dose of cytotoxic chemotherapy because of the time frame for development of neutropenia with certain agents.

Demonstrating clinical benefit of anticancer agents is challenging, particularly with delayed outcomes such as survival in the setting of multiple sequential therapies. Considering the need to shorten the duration and reduce the cost of clinical trials, much effort has been devoted to the development of biomarkers and surrogate endpoints. The National Institutes of Health (NIH) has defined a biological marker (biomarker) as a characteristic that is objectively measured and evaluated as an indicator of normal biological processes, pathogenic processes, or pharmacologic responses to a therapeutic intervention.[37] The NIH has also defined a surrogate endpoint as a biomarker that is intended to substitute for a clinical endpoint. A surrogate endpoint is expected to predict clinical benefit (or harm, or lack of benefit or harm) based on epidemiologic, therapeutic, pathophysiologic, or other scientific evidence.[37] Tumor response is probably the most common biomarker (and in many instances surrogate endpoint) in oncology patient clinical studies. Several methods for evaluating and reporting tumor shrinkage have been developed and validated. The WHO developed bidimensional tumor measurement guidelines in 1979, which have been widely

Table 29.4 Comparison of RECIST and WHO Guidelines

Component	RECIST	WHO
Characteristic	Evaluate target lesions	Evaluate measurable disease
	Maximum number of lesions: 5 per organ, up to 10 total	No maximum number of lesions
	Unidimensional measurement; longest diameter (LD) of each lesion	Bi-dimensional measurement; determine LD and greatest perpendicular diameter of each lesion; determine product (area) of each lesion
	Determine sum of LD of all target lesions	Determine sum of products of all lesions
Complete response (CR)	Disappearance of all target lesions and nontarget disease; confirmed at ≥4 weeks	Disappearance of known disease; confirmed at ≥4 weeks
Partial response (PR)	≥30% decrease in sum of LD of target lesions from baseline; confirmed at ≥4 weeks	≥50% decrease in sum of products from baseline; confirmed at ≥4 weeks
Progressive disease (PD)	≥20% increase over smallest sum observed or appearance of new lesions	≥25% increase in one or more lesions or appearance of new lesions
Stable disease (SD)	CR, PR, and PD criteria not met	Neither PR nor PD criteria met (no change)

used globally in clinical investigation for many years (Table 29.4).[38] To address issues of variability in the use of WHO criteria, the Response Evaluation Criteria in Solid Tumors (RECIST) group integrated prior response concepts into a new unidimensional approach (Table 29.4).[39] Both of these methods of tumor response evaluation are accepted by regulatory agencies, although the agencies encourage use of the same method throughout the development of a particular investigational drug.

Cytostatic agents may impart benefit by inducing tumor stasis rather than shrinkage. This form of efficacy may be more difficult to detect using tumor response as an endpoint. Stable disease (which can be defined by the tumor response methods described above) that is durable could be incorporated as an endpoint of an oncology study. Other biomarkers used to monitor the biologic activity of an agent have represented endpoints in early clinical studies. A biomarker can be evaluated prior to treatment and then again during treatment, at which time some modulation of the marker would be expected if the drug were having its intended biologic effect. Such an outcome could help provide biologic proof of principle for a molecule. Ideally, a biomarker will be in the causal path of a drug's mechanism of action or reflect an intuitive fundamental physiologic change at the cellular or tissue level. Biomarkers can play an important role in identifying a biologically active dose of an agent, and this may be different than the MTD; however, it is important to recognize that the ability of a drug to affect activity of a biomarker does not necessarily correlate with clinically meaningful activity.

Predictive (or prognostic) biomarkers are defined here as patient or tumor characteristics that could be used to predict the likelihood of a particular outcome (for example, following drug treatment). Exploratory evaluation of prospective oncology predictive biomarkers early in development may allow for identification of promising candidate markers and refinement of the assay or procedure that is required. Formal validation of a predictive biomarker would likely require a larger sample size or more formal evaluation. Estrogen receptor expression is an example of a validated predictive biomarker for responsiveness of breast cancer to antiestrogen therapy.

Dynamic imaging can play a valuable role in the development of anticancer agents. Imaging modalities, such as fluorodeoxyglucose positron emission tomography (FDG–PET), fluorodeoxy-L-thymidine (FLT)–PET, dynamic contrast-enhanced magnetic resonance imaging (DCE-MRI),[40] and vascular flow, have been used to noninvasively measure tumor metabolism or proliferation in

Table 29.5 Examples of Criteria Used To Define a Dose-Limiting Toxicity (DLT)

A DLT is defined as any of the following that can be attributed to the drug:

- Grade 3 or greater nonhematological toxicity, except grade 3 or 4 nausea, vomiting, or diarrhea that can be controlled with prophylaxis
- Grade 4 hematologic toxicity, with the following specific criteria for neutropenia: grade 4 neutropenia for five or more consecutive days or grade 3 or 4 neutropenia of any duration with sepsis or a fever greater than 38.5°C (oral)
- Any grade toxicity that in the judgment of the investigator or sponsor requires a dose reduction or removal from further study therapy
- Delayed recovery from toxicity related to treatment that delays scheduled retreatment for >14 days
- Left ventricular ejection fraction (LVEF) below 45% (or below lower limit of normal if ≥10% decline) or a 20% decline in LVEF from baseline
- An ECG that demonstrates a QTc interval ≥500 msec or increase by ≥60 msec while on therapy

response to a drug. Early incorporation of these modalities in oncology clinical development can help confirm biologic activity of an agent and provide a useful early predictor of response.

The recommended phase II doses should be derived considering the endpoint factors described in this section. The MTD may be taken forward to phase II; however, less intense regimens may also be evaluated if, for example, evidence suggests biologic or anticancer activity. Characteristics of the target population should also be taken into account.

29.3 PHASE I STUDIES

29.3.1 General Issues

A key objective of phase I oncology studies is to identify appropriate phase II doses and schedules. The relationship of the dose (and exposure) of an agent to the safety of that agent should be characterized. Considering the narrow therapeutic indices of many effective anticancer agents, and often a dose–effect relationship with respect to efficacy, a common objective of phase I cancer studies is to determine the MTD of an agent for a specific mode of administration. The MTD should take into account all side effects, any corrective action that may be required, and the extent of prior therapy to which a patient population has been exposed. The MTD determination is often guided by the incidence of dose-limiting toxicities (DLTs). DLTs are characterized by qualitative and quantitative effects of a drug on specific organ systems or general constitution. In particular, predetermined levels of drug-related AEs are set as thresholds for defining a DLT. Table 29.5 provides several examples of parameters that could be used to define a DLT.

The duration of phase I studies of oncology agents tends to be relatively long, averaging from 19 to 29 months.[41,42] Reasons for such lengthy studies include the frequent need to perform studies in a patient population with advanced cancer, the narrow therapeutic index of many oncology compounds (need to define MTD), and a lack of available surrogates for drug activity. It is also important to consider that certain classes of anticancer agents may have unique characteristics that impede accurate determination of the MTD and recommended phase II dose. For example, DLTs for antimetabolites tend to be less predictable and occur at lower dose levels compared to other classes of cytotoxic agents.[43]

Special caution is required the first time a drug is evaluated in humans. Clear algorithms for initial dose choice are available (see below). Healthy volunteers are often the most reliable subject population for evaluating pharmacokinetics and pharmacodynamics with certain biomarkers in a short time frame. Single-dose or multiple-dose studies in healthy volunteers can be performed for certain oncology agents with appropriate nonclinical profiles, with attention given to expected toxicity profile and potential for genotoxicity. Patient studies may be more appropriate for the first-in-human studies of agents with greater potential for significant toxicity. Other available standards of care often limit the ability to explore earlier lines of therapy early in the clinical development of an unproven anticancer agent. In particular, the optimal therapy of cancer is often time sensitive, requiring that proven therapies be utilized during a defined window of opportunity. For drugs with the highest risk or toxicity liability, initial human evaluation should be limited to patients with incurable, life-threatening cancer.

Determination of a safe starting dose for human studies is usually based on body surface area (BSA, usually expressed as mg/m^2), a parameter that is often used to relate toxicity of an agent between species.[44,45] A number of methods for estimating BSA for humans have been proposed. The most commonly utilized is that of DuBois: BSA = 0.007184 × weight (kg)$^{0.425}$ × height (m)$^{0.725}$, or a simplified version by Mosteller: BSA = the square root of ([height (cm) × weight (kg)]/3600).[46,47] In many cases, the oncology community has continued to utilize BSA measurements for dosing decisions, but relatively little correlation has been found between BSA and the function of organs involved in drug metabolism and disposition.[48,49] Other parameters used for dosing include dose per body weight (mg/kg) or a fixed dose. The starting dose for first-in-human studies in patients with incurable, life-threatening diseases can be calculated by applying a safety factor to the dose that is severely toxic to 10% of a rodent species (STD$_{10}$). This dose is converted to the human equivalent dose (on the basis of mg/m^2) and then a safety factor is applied (for example, one tenth the STD$_{10}$).[6,8,50,51] While the top dose or projected exposure for healthy volunteer studies should not be greater than the highest dose or exposure in animal studies, for studies involving patients with incurable, life-threatening cancer, the top dose or exposure may exceed those from animal studies if careful, incremental dose escalation is used.

29.3.2 Study Designs

A number of study designs have been utilized in phase I development of oncology agents.[41,52] These range from a more traditional approach to novel designs believed to be able to identify doses recommended for phase II studies more efficiently:

- *3+3 design* — The most commonly used method of patient cohort assignment is a "3+3" type of design,[53,54] where patients are enrolled in groups of three. This is a toxicity-guided dose-finding approach with the intent to identify the MTD based on the incidence of DLTs. If none of the three patients experiences DLT during a defined time period (for example, 1 month), then the next group of three is enrolled at the next dose level. If two or three of the three patients experience DLT, then the dose is considered to exceed the MTD and a lower dose level would be further evaluated or designated as the MTD. If one of the three experiences DLT, then the dose level is expanded by adding three more patients at the same dose level. If two or more of the six patients at that expanded dose level experience DLT, then the MTD is exceeded. Dose escalation is often patterned after a modified Fibonacci sequence, allowing large incremental increases in dose between early cohorts (e.g., 100%) and smaller increments between later cohorts (e.g., 33%).[55] This design has the advantages of being relatively straightforward with no requirement for complex calculations or statistical support. It minimizes exposing patients to excessively toxic doses of drug and has a shorter trial duration and smaller sample size compared to the continual reassessment method. It also has a long history of use and ethical committee approval. Disadvantages include: (1) dose assignments based on insufficient statistics; (2) not utilizing certain information that becomes available in the trial, a significant random component in determining the MTD (a low-dose MTD could be assigned if many dose levels between the starting dose and the MTD are used); (3) a not explicitly defined MTD that has no easily definable statistical properties; and (4) treating excess patients at dose levels with little hope of therapeutic benefit.[56]
- *Continual reassessment* — This adaptive design method attempts to improve the estimate of the MTD and reduce the number of patients treated at potentially ineffective doses. Information is propagated between dose levels to determine subsequent dose levels. Variables include dose assignment, timing of MTD identification, and the number of patients per dose. Patients are

allocated preferentially to the currently most promising dose or regimen. Termination of the study can then be based upon either achieving a predetermined number of patients at a dose within a target DLT rate for the MTD or obtaining a sufficiently narrow confidence interval for the MTD.[57,58] Advantages of this method include a more integral role of toxicity, which may result in more efficient identification of recommended phase II doses, and identifying a target dose range allowing a more seamless transition to phase II or III. Disadvantages include the statistical complexities such as determining prior distribution and parametric form[59] and possibly longer trials with more patients required.

- *Overdose control* — This method selects each dose level so the probability of exceeding the MTD is within a prespecified range.[60,61] This adaptive method utilizes all information available to determine a dose level but places a limit on the likelihood of overdose. This method may reduce the number of toxicities and still estimate the MTD with accuracy comparable to the continual reassessment method.

- *Pharmacokinetic guidance* — Safe dose escalations in humans based on measurement of drug levels in plasma, rather than on empirical escalation schemes, is the basis of this approach.[62,63] This method involves targeting a specific animal exposure (concentration × time; area under the curve [AUC]) — for example, the mouse LD_{10} (dose lethal to 10% of animals). The phase I starting dose could be 1/10 the LD_{10}. Dose escalation would be based on the exposure observed at each dose level. For example, the dose would be doubled until exposure was within 40% of the LD_{10}, then a more conventional escalation such as a modified Fibonacci sequence would be implemented. This method may allow rapid escalation to relevant exposures by fully utilizing preclinical data; however, it requires that pharmacokinetic data be available in real time. Also, toxicity in animals may not correlate with that in humans at a given exposure.

- *Accelerated titration/escalation* — This approach attempts to reduce the number of patients treated at doses that are below biologically active levels by initially utilizing single patient cohorts. These designs initially utilize large incremental dose steps (e.g., 100%). When toxicity is encountered (for example, second grade 2 toxicity or a DLT), the study resorts to cohorts of three to six patients with 40% increments between dose levels.[64] Cumulative toxicity and MTD are still important endpoints.

29.4 PHASE II STUDIES

29.4.1 General Issues

Early phase II trials in oncology development are considered important for several reasons. First, they help to identify ineffective or excessively toxic drugs using a minimum number of subjects. Second, phase II trials offer the opportunity to fine tune the recommended dose for a phase III trial population. Finally, carefully planned phase II studies offer an opportunity for regulatory approval in settings of life-threatening disease with high unmet medical need.

Most phase II studies proceed according to a one- or two-stage design, with the tumor response rate as the most widely accepted endpoint. Historically, many anticancer agents have had cytotoxic mechanisms of action. More recently, many anticancer agents have been directed at novel targets and may exhibit clinical benefit by tumor growth inhibition and not necessarily shrinkage. Because of these factors, the sequence and design of traditional phase I and II studies used for cytotoxic agents may not be appropriate for cytostatic compounds.[65] New study designs and novel approaches that could address these issues are under investigation, including randomized phase II trial designs, surrogate markers of biological activity for achieving proof of principle, new paradigms for understanding novel agents (Figure 29.1), and even the complete omission of phase II studies.

While survival remains the gold standard for clinical benefit in oncology, phase II studies are usually not appropriately controlled or are underpowered to demonstrate such a benefit. Even though it is not true for every tumor entity, many examples of a correlation between tumor response rate and improvement in survival have been observed, such as for breast and colorectal cancer.[66,67]

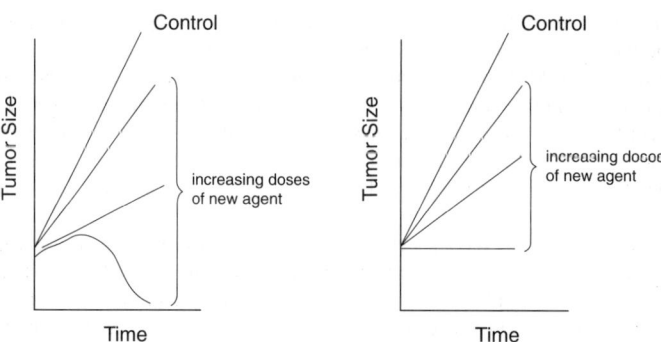

Figure 29.1   New paradigms for novel agents. (Left) Tumor regression; (right) growth delay.

Response rate is considered to be an accepted endpoint for accelerated approval by the FDA in situations where a correlation between response and survival exists.[68] Even if not associated with prolonged life, reduced tumor burden may relieve symptoms and thus improve the quality of life. Most phase II studies require patients to have a specific tumor primary site and measurable disease (as defined by one of the objective tumor response criteria (e.g., WHO or RECIST). Because responsiveness to anticancer therapy is often affected by prior therapy, it is important to consider such history. Unfortunately, tumor response does not act as an appropriate endpoint for many of the new targeted agents; therefore, new candidate endpoints are under discussion and in validation. Time to progression (TTP) or progression free survival (PFS) are frequently studied endpoints, but their acceptance by regulatory agencies varies by region, and their value is limited in a phase II setting. Endpoints involving a reduction of symptoms are considered viable endpoints for anticancer therapy and could even support full approval. Other candidate endpoints for phase II studies include target inhibition measures and changes in tumor markers; for example, cancer antigen 125 (CA125), when negative, has been accepted by the FDA as an element of a composite endpoint for ovarian cancer.[68] PET scanning and setting a threshold of percent early progressive disease (above which an agent in phase II trial should be rejected) are other endpoints. Finally, safety continues to be an important objective in phase II of oncology drug development.

Unfortunately, demonstration of activity in one tumor type does not necessarily predict for activity in others; therefore, each tumor type of interest must be studied individually in order to determine the activity of the drug in that malignancy. Finally, it is important to consider the centers at which studies are performed. Outcomes may differ between a large referral center and a community practice for reasons ranging from patient selection (i.e., willingness to travel or aggressiveness of disease dictating the opportunity to go to a referral center) to level of investment of the physician into a particular regimen.

29.4.2   Study Designs

As already discussed, the advances of new molecules that do not necessarily result in tumor shrinkage but do delay growth present a challenge for phase II trial designs. In many cases, a small, nonrandomized study with response rate as the primary endpoint will not suffice as an adequate tool for selection of a promising phase II candidate. In some cases, development has proceeded directly from phase I into phase III, thus requiring significant patient and financial resources. Innovative phase II trial designs are needed to facilitate decision-making. This section describes classic oncology phase II designs as well as novel designs emerging to better characterize novel agents.

- *Single arm (Gehan or Simon)* — These designs are typically used when the response rate is a suitable endpoint, as is true for many cytotoxic agents. In this setting, historical experiences are used to define the true response rates necessary to generate interest in pursuing a specific drug. Based on predefined target response rates, a design with two stages involving a total of 30 to 50 patients is used to determine whether an agent warrants further studies. A similar design could be used for a cytostatic agent where response rate is substituted with a clinical endpoint affected by the compound, such as early percent progressive disease or progression free survival.[69,70]
- *Multiple-arm, randomized* — Very frequently outside of oncology, phase II studies are conducted to decide which of several regimens or dose levels should be taken to the next stage of clinical testing. These experiments sometimes use a placebo or control arm. This approach was rarely used in the past in oncology, but its use is finding renewed interest.
- *Comparative* — When oncologic agents are studied in separate single-arm trials, actual differences between response rates associated with the treatments are confounded because of inherent differences between the trials; consequently, comparisons between separate single-arm trials of different treatments are not reliable. A direct comparison between more than one therapeutic option is preferred in oncology clinical development. Phase II studies are, by definition, too small to provide statistical power to yield a clinically meaningful comparison; however, phase II comparative studies allow benchmarking between an experimental therapy and a standard or more studied clinical situation with respect to many potential endpoints, including safety and efficacy. Given the limited number of patients available for phase II trials and the increasing number of new therapies being evaluated, it is critically important to conduct these trials efficiently. Some authors suggest that phase II trials are inherently comparative, with the results of the comparison determining whether to conduct a subsequent phase III trial.[71]
- *Noncomparative* — Multiple-arm randomized studies can be conducted using a Simon or Gehan two- or three-stage design in each arm separately. If possible, stratification should be performed. Arms that fail (in a multiple-stage design) should subsequently be stopped. Advantages of this approach include absence of predefined decision criterion (applicable if trying to decide on a schedule or dose not based on statistical criterion), multiple experimental arms, and multiple schedules.
- *Randomized discontinuation* — This is a staged trial design that is utilized to evaluate anticancer agents that are expected to cause stabilization of disease as their primary clinical benefit. Stage 1 consists of an open stage, where all patients receive treatment for a defined period. During this initial stage, the treatment effect in the entire population will be determined. Patients with stable disease at the end of stage 1 will be randomized in stage 2 to receive either continued active drug or a placebo, thus enabling identification of a treatment effect of prolonged stable disease.[72,73] Patients who progress while randomized to placebo can be restarted on active drug. Also, all patients achieving an objective response while on active drug would not be randomized.
- *Phase II.V (screening design)* — This design is like a phase III trial, except that it has a higher type I error (e.g., $\alpha = 0.20$) and the power to detect a larger difference with randomization to either study drug or standard of care. This design allows stopping in the event of small but true differences in outcome. If the results are positive, phase III studies with a similar design could be initiated. A drawback is that, while a positive phase II.V study may support a regulatory filing, it may not be a registrational study by itself.[54]
- *Phase II/III (Ellenberg design)* — This design compares an experimental arm with a control arm. It is suitable if a short-term surrogate endpoint exists, such as tumor response. The phase II portion should be as follows: Patients are assigned to both arms, and enrollment is stopped if the response rate in the experimental arms is less or equal to the response rate in the control arm; otherwise, the study would continue into the phase III portion.
- *Adaptive study design* — Balanced treatment allocation is the standard in many clinical research trials; however, utilization of accumulating information on the study is the hallmark of the adaptive study design. An adaptive study design is more desirable than a randomized design in instances where the disease being studied is rare and where most patients with the disease would be treated in a clinical trial. Extrapolation to some larger population is not necessary.[74]

The choice of study design depends on the type of compound, the tumor entity, and the willingness of those involved to take on risks and costs. Close collaboration between clinical oncologists and statisticians is essential in choosing the correct study design. While much more remains to be learned about cytostatic drug development, genomics plays an increasing role in identifying targets, assessing new biomarkers, and predicting safety and efficacy. Also, continued creativity in ongoing assessments of novel dose-finding and preliminary efficacy approaches will play a crucial role for future phase II study designs.

29.4.3 Importance of Patient Selection and Enrichment of Study Populations

Background information on novel therapies can be obtained from new diagnostic approaches, increased translational research, molecular imaging, genomics, and pharmacogenetics. The ability to assess biologic endpoints in the clinic is lagging despite the visible transition from cytotoxic agents to molecularly targeted drug discovery. This comprises one area that demands greater participation from clinical researchers and involvement of all departments of the sponsor in an attempt to identify enriched patient populations for phase II and even more so for phase III testing. The failure to identify subgroups of patients likely to respond will often lead to drugs performing worse than expected; therefore, it becomes especially important for the oncology research community to continuously support appropriate biologic correlative studies. The Her2/neu/Herceptin strategy emphasizes the therapeutic power of patient selection; overall survival was significantly better in patients with breast cancer expressing high levels of Her2/neu compared to a group of patients with tumors with low or no Her2/neu expression. Patient selection may ultimately lead to more successful drugs after phase II and decrease the need for large and expensive phase III trials.

29.4.4 Planning for Phase III Development

The transition from phase II to phase III requires a strategic decision based on several considerations. Significant investment in phase I and II drug development is required to provide the information necessary for phase III planning and commitment. Important issues that should be clarified in early phase development include defining study endpoints, defining the projected effect, determining whether superiority or noninferiority design is appropriate, and clarifying the toxicity profile to ensure safe administration to a larger population.

29.5 PHASE III STUDIES

Because of the complexity of cancer care and the diversity of cancer manifestations and outcomes, developing phase III studies for oncology agents is challenging.[75] In many cases, cancer standards of care must be administered within a window of time to achieve proven benefit. Patients with advanced disease also often experience considerable morbidity from their disease. For these and other reasons, studies controlled with a placebo alone arm are rare. A more common scenario is comparing an agent or regimen with an accepted standard of care. In this case, superiority is often targeted; however, noninferiority comparisons can be successful in certain settings. Double-blinded studies also may be difficult due to divergent and complex treatment schedules. Several strategies that are amenable to a double-blind or placebo-controlled approach have been employed. Administering an accepted regimen with or without the experimental agent in a randomized, placebo-controlled, double-blind fashion can be pursued. Alternatively, patients with minimal residual disease, where no accepted standard exists, could be treated with or without an experimental therapy, in a randomized double-blind, placebo-controlled study.

Defining the patient population for phase III oncology studies is very important. The nature of disease courses and outcomes across malignancies of different primaries is very heterogeneous.

Likewise, there are differences in these variables at the different disease stages and given different amounts of prior therapy. Even when a very narrow patient population is defined, there is still significant divergence in disease course and outcome. In order to minimize this heterogeneity, most phase III oncology studies limit eligibility to a specific tumor primary, disease stage, and amount of prior therapy. Selection of patients based on other variables known to be important to patient outcome should be implemented. A molecular or genetic characteristic of a tumor that may predict response to a test agent may also be used as a selection factor if supported by prior evaluation.

The approach to endpoints for phase III oncology studies is evolving.[68,76] Demonstration of survival advantage for an intervention has been the gold standard in the United States; however, in many instances, other endpoints have supported both accelerated and full regulatory approval, including response rate, time to progression, disease-free survival, symptom control, and quality of life. Alternatively, time to progression may hold greater importance in the European Union, while overall survival, response rate, symptom control, and quality of life are also considered. Unfortunately, each of these endpoints has liabilities. For example, survival outcomes can be confounded by multiple other subsequent, potentially effective therapies, including the possibility of crossover. Time to progression can be confounded by sampling biases between arms or rendered less sensitive by infrequent sampling times. In all cases, it is important to work with sites that are experienced and capable of performing controlled oncology clinical studies.

29.6 PHASE IV STUDIES

Phase IV development of oncology agents has several unique aspects. In many cases, standards of care evolve independently of product labeling in response to evolving clinical investigation and scientific data. The nature of oncology clinical care demands customization of clinical care to individual patient situations, and this has spawned numerous investigational approaches. The oncology community has a science-driven approach to patient care and therefore not only requires a clear scientific basis underlying therapies that are implemented but also must be willing to incorporate new approaches that have sound scientific basis. Because of these factors, off-label use and investigation often drive evolving standards of care in oncology.

Factors that may be evaluated in a postmarketing setting include dose level, frequency, and timing. In the phase IV setting, oncology agents are often evaluated in combination with other anticancer agents that may have unique or overlapping toxicities as well as specific drug interactions. Such combinations may also cause antagonism or synergism with respect to efficacy. It is important to characterize these issues as well as optimize such combinations in the phase IV setting.

The indications for most anticancer agents are relatively narrow, yet the majority of approved oncology agents have the ability to provide clinical benefit to patients with other stages of disease, other prior treatment histories, and across multiple malignancies. Phase IV development of oncology agents is an important setting in which to explore these other indications where patient benefit could be achieved. Again, the centers at which these studies are performed should be carefully considered to ensure that the results can be best extrapolated to the population in need.

29.7 CONCLUSIONS

Clinical development of anticancer agents has several unique characteristics compared to other therapeutic areas. The heterogeneity of tumor biology from patient to patient, the life-threatening nature of many oncology settings, and the narrow therapeutic index of many anticancer agents are just a few of the factors that make oncology drug development challenging. New molecularly targeted anticancer drugs may slow tumor growth as opposed to causing regression. With the appropriate safety profile, certain noncytotoxic anticancer agents can undergo phase I study in healthy volunteers. Identification of biomarkers and surrogate endpoints can facilitate development by enhancing understanding of drug activity at the target and possibly allowing preselection of more appropriate patient populations. The future of oncology therapy will likely see less dependence on tumor histology or tumor primary site and more dependence on the molecular or genetic signature of a tumor.

REFERENCES

1. American Joint Committee on Cancer, *AJCC Cancer Staging Manual*, 6th ed., Springer-Verlag, New York, 2003.
2. Chabner, B.A. and Longo, D.L., *Cancer Chemotherapy and Biotherapy*, 3rd ed., Lippincott Williams & Williams, Philadelphia, 2001.
3. DeVita, V.T., Hellman, S., and Rosenberg, S.A., *Cancer: Principles and Practice of Oncology*, 6th ed., Lippincott Williams & Williams, Philadelphia, 2001.
4. Clinton, W. and Gore, A., Reinventing the regulation of cancer drugs: accelerating approval and expanding access, in *National Performance Review*, National Partnership for Reinventing Government, Washington, D.C., 1996.
5. Burtles, S.S. et al., Revisions of general guidelines for the preclinical toxicology of new cytotoxic anticancer agents in Europe: the Cancer Research Campaign (CRC) Phase I/II Clinical Trials Committee and European Organization for Research and Treatment of Cancer (EORTC) New Drug Development Office, *Eur. J. Cancer*, 31A(3), 408–410, 1995.
6. DeGeorge, J.J. et al., Regulatory considerations for preclinical development of anticancer drugs, *Cancer Chemother. Pharmacol.*, 41(3), 173–185, 1998.
7. JPMA, *Pharmaceutical Administration and Regulations in Japan*, English Regulatory Information Task Force, Japan Pharmaceutical Manufacturers Association, Tokyo, 2002, pp. 1–106.
8. Grieshaber, C.K. and Marsoni, S., Relation of preclinical toxicology to findings in early clinical trials, *Cancer Treat. Rep.*, 70(1), 65–72, 1986.
9. Schurig, J.E. and Bradner, W.T., Small animal toxicological studies of anticancer drugs, in *Fundamentals of Cancer Chemotherapy*, Hellman, K. and Carter, S.K., Eds., McGraw-Hill, New York, 1987, pp. 248–261.
10. Lowe, M., Large animal toxicological studies of anticancer drugs, in *Fundamentals of Cancer Chemotherapy*, Hellman, K. and Carter, S.K., Eds., McGraw-Hill, New York, 1987, pp. 236–247.
11. Johnson, J.I. et al., Relationships between drug activity in NCI preclinical *in vitro* and *in vivo* models and early clinical trials, *Br. J. Cancer*, 84(10), 1424–1431, 2001.
12. Weinstein, J.N. et al., An information-intensive approach to the molecular pharmacology of cancer, *Science*, 275(5298), 343–349, 1997.
13. Yamori, T., Panel of human cancer cell lines provides valuable database for drug discovery and bioinformatics, *Cancer Chemother. Pharmacol.*, 52(Suppl. 1), S74–S79, 2003.
14. Takimoto, C.H., Anticancer drug development at the U.S. National Cancer Institute, *Cancer Chemother. Pharmacol.*, 52(Suppl. 1), S29–233, 2003.
15. Brown, J.M., NCI's anticancer drug screening program may not be selecting for clinically active compounds, *Oncol. Res.*, 9(5), 213–215, 1997.
16. Voskoglou-Nomikos, T., Pater, J.L., and Seymour, L., Clinical predictive value of the *in vitro* cell line, human xenograft, and mouse allograft preclinical cancer models, *Clin. Cancer Res.*, 9(11), 4227–4239, 2003.
17. Langdon, S.P. et al., Preclinical phase II studies in human tumor xenografts: a European multicenter follow-up study, *Ann. Oncol.*, 5(5), 415–422, 1994.
18. Newell, D.R., Flasks, fibres and flanks: pre-clinical tumour models for predicting clinical antitumour activity, *Br. J. Cancer*, 84(10), 1289–1290, 2001.
19. Rowinsky, E.K. et al., Sequence-dependent cytotoxic effects due to combinations of cisplatin and the antimicrotubule agents taxol and vincristine, *J. Cancer Res. Clin. Oncol.*, 119(12), 727–733, 1993.
20. Jekunen, A.P. et al., Synergistic interaction between cisplatin and taxol in human ovarian carcinoma cells *in vitro*, *Br. J. Cancer*, 69(2), 299–306, 1994.

21. Cohen, M.H. et al., FDA drug approval summary: gefitinib (ZD1839) (Iressa) tablets, *Oncologist*, 8(4), 303–306, 2003.

22. Johnson, E.D.H., Zhv, J., and Schiller J. et al., ECOG 1594, a randomized phase III trial in metastatic non-small cell lung cancer (NSCLC): outcome of PS2 patients, an Eastern Cooperative Oncology Group trial [abstract], *Proc. Am. Soc. Clin. Oncol.*, 18, 416a, 1999.

23. Oken, M.M. et al., Toxicity and response criteria of the Eastern Cooperative Oncology Group, *Am. J. Clin. Oncol.*, 5(6), 649–655, 1982.

24. Gridelli, C. and Hainsworth, J., Meeting the chemotherapy needs of elderly and poor performance status patients with NSCLC, *Lung Cancer*, 38(Suppl. 4), 37–41, 2002.

25. Lee, K.W. et al., Doxorubicin-based chemotherapy for diffuse large B-cell lymphoma in elderly patients: comparison of treatment outcomes between young and elderly patients and the significance of doxorubicin dosage, *Cancer*, 98(12), 2651–2656, 2003.

26. Langer, C.J. et al., Cisplatin-based therapy for elderly patients with advanced non-small-cell lung cancer: implications of Eastern Cooperative Oncology Group 5592, a randomized trial, *J. Natl. Cancer Inst.*, 94(3), 173–181, 2002.

27. Schild, S.E. et al., The outcome of combined-modality therapy for stage III non-small-cell lung cancer in the elderly, *J. Clin. Oncol.*, 21(17), 3201–3206, 2003.

28. Hammerlein, A., Derendorf, H., and Lowenthal, D.T., Pharmacokinetic and pharmacodynamic changes in the elderly: clinical implications, *Clin. Pharmacokinetics*, 35, 49–64, 1998.

29. Baker, S.D. and Grochow, L.B., Pharmacology of cancer chemotherapy in the older person, *Clin. Geriatr. Med.*, 13, 169–183, 1997.

30. Repetto, L., Greater risks of chemotherapy toxicity in elderly patients with cancer, *J. Supportive Oncol.*, 1(Suppl. 2), 18–24, 2003 (www.supportiveoncology.net).

31. Beers, M.H., Explicit criteria for determining potentially inappropriate medication use by the elderly: an update, *Arch. Intern. Med.*, 157(14), 1531–1536, 1997.

32. Smith, M. et al., Conduct of phase I trials in children with cancer, *J. Clin. Oncol.*, 16(3), 966–978, 1998.

33. Bernstein, M.L., Reaman, G.H., and Hirschfeld, S., Developmental therapeutics in childhood cancer: a perspective from the Children's Oncology Group and the U.S. Food and Drug Administration, *Hematol. Oncol. Clin. North Am.*, 15(4), 631–55, 2001.

34. WHO, *Handbook of Reporting Results of Cancer Treatment*, World Health Organization, Geneva, 1979.

35. Green, S. and Weiss, G.R., Southwest Oncology Group standard response criteria, endpoint definitions and toxicity criteria, *Invest. New Drugs*, 10(4), 239–253, 1992.

36. Cancer Therapy Evaluation Program, *Common Terminology Criteria for Adverse Events*, Version 3.0, 2003 (http://ctep.cancer.gov).

37. Group, B.D.W., Biomarkers and surrogate endpoints: preferred definitions and conceptual framework, *Clin. Pharm. Ther.*, 69(3), 89–95, 2001.

38. Miller, A.B. et al., Reporting results of cancer treatment, *Cancer*, 47(1), 207–214, 1981.

39. Therasse, P. et al., New guidelines to evaluate the response to treatment in solid tumors: European Organization for Research and Treatment of Cancer, National Cancer Institute of the United States, National Cancer Institute of Canada, *J. Natl. Cancer Inst.*, 92(3), 205–216, 2000.

40. Choyke, P.L., Dwyer, A.J., and Knopp, M.V., Functional tumor imaging with dynamic contrast-enhanced magnetic resonance imaging, *J. Magn. Reson. Imaging*, 17(5), 509–520, 2003.

41. Eisenhauer, E.A. et al., Phase I clinical trial design in cancer drug development, *J. Clin. Oncol.*, 18(3), 684–692, 2000.

42. Eckhardt, S.G. et al., *The Continual Reassessment Method (CRM) for Dose Escalation in Phase I Trials in San Antonio Does Not Result in More Rapid Study Completion*, Abstract #627, American Society of Clinical Oncology Annual Meeting, Atlanta, GA, May 15–19, 1999.

43. Seymour, L. and Eisenhauer, E., A review of dose-limiting events in phase I trials: antimetabolites show unpredictable relationships between dose and toxicity, *Cancer Chemother. Pharmacol.*, 47(1), 2–10, 2001.

44. Pinkel, D., The use of body surface area as a criterion of drug dosage in cancer chemotherapy, *Cancer Res.*, 18(7), 853–856, 1958.

45. Freireich, E.J. et al., Quantitative comparison of toxicity of anticancer agents in mouse, rat, hamster, dog, monkey, and man, *Cancer Chemother. Rep.*, 50(4), 219–244, 1966.

46. DuBois, D. and DuBois, E., A formula to estimate the approximate surface area if height and weight be known, *Arch. Internal Med.*, 17, 863–871, 1916.

47. Mosteller, R.D., Simplified calculation of body-surface area, *N. Engl. J. Med.*, 317(17), 1098, 1987.
48. Sawyer, M. and Ratain, M.J., Body surface area as a determinant of pharmacokinetics and drug dosing, *Invest. New Drugs*, 19(2), 171–177, 2001.
49. Baker, S.D. et al., Role of body surface area in dosing of investigational anticancer agents in adults, 1991–2001, *J. Natl. Cancer Inst.*, 94(24), 1883–1888, 2002.
50. Reigner, B.G. and Blesch, K.S., Estimating the starting dose for entry into humans: principles and practice, *Eur. J. Clin. Pharmacol.*, 57(12), 835–845, 2002.
51. Penta, J.S., Rosner, G.L., and Trump, D.L., Choice of starting dose and escalation for phase I studies of antitumor agents, *Cancer Chemother. Pharmacol.*, 31(3), 247–250, 1992.
52. Ahn, C., An evaluation of phase I cancer clinical trial designs, *Stat. Med.*, 17(14), 1537–1549, 1998.
53. Dixon, W.J., The up and-down method for small samples, *Am. Stat. Assoc. J.*, 60, 967–978, 1965.
54. Simon, R., Clinical trials in cancer, in *Cancer: Principles and Practice of Oncology*, DeVita, V.T., Hellman, S., and Rosenberg, S.A., Eds., Lippincott Williams & Wilkins, Philadelphia, 2001, pp. 521–548.
55. Schneiderman, M.A., Mouse to man: statistical problems in bringing a drug to clinical trial, in *Proceedings of the Fifth Berkeley Symposium on Mathematical Statistical Probability*, University of California, Berkeley, 1967, p. 855.
56. Berry, D.A., Statistical innovations in cancer research, in *Case Studies in Bayesian Statistics*, Gatsonis, C. and Kass, R.E., Eds., Springer-Verlag, Berlin, 2001.
57. O'Quigley, J., Shen, L.Z., and Gamst, A., Two-sample continual reassessment method, *J. Biopharm. Stat.*, 9(1), 17–44, 1999.
58. Heyd, J.M. and Carlin, B.P., Adaptive design improvements in the continual reassessment method for phase I studies, *Stat. Med.*, 18(11), 1307–1321, 1999.
59. Dent, S.F. and Eisenhauer, E.A., Phase I trial design: are new methodologies being put into practice?, *Ann. Oncol.*, 7(6), 561–566, 1996.
60. Babb, J., Rogatko, A., and Zacks, S., Cancer phase I clinical trials: efficient dose escalation with overdose control, *Stat. Med.*, 17(10), 1103–1120, 1998.
61. Cheng, J.D. et al., Individualized patient dosing in phase I clinical trials: the role of escalation with overdose control in PNU-214936, *J. Clin. Oncol.*, 22(4), 602–609, 2004.
62. Collins, J.M., Grieshaber, C.K., and Chabner, B.A., Pharmacologically guided phase I clinical trials based upon preclinical drug development, *J. Natl. Cancer Inst.*, 82(16), 1321–1326, 1990.
63. Graham, M.A. and Workman, P., The impact of pharmacokinetically guided dose escalation strategies in phase I clinical trials: critical evaluation and recommendations for future studies, *Ann. Oncol.*, 3(5), 339–347, 1992.
64. Simon, R. et al., Accelerated titration designs for phase I clinical trials in oncology, *J. Natl. Cancer Inst.*, 89(15), 1138–1147, 1997.
65. Korn, E.L. et al., Clinical trial designs for cytostatic agents: are new approaches needed?, *J. Clin. Oncol.*, 19(1), 265–272, 2001.
66. Slamon, D.J. et al., Use of chemotherapy plus a monoclonal antibody against HER2 for metastatic breast cancer that overexpresses HER2, *N. Engl. J. Med.*, 344(11), 783–792, 2001.
67. Hurwitz, H. et al., Bevacizumab (a monoclonal antibody to vascular endothelial growth factor) prolongs survival in first-line colorectal cancer (CRC): results of a phase III trial of bevacizumab in combination with bolus IFL (irinotecan, 5-fluorouracil, leucovorin) as first-line therapy in subjects with metastatic CRC, in *Proceedings of the 39th American Society of Clinical Oncology Annual Meeting*, Chicago, IL, May 31–June 3, 2003.
68. Johnson, J.R., Williams, G., and Pazdur, R., End points and United States Food and Drug Administration approval of oncology drugs, *J. Clin. Oncol.*, 21(7), 1404–1411, 2003.
69. Simon, R., Wittes, R.E., and Ellenberg, S.S., Randomized phase II clinical trials, *Cancer Treat. Rep.*, 69(12), 1375–1381, 1985.
70. Simon, R., Designs for efficient clinical trials, *Oncology (Huntingt.)*, 3(7), 43–49, 51–53, 1989.
71. Estey, E.H. and Thall, P.F., New designs for phase 2 clinical trials, *Blood*, 102(2), 442–448, 2003.
72. Kopec, J.A., Abrahamowicz, M., and Esdaile, J.M., Randomized discontinuation trials: utility and efficiency, *J. Clin. Epidemiol.*, 46(9), 959–971, 1993.
73. Rosner, G.L., Stadler, W., and Ratain, M.J., Randomized discontinuation design: application to cytostatic antineoplastic agents, *J. Clin. Oncol.*, 20(22), 4478–4484, 2002.

74. Berry, D.A. and Eick, S.G., Adaptive assignment versus balanced randomization in clinical trials: a decision analysis, *Stat. Med.*, 14(3), 231–246, 1995.

75. Roberts, Jr., T.G., Lynch, Jr., T.J., and Chabner, B.A., The phase III trial in the era of targeted therapy: unraveling the "go or no go" decision, *J. Clin. Oncol.*, 21(19), 3683–3695, 2003.

76. CPMP, *Note for Guidance on Evaluation of Anticancer Medicinal Products in Man*, CPMP/EWP/205/95, Committee for Proprietary Medicinal Products, European Agency for the Evaluation of Medicinal Products, London, 2001.

PART XII

Assessment of Antiinflammatory and Pain Drugs

CHAPTER 30

Analgesics

Christopher L. Wu, Robert W. Hurley, and Joseph W. Stauffer

CONTENTS

30.1 INTRODUCTION

Uncontrolled pain is a significant global public health problem, as over one third of the world's population suffers from persistent pain.[1] In the United States alone, pain-related costs are estimated at $100 billion annually.[1] Common pain conditions (e.g., arthritis, backache, headache, musculo-skeletal pain) are experienced by up to 13% of the total U.S. workforce at any given time, with the costs of lost productive time estimated at $61.2 billion annually.[2] On an individual level, uncontrolled pain results in significant distress that can dominate and disrupt a person's life.[3] Federal policymakers, including the U.S. Congress, which declared this decade as the "decade of pain control and research," and the Joint Commission on Accreditation of Healthcare Organizations (JCAHO), which has implemented and enforced new guidelines for pain management, have placed increasing emphasis on adequate treatment of pain.[4] Currently available analgesic therapies are not especially efficacious in treating certain types of pain (e.g., neuropathic) due in part to the presence of intolerable side effects from these medications. Over the past two decades, tremendous strides have been made in our understanding of the molecular and cellular mechanisms of pain. Although pain is a subjective phenomenon and incorporates both the neurobiology of nociception and psychosocial input, elucidation of the specific molecules involved in the processes of nociception will allow targeted development of new analgesic agents that may have greater analgesic efficacy with fewer side effects. Successful development of new analgesic agents requires an understanding of the regulatory issues and proper methodology in designing clinical trials including assessment of appropriate endpoints.

30.2 GENERAL CONSIDERATIONS

Analgesic drug development for the treatment of pain may be relatively difficult compared to other drugs. Unlike other disease states where definitive endpoints can be obtained (e.g., death for cancer drug development), pain *per se* is a relatively subjective symptom, and the proper methods to assess the efficacy of analgesics are the subject of some controversy. Further complicating analgesic drug development is the fact that "pain" encompasses a broad spectrum of conditions of differing etiologies. Although pain is typically categorized based on the duration (acute vs. chronic) or etiology (nociceptive, visceral, neuropathic), the actual delineations between categories are not as precise. Some of the parameters used in analgesic drug development will be different for different categories (e.g., animal models or clinical endpoints), with the most significant differences occurring between drugs developed for acute (e.g., postoperative, blunt trauma, acute visceral) and chronic pain. Further complicating this picture is the fact that many animal models used to study acute and chronic pain preclinically do not necessarily translate as predictive models for the human condition. The U.S. Food and Drug Administration (FDA) has published a guideline for the clinical evaluation of analgesic drugs;[5] however, this guideline has been withdrawn (per August 5, 2003, *Federal Register* notice; www.fda.gov/cder/guidance/guidance.htm). It is possible that this guidance, which primarily focused on drug development for acute pain, may be revised in part to include recent recommendations for outcome assessments in clinical trials evaluating the efficacy and effectiveness of analgesics for the treatment of chronic pain.[6] Despite the withdrawal of the FDA's guidance for the clinical evaluation of analgesic drugs, this document still provides some solid fundamental concepts in analgesic drug development, especially for drugs designed for the treatment of acute pain. The principles of this guidance and other multidisciplinary guidelines are incorporated in this chapter.

30.2.1 Assessment of Pain

Because pain is a subjective phenomenon, the severity of pain is typically assessed with self-reported measures (see Table 30.1). Several commonly used pain rating systems are available that should be used concurrently during analgesic drug development. Pain should be assessed at rest,

Table 30.1 Assessment of Analgesia

Area under the curve (AUC or TOTPAR)
Core outcomes (see Section 30.2.2)
Duration of analgesia
Likert-type scales
Numbers needed to treat (NNT)
Numeric rating scale (NRS)
Onset of analgesia
Pain intensity difference
Pain relief
Percentage pain relief
Sum of pain intensity differences (SPID)
Visual analog scale (VAS)

with appropriate activity (e.g., ambulation, cough), at baseline (prior to analgesic drug administration), and at regular intervals adapted to the anticipated time–effect characteristics of the analgesic drug under evaluation. Assessment intervals should be chosen such that the onset of analgesic effect, peak analgesic effect, and duration of analgesic effect can be determined. Although many of the pain assessment issues in this section are applicable to both acute and chronic pain analgesic drug development, additional considerations for the assessment of pain for chronic pain analgesic drug development are discussed later (see Section 30.2.2.1).

Many of the assessments of pain are unidimensional instruments. Some of the most commonly used instruments include the visual analog scale (VAS), numeric rating scale (NRS), and categorical/Likert scale. The VAS is a written assessment that typically utilizes a horizontal, unmarked, 100-mm line with the left end marked as "no pain" and the right end marked as "worst pain imaginable." Subjects put a mark on the line corresponding to their level of pain. Although a vertical line can also be used and should provide similar results, the vast majority of studies utilize a horizontal line. It is important not to have other marks on the line, as they could unduly influence a subject's rating of pain. The VAS provides continuous data (assuming normally distributed data) and should be analyzed statistically as such, despite the controversy over whether the VAS is actually a linear or proportional measure. The NRS can be applied in either written or verbal form and typically utilizes a rating from 0 (corresponding to "no pain") to 10 (corresponding to "worst pain imaginable"). Likert scales are typically four- or five-item instruments (e.g., ratings of "none," "mild," "moderate," "severe") that attempt to quantify pain. Technically, NRS and Likert responses are categorical, not normally distributed, and should be analyzed accordingly, although some investigators will treat NRS results as continuous variables. All items on a Likert scale have the same weight in the summating procedure. Because both the NRS and Likert scales may be applied verbally, these may be occasionally referred to as "verbal rating scales."

Data from VAS or NRS can be transformed into other ratings to assess analgesia. These rating include percentage pain reduction, numbers needed to treat (NNT), and area under the curve (AUC). The AUC or total area under the pain relief curve (TOTPAR) is a summary measure that integrates serial assessments of a subject's pain over the duration of the study. Peak effects for pain intensity, pain intensity difference, and pain relief can be derived from AUC data.[5] The area under the pain relief vs. time curve can be used to derive the proportion of patients experiencing typically 50% pain relief over a specified time frame and the NNT for 50% pain relief of the analgesic drug being evaluated. Patients can be asked directly to assess their percentage pain reduction or pain relief, although percentage pain reduction can also be calculated by taking the difference between pre- and post-treatment pain divided by the pretreatment pain. Good overall agreement has been found between the two methods with regard to determining the percentage of pain reduction.[7]

The study design for analgesic drugs (e.g., sample size calculations, interpretation of analgesic drug trial data) should be based on clinically meaningful reductions in pain; however, because the typical pain assessment (i.e., VAS or NRS) does not have any intrinsic meaning, the clinical importance of a decrease in pain scores alone is difficult to evaluate. Relatively recent data on patients with acute pain suggest that the minimal change in the NRS that is noticeable is approximately 20%, with clinically meaningful reductions of 35% and 44% as the baseline intensities for moderate and severe pain, respectively.[8] Such findings differ slightly from studies in chronic and cancer pain patients where a 30 to 33% decline in VAS was determined to be a clinically important difference to patients.[9,10] Of note is that the global impression of change in pain was shown to be the same across diverse chronic pain disorders.[9] Complicating these findings is the fact that the meaning of a change in NRS depends on the baseline pain intensity, with a larger change required for a higher baseline pain severity.[8] A clinically perceptible minimal change in VAS or NRS may not be sufficient to evaluate analgesic effectiveness, whereas the typical 50% cutoff used for NNT calculations may be too stringent.[8]

30.2.2 Core Outcome Domains for Analgesic Trials

One of the concerns regarding regulatory guidance in analgesic trials is the relative paucity of recommendations for chronic pain drug development. Unlike acute pain, chronic pain is generally considered more resistant to currently available analgesic therapies and is multidimensional in nature, affecting all aspects of a person's life. To comprehensively assess the efficacy of an analgesic in the treatment of chronic pain, several core domains should be assessed with valid, psychometrically developed instruments.[6] The investigator should give strong consideration to assessing these domains during analgesic drug development (especially for chronic pain), although these core domains are not a requirement for regulatory approval and may be excluded in some instances.[6] The domains assessed should be congruent to the purpose of the trial, the drug evaluated, the type of pain studied, and specific patient population. Finally, available generic instruments (lacking in responsiveness but allow comparisons of the effect across different diseases) and disease-specific instruments (likely to reveal clinical improvement for that particular disease but results may not be generalizable to a broader population) have advantages and disadvantages in assessing these core domains; however, a combination of both generic- and disease-specific instruments will most likely provide a comprehensive evaluation of analgesic efficacy for chronic pain.

30.2.2.1 Pain

In addition to the considerations previously described (see Section 30.2.1), assessment of chronic pain should include measures other than a unidimensional VAS or NRS rating. Some of these may include the intensity, location, specific descriptors, and qualities associated with chronic pain.[6] Although several validated multidimensional instruments to assess chronic pain are available, the McGill Pain Questionnaire and Brief Pain Inventory may be advantageous, as these have been widely used in clinical trials and are available in many multilingual versions.[11] Another multidimensional instrument used to assess chronic pain is the Multidimensional Pain Inventory (MPI).[12]

30.2.2.2 Physical Functioning

Physical functioning is an important endpoint in analgesic trials for chronic pain and should be considered one of the core domains assessed in all clinical trials of chronic pain.[6] Assessing physical function includes measuring diverse aspects such as activities of daily living (ADL), such as household chores, work, and self-care; strength; and endurance. Two different levels of activity should be assessed in the domain of physical functioning: self-care behaviors (e.g., ADLs) and social-role functioning. The effect of pain on ADLs should be considered a core domain, however, whereas its effect on social functioning is more likely to be considered a supplemental domain.[6]

30.2.2.3 Emotional Functioning

The effect of chronic pain on emotional functioning is well recognized, as chronic pain is frequently associated with depression, anxiety, and irritability.[6] Assessment of emotional functioning should be considered a core outcome in analgesic drug development for chronic pain.[6] Several generic (e.g., Medical Outcomes Study SF-36) and specific (e.g., Profile of Mood States, or POMS) instruments are available for assessing emotional functioning and have been used to assess the efficacy of analgesic agents for chronic pain.[13]

30.2.2.4 Rating of Global Improvement

Limiting assessments to individual outcomes, such as pain, may not adequately capture the overall evaluation or global impression of the analgesic drug by the patient. Although the use of global ratings in assessing analgesic efficacy is controversial due in part to its lack of responsiveness (discriminatory ability to detect small changes) and methodologic issue (e.g., recall bias), participant ratings of global improvement and satisfaction are important in that patients are more likely to comply and adhere to analgesic therapy if they generally feel more positively toward the drug.[6] Despite the limitations of global ratings, recent studies have provided evidence for the validity of global ratings in chronic pain trials, and it is recommended that at least one rating of global improvement be concurrently used with individual outcomes when assessing the efficacy of analgesic agents.[9,14] Care should be taken when designing global questionnaires or scales, as these might be written in such a way that unfair bias can arise either for or against the compound under study.

30.2.2.5 Symptoms and Adverse Events

The evaluation of symptoms and adverse events plays an important role in the acceptance (and ultimately treatment adherence and overall therapeutic efficacy) of an analgesic drug.[6] Relatively common side effects (e.g., nausea, emesis, sedation, headache, pruritus, constipation, urinary retention) should always be assessed. Typically, only the percentage of subjects experiencing a specific side effect is assessed during analgesic drug development; however, an assessment of severity (e.g., VAS nausea), importance of the symptom to the subject, and changes in these parameters over time is also recommended.[6]

30.2.3 Study Design-Related Issues

Proper study design and interpretation are critical in analgesic drug development. Particular study design issues related to the specific phase of drug development are discussed in the relevant sections. In this section, we provide some general suggestions, many of which are based on prior FDA recommendations[5] for proper study design during analgesic drug development.

- *Crossover vs. parallel design* — Crossover designs (where subjects serve as their own controls) reduce intersubject variability (which can be quite considerable in analgesic trials) and in general maximize efficient use of study subjects. The disadvantages of crossover designs include potential carryover effects (both pharmacologic or psychological) of the analgesic drug, problems with trend effect in the underlying source of pain (i.e., pain may not be steady during the testing interval), and dropouts leading to loss of data which may lead to bias when dropouts are unequally distributed.[5] Analgesic trials using a crossover design require patients with recurring pain of the same intensity before each treatment. Although a carryover effect may occur, the crossover design does allow for some evaluation of this effect.[5] Parallel designs do not have any carryover effect among study treatments, as patients are utilized only once for the study purposes; however, studies that utilize a parallel design require a relatively large homogenous subject population in part to address the intersubject variability in responses to analgesic drugs.

- *Placebo and controls* — Efficacy of a particular dose of an analgesic agent may be established by showing analgesic superiority over placebo, although a negative result might indicate that an inappropriate dose for the analgesic drug was chosen.[5] Placebos can be either active (e.g., normal saline) and inactive (e.g., diphenhydramine). Use of both types of placebo may be helpful in determining analgesic superiority (see discussion on blinding below) and may ultimately influence the labeling of the product.[5] In addition, new analgesic drugs are typically compared to an appropriate, already accepted and approved standard analgesic agent. To determine the dose–response curve of a new analgesic drug, it is usually tested in several doses compared to an appropriate analgesic standard (usually with a similar mechanism of action to the test drug). Common examples of standard analgesics are morphine, aspirin, ibuprofen, acetaminophen, and codeine. Certainly more than one standard analgesic agent may be used, typically with "high-standard" (presumably with greater analgesic efficacy) and "low-standard" analgesics relative to the new analgesic drug. Currently, a head-to-head comparison of analgesic drugs is not generally required to establish pivotal efficacy for gaining marketing approval in the United States; however, this is not necessarily the case in Europe, where noninferiority trials between the study drug and established gold standard are more the norm.
- *Randomization* — By ensuring that known and unknown factors are equally distributed among the groups, proper randomization (individual patient or treatment sequences) reduces selection bias and is critical to trials in analgesic drug development. The process of randomization should be clearly explained in the methodology. For treatment sequences requiring several drug administrations (as might occur in a crossover design), block randomization of treatment sequences is preferable.
- *Blinding* — Because of the subjective nature of pain, blinding is especially important in analgesic drug development trials. Double-blind trials, with both the investigator and subject unaware of the treatment administered, should be standard practice. Unblinding of a study may inadvertently occur as a result of side effects from the analgesic drug, particularly if an inactive placebo is utilized. Having the investigators and subjects guess which treatment was administered is important to assess the robustness of blinding.
- *Assays* — It is generally necessary to incorporate a method of verifying assay sensitivity in every study undertaken, as a study that does not contain some measure of assay sensitivity generally does not provide substantial evidence for the efficacy of the analgesic being evaluated.[5] In cases where placebo is not possible or practical, estimation of the relative potency of test drug compared to the standard analgesics may be used.[5]

Finally, as suggested in the Consolidated Standards of Reporting Trials (CONSORT),[15] participant disposition should also be detailed. Details should be provided on all subjects screened (including those screened not enrolled), extent and reasons for treatment nonadherence, protocol violations (e.g., use of concomitant medications), premature subject withdrawal (and reasons for withdrawal), and loss to follow-up.[6] Specifically, the number of withdrawals related to each side effect or symptoms should be noted. Assessing participant disposition during analgesic drug development is important, as analgesic efficacy is ultimately determined by a subject's adherence to the treatment regimen.

30.3 PRECLINICAL STUDIES

Preclinical trials in drug development for analgesics are essential, as an increasing number of potential agents may be developed as analgesics. For analgesic trials, animal studies are useful to determine the category (e.g., narcotic-like, narcotic antagonist properties, peripherally acting agents) of analgesics into which the test drug falls, as standards of comparison in subsequent clinical trials and identification of adverse events will depend in part on the categorization of the drug.[5] In addition, appropriate animal studies should be performed to determine pharmacokinetic and pharmacologic activity and toxicology and tetrology profiles. We will briefly review the possible targets for analgesic agents as well as the pros and cons of various commonly used animal models of pain.

30.3.1 Neurobiology of Nociception

With the recent major advances in identifying a myriad of new molecular and cellular processes involved in the process of nociception, investigators and pharmaceutical firms have many new targets for novel analgesic therapies. Although it may seem simplistic to develop an antagonist against one of these nociceptive targets, investigators must recognize that the neurobiology of nociception is extremely complex, with redundancy and plasticity such that no "final common pathway" exists for the process of nociception. However, understanding the neurobiology of nociception is crucial when contemplating which nociceptive processes to target in the development of novel analgesic compounds (Table 30.2).[16–37] This section provides a brief overview of the neurobiology of nociception, although greater details of these processes are provided in the references noted.[16–37]

30.3.1.1 Primary Afferents and Peripheral Nerve Neurotransmitters

A variety of mechanical, thermal, or chemical stimuli can result in the sensation of pain. Information about these painful or noxious stimuli is carried to higher brain centers by receptors and neurons that are distinct from those that carry innocuous somatic sensory information. Small-diameter $A\delta$ and C fibers primarily transmit nociceptive information, but a subset of $A\delta$ and C fibers are thermoreceptors that transmit nonpainful cold and warm information, respectively.[38] Neurotransmission by the $A\delta$ and C fibers is performed by numerous peptides and amino acids. Substance P (SP) was the first peptide to be defined as specific to the small-diameter primary afferents, and it is released by noxious thermal, mechanical, and chemical stimulation of the periphery.[39–41] Exogenous application of SP into the spinal cord results in dorsal horn neuron activity[42] and behavioral responses consistent with pain.[43] Neurokinin-1 (NK-1) is the receptor for SP and is found on superficial and deep neurons in the dorsal horn of the spinal cord.[44] Other peptides present in the small-diameter afferents include calcitonin growth-related protein (CGRP), galanin, vasoactive intestinal polypeptide (VIP), and somatostatin (SST); however, their role in the modulation of nociceptive transmission is less well understood.

In addition to these peptides, the excitatory amino acid glutamate is also present within small-diameter primary afferents; it is released by noxious stimulation[45] and activates the second-order dorsal horn neurons.[46] The effects of glutamate are predominantly mediated by three receptor classes: alpha-amino-3-hydroxy-5-methyl-4-isoxazolepropionic acid (AMPA)/kainate, N-methyl-D-aspartate (NMDA), and metabotropic glutamate receptors (mGluR). AMPA receptors are found on postsynaptic neurons predominantly within the superficial dorsal horn.[47] NMDA receptors are found both pre- and postsynaptically (i.e., on nociceptive primary afferents and apposing second-order neurons within the superficial and deep dorsal horn).[48] The mGluR receptors are predominantly found postsynaptically on the cell body and dendrites of dorsal horns neurons. The primary afferent presynaptic nerve terminal in the spinal cord is a potential therapeutic target. It possesses numerous receptor systems that can enhance transmission by increasing transmitter release, including all the excitatory amino acid receptors, voltage-gated calcium channels, and purinergic receptors, as well as systems that inhibit transmission by reducing transmitter release, such as the α_2-adrenergic, glycinergic, serotoninergic, and opioid receptors (μ and δ, predominantly) and GABAergic (GABA$_B$) receptors.[49–51]

30.3.1.2 Spinal Cord and Supraspinal Structures

The primary afferents release neurotransmitters activating the second-order projection neurons of the spinal cord. Second-order neurons of the dorsal horn possess a wide variety of neurotransmitter receptors. A subset of these receptors causes depolarization of the dorsal horn neuron and functions to increase nociceptive pain transmission. These include the excitatory amino acid receptors,

Table 30.2 Possible Novel Targets for Analgesic Drug Development

Target	Classification	Preclinical Target	Phase I	Phase II	Beyond Phase II[a]
Acetylcholine	Receptor	Muscarinic (M1–5) Nicotinic	Neostigmine (IT)	—	Botulinum toxin
Adenosine	Receptor	Subtypes A1–3 Adenosine kinase	—	—	—
Adrenergic	Receptor	Subtypes alpha$_{1-2}$	—	Clonidine (IT)	Clonidine
Calcium channel	Ion channel	Types L, T, N, P, Q, R	—	Ziconotide	Topiramate Pregabalin
Cannabinoid	Receptor	Types CB1 and 2	Dexanabinol	Dronabinol	—
Cyclooxygenase	Enzyme	Subtypes COX 1–III	Ketorolac (IT)	Etoricoxib	Parecoxib Valdecoxib Etrocoxib
GABA	Receptor	Subtypes GABA-A/B/C	—	—	—
Glutamate	Receptor	Metabotropic (mGluR1-8) Ionotropic glutamate (AMPA, kainite)	—	LY-293558	—
Kinins	Receptor	Neurokinin (NK1–3) Bradykinin (BK1, 2) Cholecystokinin (CCKa, b)	Devazepdide L-365,260	—	—
NMDA	Receptor	Subtype: glycine-B, NR2B	—	CNS 5161	Memantine Ketamine Dextromethorphan
Opioid	Receptor Mu, delta, kappa ORL1	Neuropeptide nociceptin/Orphanin FQ	—	—	See Table 30.3 for clinically used opioids
Serotonin	Receptor Subtypes: 5-HT1-7	—	—	—	—
Sodium channel	Ion channel	Tetrodoxtin sensitive (I, II, IIA, III, PN1, VI) Tetrodoxtin insensitive (PN3/SNS, SNS2, Nav)	—	Tetrodotoxin	Lamotrigine Oxcarbazaepine
Vanilloid	Receptor	VR1	—	—	—
Others	Intracellular enzyme Membrane protein	PKA, PKC-gamma, nitric oxide P2X3	—	—	—

[a] Includes phase II, phase IV, and already approved drugs. Not all drugs have regulatory approval for analgesic indications but may have been shown to have analgesic efficacy in off-label uses.

Note: COX, cyclooxygenase; GABA, gamma aminobuytyric acid; IT, intrathecal; PK, phosphokinase.

Source: Data for this table were obtained from several references,[16–37] and Nitu and colleagues[4] were particularly useful.

NMDA, AMPA/kainite, mGluR, and the SP receptor, NK-1. Activation of other receptors results in hyperpolarization of the postsynaptic neuron, thereby inhibiting transmission of noxious stimuli. These include the opioid receptors, γ-aminobutyric acid A (GABA$_A$) receptors, and serotonin receptors. Neurotransmission by the second-order neurons of the dorsal horn on bulbar or thalamic targets is primarily performed by glutamate, resulting in depolarization of postsynaptic AMPA- and NMDA-receptor-containing neurons.[52] These neurons also contain numerous peptide neurotransmitters, including cholecystokinin (CCK), VIP, SP, and dynorphin.[53] Finally, numerous neurotransmitters are involved in descending inhibition including serotonin, enkephalin, GABA, glutamate, and SP.[54–57] The dorsolateral pontine tegmentum (DLPT) contains all of the noradrenergic neurons that project to the rostral ventromedial medulla (RVM) and the spinal cord.[58,59] In animal models, electrical stimulation of the DLPT sites produces analgesia[60,61] that is mediated by the α_2-adrenergic receptor.[61]

30.3.2 Animal Models of Pain

Despite the fact that cellular and molecular studies have conclusively demonstrated the role of these targets in the process of nociception, investigators must properly test these compounds in animals prior to performing any human trials. Animal models provide pivotal information on which clinical trials are based. Although several standard animal models mimic different pain states, each model is created with distinct mechanisms, and the results of these tests should be interpreted within the context of that specific model.[62] Animal models of pain are typically behavioral in nature and share common weaknesses; for example, the neural basis of the behavioral tests is poorly understood, test responses are monitored around a nociceptive threshold that is most likely less than that of clinical pain, many models lack a stimulus–response relationship, and assessing threshold responses to stimuli is difficult.[63] Nevertheless, currently available animal models are essential in the development of new analgesic agents, and understanding the relevant details of important models is critical for the proper interpretation of preclinical trial data in preparation for clinical trials.

The numerous animal models of nociception attempt to reproduce the wide variety of human pain syndromes based on the etiology as well as chronicity of the injury. Pain studies in animals can be divided into broad categories based on the animal's type of injury, the stimulus used to elicit a response, and the animal's response to the injury. Animals involved in the studies of acute pain typically do not have any previous injuries, whereas those for chronic pain syndromes have injuries of an inflammatory or neuropathic nature. Testing the animal's nociceptive threshold is performed by examining the animal's response to mechanical, thermal, or chemical stimuli. The majority of behavioral models of nociceptive processing involve the use of mice or rats, and the following discussion will involve such models.

30.3.2.1 Stimuli

Stimuli from each sensory modality have been used to emulate a painful sensory experience in the world outside of the laboratory. Thermal stimulation has been the most common nociceptive stimulus. It has been used as a model of nociceptive responsiveness in naïve animals to represent baseline nociceptive thresholds as well as in injured animals to represent altered nociceptive responsiveness. The stimulus is most often applied to the tail or hindpaw of the animal, and the time it takes for the animal to withdraw the affected body part from the nociceptive stimulus represents the animal's withdrawal latency. This baseline latency can then be compared with subsequent withdrawal latencies after experimental conditions have been changed. The thermal stimulus is most commonly delivered by a high-intensity light bulb with a focused beam of light on the desired anatomic site.[64–66] Other models use a thermistor attached to the animal's tail or hindpaw or a large metal plate upon which the animal is placed through which hot water is circulated to produce a nociceptive stimulus.[67] Less commonly, a cold stimulus is used to produce a nociceptive response.[68] These modes of acute nociceptive stimulation can produce prolonged injuries to the animals; however, the time and intensity of the stimulus have been standardized in the literature so tissue damage and long-term injury do not occur.

Like thermal stimulation, mechanical stimulation can be used to determine baseline thresholds in uninjured animals and altered thresholds in chronically injured animals. Standard stimulation using a pressure is applied to calibrated callipers or a compression device that can deliver the same amount of force repeatedly. Most commonly, the stimulus is applied gradually with increasing force to the tail or hindpaw and the time to removal of the body part is recorded as the withdrawal latency. Mechanical allodynia can be tested using Von Frey testing, in which a succession of calibrated filaments of increasing tensile strength is applied to the animal. The pressure applied by the Von Frey filaments is not noxious in the naïve animal and is therefore used only in animals with altered thresholds from previous injury. Although the above models of mechanical stimulation test primarily cutaneous stimulation, visceral nociceptive thresholds can be determined using distension of hollow visceral organs such as the colon with distensible balloons.[69]

30.3.2.2 Inflammatory Models

The majority of inflammatory pain models involve the injection of a chemical or immunologic irritant into the dermis, subcutaneous fat, or joint of an animal. The most commonly used chemical stimulus that produces both spontaneous and elicited pain behavior is the formalin test, in which a small volume of a 37% formaldehyde solution is intradermally injected into the dorsal surface of the hindpaw of a rodent. The animal's nociceptive behaviors, including posturing, flinching, and biting, are observed for typically 60 minutes following injection. Standard concentrations of dilute formalin injected in this manner produce a characteristic biphasic pattern of pain behavior involving intense activity followed by quiescence and then again the reappearance of flinching, posturing, and biting.[70] Similar to the formalin test, intradermal injection of bradykinin, substance P, or capsaicin to the hindpaw produces mechanical and thermal allodynia and hyperalgesia lasting for less than 4 hours.[71] The subcutaneous injection of carrageenan[64] or complete Freund's adjuvant produces longer term injuries of a mixed chemical and resultant inflammatory nature. For example, the edema and hyperalgesia produced after injection of carrageenan into the plantar surface of the hindpaw is relatively transient (~1 day),[72] whereas that produced by complete Freund's adjuvant (CFA) is substantially longer (>14 days).[73] The extended duration of CFA-induced inflammation enables characterization of alterations in nociceptive threshold and drug effects of these animals during different stages of development of inflammation; therefore, this model may approximate the extended duration of many chronic pain syndromes in humans more closely.[74]

30.3.2.3 Neuropathic Models

The three standard models of nerve injury include chronic constriction injury (CCI) by loose ligation of the sciatic nerve,[75] tight ligation of the partial sciatic nerve (PSL),[76] and tight ligation of spinal nerves (SNL).[77] All three methods of peripheral nerve injury produce behavioral signs of chronic- and acute-evoked pain with similar time courses; however, there are considerable differences in the magnitude of each nociceptive component between models. Signs of mechanical allodynia as assessed by Von Frey filaments have been found to be the largest in the SNL injury and smallest in the CCI model. Behavioral signs representing ongoing pain as assessed by spontaneous nociceptive behaviors are more prominent in the CCI model than in the other two. Although the behavioral signs of neuropathic pain tend to decrease after sympathectomy in all three models, the change is most apparent in the SNL model. Studies suggest that these three rat models have contrasting features, yet all are useful neuropathic pain models, possibly representing different populations of human patients with neuropathic pain.[78]

30.3.2.4 Disease Models

Although all animal models are intended to reproduce human pain conditions in the form of similar etiology or eliciting stimulus, few duplicate injuries seen in common clinical scenarios. Recently, animal models of postoperative incisional pain and bone pain associated with cancer have been developed. In the post-incisional pain model,[79] a small longitudinal incision is made through the skin, fascia, and muscle of the plantar aspect of the hindpaw in anesthetized rats. Mechanical response thresholds are determined using Von Frey filaments at different areas around the wound before surgery and on subsequent days. Spontaneous pain behaviors are assessed using a cumulative pain score based on the weight-bearing behavior of the animals. This model produces a reliable and quantifiable mechanical hyperalgesia lasting for several days after surgery. Characterization of this model has revealed results very similar to those obtained in human postoperative pain studies.[80] Bone pain associated with primary as well as metastatic disease is common and excruciating in patients with cancer. Mechanisms that give rise to bone cancer pain have been studied using a mouse model with intramedullary injection and containment of osteolytic sarcoma cells in the femur. These tumor cells induced bone destruction as well as ongoing and movement-evoked pain behaviors similar to those found in patients with bone cancer pain.[81] Interestingly, the reorganization of the spinal cord after this injury is significantly different from that observed in mouse models of chronic neuropathic or inflammatory pain.[82]

30.4 CLINICAL STUDIES

30.4.1 Phase I

In general, phase I trials include the initial introduction of an analgesic drug into humans after preclinical studies are successfully completed. The main purpose of phase I trials is to evaluate the new analgesic agent for side effects or evidence of organ toxicity.[5] Typically, phase I trials are conducted in normal adult subjects in a closely monitored institutionalized (inpatient) setting. Outpatients, women of child-bearing age, children, and patients with significant coexisting diseases are typically excluded. In addition, patients taking concomitant drug therapy should be excluded. The new analgesic agent is administered over a relatively wide dose range with the duration of administration appropriate for phase II studies of analgesic efficacy. Initial phase I trials are a series of single-dose, randomized, controlled trials of increasing analgesic drug dosage with approximately 10 to 12 subjects evaluated at each dose. Dose formulations at this stage may include intravenous or oral solutions, capsules, or tablets. Usually, the goal is to establish a maximum tolerated dose (in part based on multiple-dose ranging experiments in rodent and nonrodent species) in these healthy subject volunteers.

A comprehensive history recording and physical examination with extensive laboratory testing should be conducted in part to screen out subjects with significant medical abnormalities. Typical laboratory testing might include a complete blood chemistry tests with platelet count, urinalysis, serum creatinine and blood urea nitrogen, liver function tests, fasting blood glucose, electrocardiogram, and glucose-6-phosphate dehydrogenase (G6PD) deficiency screen for subjects scheduled for multiple drug administration. Other tests may also be indicated. Vital signs and organ function should be closely monitored during the study.

In general, studies to determine absorption (e.g., blood levels and urinary excretion curves), metabolism, distribution, and plasma binding should be undertaken as soon as technically feasible although testing for therapeutic effect does not necessarily need to be delayed.[5] Certain phase I trials (e.g., pharmacokinetics in subpopulations, repeated-dose/multiple-daily-dose studies) are undertaken late in the clinical development of a new analgesic and, despite the timing, these trials (which are crucial to determine the proper use of the analgesic drug and will influence the labeling of the drug) are considered phase I studies.[5]

Occasionally, a new analgesic drug may be withdrawn after phase I testing. Some potential reasons for withdrawal during phase I are intolerable side effects (e.g., severe, nausea, vomiting, sedation), significant adverse events (e.g., severe hypotension, cardiac arrest), or evidence of significant organ toxicity (e.g., liver or renal failure), in addition to increasing regulatory concern and scrutiny regarding QT prolongation. Assessing QT prolongation in phase I trials is crucial for any new analgesic drug (www.fda.gov/ohrms/dockets/ac/03/briefing/pubs%5Cshah.pdf) and may be a reason for drug withdrawal during phase I trials. Finally, genetic polymorphisms (e.g., CYP2D6 deficiencies) that may impact blood levels, and ultimately the dose–response curves in phase II will be highly scrutinized in phase I. Although these deficiencies may be more relevant to the development of analgesic drugs for chronic pain, drug exposures in these subpopulations may impact clinical safety and efficacy responses and may influence the decision as to whether or not a new analgesic drug can be developed beyond phase I or II.

30.4.2 Phase II

In phase II trials, analgesic agents are tested for effectiveness and relative safety in a closely monitored setting. Phase II trials should result in information regarding how the new analgesic drug compares vs. standard analgesics with respect to side effects, onset of analgesia, peak analgesia, and duration of analgesia.[5] Initial phase II trials evaluate the new analgesic drug over a range of doses and should include subjects that are free of coexisting diseases and concomitant medications. Subjects' etiology of pain should be relatively homogeneous, as examining subjects with pain of mixed etiologies will invariably decrease assay sensitivity and make it difficult to interpret results.[5]

Appropriate pain models (e.g., nociceptive/musculoskeletal, neuropathic, visceral) and routes of administration (e.g., oral, intravenous, transdermal) should be used and mirror the indication for which the drug will ultimately be approved. Several pain models should be used, as "substantial evidence" for analgesic efficacy requires replicate data of efficacy in at least two pain models.[5] The entire dose–response curve of the new analgesic should be examined, as this will be the basis for selecting the dose used in later phase II and phase III trials. The new analgesic should be tested against analgesic standards that have a similar mechanism of action. Although most studies use 30 to 50 subjects per group for parallel phase II analgesic trials, this number may change depending on the sample size assumptions that are considered clinically relevant.[5]

The main endpoints used in phase II trials have been described earlier (see Sections 30.2.1 and 30.2.2). Other analgesic endpoints, including onset of analgesia and duration of analgesia, are also commonly used for phase II trials. Onset of analgesia can be assessed by using a stopwatch to measure the time to first detection of pain relief, asking the subject to estimate when relief first occurred, or measuring pain relief and pain intensity at regular intervals.[5] Duration of analgesia is commonly assessed by measuring the time from administration of the study drug to time required for the pain to return to baseline, the time until the subjects requests remedication, the time when 50% of subjects remedicated, or the percentage of subjects who did not remedicate at any given time interval.[5]

Many of the study design and methodologic issues in phase II trials were addressed in Section 30.2.3. Although phase II trials are not designed to determine "safety" *per se*, the side-effect data must be meticulously obtained and closely examined, in part, to determine the presence of a dose–response relationship or unusual events. Potential reasons for delays in approval for phase II trials include insufficient doses examined, inappropriate pain models, or evidence of significant organ toxicity (e.g., hematologic, hepatic, renal). Exploration of appropriate subject populations and a wide dynamic dose range are critical for establishing confidence for the much larger trials required for phase III trials. Understanding the statistical effect sizes and confidence intervals from phase II data may be extremely helpful prior to initiating phase III trials, which can be very costly.

30.4.3 Phase III

After the analgesic effectiveness has been established, well-documented controlled and uncontrolled phase III clinical trials are undertaken to obtain additional evidence of analgesic effectiveness for specific indications and drug-related side effects. In phase III trials, the analgesic drug is tested under a variety of disease states and therapeutic regimens to determine "clinical acceptability" by substantial numbers of patients and physicians.[5] If the analgesic agent has an oral formulation, studies on outpatients should also be conducted. If the analgesic drug is to be administered on a chronic basis, appropriate laboratory tests should be obtained at regular intervals.

Patients chosen for phase III trials should not be excluded on the basis of age, gender, concomitant medications, or coexisting diseases. The analgesic effectiveness of the new drug should be evaluated in several types of pain (which will justify "general purpose" analgesic labeling), although suitably targeted studies should be undertaken if specific labeling indications are anticipated (e.g., obstetric analgesia).[5] Multiple-dose (either PRN or fixed dosing), short-term therapy with the analgesic drug should be designed. Dosing and dosing intervals in phase III trials should be based on the results of phase II trials. The dosing intervals for phase II trials are those tentatively identified for the package insert and should be comparable to those produced by approved standard analgesics.[5] Finally, phase III trials should include analysis of data on analgesic efficacy, safety, and dosing frequency. Although variability in assay sensitivity with multiple- or repeat-dose regimens may increase, these models reflect the administration of a drug under more clinically relevant circumstances.[5] (See Table 30.3 and Table 30.4.)

30.5 SPECIAL POPULATIONS

30.5.1 Chronic Pain (Including Cancer and Neuropathic Pain)

Chronic pain is a multidimensional disease where straightforward assessment of analgesic efficacy (as might be expected for analgesic drug development for acute postoperative pain) only provides limited information on the overall analgesic efficacy, acceptability, and safety of the drug. As described earlier (Section 30.2.2), only assessment using a comprehensive set of outcomes will allow for the true determination of the long-term analgesic efficacy for the treatment of chronic pain. Although updated guidelines from the FDA for the evaluation of analgesic drugs for chronic pain are not yet available, other recommendations for the evaluation of analgesic drugs are available.[6] In previous guidance, the FDA suggested that new opioid and opioid-antagonist agents be assessed for evidence of tolerance development and physical dependence with clinical pharmacology studies to assess behavioral, subjective, and physiological responses in comparison to an appropriate analgesic standard.[5]

30.5.2 Geriatric Pain

The increasing emphasis on geriatric medicine is due to the fact that the elderly will account for approximately 20% of the U.S. population by 2020 (up from 12.5% currently) and 38% of all healthcare spending (approximately 5% of the U.S. gross domestic product).[83] It has been estimated that 55% of the elderly experience pain on a daily basis, and the prevalence of persistent pain may be as high as 80%.[4] Although experimental data suggest that older subjects have a different threshold for nociception compared to younger patients, cognitive and psychomotor parameters must be accounted for when assessing experimental nociception in the elderly.[84] In terms of analgesic drug development, older patients generally require lower doses of analgesic medications, such as opioids. In addition, elderly subjects may have decreased metabolic and elimination capabilities compared to younger patients. During analgesic drug development, pharmacokinetic studies (phase I) and clinically relevant trials (phase III) should be conducted with this population in mind.

Table 30.3 Examples of Common Analgesic Drugs in Clinical Practice

Class of Drug	Generic Names (Trade Names)	Mechanisms of Action	Adverse Reactions[a]	Contraindications[a]
Opioids	Morphine (MS Contin®) Hydromorphone (Diluadid®) Fentanyl (Actiq®)	Activation of μ receptor (spinal and supraspinal)	Nausea, vomiting, pruritus, urinary retention, sedation, paralytic ileus, respiratory depression	Allergy to opioid, respiratory depression, paralytic ileus, severe asthma or hypercarbia
NSAID	Ibuprofen (Motrin®, Advil®) Celecoxib (Celebrex®) Rofecoxib (Vioxx®)	Inhibition of PG synthesis via inhibition of COX	Hepatic, renal, GI, hematologic, fluid retention/edema	Allergy to NSAID, asthma-urticaria with aspirin or other NSAIDs
Local anesthetic	Lidocaine (Lidoderm®) Ropivacaine (Naropin®) Levobupivacaine (Chriocaine®).	Blocks conduction of nerve impulses via sodium channel inhibition	Toxicity including seizures and cardiac arrest	Allergy to local anesthetics
Anticonvulsant	Gabapentin (Neurontin®)	Unknown	Sedation, fatigue, nystagmus, weight gain, dizziness, diplopia	Allergy to anticonvulsants
Serotonin antagonist	Sumatriptan (Imitrex®) Frovatriptan (Frova®) Zolmitriptan (Zomig®)	Agonist for serotonin subtype causing vasoconstriction	Cerebrovascular, cardiac, GI, hypertension	Allergy, patients with ischemic, vascular, or cerebrovascular disease, uncontrolled hypertension, or taking MAO inhibitors

[a] General adverse reactions and contraindications are listed; see individual agents for specific adverse reactions and contraindications.

Note: COX, cyclooxygenase; GI, gastrointestinal; MAO, monoamine-oxidase inhibitor; NSAID, nonsteroidal antiinflammatory drug; PG, prostaglandin.

Table 30.4 Examples of Recently Approved New Analgesic Agents

Analgesic, Year Approved (U.S.)[a]	Sponsor	General Class of Drug	Indication
Bromfenac (Duract®), 1995	Wyeth-Ayerest Laboratories	NSAID	Short-term (< 10 days) management of pain
Tramadol (Ultram®), 1995	Johnson Pharmaceuticals	Other	Short-term management of acute pain
Etodolac (Lodine® XL), 1996	Wyeth-Ayerest Laboratories	NSAID	Osteoarthritis and rheumatoid arthritis
Ropivacaine (Naropin®), 1996	Astra USA, Inc.	Local anesthetic	Local/regional anesthesia for surgery, postoperative pain management and obstetrical procedures
Zolmitriptan (Zomig®), 1997	Zeneca, Ltd.	Serotonin agonist	Migraine headaches
Sumatriptan (Imitrex®), 1997	Glaxo Wellcome, Inc.	Serotonin agonist	Migraine headaches
Celecoxib (Celebrex®), 1998	G.D. Searle	NSAID	Osteoarthritis and rheumatoid arthritis
Oral transmucosal fentanyl (Actiq®), 1998	Anesta Corporation	Opioid	Breakthrough cancer pain in patients who are already receiving and who are tolerant to opioid therapy
Rofecoxib (Vioxx®), 1999	Merck & Company	NSAID	Osteoarthritis, acute pain, and primary dysmenorrhea
Levobupivacaine (Chirocaine®), 1999	Darwin Discovery, Ltd.	Local anesthetic	Surgical anesthesia and pain management
Lidocaine (Lidoderm®), 1999	Hind Health Care	Local anesthetic	Pain in post-herpatic neuralgia
Frovatriptan (Frova®), 2001	Elan Pharma International, Ltd.	Serotonin agonist	Migraine headaches
Valdecoxib (Bextra®), 2001	G.D. Searle	NSAID	Osteoarthritis, rheumatoid arthritis, and primary dysmenorrhea
Gabapentin (Neurontin®), 2002	Parke Davis Pharmaceuticals	Anticonvulsant	Management of postherpetic neuralgia

[a] Generic name (trade name).

Note: NSAID: nonsteroidal antiinflammatory drug.

30.6 SUMMARY

With our increased knowledge of the process of nociception, the untapped potential for new analgesic drug development is enormous. Numerous targets are available for analgesic drug development and data from many preclinical trials are promising,[85] however, to fully developing a new analgesic agent is challenging as many methodologic issues are involved. These include analgesic assessments, animal models, and study design-related issues that must be meticulously and properly addressed at each step of the regulatory process. In addition to those that address analgesic drug development for acute pain, newer guidelines or guidance should be developed for the evaluation of analgesic for chronic pain. Despite all the hurdles, development of new analgesic agents will continue to be a valuable endeavor as the burden of pain is considerable at both an individual and societal level.

REFERENCES

1. Stucky, C.L. et al., Mechanisms of pain, *Proc. Natl. Acad. Sci. USA*, 98(21), 11845–11846, 2001.
2. Stewart, W.F. et al., Lost productive time and cost due to common pain conditions in the U.S. workforce, *JAMA*, 290(18), 2443–2454, 2003.
3. Scholz, J. and Woolf, C.J., Can we conquer pain?, *Nat. Neurosci.*, 5(Suppl.), 1062–1067, 2002.
4. Nitu, A.N. et al., Emerging trends in the pharmacotherapy of chronic pain, *Expert Opin. Investig. Drugs*, 12(4), 545–559, 2003.
5. CDER, *Clinical Evaluation of Analgesic Drugs*, Center for Drug Evaluation and Research, U.S. Food and Drug Administration, Washington, D.C., 1992 (withdrawn 2003) (www.fda.gov/cder/guidance/old041fn.pdf).
6. Turk, D.C. et al., Core outcome domains for chronic pain clinical trials: IMMPACT recommendations, *Pain*, 106(3), 337–345, 2003.
7. Cepeda, M.S. et al., Agreement between percentage pain reductions calculated from numeric rating scores of pain intensity and those reported by patients with acute or cancer pain, *Pain*, 106(3), 439–442, 2003.
8. Cepeda, M.S. et al., What decline in pain intensity is meaningful to patients with acute pain? *Pain*, 105(1–2), 151–157, 2003.
9. Farrar, J.T. et al., Clinical importance of changes in chronic pain intensity measured on an 11-point numerical pain rating scale, *Pain*, 94(2), 149–158, 2001.
10. Farrar, J.T. et al., Clinically important changes in acute pain outcome measures: a validation study, *J. Pain Symptom Manage.*, 25(5), 406–411, 2003.
11. Caraceni, A. et al., Pain measurement tools and methods in clinical research in palliative care: recommendations of an Expert Working Group of the European Association of Palliative Care, *J. Pain Symptom Manage.*, 23(3), 239–255, 2002.
12. Wittink, H. et al., Comparison of the redundancy, reliability, and responsiveness to change among SF-36, Oswestry Disability Index, and Multidimensional Pain Inventory, *Clin. J. Pain*, 20(3), 133–142, 2004.
13. Stacey, B.R. and Glanzman, R.L., Use of gabapentin for postherpetic neuralgia: results of two randomized, placebo-controlled studies, *Clin. Ther.*, 25(10), 2597–2608, 2003.
14. Fischer, D. et al., Capturing the patient's view of change as a clinical outcome measure, *JAMA*, 282(12), 1157–1162, 1999.
15. Moher, D. et al., The CONSORT statement: revised recommendations for improving the quality of reports of parallel-group randomized trials, *Ann. Intern. Med.*, 134(8), 657–662, 2001.
16. Wu C.L. et al., Gene therapy for the management of pain. Part I. Methods and strategies, *Anesthesiology*, 94(6), 1119–1132, 2001.
17. Wu C.L. et al., Gene therapy for the management of pain. Part II. Molecular targets, *Anesthesiology*, 95(1), 216–240, 2001.
18. Gribkoff, V.K., The therapeutic potential of neuronal KCNQ channel modulators, *Expert Opin. Ther. Targets*, 7(6), 737–748, 2003.

19. Humphrey, J.M., Medicinal chemistry of selective neurokinin-1 antagonists, *Curr. Top. Med. Chem.*, 3(12), 1423–1435, 2003.

20. Zaveri, N., Peptide and nonpeptide ligands for the nociceptin/orphanin FQ receptor ORL1: research tools and potential therapeutic agents, *Life Sci.*, 73(6), 663–678, 2003.

21. North, R.A., The P2X3 subunit: a molecular target in pain therapeutics, *Curr. Opin. Investig. Drugs*, 4(7), 833–840, 2003.

22. Smith, P.F., Therapeutic *N*-methyl-D-aspartate receptor antagonists: will reality meet expectation?, *Curr. Opin. Investig. Drugs*, 4(7), 826–832, 2003.

23. Lopez-Rodriguez, M.L. et al., VR1 receptor modulators as potential drugs for neuropathic pain, *Mini Rev. Med. Chem.*, 3(7), 729–748, 2003.

24. Pin J.P. and Acher, F., The metabotropic glutamate receptors: structure, activation mechanism and pharmacology, *Curr. Drug Target CNS Neurol. Disord.*, 1(3), 297–317, 2002.

25. Croxford, J.L., Therapeutic potential of cannabinoids in CNS disease, *CNS Drugs*, 17(3), 179–202, 2003.

26. Sawynok, J., Topical and peripherally acting analgesics, *Pharmacol. Rev.*, 55(1), 1–20, 2003.

27. Patrignani P. et al., Clinical pharmacology of etoricoxib: a novel selective COX2 inhibitor, *Expert Opin. Pharmacother.*, 4(2), 265–284, 2003.

28. Palmer S.L. et al., Cannabinergic ligands, *Chem. Phys. Lipids*, 121(1–2), 3–19, 2002.

29. Szekely, J.I. et al., The role of ionotropic glutamate receptors in nociception with special regard to the AMPA binding sites, *Curr. Pharm. Des.*, 8(10), 887–912, 2002.

30. Cox, B., Calcium channel blockers and pain therapy, *Curr. Rev. Pain*, 4(6), 488–498, 2000.

31. Trujillo, K.A., Are NMDA receptors involved in opiate-induced neural and behavioral plasticity? A review of preclinical studies, *Psychopharmacology (Berlin)*, 151(2–3), 121–141, 2000.

32. Staats, P.S. et al., Intrathecal ziconotide in the treatment of refractory pain in patients with cancer or AIDS: a randomized controlled trial, *JAMA*, 291(1), 63–70, 2004.

33. Fisher, K. et al., Targeting the *N*-methyl-D-aspartate receptor for chronic pain management: preclinical animal studies, recent clinical experience and future research directions, *J. Pain Symptom Manage.*, 20(5), 358–373, 2000.

34. Chizh, B.A., Novel approaches to targeting glutamate receptors for the treatment of chronic pain: review article, *Amino Acids*, 23(1–3), 169–176, 2002.

35. Willis, W.D., Role of neurotransmitters in sensitization of pain responses, *Ann. N.Y. Acad. Sci.*, 933, 142–156, 2001.

36. Kowaluk, E.A. et al., Adenosine kinase inhibitors, *Curr. Pharm. Des.*, 4(5), 403–416, 1998.

37. Eisenach, J.C., Muscarinic-mediated analgesia, *Life Sci.*, 64(6–7), 549–554, 1999.

38. Darian-Smith, I., Thermal sensibility, in *Handbook of Physiology*, Darian-Smith, I., Brookhart, J.M., and Mouncastle, V.B., Eds., American Physiological Society, Bethesda, MD, 1984, pp. 879–914.

39. Oku, R. et al., Release of substance P from the spinal dorsal horn is enhanced in polyarthritic rats, *Neurosci. Lett.*, 74(3), 315–319, 1987.

40. Tiseo, P.J. et al., Differential release of substance P and somatostatin in the rat spinal cord in response to noxious cold and heat: effect of dynorphin A(1-17), *J. Pharmacol. Exp. Ther.*, 252(2), 539–545, 1990.

41. Oh, S.B. et al., Chemokines and glycoprotein120 produce pain hypersensitivity by directly exciting primary nociceptive neurons, *J. Neurosci.*, 21(14), 5027–5035, 2001.

42. Salter, M.W. and Henry, J.L., Responses of functionally identified neurones in the dorsal horn of the cat spinal cord to substance P, neurokinin A and physalaemin, *Neuroscience*, 43(2–3), 601–610, 1991.

43. Malmberg, A.B. and Yaksh, T.L., Hyperalgesia mediated by spinal glutamate or substance P receptor blocked by spinal cyclooxygenase inhibition, *Science*, 257(5074), 1276–1279, 1992.

44. Stucky, C.L. et al., Time-dependent changes in Bolton–Hunter-labeled ^{125}I-substance P binding in rat spinal cord following unilateral adjuvant-induced peripheral inflammation, *Neuroscience*, 57(2), 397–409, 1993.

45. Jeftinija, S. et al., Excitatory amino acids are released from rat primary afferent neurons *in vitro*, *Neurosci. Lett.*, 125(2), 191–194, 1991.

46. Aanonsen, L.M. et al., Excitatory amino acid receptors and nociceptive neurotransmission in rat spinal cord, *Pain*, 41(3), 309–321, 1990.

47. Dougherty, P.M. et al., The role of NMDA and non-NMDA excitatory amino acid receptors in the excitation of primate spinothalamic tract neurons by mechanical, chemical, thermal, and electrical stimuli, *J. Neurosci.*, 12(8), 3025–3041, 1992.

48. Liu, H. et al., Evidence for presynaptic *N*-methyl-D-aspartate autoreceptors in the spinal cord dorsal horn, *Proc. Natl. Acad. Sci. USA*, 91(18), 8383–8387, 1994.

49. Glaum, S.R. et al., Inhibitory actions of mu- and delta-opioid receptor agonists on excitatory transmission in lamina II neurons of adult rat spinal cord, *J. Neurosci.*, 14(8), 4965–4971, 1994.

50. Hammond, D.L. and Bonica, J.J., Role of spinal GABA in acute and persistent nociception, *Reg. Anesth. Pain Med.*, 26(6), 551–557, 2001.

51. Stone, L.S. et al., Differential distribution of alpha2A and alpha2C adrenergic receptor immunoreactivity in the rat spinal cord, *J. Neurosci.*, 18(15), 5928–5937, 1998.

52. Blomqvist, A. et al., Evidence for glutamate as a neurotransmitter in spinothalamic tract terminals in the posterior region of owl monkeys, *Exp. Brain Res.*, 108(1), 33–44, 1996.

53. Leah, J. et al., Neuropeptides in long ascending spinal tract cells in the rat: evidence for parallel processing of ascending information, *Neuroscience*, 24(1), 195–207, 1988.

54. Skagerberg, G. and Bjorklund, A., Topographic principles in the spinal projections of serotonergic and non-serotonergic brainstem neurons in the rat, *Neuroscience*, 15(2), 445–480, 1985.

55. Antal, M. et al., Direct evidence of an extensive GABAergic innervation of the spinal dorsal horn by fibres descending from the rostral ventromedial medulla, *Neuroscience*, 73(2), 509–518, 1996.

56. Bowker, R.M. et al., Peptidergic neurons in the nucleus raphe magnus and the nucleus gigantocellularis: their distributions, interrelationships, and projections to the spinal cord, *Prog. Brain Res.*, 77, 95–127, 1988.

57. Menetrey, D. and Basbaum, A.I., The distribution of substance P-, enkephalin-, and dynorphin-immunoreactive neurons in the medulla of the rat and their contribution to bulbospinal pathways, *Neuroscience*, 23(1), 173–187, 1987.

58. Kwiat, G.C. and Basbaum, A.I., The origin of brainstem noradrenergic and serotonergic projections to the spinal cord dorsal horn in the rat, *Somatosens. Mot. Res.*, 9(2), 157–173, 1992.

59. Clark, F.M. and Proudfit, H.K., Projections of neurons in the ventromedial medulla to pontine catecholamine cell groups involved in the modulation of nociception, *Brain Res.*, 540(1–2), 105–115, 1991.

60. Proudfit, H.K., Pharmacologic evidence for the modulation of nociception by noradrenergic neurons, *Prog. Brain Res.*, 77, 357–370, 1988.

61. Yeomans, D.C. et al., Antinociception induced by electrical stimulation of spinally projecting noradrenergic neurons in the A7 catecholamine cell group of the rat, *Pain*, 48(3), 449–461, 1992.

62. Wang, L.X. and Wang, Z.J., Animal and cellular models of chronic pain, *Adv. Drug Deliv. Rev.*, 55(8), 949–965, 2003.

63. Le Bars, D. et al., Animal models of nociception, *Pharmacol. Rev.*, 53(4), 597–652, 2001.

64. Hargreaves, K. et al., A new and sensitive method for measuring thermal nociception in cutaneous hyperalgesia, *Pain*, 32(1), 77–88, 1988.

65. Dirig, D.M. et al., Characterization of variables defining hindpaw withdrawal latency evoked by radiant thermal stimuli, *J. Neurosci. Methods*, 76(2), 183–191, 1997.

66. D'Amour, F.E. and Smith, D.L., A method for determining loss of pain sensation, *J. Pharmacol. Exp. Ther.*, 72, 74–79, 1941.

67. Woolfe, G. and MacDonald, A.D., The evaluation of the analgesic action of pethidine hydrochloride (Demerol), *J. Pharmacol. Exp. Ther.*, 80, 300–307, 1944.

68. Choi, Y. et al., Behavioral signs of ongoing pain and cold allodynia in a rat model of neuropathic pain, *Pain*, 59(3), 369–376, 1994.

69. Anderson, R.H. et al., A distension control device useful for quantitative studies of hollow organ sensation, *Physiol. Behav.*, 41(6), 635–638, 1987.

70. Dubuisson, D. and Dennis, S.G., The formalin test: a quantitative study of the analgesic effects of morphine, meperidine, and brain stem stimulation in rats and cats, *Pain*, 4(2), 161–174, 1977.

71. Oh, S. et al., Chemokines and glycoprotein120 produce pain hypersensitivity by directly exciting primary nociceptive neurons, *J. Neurosci.*, 21(14), 5027–5035, 2001.

72. Hurley, R.W. et al., Gabapentin and pregabalin can interact synergistically with naproxen to produce antihyperalgesia, *Anesthesiology*, 97(5), 1263–1273, 2002.

73. Hurley, R.W. and Hammond, D.L., The analgesic effects of supraspinal mu and delta opioid receptor agonists are potentiated during persistent inflammation, *J. Neurosci.*, 20(3), 1249–1259, 2000.

74. Colpaert, F.C., Evidence that adjuvant arthritis in the rat is associated with chronic pain, *Pain*, 28(2), 201–222, 1987.

75. Bennett, G.J. and Xie, Y.K., A peripheral mononeuropathy in rat that produces disorders of pain sensation like those seen in man, *Pain*, 33(1), 87–108, 1988.

76. Seltzer, Z. et al., Autotomy behavior in rats following peripheral deafferentation is suppressed by daily injections of amitriptyline, diazepam and saline, *Pain*, 37(2), 245–250, 1989.

77. Kim, S.H. and Chung, J.M., An experimental model for peripheral neuropathy produced by segmental spinal nerve ligation in the rat, *Pain*, 50(3), 355–363, 1992.

78. Kim, K.J. et al., Comparison of three rodent neuropathic pain models, *Exp. Brain Res.*, 113(2), 200–206, 1997.

79. Brennan, T.J. et al., Characterization of a rat model of incisional pain, *Pain*, 64(3), 493–501, 1996.

80. Zahn, P.K. et al., Mechanisms for pain caused by incisions, *Reg. Anesth. Pain Med.*, 27(5), 514–516, 2002.

81. Schwei, M.J. et al., Neurochemical and cellular reorganization of the spinal cord in a murine model of bone cancer pain, *J. Neurosci.*, 19(24), 10886–10897, 1999.

82. Honore, P. et al., Murine models of inflammatory, neuropathic and cancer pain each generates a unique set of neurochemical changes in the spinal cord and sensory neurons, *Neuroscience*, 98(3), 585–598, 2000.

83. Anderson G.F. and Hussey, P.S., Population aging: a comparison among industrialized countries, *Health Aff.*, 19(3), 191–203, 2000.

84. Pickering, G. et al., Impact of age, gender and cognitive functioning on pain perception, *Gerontology*, 48(2), 112–118, 2002.

85. Ridgway, D., Analgesics for acute pain: meeting the United States Food and Drug Administration's requirements for proof of efficacy, *Clin. J. Pain*, 20(3), 123–132, 2004.

PART XIII

Assessment of Biopharmaceuticals

CHAPTER 31

Vaccines

Chi-Jen Lee, Lucia H. Lee, Christopher L. Wu, and Benjamin R. Lee

CONTENTS

31.1 INTRODUCTION

Disease prevention using vaccination strategies has been an important public health achievement. Successful vaccination has eradicated smallpox and eliminated poliomyelitis in many areas of the world. A 90 to 100% decline in mortality and morbidity of several childhood infections has occurred since the introduction of vaccines and implementation in routine childhood immunization schedules. The use of appropriate vaccines has prevented 150,000 and 750,000 deaths per year from poliomyelitis and measles, respectively. New technologies including recombinant DNA approaches, peptide synthetic chemistry, and new immunomodulating adjuvants have contributed to the development of novel vaccines and improvement of existing vaccines.

Vaccines represent only a small proportion of the global drug market, but they occupy a significant position in terms of public health importance. Many vaccines are listed as essential medicines and are indispensable elements of health programs. More than 60% of all vaccine doses produced worldwide are purchased and distributed through international organizations, including the United Nations Children's Fund (UNICEF), World Health Organization (WHO), and Pan-American Health Organization (PAHO). The majority of vaccine manufacturers are health research institutes and government agencies. Compared to the vaccine supply of international organizations and governments, the commercial vaccine market accounts for only 14% of the total vaccine distribution but 75 to 80% of the value.[1]

Recent advances in biotechnology and molecular immunology have provided a more optimistic outlook for vaccine manufacturers. The vaccine market in the early 1990s was estimated at approximately US$2 billion. It is generally anticipated that in the early 2000s, the commercial vaccine market will reach a sales value twice to three times that of the early 1990s and that average annual growth rates will be above 10%.

It has been reported that, in the 1980s, the average period required to develop a new drug (new chemical entity) from preclinical research to product licensure was 12 years.[2,3] A similar pattern applies for biological and chemical products. Preclinical research and development require 2 to 4 years, clinical trials 5 to 7 years, and license application 2 to 3 years.[4,5] Thus, clinical trials clearly have become a major expense in vaccine research and development.

Following preclinical research of a vaccine candidate, clinical trials are conducted to establish acceptable safety and to assess immune response to demonstrate efficacy. In addition, consistency of production should be demonstrated by showing comparable clinical responses to different vaccine lots. Factors impacting trial costs include selection of the study population, the number of subjects required to detect potential adverse reactions, and the documentation required to ensure quality assurance. Manufacturers tend to outsource these responsibilities to contract research organizations (CROs).

Rapid changes in population distributions have introduced potential differences in safety, immunogenicity, and efficacy among populations; thus, safety and immunogenicity data should be obtained from the specific population in which the clinical trials are performed. This globalization approach has been used in the development of pneumococcal 9- and 11-valent conjugate vaccines designed to benefit individuals in the United States and foreign countries, as well as specific high-risk population (e.g., Eskimos and Native Americans).

Another factor impacting trial conditions is the number of subjects required to demonstrate a statistically meaningful difference in safety and efficacy of an investigational vaccine compared to a control vaccine. For example, a tetravalent recombinant rotavirus vaccine was licensed in August 1998. Clinical trials for the candidate vaccine, which included more than 10,000 recipients, were sufficient to show efficacy but were not adequate to detect intussusception as a potential safety concern.[6] The Centers for Disease Control and Prevention (CDC) recommended post-licensure surveillance on this adverse event, and by June 1999, following distribution of 1.8 million doses of vaccine, increased occurrences of intussusception related to vaccination were observed in vaccine recipients. For this reason, the manufacturer voluntarily withdrew the vaccine from the market in 2000. Since then, the FDA has considered requiring expanded phase III trials for subsequent development of any live rotaviral vaccine to alleviate concerns about vaccine-associated intussusception.

Vaccine protection, measured in a clinical efficacy trial, can sometimes be correlated with specific immune responses. The identification of an immune correlate can facilitate planned trials, as fewer study participants are needed and the duration of the trial is not as long. Vaccine efficacy is traditionally defined as a reduction in the infection rate following the immunization. It is estimated by the rate of prevention of disease after deliberate challenge with virulent microorganisms or by induction of immunogenicity when a specific immune response is shown to prevent infection. Efficacy is generally evaluated in prospective randomized, controlled studies. Double-blind trials with placebo controls are necessary to minimize bias in patient assignment and in evaluation of immune responses.

Initial assessment of immune responses following vaccination occurs in phase I and II trials. One measure of a vaccine to elicit the intended immunogenic response is serum antibody concentrations. Usually, range doses and several administration routes are valuated to decide the final dose and dosing regimen. Phase III trials to assess efficacy are conducted after early-phase trials have produced preliminary results on the safety and immunogenicity of the vaccine. The appropriate size of phase III vaccine trials depends on various factors, including the primary outcome measure, disease rate, and acceptable error rates. Sample sizes necessary to study efficacy based on levels of immune response are usually smaller than those required to evaluate prevention of clinical disease, and vaccines to prevent common diseases can be evaluated in smaller trials than vaccines to prevent rare diseases. For example, the efficacy of varicella vaccine was established in a clinical trial that included fewer than 1000 subjects. In contrast, the field trial of the Salk polio vaccine required nearly half a million children to accurately evaluate the efficacy of the vaccine.

Safety evaluation is a critical concern in all phases of vaccine development, from phase I through phase IV. Phase I trials are frequently designed as dose-finding studies and often include objectives to assess clinical laboratory toxicity and serious adverse events, antibody titers, allergic reactions, and local reactions such as erythema, induration, pain, and tenderness. For live bacterial or viral recombinant vaccines, safety assessments are initially examined in an inpatient facility to permit close observation and reporting of signs and symptoms, as vaccine strains can potentially be transmitted to household contacts. Phase II trials, often placebo controlled, are designed to further evaluate safety and provide a preliminary estimate of vaccine impact on important health outcomes such as infection, hospitalization, or absenteeism for school or employment. Phase III trials confirm the efficacy of the selected vaccine dose and dosing regimen and also include objectives to assess duration of protection.

As more vaccines are used for the pediatric immunization and the incidence of serious infectious diseases has declined, public expectation of fewer vaccine-associated adverse events has become the norm. As a result, the prelicense safety evaluation has been expanded and performed extensively.[7]

31.2 VACCINE DEVELOPMENT IN THE TWENTY-FIRST CENTURY

In 1985, the Institute of Medicine (IOM) published two reports that have served as a basis for the development of vaccines against many infectious diseases considered major threats to public health.[8,9] Several of the recommended vaccines in that report have been licensed; Table 31.1 lists vaccines recently licensed in the United States. In 1995, the National Institutes of Health (NIH) asked the IOM to review progress made since the 1985 vaccine reports in order to recommend new priorities for vaccine development. Several differences between the vaccine project published in 1985 and projects recommended in 1995 can be observed:

- New projects focused on vaccines related to domestic public health importance; no international concerns were included.
- Vaccines were recommended based on the assumption that they could be licensed within the next two decades.
- New projects emphasized therapeutic vaccines directed against chronic diseases, such as autoimmune diseases and cancers.
- Vaccines for the prevention of human immunodeficiency virus (HIV) were not included; it was suggested that they should be considered separately.

Table 31.2 lists the vaccine candidates recommended in 1995 by the IOM for development in the United States.

Infectious diseases cause approximately one third of all deaths in the world each year. Vaccines would be the most cost effective means to prevent these deaths; however, either existing vaccines are not available in certain areas or, more frequently, no suitable vaccines against the diseases exist. The problem is particularly critical in developing countries, where only five vaccines against the 20 most important diseases that cause mortality are in widespread use; that is, each year about 8.2 million people die in developing nations even though vaccines exist that could potentially prevent their mortality. Thus, the need to develop and apply new and improved vaccines in many areas of the world is great.

The International Vaccine Institute (IVI) was a project of the Children's Vaccine Initiative (CVI), sponsored by the World Bank, WHO, UNICEF, and the Rockefeller Foundation, to develop new vaccines and upgrade existing vaccines for developing countries. The Institute's strategic plan focused primarily on the Commencement Phase (1997 to 2000), which was intended to lay the

Table 30.1 Recently Licensed Vaccines in the United States

Vaccine Product	Trade Name	License Approval Date	Manufacturer
DTaP Vaccines/Combinations			
DTaP–HBV–IPV	Pediarix®	12/13/02	GlaxoSmithKline
DTaP	Daptacel®	05/14/02	Aventis Pasteur
DTaP (reduced thimerosal)	Tripedia®	03/07/01	Aventis Pasteur
DTaP (fifth dose)	Infanrix™	07/07/03	GlaxoSmithKline
DTaP	Certiva™	07/29/98	North American Vaccine
Pneumococcal Conjugate			
Invasive pneumococcal disease	Prevnar®	02/17/00	Wyeth–Ayerst
Otitis media	Prevnar®	10/01/02	Wyeth–Ayerst
Hepatitis A, B Vaccines/Combinations			
Hepatitis A–hepatitis B	Twinrix®	05/11/01	GlaxoSmithKline
Hepatitis A, extended timing of booster (6–18 months)	VAQTA®	09/04/02	Merck
HibOMP–hepatitis B	COMVAX®	10/02/96	Merck
Hepatitis B, preservative free	RECOMBIVAX®	08/27/99	Merck
Influenza	FluMist®	06/17/03	Medimmune
Typhoid			
Live oral, Ty21a	Vivotif Berna®	12/15/89	Berna Biotech
Vi-PS	Typhim Vi™	11/28/94	Aventis Pasteur
Japanese B encephalitis	JE-VAX®	12/10/92	Aventis Pasteur
Haemophilus B Conjugate			
PRP-CRM197	HibTITER®	12/21/88	Lederle Laboratories
PRP-OMPC	PedvaxHIB®	12/20/89	Merck
PRP-T	ActHIB®	03/30/93	Aventis Pasteur
	OmniHIB®	—	GlaxoSmithKline
Varicella	VARIVAX®	03/17/95	Merck
Rotavirus	RotaShield®	08/31/98	Wyeth Laboratories

groundwork for the Institute and Operation Phase (2001 onward), which was designed to conduct extensive vaccine research and development. The Institute emphasized the importance of vaccine development to reducing the burden of disease, especially in Asia. Based on practical considerations, the IVI plans to focus on two groups of vaccines over the next several years. Work on group I vaccines was initiated immediately, while work on vaccines selected from group II will begin as resources become available:

- Group I vaccines — *Haemophilus influenzae* type b, *Streptococcus pneumoniae*, *Neisseria meningitides*
- Group II vaccines
  - Respiratory infection – tuberculosis
  - Gastrointestinal tract diseases — cholera, rotavirus, *Shigella*, typhoid, hepatitis B and combinations, human immunodeficiency virus
  - Vectorborne diseases — malaria, Japanese encephalitis, Dengue

Developing countries bear a disproportionate share of infectious disease incidences. In addition, vaccines do not yet exist against many of the important "killer diseases," and even when vaccines exist many of them are not available to the general population. Biotechnology and molecular

Table 31.2 Vaccine Candidates for Development in the United States

Respiratory Infection

Influenzae A and B, cytomegalovirus (CMV), *Streptococcus pneumoniae*, respiratory syncytial virus, *Mycobacterium tuberculosis*, group A *Streptococcus*

Gastrointestinal Tract Infection

Rotavirus, shigella, enterotoxigenic *Escherichia coli*, *Helicobacter pylori*, hepatitis C

Sexually Transmitted Diseases

Neisseria gonorrhea, chlamydia, herpes simplex virus, human papilloma virus

Autoimmune and Chronic Diseases (Therapeutic Vaccine)

Rheumatoid arthritis, multiple sclerosis, melanoma, Alzheimer's disease, insulin-dependent diabetes

Others

Borrelia burgdorferi (Lyme disease), Epstein–Barr virus (infectious mononucleosis), group B *Streptococcus*, *Neisseria meningitides*, group B *Coccidiodes immitis*

immunology have developed and advanced in an extraordinary way since the 1980s. These advances have occurred because of the development of molecular approaches to cloning and characterization of virulence factors of specific pathogens and because of the better understanding of the cellular and molecular interaction that follow host responses to immunization or infection with a specific pathogen. Furthermore, rapid progress has been made on mucosal immunity and vaccine delivery systems. The mammalian mucosal immune system involves an integrated network of tissues, lymphoid cells, and effector molecules. The induction of peripheral immune responses by parenteral vaccination does not induce significant mucosal immunity. In contrast, induction of mucosal immune responses can result in protective immunity in the local and systemic compartments.

Mucosal surfaces are enormous, approximately 300 to 400 m². The major antibody isotype in external secretion is immunoglobulin A (IgA); approximately 40 mg of IgA per kilogram of body weight is made in mucosal effector tissues each day, particularly in the gastrointestinal tract. The use of vaccines that induce protective mucosal immunity thus becomes attractive as most infectious agents enter the body via mucosal surfaces. At present, of 30 categories of vaccines, toxoids, and proteins licensed for use in the United States, only 4, including oral poliovirus (OPV), rotavirus, adenovirus, and typhoid, are administered orally and none is given intranasally. Mucosal immunity can be induced by immunogenic stimulation of mucosal-associated lymphoid tissue (MALT), which produces secretary IgA (S-IgA) and IgG antibodies. S-IgA may inhibit the adherence and invasion of mucosal pathogens and neutralize the virulent enzymes and toxin.[10,11]

Most vaccine antigens produce only weak immune responses when given by themselves, either parenterally or orally. The induction of an effective immune response usually requires the addition of an adjuvant, which is a substance to enhance the immune response. Adjuvants affect many aspects of antibody responses, including the kinetics, duration, quantity, isotype, avidity, and generation of protective immunity. A number of major breakthroughs have occurred within the context of novel vaccine delivery systems. These include the application of lipid- or detergent-based adjuvants such as liposomes, immune-stimulating complexes (ISCOMS), and microspheres coated with biodegradable polymer (e.g., DL-lactide-coglycolide). Important advances have also been made in the development and use of viruses for the delivery of foreign antigens. Vaccinia virus has been successfully used for several antigens and cytokines, and recombinant adenovirus for delivery to the mucosal tissues of the gastrointestinal tract as well as to the upper respiratory tract and lung. Delivery of vaccines by intranasal immunization has shown that this is an effective route for the induction of respiratory and parenteral immune responses. Adenovirus vectors have been used not only as a means for mucosal immunization but also as potential vectors to transfer the corrective gene DNA for the treatment of cystic fibrosis.

Preventing infections in neonates and young infants by immunization of pregnant women is a concept conceived many years ago. The rationale for maternal immunization during pregnancy is based on the observations that maternal immunization before or during pregnancy would induce high concentrations of specific antibodies that would be transferred across the placenta, thereby passively protecting the infant. In addition, active immunization of the infant could induce a booster effect if the mother was immunized during pregnancy. This approach has been extensively studied for the prevention of diphtheria, tetanus, and pertussis infections in infants. Maternal immunization for the prevention of infection in the infants is used routinely for neonatal tetanus. WHO has recommended that this approach be extended for the prevention of diseases caused by other pathogens.

The possibility of maternal immunization for the prevention of several infectious diseases, including group B *Streptococcus* (GBS), *Haemophilus* type b, meningococcal groups A and C, *Streptococcus pneumoniae*, and viral pathogens (e.g., hepatitis B virus, influenza virus, respiratory syncytial virus), has been extensively studied. Despite considerable research data supporting the feasibility, safety, and cost-effectiveness of this approach, the medical community and manufacturers are reluctant to enforce it. Obstacles to this approach involve ethical, legal, and sociological concerns, but the issue concerning the liability of vaccine manufacturers has been the overriding factor for the slow progress in the United States.

31.3 GLYCOCONJUGATE VACCINES

Encapsulated bacterial pathogens still cause the most prevalent and serious infections in the United States and many other areas of the world. The mortality and morbidity of bacteremia, meningitis, and pneumonia due to these organisms are particularly high in children, the elderly, and immuno-deficient patients. Several factors, including the high mortality and morbidity, endemic and epidemic diseases, and expanding incidence of antibiotic-resistance strains, have emphasized the importance of vaccine development for the prevention of bacterial infections.

Capsular polysaccharides (PSs) are cell-surface polymers consisting of oligosaccharide repeating units. These PSs are the main virulence factor responsible for the pathogenesis of encapsulated bacteria. Most adult animal sera contain antibodies against PS antigens of various pathogenic bacteria; for example, antibodies to pathogens (e.g., *Haemophilus* type b; meningococcal groups A, B, and C; pneumococcal type 3) were detected in animals as they grew or in human adults who had never had contact with these organisms. The possible antigenic sources of these serum protective antibodies have been identified and found to be derived from cross-reactive antigens distributed in intestinal and pharyngeal bacteria.

Capsular PSs are involved in interactions with the immune system to produce protective immunity. These PSs are highly polar and hydrophilic and interfere with cell-to-cell interactions with phagocytes. The ability of host phagocytes to ingest and kill invading pathogens requires coating of the bacteria by specific antibodies and complement. This process, known as *opsonization*, results in phagocytosis, which destroys invading bacteria. Antibodies bound to capsule may act as bacterial cell to phagocytic cell ligands or as complement activator. Anticapsular antibodies increase the rate of clearance of pneumococci, primarily through the activation of the classical complement pathway. In contrast, these antibodies destroy *Haemophilus* type b through the lysis of bacteria.

The antibody response to capsular PSs is independent of control by the thymus (TI), whereas the response to protein antigens is thymus dependent (TD), requiring T-lymphocytes for both its induction and regulation. Both amplifier and helper T-cells are CD4+ and CD8–, and both positively enhance the antibody response, which in mice is primarily IgG3. Amplifier T-cells expand an already ongoing antibody response. In contrast, suppressor T-cells, which are CD4– and CD8+,

Table 31.3 Characterization of Hib Conjugate Vaccines

Vaccine	HbOC	PRP-OMPC	PRP-T	PRP-T
Manufacturer	Wyeth-Lederle	Merck	Aventis Pasteur	GlaxoSmithKline
Trade name	HibTITER	PedvaxHib	ActHIB	OmniHIB
Approval date	12/21/88	12/20/89	3/30/93	—
Carrier protein	CRM197	OMPC	TT	TT
Saccharide size	Oligosaccharide	PS	PS	PS
Spacer	None	Bigeneric spacer	6 carbon spacer	—
PS (μg/0.5 mL dose)	10	15	10	—
Immunogenicity	High in children 18 to 24 months and older; strong Ab response in infants with first dose	High in children and adults	High	Similar to HbOC
Recommended vaccination	2, 4, 6, and 12–15 months	2, 4, and 12–15 months	2, 4, 6, and 12–15 months	—

Note: HbOC, *Haemophilus* b oligosaccharide conjugate; OMPC, outer membrane protein conjugate; PRP, polyribosyl ribitol phosphate; PRP-T, *Haemophilus influenzae* capsular polysaccharide tetanus conjugate vaccine (PRP-T); PS, polysaccharide; TT, tetanus toxoid.

inhibit B-cell proliferation after antigenic binding. Activated suppressor T-cells are influenced by lymphokines produced by helper T-cells. Interleukins IL-2, IL-4, and IL-5 and interferon-γ are required for the activation or clonal expansion of suppressor T-cells.

The immune system of infants differs from that of adults in both its lack of previous antigenic exposure and its functional immaturity. Infants obtain IgG almost exclusively through transplacental passage, and endogenous immunoglobulin is largely restricted to IgM antibody. In contrast, rodents acquire maternal antibodies both before and after birth. Immune response to most bacterial PS antigens is poor in children less than 2 years of age. This lack of responsiveness to PS antigens makes the period between 6 to 24 months of age particularly susceptible to high incidence rates of *Haemophilus* type b, meningococcal, and pneumococcal infections. Chemical coupling of a PS to a carrier protein to form a glycoconjugate greatly improves the immunogenicity of a PS. For example, the 7-valent pneumococcal conjugate vaccine, Prevnar®, appears to be highly effective in preventing invasive disease in young children and to have a significant impact on the otitis media.[12]

At present, licensed bacterial glycoconjugate vaccines of *Haemophilus* type b, meningococcal group C, and 7-valent pneumococcal types are available for the immunization of young children to prevent bacterial infection. Four *Haemophilus influenzae* type b (Hib) conjugate vaccines have been developed and have undergone extensive clinical studies. The vaccines all use the same polysaccharide (polyribosylribitol phosphate [PRP]) but otherwise differ in the size of the PS, the protein carrier, and the type of linkage as well as the type of immune response induced. Table 31.3 shows the characterization of Hib conjugate vaccines.

Haemophilus influenzae type b oligosaccharide conjugate (HbOC) vaccine differs from other Hib conjugate vaccines in that it uses oligosaccharides of approximately 20 PRP repeating units which are covalently linked, without a spacer, to the protein CRM197, a nontoxic variant of diphtheria toxin. In young children, immunogenicity is age dependent, and two or three doses are required. An initial dose at 2 months of age does not induce an antibody response, but a significant response is induced to the second dose at 4 months of age. After a third dose at 6 months of age, high antibody levels are produced in almost all infants. Preexisting maternally acquired antibody does not affect the immune response to HbOC. Antibodies induced by HbOC are predominantly IgG$_1$ and are bactericidal.

The PRP–OMPC (polyribosylribitol phosphate–outer membrane protein complex) vaccine differs markedly in both composition and immunogenicity from other Hib conjugate vaccines. It links medium lengths of PRP by a bigeneric spacer molecule to protein components of meningococcal serogroup B outer membrane vesicles. It induces an immune response that is less age dependent than the response to other Hib conjugate vaccines. Most adults and children respond to a single vaccine dose by producing high levels of antibody. A booster response is seen in older children but is not clearly seen in young infants with a second or third dose. The decay of antibody levels between 4 and 12 months of age is a concern with this vaccine. About one fourth of vaccine recipients have levels of less than 0.15 mg/mL a year after completing their primary immunization series. Responses to PRP–OMPC are not affected by maternally acquired or passively administered antibody. It is also immunogenic in high-risk populations who have had poor responses to PRP vaccine. The antibody induced by PRP–OMPC is primarily IgG_1 and is opsonophagocytic and bactericidal. More recently, a hepatitis B–PedvaxHIB combination vaccine (COMVAX®) was licensed and used to reduce the number of injections required to immunize infants.

Among the first PRP–protein conjugate vaccines developed at the National Institutes of Health was PRP-T, which is now manufactured by Aventis Pasteur (ActHIB®) and by GlaxoSmithKline (OmniHIB®). The vaccine contains large PS that is extracted from culture supernatant and linked by a six-carbon spacer to tetanus toxoid carrier. The immune response to PRP-T is similar to that of HbOC. A single dose of the vaccine is highly immunogenic in adults and in older children. In most infants administered a first dose between 2 and 4 months of age, no response is seen; however, second and third doses at 2-month intervals induce high antibody concentrations in serum. Geometric mean antibody concentrations of 5 to 10 μg/mL are achieved after a three-dose immunization, and high antibody levels usually persist a year after injection. As with other Hib conjugate vaccines, the antibodies induced are primarily IgG_1 and immunogenic in high-risk populations.

Haemophilus influenzae type b conjugate vaccine technology has been widely applied for vaccine development to prevent diseases caused by other encapsulated bacteria, including *Pneumococcus*, *Meningococcus*, and group B *Streptococcus*. The lessons learned from preventing Hib disease have important implications for the prevention of these and other bacterial infection.

31.3.1 Pneumococcal Conjugate Vaccines

The 23-valent pneumococcal polysaccharide (PS) vaccine is effective against bacteremic pneumococcal disease in adults and is cost effective for routine immunization of the elderly; however, the PS vaccine is not sufficiently immunogenic in infants and young children. Chemical coupling of a PS to a carrier protein to form a PS–protein conjugate greatly improves the immune responses of a PS. In addition to the glucoconjugate, other approaches to enhancing protective immunity that have been investigated include pneumococcal proteins, DNA vaccines, and the use of adjuvants. The 7-valent pneumococcal conjugate vaccine, Prevnar®, is highly effective in preventing invasive disease in young children and appears to have a significant impact on the incidence of otitis media requiring pressure-equalization (PE) tube placement.[13] Each PS of serotypes 4, 6B, 7F, 9V, 14, 18C, 19F, and 23F is conjugated individually to the carrier protein CRM197.

Over the past several years, manufacturers have developed pneumococcal conjugate vaccines using different approaches. These vaccines differ in the number of contained serotypes, the carrier proteins, and their conjugation methods. Table 31.4 describes the characterization of pneumococcal conjugate vaccines prepared by manufacturers for clinical trials. The number of serotypes included in the vaccine candidates in clinical trials ranges from 7 to 11. In addition to 7-valent vaccine, Wyeth Lederle has also prepared a 9-valent candidate that includes types 1 and 5 in the vaccine. GlaxoSmithKline and Aventis Pasteur have included types 1, 3, 5, and 7F in their 11-valent vaccines. The amount of PS for each conjugate also differs between the vaccines, ranging from 1 to 10 μg/type.

Table 31.4 Characterization of Pneumococcal Conjugate Vaccines

	Manufacturer			
	Wyeth-Lederle	**Merck**	**Aventis Pasteur**	**GlaxoSmithKline**
Serotype	7-valent (4, 6B, 9V, 14, 18C, 19F, 23F)	7-valent (4, 6B, 9V, 14, 18C, 19F, 23F)	7-valent + 1, 3	7-valent + 1, 3, 5, 7F
Carrier	CRM197 protein D	MOMP	DT, TT	*Haemophilus influenzae*
Conjugation method	Reductive amination	Bigeneric linker	Covalently coupled with ADH	NA
PS content (µg/dose) per serotype	2–4	1–3.5	1–10	1
Adjuvant	Aluminum phosphate	Aluminum hydroxide	—	—

Note: ADH, adipic acid dihydrazide; DT, diphtheria toxoid; MOMP, meningococcal outer membrane protein; TT, tetanus toxoid; NA, not available.

Although it would be preferable to include a larger number of different PSs in a conjugate vaccine, the increased amount of carrier protein in the final vaccine may impair the antibody response to the PS antigen.[14,15] Few different proteins similar to carrier in Hib conjugates have been used in pneumococcal conjugate vaccines. Wyeth Lederle continues using CRM197, a nontoxic mutant of diphtheria toxin. The Aventis Pasteur vaccine candidate has two different carriers. The PSs from types 3, 6B, 14, and 18C are conjugated to diphtheria toxoid, whereas those from types 1, 4, 5, 7F, 9V, 19F, and 23F are conjugated to tetanus toxoid. Merck uses meningococcal outer membrane protein. In contrast, GlaxoSmithKline has used *Haemophilus influenzae* protein D.

The conjugation methods used in the Hib conjugate vaccines have been applied in preparing pneumococcal conjugates. Wyeth Lederle first activates the PS by reaction with sodium periodate. The CRM197 is then coupled to the PS through reductive amination. Merck uses a bigeneric linker to couple PS to carrier protein. The PSs are derivatized to introduce amino groups, which are subsequently converted to bromoacetyl groups, and the meningococcal outer membrane protein (MOMP) is derivatized to introduce thio groups. The thiolated protein is coupled to the bromoacetylated PS to form the conjugate. Aventis Pasteur covalently links each PS to either tetanus toxoid or diphtheria toxoid using an adipic acid dihydrazide (ADH) linker technique. PSs are activated and derivatized with ADH and cyanoborohydride. The activated, derivatized PSs are coupled to the carrier protein with a carbodiimide. The conjugation method for GlaxoSmithKline's candidate vaccine has not been reported.

Infants less than 2 years old are the main target group for pneumococcal conjugate vaccines. Most clinical trials for three-dose immunization at 2, 4, and 6 months of age followed by a booster dose at 12 to 15 months have focused on the safety and immunogenicity of candidate vaccines in infants. It appears that three doses may be needed for optimum immune responses to PncOMPC and PncCRM vaccines in infants. For the PncT vaccine, no dose dependency was observed after the primary immunization, whereas the booster response was highest in the group primed with the lowest dose of the conjugate vaccine.[16] In contrast, in PncD vaccine, the highest dose induced the highest response after primary immunization, but the booster response was greatest in the group primed with the lowest dose.[17]

Pneumococcal conjugate vaccines raise several issues. The main issue is the potential for replacement disease with non-vaccine serotypes that may affect the benefit observed from reduction in disease caused by vaccine types. Several pneumococcal proteins, including pneumococcal surface protein A (PspA), pneumococcal surface adhesin A (PsaA), pneumolysin (Ply), autolysin (Aly), and hemin-binding protein are considered promising vaccine antigens, or carrier proteins for pneumococcal conjugates.

Table 31.5 Characterization of Meningococcal Group C Conjugate Vaccines

	Vaccine		
	Meningitec™	Menjugate®	NeisVac-C®
Manufacturer	Wyeth Ayerst	Chiron	Baxter
Carrier	CRM197	CRM197	Tetanus toxoid (TT)
Group C polysaccharide (PS)	O-acetylated	O-acetylated	De-O-acetylated
10 µg of group C PS conjugated to	15 µg CRM197	11–25 µg CRM197	10–20 TT
Adjuvant	$AlPO_4$	$Al(OH)_3$	$Al(OH)_3$
Conjugation method	Reductive amination	Group C PS partially hydrolyzed at low pH; CRM attached to bis-N-hydroxysuccinamide ester of adipic acid	Group C PS is deacetylated then reacetylated; conjugated to TT by reductive amination
Remarks	Contains sodium chloride; single-dose preparation; liquid suspension; vial	Contains mannitol, sodium-phosphate buffer; single-dose, freeze-dried, vial reconstituted with diluent	Contains sodium chloride; single-dose, prefilled syringe

31.3.2 Meningococcal Group C Conjugate Vaccines

Meningococcal group C conjugate vaccines are currently licensed from three manufactures in Europe and Canada. Table 31.5 lists meningococcal group C conjugate vaccines prepared from different manufacturers. Meningitec™ (Wyeth Ayerst) is prepared by the activation of group C PS with sodium periodate and conjugation of activated oligosaccharide to CRM197 by reductive amination. Menjugate® (Chiron) is also conjugated group C oligosaccharide to CRM197; however, Menjugate® is prepared from group C PS that has been partially hydrolyzed at low pH and size fractionated before being conjugated to carrier protein through a bis-N-hydroxysuccinamide ester of adipic acid. In contrast, in synthesis of NeisVac-C® (Baxter), the group C PS is first deacetylated with sodium hydroxide, then the amino groups are reacetylated with acetic anhydride. Following activation with sodium periodate, the de-O-acetylated oligosaccharide is conjugated directly to the tetanus toxoid by reductive amination. The single dose of these three vaccines does not contain any preservative. In contrast, the multivials prepared by Chiron use phenoxyethanol as a preservative.

The conjugate vaccines elicited more effective anti-PS IgG antibody than PS vaccines with respect to higher avidity or the ability to induce complement-mediated bactericidal activity. Conjugate vaccines also induce a population of long-lasting B cells capable of responding to PS and produce long-lasting immunologic memory. Children 12 months to 5 years of age given a single dose of the Chiron or Wyeth Ayerst conjugate vaccines develop serum bactericidal antibody titers of 1:8 to 1:64 when measured with rabbit complement.

Meningococcal conjugate vaccines have been licensed in many European countries and in Canada, but not in the United States. In the United Kingdom, group C conjugate vaccine is recommended for all children from 2 months of age, adolescents, and adults up to 23 years of age. In the United States, it is considered that routine vaccination of toddlers with a combined group C and Y vaccine would have the greatest health benefit per dose of vaccine administered. A polyvalent pneumococcal conjugate vaccine that also contains conjugated meningococcal group C conjugate vaccine is under clinical trials by Wyeth Ayerst for use in infants. Application of these vaccines to routine immunization of young children and older high school or college students could have an important impact on reducing incidence of meningococcal disease.

31.4 VACCINES INVOLVED IN INDUCING MUCOSAL IMMUNITY

At present, more than 25 vaccines have become available for human use. With the exception of vaccines against poliomyelitis (Sabin oral polio vaccine [OPV]), typhoid, cholera, adenovirus, and live rotavirus vaccine, all currently available vaccines are licensed for use only through subcutaneous or intramuscular injection. In an effort to reduce the incidence of vaccine-associated paralytic polio, a switch from OPV to inactivated polio vaccine (IPV) was recommended for routine use in the United States. The recently licensed rotavirus vaccine was withdrawn in 2000 because of its association with intussusception in vaccine recipients.

The mucosal surfaces of the gastrointestinal and respiratory tracts represent the main entry point for most human pathogens. Direct inoculation of pathogens into the blood stream and sexual contact are other important routes of infection. The mucosal surfaces represent a critical component of the human immune system. The major antibody isotype in external secretions is secretory IgA (S-IgA). Approximately 40 mg of IgA per kg body weight is secreted daily. The major effector cells in the mucosal surfaces are not IgA B-cells, but T-lymphocytes of CD4+ as well as CD8+ phenotypes. T-lymphocytes may represent up to 80% of the entire mucosal lymphoid cell population.

The immune system operating on external mucosal surfaces consists of gut-associated lymphoid tissue (GALT), the lymphoid structures associated with bronchoepithelius and lower respiratory tract (BALT), ocular tissue, salivary glands, tonsils and nasopharynx (NALT), larynx (LALT), middle ear cavity, genital tracts, mammary glands, and products of lactation. The lymphoid follicles in the GALT and BALT are considered the main inductive sites of mucosal immune response. The common features of all inductive mucosal sites include an epithelial surface containing M cells (cells with microfold). In addition to M cells, mucosal epithelium contains mucin-producing glandular cells, lymphocytes, plasma cells, dendritic cells, and macrophages. The mucosal epithelial cells express polymeric immunoglobulin receptor (pIgR) and secretory component, major histocompatibility complex (MHC) class I and II molecules, adhesion molecules, and a variety of cytokines.

The dendritic cells are associated with potentiation of immune response and promote development of active immunity. They are potent antigen-presenting cells (APCs) and are critical in initiating primary immune responses and the generation of T-cell-dependent B-cell responses. The APC function is attributed in part to their ability to express costimulatory molecules (CD80 and CD86) and other accessory ligands necessary for upregulation of immune response. The complex of IgA and pIgR is referred to as S-IgA. Following exposure to an antigen and its uptake through the M cells, the degree of activation of T-cells, dendritic cells, and B-cells, especially of the IgA isotype, is variable. S-IgA at mucosal surfaces inhibits the adherence and invasion of mucosal pathogens and neutralizes virulence factors.[18,19]

Oral immunization with cholera toxin (CT) results in antibody response in saliva and genital tract secretions. On the other hand, intragastric immunization results in IgA antibody responses restricted to the small intestine. Intranasal immunization results in development of antibody response in the mammary glands and genital tract. Oral immunization with live *Chlamydia trachomatis* induces IgA response in the genital tract, lungs, and intestine. These observations suggest that after the initial immunization at the inductive sites in GALT or BALT, reexposure to the antigen at the distant mucosal site results in enhanced immune response. Intranasal immunization of mice with pneumococcal surface protein A or a capsular polysaccharide–protein conjugate has been shown to induce effective mucosal as well as systemic immune responses and long-lasting protection against nasopharyngeal carriage and bacterial challenge. The resistance to carriage was directly dependent on mucosal rather than serum antibody activity. Intranasal immunization was also highly effective against systemic infections following intravenous, intratracheal, or intraperitoneal challenge.[20] Moreover, mice that received intranasal immunization with pneumococcal type 9V polysaccharide conjugated with inactivated pneumolysin produced high 9V PS IgG and IgA antibodies in their serum, spleen, intestine, lung, Peyer's patch, and fecal extract samples. Mice immunized with this glycoconjugate also exhibited opsonophagocytic activity and rapid bacterial clearance from blood and provided homologous and cross-protection against challenge with virulent pneumococci.[21] These studies indicate that intranasal immunization with glycoconjugate vaccines may serve as an alternative and convenient approach for prevention of pneumococcal infection.

Nasal immunization has been used successfully with live influenza A and B virus vaccines in both children and adults.[22,23] It appears that nasal immunization may be superior to oral or intestinal immunization for inducing antibody response in the genital tract. Both the nasal and oral immunization routes appear to be effective in inducing antibody response in the milk and mammary glands.

More recent studies have focused on immunization by mixed mucosal routes or a combination of mucosal and parenteral routes of immunization. Comparative studies following injection with cholera vaccine in Pakistani and Swedish women showed that Pakistani women who had prior natural mucosal infection with cholera exhibited a significant rise in IgA antibody titer in milk and saliva. In contrast, Swedish women with no prior exposure to cholera did not exhibit an increase in antibody response in the mucosal secretions.[24] Mucosal immune responses have also been enhanced by parenteral priming followed by oral booster immunization in *Shigella*, *Neisseria gonorrheae*, *Streptococcus pneumoniae*, *Vibrio cholerae*, and poliovirus. Enhancement of mucosal immune response can thus be achieved by parenteral or mucosal priming with infectious agents.

Many mucosal adjuvants have been tested to enhance the immunogenicity of mucosally administered antigens, including cholera toxin B subunit, *Escherichia coli* heat-labile toxin, lectins and polyelectrolytes, ISCOMs, low-oil emulsion (MF-59), lipid A, lysophosphatidyl glycerol, and cytokines. Antigens in general induce weak or insufficient immune responses when administered mucosally. Adjuvants influence almost every aspect of immune response to an antigen. The most potent adjuvants to date are the protein enterotoxins of *Vibrio cholerae* (CT) and the heat-labile toxin (LT) of enterotoxigenic *E. coli*. The two toxins have about 80% sequence homology and exhibit significant immunologic cross-reactivity. CT binds to M cells and to the GM_1-ganglioside receptors on the mucosal epithelium. Either free or conjugate CTB subunits can act as adjuvants in intranasal immunization; however, unconjugated CTB is not effective as an adjuvant in oral immunization. In contrast, unconjugated holotoxin can exhibit a high level of adjuvant effect for antigens administered orally. In general, this adjuvant activity of native CT is directly related to the enterotoxicity. It is difficult to separate toxigenic effects from adjuvant effects.

Immunoprophylaxis by the mucosal immunity is an important approach to controlling mucosally acquired infections. The ability to induce a systemic and secretary immune response following immunization is determined by various factors, including the nature of the antigens, route of administration, and adjuvants used. The strategies for potential vaccines involved in inducing mucosal immunity include development of nonreplicating subunit vaccines, DNA vaccines, plant and other recombinant products, applying effective mucosal adjuvants and vaccine delivery systems designed to conserve the functional integrity, and delivering antigens to the mucosal immune system. A mucosally delivered vaccine represents a painless way to provide vaccine antigens in a single dose or a combination of multiple antigens against more than one infectious disease. Such vaccines may be preferred over the vaccines administered by injection and could be more effective in preventing systemic illness as well as mucosal infections during subsequent natural challenge with pathogens.

REFERENCES

1. European Vaccine Manufacturers, *Study on Vaccines for Human Use and Their Rational Use in Europe and Worldwide*, European Federation of Pharmaceutical Industries Association (EFPIA), Brussels, 1994.
2. Lis, Y. and Walker, S.P., Novel medicine marketed in the UK (1960–87), *Br. J. Clin. Pharmacol.*, 28, 333–343, 1989.
3. Di Masi, J.A., Hansen, R.W., Grabowski, H.G. et al., Cost of innovation in the pharmaceutical industry, *J. Health Econ.*, 10, 107–142, 1991.

4. Joglekar, P. and Paterson, M.L., A closer look at the returns and risks of pharmaceutical R&D, *J. Health Econ.*, 5, 153–177, 1986.

5. Struck M.M., Biopharmaceutical R&D success rates and development times, *Biotechnology*, 12, 674–677, 1994.

6. Jacobson, R.M., Adegbenro, A., Pankratz, V.A., and Poland, G.A., Adverse events and vaccination: the lack of power and predictability of infrequent events in pre-licensure study, *Vaccine*, 19, 2428–2433, 2001.

7. Foulkes, M.A. and Ellenberg, S.S., Vaccine efficacy and safety evaluation, in *The Jordan Report 20th Anniversary: Accelerated Development of Vaccines 2002*, National Institute of Allergy and Infectious Diseases, National Institutes of Health, U.S. Department of Health and Human Services, Washington, D.C., 2002, pp. 63–68.

8. Institute of Medicine, *New Vaccines Development: Establishing Priorities*. Vol. 1. *Diseases of Importance in the United States*, National Academy Press, Washington, D.C., 1985.

9. Institute of Medicine, *New Vaccines Development: Establishing Priorities*. Vol. 2. *Diseases of Importance in Developing Countries*, National Academy Press, Washington, D.C., 1985.

10. Mestecky, J., Michalek, S.M., Moldoveanu, Z. et al., Route of immunization and antigen delivery systems for optimal mucosal immune responses in humans, *Behring Inst. Mitt.*, 98, 33–43, 1997.

11. Wu, H.Y., Nahm, M.H., Guo, Y. et al., Intranasal immunization of mice with PspA (pneumococcal surface protein A) can prevent intranasal carriage, pulmonary infection, and sepsis with *Streptococcus pneumoniae*, *J. Infect. Dis.*, 175, 839–846, 1997.

12. Lee, C.J., Lee, L.H., Lu, C.S. et al., Bacterial polysaccharides as vaccines: immunity and chemical characterization, in *The Molecular Immunology of Complex Carbohydrates*, Vol. 2, Wu, A.M., Ed., Kluwer Academic, Norwell, MA, 2001, pp. 453–471.

13. Black, S., Shinefield, H., Fireman, B. et al., Efficacy, safety and immunogenicity of heptavalent pneumococcal conjugate vaccine in children, *Pediatr. Infect. Dis. J.*, 19, 187–195, 2000.

14. Fattom, A., Cho, Y.H., Chu, C. et al., Epitopic overload at the site of injection may result in suppression of the immune response to combined capsular polysaccharide conjugate vaccine, *Vaccine*, 17, 126–133, 1999.

15. Dagan, R., Eskola, J., Leclerc, C. et al., Reduced response to multiple vaccine sharing common protein epitopes that are administered simultaneously to infants, *Infect. Immun.*, 66, 2093–2098, 1998.

16. Ahman, H., Kayhty, H., Vuorela, A. et al., Dose dependency of antibody response in infants and children to pneumococcal polysaccharides conjugated to tetanus toxoid, *Vaccine*, 17, 2726–2732, 1999.

17. Ahman, H., Kayhty, H., Lehtonen, H. et al., *Streptococcus pneumoniae* capsular polysaccharide–diphtheria toxoid conjugate vaccine is immunogenic in early infancy and able to induce immunologic memory, *Pediatr. Infect. Dis. J.*, 17, 211–216, 1998.

18. Mestecky, J., Michalek, S.M., Moldoveanu, Z. et al., Routes of immunization and antigen delivery system for optimal mucosal immune responses in humans, *Behring Inst. Mitt.*, 98, 33–43, 1977.

19. Steinmetz, L., Comparative *in vivo* analysis of IgA- and IgG-mediated mucosal defense against pathogens, *Behring Inst.*, 98, 53–55, 1997.

20. Wu, H.Y., Nahm, M.H., Guo, Y. et al., Intranasal immunization of mice with PspA (pneumococcal surface protein A) can prevent intranasal carriage, pulmonary infection, and sepsis with *Streptococcus pneumoniae*, *J. Infect. Dis.*, 175, 839–846, 1977.

21. Lee, C.J., Lee, L.H., and Frasch, C.E., Protective immunity of pneumococcal glycoconjugates, *CRC Crit. Rev. Microbiol.*, 29(4), 1–17, 2003.

22. Belshe, R.B., Mendelman, P.M., Treanor, J. et al., The efficacy of live attenuate, cold-adopted, trivalent, intranasal influenza virus vaccine in children, *N. Engl. J. Med.*, 338, 1405–1412, 1998.

23. Kuno-Sakai, H., Kimura, M., Ohta, K. et al., Developments in mucosal influenzae virus vaccines, *Vaccine*, 12, 1303–1308, 1994.

24. Svennerholm, A.M., Hanson, L.A., Holmgren, J. et al., Different secretor immunoglobulin A antibody responses to cholera vaccination in Swedish and Pakistani women, *Infect. Immun.*, 30, 427–430, 1980.

CHAPTER 32

Herbal Products as Complementary and Alternative Medicine

Chi-Jen Lee, Lucia H. Lee, Christopher L. Wu, and Benjamin R. Lee

CONTENTS

32.1 INTRODUCTION

Many Western medicines contain natural products or their extracts, and a resurgence of interest in these products has recently occurred, particularly with regard to Oriental medicines. Herbal products, including traditional Chinese medicines and Kampo drugs, have been used for centuries in Asian countries to prevent a variety of ailments, thus indirectly reducing treatment costs through disease prevention. The World Health Organization (WHO) has urged member countries to develop new medicines that combine the ancient arts of herbs with modern pharmaceutical sciences. Oriental medicines are a widely accepted means of healing even in high-technology societies in Asia. In Japan, Taiwan, China, Korea, and other Asian nations, the old and new medicines have been practiced in parallel since the 1970s. In many scientific laboratories, researchers use advanced technology to analyze the properties of herbs to search for active ingredients. Intensive research programs on plant medicines have been conducted in Japan, China, Germany, and other areas; however, to most Westerners, herbal products are mysterious medicines because the active components are often poorly characterized and the mechanisms of action frequently misunderstood.

Many ancient and modern cultures have used plant components for medicinal purposes. Many current drugs manufactured by the pharmaceutical industry are derived from plants. For example, quinine, ephedrine, atropine, codeine, and salicylic acid are all derived from plants that were known to be effective in the treatment of certain diseases long before chemists isolated their active ingredients and synthesized similar chemical compounds.

Complementary and alternative medicine, as defined by the National Center for Complementary and Alternative Medicines (NCCAM), part of the National Institutes of Health (NIH) established in 1999, is a group of diverse medical and healthcare systems, practices, and products that are not currently considered to be part of conventional medicine. Plants and their products make up an important research area for NCCAM. About 25% of the economic market for dietary supplements in the United States consists of botanicals.

The increasing use of medicinal herbs in recent years reflects the growing public interest in alternatives to conventional medicine. Herbal medicines continue to be a major market in U.S. pharmacies and constitute a multibillion dollar industry. In 2002, American consumers spent $49.6 billion on dietary supplement sales and payments to alternative healthcare providers. Although approximately 1500 botanicals are sold as dietary supplements or ethnic traditional medicines, herbal products are not subject to U.S. Food and Drug Administration (FDA) premarket testing to ensure their safety and efficacy. NCCAM will spend an estimated $103.5 million in 2005 to fund scientific studies of alternative and complementary medicines and treatments. Government funding for the center rose from $50 million in 1999 to $117 million in 2004.

Recent interests in the search for effective therapeutic agents derived from plants have focused on oriental herb medicine. In 1957, healthcare personnel working in the Jiansu province in China became aware of the high incidence of childless families among people consuming large amounts of crude cottonseed oil. Women who were brought up on a diet of cottonseed oil but married men outside the region were raising children at normal rates, while those who married men from the same region remained childless. In 1971, a Chinese research team studied the effect of the cottonseed oil extract (gossypol) on the reproductive performance of male rats. It was observed that subsequent mating of male rats treated with the extract produced no offspring. After withdrawal of the extract, fertility was restored 3 to 5 weeks later. The investigators concluded that the extract of cottonseed oil is an effective oral male contraceptive.

In 1992, the FDA approved taxol, a chemical compound isolated from the Pacific yew tree (*Taxus brevifolia*), for the treatment of ovarian cancer. In 1994, the FDA approved taxol for therapeutic use in patients with metastatic breast cancer unresponsive to other treatments. Taxol was discovered during the screening program conducted by the National Cancer Institute between 1958 and 1980, in which extracts of over 35,000 plant species were tested for anticancer activity. Intensive research on the chemical synthesis of taxol, *Taxus* needle extractions, cultivation of *Taxus* plants, identification of drug analogs, and cell culture production has been conducted to increase the supply of taxol for clinical trials.[1]

Many people with cancer take herbs and other alternative therapies, hoping they will help treat their diseases. Types of alternative therapies commonly used include vitamins and minerals, anti-oxidants, enzymes, amino acids, animal extracts, hormones, herbs, and other dietary supplements. People take these products for various reasons, such as the desire to actively participate in treatment and to improve nutrition. In many cases, friends or family members encourage cancer patients to try the herbal products; however, while many dietary supplements may be taken as cancer cures, extensive studies are required to establish the efficacy of these products against the disease.

32.2 CLINICAL TRIALS ON HERBAL PRODUCTS

Some basic differences in the practice of traditional Chinese medicine (TCM) and Western medicine can be identified. In most conditions, Western medicines are based on the one-drug/one-disease model; that is, the same medication is prescribed to all patients diagnosed with the same illness. In TCM, each patient is prescribed an individual formulation based on an evaluation of patient's health conditions and the environment. Adhering to the current design of clinical trials for chemical drugs could prove difficult when conducting trials for TCM; however, many double-blinded, randomized, placebo-controlled studies have been conducted for heterogeneous herbal products. Such studies are important for providing evidence that demonstrates the efficacy and safety of herbal products to the medical community and regulatory agencies.

The basic principle and design of clinical trials for herbal products should be the same as those for chemical drugs. The population size should be large enough to allow accurate and clear evaluation of results by statistical analysis. No single protocol can be used for all clinical trials, and several points should be considered before conducting costly and time-consuming studies:

- Such clinical trials must select well-defined clinical endpoints and surrogate markers. Current good clinical practices (CGCPs) should be followed and enforced.
- Specific regulations relevant to the intended market should be followed.
- Herbal products are regulated differently from country to country; many countries have published guidelines on the regulation of plant medicines, and selling products in these markets requires a thorough understanding of such regulations.
- The selection of products should consider products intended for diseases with no effective treatment by conventional drugs or current treatment with severe side effects.

A few well-known clinical trials have been conducted using TCM formulations for atopic eczema for adults[2] and children.[3] These studies used 40 patients, equally divided into a trial group and a control group. The herbal formulation and the placebo were similar to each other in taste and appearance. The herbal products used consisted of 10 herbs (*Ledebouriella seseloides*, *Potentilla chinensis*, *Clematis armandii*, *Rehmannia glutinosa*, *Paeonia lactiflora*, *Lophatherum gracile*, *Dictamus dasycarpus*, *Tribulus terrestris*, *Glycyrrhiza globra*, and *Schizonepeta tenuifolia*) administered by oral infusion for 20 weeks. The results in both adults and children showed that significant improvements were observed in those receiving active treatment compared to those given placebo. At the end of 1 year, most children in the treated group were able to discontinue or reduce the dosage of medicine required to treat the eczema.[4]

Bupleurum Combination (minor, Sho-saiko-to) is a formulation of seven herbs (*Bupleurum chinense*, *Panax ginseng*, *Glycyrrhiza uralensis*, *Zingiber officinale*, *Zinzyphus vulgaris*, *Scutellaria baicalensis*, and *Pinellia ternata*) studied in a double-blind, placebo-controlled trial conducted at 21 university hospital and medical facilities in Japan.[5,6] During the 8-month period from June 1994 to January 1995, 220 patients with allergic rhinitis were enrolled, divided into two groups, and treated with this herbal formulation or with a placebo for 2 weeks. The results showed that a consistently higher degree of symptomatic relief was observed in the treated group compared to the controls for symptoms of allergic rhinitis including sneezing, runny nose, and stuffy nose. Furthermore, unlike common antihistamine drugs, the herb product did not cause drowsiness.

Research projects in herbal products conducted in NCCAM cover a wide range from laboratory-based research studying the effects of herbal products on the body to large clinical trials testing their safety and effectiveness in people. Exploring how and why botanicals act in the body is a key step in evaluating their safety and effectiveness. Recent NCCAM-sponsored research has led to important insights about botanicals with regard to:

- *Potential interactions between herbs and chemical drugs* — Clinical studies have found that both St. John's wort and PC SPES (a botanical mixture marketed for prostate health until the FDA warned consumers to stop its use because it contained an unlabeled prescription drug) affect the activity of a key enzyme in the liver. This, as a result, affects the metabolism of some drugs by the body, causing some of them to be less effective and others more toxic.
- *Benefits for the treatment of diseases* — A study in 2003 found that an extract from the root of Chinese skullcap (Huang Qin) strongly inhibited cancer cell growth in the laboratory, especially cells present in head and neck cancers that were resistant to multidrug chemotherapy. Many polysaccharides isolated from fungi and higher plants exhibit immunostimulating and antitumor activities in certain cancer patients.

- *Ineffectiveness and lack of benefit in medical application* — Many herbal products do not deliver on claims made for them. For example, in December 2003, a study showed that an Echinacea preparation did not lessen the symptoms or duration of colds in children. The study included 500 children, ages 2 to 11 years, who were given Echinacea when they started to have symptoms of a cold.

In fiscal year 2003, NCCAM spent $24.8 million on research related to botanicals. In 2004, research on botanicals continues to be a very active area, and phase III clinical trials sponsored by NCCAM are progressing on several botanicals, such as ginseng and ginkgo. Over 60 million Americans use herbal medicines; of these, one fourth also take prescription drugs. Physicians are often unaware of herbal use and of possible drug–herb interactions in their patients. Ginseng and ginkgo, enhancers of physical and mental performance, are two of the most widely taken herbals. A double-blinded, randomized, prospective study has been proposed to study the effects of ginseng and ginkgo on (1) disposition of probe drugs, (2) cognitive function, and (3) glutathione-*S*-transferase and quinine reductase enzymes implicated in the chemoprevention of cancer.

32.3 IMMUNOMODULATING POLYSACCHARIDES ISOLATED FROM FUNGI AND HIGHER PLANTS

Immunomodulating and antitumor activities have been observed in the polysaccharide (PS) fractions of fungi and higher plants. These polysaccharides have been tested in animal models and in human clinical trials to treat selected tumors. The mechanisms of the immunostimulating and antitumor activities of these polysaccharides are thought to involve the functions related to amplification of phagocytosis, activation of macrophages, T-lymphocytes and complement, and enhancement of cytokine production and cell-mediated immune response.[7]

The immunity of the body decreases with age, which is thought to be associated with a consequent decreased recognition of antigens and perhaps an increased frequency of diseases such as arthritis, diabetes, and cancer in the elderly. Because immunomodulating polysaccharides can stimulate the immune response, PSs may potentially help to prevent these types of diseases. As a result, overall quality of life and ultimately the survival rate of the elderly population might also be improved.

Immunostimulating polysaccharides have been isolated and purified from many fungi and plants. In 1969, a polysaccharide with a marked antitumor activity was isolated from the edible mushroom *Lentinus edodes* (Hsiang-Ku) and named lentinan.[8] Likewise, *Ganoderma* (Lingzhi, Ling-chih), a medicinal fungus, is recognized as a valuable tonic remedy in China. Commercial products that include *Ganoderma* as an ingredient (e.g., health foods) have been widely used in Asian countries. Recently, such health foods have become popular in the United States. The primary immunostimulating fungal polysaccharides are shown in Table 32.1.

Lentinan is one of the most thoroughly studied fungal polysaccharides. The structure of lentinan consists of a repeating units of five β-(1–3) glucopyranoside linkages and two β-(1–6) glycopyranoside branch chains that exist mainly as a right-handed, triple-helical structures in a solid state, with possible hydrogen bonds between adjacent glucose units. Lentinan has a molecular weight of up to 10^6 kDa.[9–11] It is relatively nontoxic. The LD_{50} in mice and rats is estimated to be 250 to 500 mg/kg by intravenous administration and greater than 2500 mg/kg by intraperitoneal, subcutaneous, or oral routes. Lentinan exhibits marked immunostimulating and antitumor activities in animal experiments. A multicenter clinical study of lentinan used in combination with cytostatic agents was conducted in patients with advanced unresectable and recurrent gastric cancer. Participants receiving chemotherapy and lentinan were observed to have a prolonged survival rate (297 days vs. 199 days) and improved quality of life.[12]

Polysaccharide K (PSK), or krestin, is a protein-bound β-glucan containing approximately 25% protein; PSK and a polysaccharide peptide known as PSP were isolated from *Coriolus versicolor*.

Table 32.1 Immunostimulating Fungal Polysaccharides

Product	Scientific Name	Active Components	Activities
Lentinus (Hsiang-ku)	*Lentinus edodes* *Coriolus versicolor*	PS (lentinan) PSK (krestin) PSP	Enhances immune functions Stimulates cytokine production CSF, IL-1, TNF-γ
Ganoderma (Lingzhi Ling-chih)	*Ganoderma lucidum*	PS (G–A)	Enhances immune functions; antitumor activity
Hoelen (Fuling)	*Poria cocos*	PS, pachymaran	Antitumor activity; enhances phagocytic activity and production of TCGF
Polyporus (Zhuling, Chu-ling)	*Polyporus umbellatus* (*Grifola umbellate*)	GU2, GU3, GU4	Regulates and stimulates immune system; transforms cancer cells into normal cells; stimulates phagocytic activity; increases cAMP in sarcoma 180 cells; improves lung cancer survival rate
Ascomyces (Tung-chung-hsia-tsao)	*Cordyceps ophioglossoides*	CO-1 (galactomannan)	Inhibits tumor cell growth
Trichlomataceae (Shuh-hua)	*Schizophyllum commune*	Schizophyllan	Antitumor activity; stimulates IL-2 production

Note: cAMP, cyclic adenosine monophosphate; CSF, colony-stimulating factor; G, glucose; G-A, arabinogalactan; GU, *Grifola umbellate*; IL, interleukin; PS, polysaccharide; PSK, polysaccharide K; PSP, polysaccharide peptide; TCGF, T-cell growth factor (IL-2); TNF, tumor necrosis factor.

PSP has a molecular weight of approximately 100 kDa and contains glutamic and asparatic acids in its polypeptide components, as well as the neutral amino acids leucine and valine. The structure of the main glucoside portion is β-glucan, which includes α-1,4 and β-1,3 glucoside linkages, and branched chains including 1–3, 1–4, and 1–6 bonds. Also, branches at the 3 and 6 positions occur in a ratio of one per several 1–4 linkages. The primary monomer of the PS portion is glucose, with decreasing percentages of mannose, xylose, galactose, and fructose. The presence of fructose in PSK and rhamnose and arabinose in PSP distinguishes the two protein-bound polysaccharides, which are otherwise chemically similar. PSK is a promising potential adjuvant cancer therapy agent. PSP is thought to contribute to prolonging the 5-year survival of patients with cancers of the stomach, colon rectum, esophagus, nasopharynx, lung, and breast. PSK is thought to increase leukocyte activation and induction of cytokines. Natural killer and lymphocyte-activated killer cell activation has been demonstrated *in vivo* and *in vitro*. Thus, PSK can be applied as a potential antitumor and immunostimulating agent. PSK exhibits antioxidant capabilities, which may play a role as a tissue chemo- and radioactive-protector when used in combination with chemotherapy or radiotherapy for the treatment of cancer. PSK may inhibit carcinogenesis by direct inhibition of various carcinogens on vulnerable cell lines.[13]

Ganoderma (Lingzhi, Ling-chih, rheishi) has been used in China as an herbal drug (*Fu-cheng Ku-pen* ["supporting the vital force and securing the root"]) for thousands of years. Its major components with pharmacological activities include triterpenses and polysaccharides. *Ganoderma lucidum* polysaccharide (GL-PS) has been reported to exhibit remarkable activities in modulating immune functions and inhibiting tumor growth.[14,15] Extensive immunomodulating effects, including promoting the function of mononuclear phagocytes and humoral as well as cellular immunity, have been observed. A water-soluble, antitumor PS, GL-1, which has a molecular weight of 40 kDa, was isolated from the fruit bodies of *Ganoderma lucidum*. GL-1 is a D-glucopyranosyl with α and β(1–4), β(1–6), and β(1–3) linkages. The nondialyzable fraction, GL-2, has a molecular weight of 38 kDa and exhibits only glucose on acid hydrolysis. GL-3 has a molecular weight of 37 kDa.

Similar inhibitory activity (95.6 to 98.5%) on the growth of the Sarcoma 180 tumor cell was observed in GL-1, GL-2, and GL-3 when injected intraperitoneally (20 mg/kg) for 10 days.[16] In addition, seven polysaccharides (PSG1 to PSG7) have been isolated from *G. lucidum* spores. All polysaccharides exist naturally as glucan, but each glucan has a different sugar chain structure, which contributes to a unique glycosyl linkage and sugar chain conformation. Purified PS fractions of PSG2, PSG4, PSG5, and PSG6 exhibit immunostimulating activity, while PSG3 and PSG7 have no obvious effect on T- and B-lymphocytes proliferation.

Treatment of advanced-stage cancer patients with Ganopoly, a *Ganoderma lucidum* polysaccharide extract, at an oral dosage of 1800 mg three times daily for 12 weeks increased the plasma concentration of interleukin-2 (IL-2), IL-6, and interferon gamma (IFN-γ), as well as natural killer (NK) cell activity. Also, IL-1 and tumor necrosis factor alpha (TNF-α) levels were decreased.[17]

Other fungal polysaccharides with immunostimulating and antitumor activities have been isolated from hoelen (Fuling), *Polyporus* (Chu-ling, Zhuling), *Ascomyces* (Tung-chung-hsia-tsao), and other herbs. In general, polysaccharides from higher plants are complex heteroglycans. Many antitumor polysaccharides are soluble D-glucans and are not quickly hydrolyzed by D-glucanases. Many of these herbs are frequently used in combination to promote longevity in traditional Chinese medicine. Because their actions are mild, prolonged use may be necessary to achieve the desired effects. No major side effects occur if these preparations are used properly.

One of the most widely used Chinese medicines is angelica, the root of *Angelica sinensis*, among others of the same family (e.g., *A. gigas* and *A. acutiloba*), which is taken for its antiulcer activity. The polysaccharide fractions from angelica (AP) prevent gastric mucosal damage, and its preventive effect is dose dependent. Simultaneous administration of AP and prostaglandin E2 reduces mucosal myeloperoxidase activity. AP has a direct stimulating effect on gastric epithelial cells for wound healing. A polysaccharide isolated from *A. autiloba* (Tang-kuei) has been reported to induce interferon, stimulate B-lymphocytes, mediate antitumor activity against Ehrlich ascites, and activate polyclonal B cells and complement. Polysaccharide isolated from angelica contains rhamnose, glucose, galactose, fructose, arabinose, xylose, and mannose. Mice injected with angelica PS (0.2 to 1.0 mg/dose, i.p.) followed by administration of pneumococcal type 9V PS–protein conjugate (5 μg/dose, i.p.) produced higher serum levels of 9V PS immunoglobulin G (IgG) and IgM antibodies than the untreated control group. Mice treated with angelica PS exhibit more rapid bacterial clearance from blood after challenge with virulent-type 19F pneumococci. In addition, in mice immunized with type 9V PS glycoconjugate, the treatment of angelica PS induced significantly higher levels of TNF-α, IL-2, and IL-4 than occurred in the control group. These results indicate that the stimulating effects of herb polysaccharides might contribute to the protective effects of a bacterial glycoconjugate through the enhancing activities of cytokines and immune response.[18]

Polysaccharide fractions have been obtained from other higher plants, many of which show antitumor and immunostimulating activities in animals. The possible mechanisms of action of polysaccharides from higher plants include lymphoproliferation; increased colony-stimulating factors and interferon production; and stimulation of NK cells, T-cells, B-cells, macrophages, and complement systems. These higher plants include *Radix astragali* (Huangqi), *Panax ginseng* (Ginseng), and *Cnidium rhizome* (Chuan-kung), among others. The primary immunostimulating plant polysaccharides are described in Table 32.2.

32.4 DEVELOPMENT AND EVALUATION OF HERBAL PRODUCTS

Herbal products are mainly recognized as health supplements intended to promote overall well-being rather than treat specific health conditions or diseases. In the United States, an herbal product is not considered a drug and thus is not subject to the same regulations for drugs or biologics. Currently, a system to evaluate the safety, stability, and manufacturing consistency of herbal products has not yet been established. If herbal products are intended for the treatment or prevention

Table 32.2 Immunostimulating Plant Polysaccharides

Product	Scientific Name	Active Components	Main Activity
Angelicae	Angelica sinensis	Polysaccharides (AR-arabinogalactan IIa), AR-4 IIa, AR IIb-1, AR IIb-2c	Activation of complement
Astragalus	Astragalus mongholicus	Polysaccharides	Intensifies phagocytosis
	Radix astragali	Polysaccharides	Restores hematopoietic function
	Bupleurum falcatum	BR-5-1	Activation of complement
Ginseng	Panax ginseng	Ginsenosides, panaxosides, panaxatriol	Enhances phagocytosis of macrophages; promotes lymphocytic transformation
Cnidii (Chuan-kung)	Cnidii rhizoma	Polysaccharides	Stimulate cytokine production
Radix codonopsis (Dangshen)	Codonopsis pilosula	Polysaccharides	Immunostimulating and antitumor activities
Fructus lycii (Gouqizi)	Lycium barbarum	Polysaccharides	Enhances IL-2 and protein kinase C and antitumor activities
Ciwujia	Acanthopanax chiisqnensis, A. senticosus	Polysaccharides	Enhances phagocytosis of macrophages and antitumor activity

of a specific disease, however, then the same requirements for preclinical and clinical studies and quality assurance that apply to drugs would have to be met. Also, a proven pharmacological effect would have to be demonstrated in well-controlled clinical trials. In many cases, the therapeutic indications listed on the label of an herbal product are based not on accepted scientific methods of biochemical analyses, animal studies, and clinical trials but on limited subjective observations and anecdotal experiences.[19] The development and evaluation of herbal products can be approached in a manner similar to drug development, with an emphasis on characterization of purified active component, well-controlled clinical trials, and quality control testing.[20–22]

32.4.1 Manufacturing Process

Product development begins with the preparation of raw materials and purification and characterization of the active components. Standard operating procedures (SOPs) should be established to ensure consistent herbal growth and harvest conditions, in addition to processes to maintain the stability of the active component during prolonged storage. Characterization of the raw herbs further ensures that a uniform, stable product will be available for large-scale production of the herbal product. Similarly, quality control testing provides additional assurances that the active herbal component can be identified by morphological and chemical characteristics and that the final product is free of microbial and chemical contamination. The principles and conditions similar to the regulatory guidance of CGMPs should be established for the manufacturing process and enforced.

32.4.2 Clinical Trials

In general, the approaches to clinical trials for an herbal product would be similar to an evaluation of any chemical drug. If no adverse safety or toxicity is observed in preclinical animal studies, then a phase I trial to examine the safety of an herbal product in humans can proceed. Because herbal products would likely be used in combination with another drug, inclusion of an appropriate control group is critical to demonstrating specific therapeutic effects. Phase II trial results would evaluate the therapeutic effectiveness in patients, further characterize the overall safety profile, and enable selection of an optimal dosing regimen for phase III trials. Phase III trial results would provide the essential data required to demonstrate the effectiveness and safety of the product. All trials from phase I to phase IV should be conducted according to CGCP regulations.

32.4.3 Quality Control of Products

Detailed specifications regarding the herbal active components, final formulation, and extract products should be established, as well as the control test methods for assessing product quality. Analytical testing of the completed lot of a final product should be performed before releasing the lot for commercial use. Similarly, inspection should be conducted for incoming raw materials and at various stages during the manufacturing processes, such as during packaging, labeling, and lot-release testing.

   In summary, a comprehensive process that allows evaluation and production of well-characterized, high-quality herbal products could serve as a basis for wider acceptance of therapeutic indications for these products by the international medical community and regulatory agencies.[23]

REFERENCES

1. Borman, S., Scientists mobilize to increase supply of anticancer drug taxol, *Chem. Eng. News*, September 2, 1991, p. 11.

2. Schechan, M.P., Rustin, M.H.A., Atherton, D.A. et al., Efficacy of traditional Chinese herbal therapy in adult atopic dermatitis, *Lancet*, 340, 13–17, 1992.

3. Sheehan, M.P. and Atherton, D.J., A controlled trial of traditional Chinese medicinal plants in widespread non-exudative atopic eczema, *Br. J. Dermatol.*, 126, 179–184, 1992.

4. Sheehan, M.P. and Atherton D.J., One-year follow up of children treated with Chinese medicinal herbs for atopic eczema, *Br. J. Dermatol.*, 130, 488–493, 1994.

5. Oka, H., Yamamoto, S., Kuroki, T. et al., Prospective study of chemoprevention of hepatocellular carcinoma with Sho-saiko-to, *Cancer*, 76, 743–749, 1995.

6. Yano, H., Mizoguchi, A., Fukuda, K. et al., The herbal medicine Sho-saiko-to inhibits proliferation of cancer cell lines by inducing apoptosis and arrest at the G_0/G_1 phase, *Cancer Res.*, 54, 448–454, 1994.

7. Lee, C.J., *Managing Biotechnology in Drug Development*, CRC Press, Boca Raton, FL., 1996, pp. 118–126.

8. Chihara, G., Hamuro, J., Maeda, Y. et al., Fractionation and purification of the polysaccharides with marked antitumor activity, especially lentinan, from *Lentinus edodes* (Berk.) Sing. (an edible mushroom), *Cancer Res.*, 30, 2776–2781, 1970.

9. Chihara, G., Hamuro, J., Maeda, Y. et al., Antitumor polysaccharide derived chemically from natural glucan (pachymaran), *Nature*, 225, 943–944, 1970.

10. Lien, E.J., Fungal metabolites and Chinese herbal medicine as immunostimulants, *Prog. Drug Res.*, 34, 395–420, 1990.

11. Bluhm, T.L. and Sarko, A., The triple helical structure of lentinan, a linear $\beta(1–3)$-D-glucan, *Can. J. Chem.*, 55, 293–299, 1977.

12. Nakano, H., Namatame, K., Nemato, H. et al., A multi-institutional prospective study of lentinan in advanced gastric cancer patients with unresectable and recurrent diseases: effect on prolongation of survival and improvement of quality of life, *Hepatogastroenterology*, 46, 2662–2668, 1999.

13. Fisher, M. and Yang, L.X., Anticancer effects and mechanisms of polysaccharide-K (PSK): implication of cancer immunotherapy, *Anticancer Res.*, 22, 1737–1754, 2002.

14. Lin, Z.B., Pharmacological activities of Lingzhi, in *Modern Research of* Ganoderma lucidum, 2nd ed., Lin, Z.B., Ed., Beijing Medical University Press, Beijing, 2001, pp. 219–283.

15. Leung, S.W.S., Yeung, K.Y., Siow Ricky, Y.L. et al., Lingzhi (*Ganoderma*) research: the past, present and future perspectives, in Ganoderma: *Genetics, Chemistry, Pharmacology and Therapeutics*, Lin, Z.B., Ed., Beijing University Press, Beijing, 2002, pp. 1–9.

16. Miyazaki, T. and Nishijima, M., Studies on fungal polysaccharides. XXVII. Structural examination of water-soluble, antitumor polysaccharide of *Ganoderma lucidum*, *Chem. Pharm. Bull.*, 29(12), 3611–3616, 1981.

17. Zhou, G.Y., Jiang, S., Huang, M. et al., Effects of ganopoly (a *Ganoderma lucidum* polysaccharide extract) on the immune functions in advanced-stage cancer patients, *Immunol. Invest.*, 32(3), 201–215, 2003.

18. Lee, C.J., Koizumi, K., Koizumi, M. et al., Immunomodulating effects of polysaccharides isolated from herbal products, *J. Trad. Med.*, 16, 175–182, 1999.

19. Wood, A.J.J. and De Smet, P., Herbal remedies, *N. Eng. J. Med.*, 347, 2047–2056, 2002.

20. Mitscher, L.A., Pillai, S., and Shankel, D.M., Some transpacific thoughts on the regulatory need for standardization of herbal medical products, *J. Food Drug Anal.*, 8(4), 229–234, 2000.

21. CDER, *Guidance for Industry: Botanical Drug Products*, Center for Drug Evaluation and Research, U.S. Food and Drug Administration, Rockville, MD, 2001, pp. 1–48 (http://www.fda.gov/cder/guidance).

22. Wu, K.M., Degeorge, J.G., Atrkchi, A. et al., Regulatory science: a special update from the United States Food and Drug Administration: preclinical issues and status of investigation of botanical drug products in the United States, *Toxicol. Lett.*, 111, 199–202, 2000.

23. Lee, C.J., Huo, Y.S., Lee, L.H. et al., Immunomodulating fungal and plant polysaccharides: biochemistry, immunologic activity and clinical application, *J. Trad. Med.*, 21(2), 67–80, 2004.

CHAPTER **33**

Biotechnology-Derived Pharmaceuticals

Chi-Jen Lee, Lucia H. Lee, Christopher L. Wu, and Benjamin R. Lee

CONTENTS

33.1 INTRODUCTION

Since 1982, when the first recombinant human insulin was licensed for therapeutic use, 50 additional pharmaceuticals and vaccines have been developed by biotechnology companies and approved by regulatory agencies. Advances in molecular biology, genomics, and proteomics, as well as innovations in pharmaceutical sciences have led to a rapid increase in the number of large-molecule pharmaceuticals for medical use. The human genome project has resulted in the identification of 30,000 human genes. The application of this new information to create new diagnostics, vaccines, and therapeutics holds great promise for the future of medical care. Biopharmaceuticals have revolutionized the prevention and treatment of diseases that currently are incurable or difficult to treat, such as cancer and cardiovascular, autoimmune, and genetic diseases; however, the complexity of the science and technology of biopharmaceuticals has resulted in challenges with regard to ensuring product quality, safety, and efficacy. In contrast to small-molecule drugs, which are chemically synthesized and whose structures are defined, biological products are derived from living sources, including humans, animals, plants, and microorganisms, using complicated manufacturing processes. These heterogeneous mixtures of large molecules are difficult to characterize, often display species specificity and various pharmacologic activities, are immunogenic, tend to be heat sensitive, and are susceptible to microbial contamination.

Despite these difficulties and challenges, a drive is currently underway to facilitate development in order to gain competitive advantages and maximize returns on investment. Early entry to human clinical trials is crucial to the biologic development process; however, the regulation of these products should be based on sound science, regulations, and their safety and efficacy profiles.

Approval of these products, similar to that of chemical drugs, requires research, policy development, review, and compliance activities. These activities can add value to a product and prevent conducting inappropriate clinical trials and the need to repeat studies later in the development process.

33.2 RECOMBINANT DNA TECHNOLOGY
AND ITS DERIVED PRODUCTS

The major classes of biopharmaceuticals include recombinant proteins, monoclonal antibodies (MAbs), vaccines, blood products, and gene transfer products. The progress in rDNA technology has made it possible to isolate DNA from a human gene and recombine it with the DNA of an unrelated prokaryotic or eukaryotic host within a plasmid expression vector. Transformation of the producer cells with these expression plasmids leads to the production of active human proteins in these host species. Hormones, blood clotting factors, enzymes, growth factors, and cytokines have been produced by this technology and licensed for use in disease treatment. Several other important therapeutic proteins, such as human thrombopoietin (TPO), and vaccines are in clinical development.[1-3]

Recombinant DNA technology involves isolating specific gene DNA that contains the genetic code for a desired protein and inserting it into a cell that can reproduce the protein rapidly and produce large quantities of the desired protein. *Escherichia coli*, yeast, and mammalian cells such as Chinese hamster ovary (CHO) and human myeloma cells are used most commonly to reproduce human proteins. These cells can be genetically manipulated easily to multiply and divide rapidly, and they produce large quantities of protein. *E. coli* cells are genetically simple, well analyzed, and less expensive than other cell types, but they cannot perform some complicated biochemical reactions, such as glycosylation, that are characteristic of more advanced mammalian cells. The isolated gene DNA is inserted to a plasmid and transformed into the host cell. A plasmid is a circular strand of DNA that can replicate inside a host cell. The human gene is spliced to the plasmid by DNA ligase to form the recombinant DNA molecule. The host cell takes the DNA molecule, and the plasmid-containing human gene is replicated in the host cell to produce the desired protein. The protein is secreted, purified, and formulated into the therapeutic product. Recombinant proteins can be produced in their native form, as analogs of the native protein, in truncated form, or as modified native proteins via polyethylene glycosylation, deglycosylation, or asialation to alter their activity.[4-6]

Over the past several years, a number of monoclonal antibodies have been approved or are in the late stages of development for therapeutic use in such areas as cancer, transplant rejection, autoimmune disease, allergy, and viral infection.[7-10] The ability to produce a recombinant molecule with low immunogenicity and to design a molecule to achieve a specific function has allowed the development of MAbs tailored for specific clinical applications. These antibodies are truncated, dissected into minimal binding fragments, and rebuilt into multivalent high-avidity drugs. Furthermore, MAbs and their fragments have been fused with enzymes for prodrug therapy, toxins and radiochemicals for cancer targeting, viruses for gene therapy, and lipids for improved systemic delivery.[11,12]

Conventional vaccines involve live attenuated microorganisms, inactivated whole cells, and subunit preparations for prevention of infectious diseases; however, recent advances in molecular immunology and our understanding of disease processes and the mechanisms of protective immunity have facilitated the development of new, rationally designed vaccines for preventive and therapeutic use in various indications, including infectious diseases, cancer, allergy, contraception, and bioterrorism.[13,14] These new vaccines include synthetic peptide and recombinant protein vaccines, glycoconjugates, genetically attenuated bacterial and viral pathogens, detoxified toxins, antigens expressed in transgenic plants, and DNA vaccines.[15-19] Several biotechnology-derived products have been licensed (see Table 33.1).

Gene transfer products were originally devised to treat genetic diseases, such as severe combined immune deficiency (SCID), hemophilia, or cystic fibrosis, by replacing a defective gene. They have been developed for prophylactic and therapeutic indications, including enhancement of tumor-specific immunity, prevention or treatment of infectious diseases, immunomodulation to treat allergy and autoimmunity, and facilitating gene-directed enzyme prodrug cancer therapy.[20–23] Two transfer vectors — bacterial plasmid DNA and live virus — have been used most commonly for genetically engineered products to express specific proteins. Plasmid DNA is administered in saline as naked DNA or complexed with a carrier. Viral vectors are generally replication deficient.[24,25] Live attenuated bacterial vectors are also used.[26] Extensive research has been focused on reducing vector immunogenicity, achieving more specific vector targeting, increasing the efficiency of vector uptake and nuclear targeting, and obtaining prolonged gene expression.[27]

33.3 EVALUATION OF GENE THERAPY AND DNA VACCINES

33.3.1 Gene Therapy

Since the β-globin gene, the first disease-associated gene, was cloned, it has become possible to isolate, sequence, and analyze genes causally related to most heritable and acquired diseases. For example, genes associated with cystic fibrosis, Duchenne muscular dystrophy, and SCID have been identified, isolated, and characterized. In the diagnosis and treatment of cancers, the discovery of oncogenes, tumor suppressor genes, and oncogenic viruses has contributed significantly to our understanding of the molecular mechanisms and development of particular types of cancers.

Investigators have applied this new information on molecular genetics and pathology to create innovative approaches to gene therapy. Gene therapy is a treatment directed at the gene expression level to replace defective genetic material or alter the phenotype of target cells for the purpose of preventing or curing a particular disease. Currently, only somatic cell gene therapy is being considered. The target cells are isolated from the body, grown in culture, genetically manipulated, and then returned to the patient from whom the original cells were removed. Gene transfer in humans is mainly performed in bone marrow and skin cells because only these cells can be cultivated in tissue culture.

The first application of human gene therapy was conducted in 1990, when a 4-year-old girl received autologous T-cells that were genetically modified to express adenosine deaminase (ADA) to correct this genetic deficiency. The T-lymphocytes were isolated, a normal ADA gene was introduced using a retroviral vector, and the cells were then returned to the girl. The immune responses of the patient significantly improved, thus reducing the incidence of infections and allowing her to lead a more normal life.[28]

Genetically modified lymphocytes have been transferred to patients with advanced cancer. Tissue-infiltration lymphocytes (TILs) are T-cells that are isolated from the infiltrating solid tumors and can kill tumors when grown in large number together with interleukin-2 (IL-2) in tissue culture. When the TILs are isolated from malignant melanomas and cultured in tissue culture by IL-2, genetically modified using a retroviral vector carrying the neomycin-resistant gene, and returned to the patient, they cause regression of the melanoma in 35 to 40% of patients.[29]

The use of gene transfer therapy will continue to grow as new information is obtained from results of the Human Genome Project. More than 200 active gene therapy investigational new drug (IND) applications are currently in effect. Conquering diseases such as cystic fibrosis, cancers, heart diseases, hemophilia, and many others is the goal of many of these clinical trials. To date, no gene therapy product has been licensed for commercial use, but the promise of this technology is optimistic and encouraging. The need to support the basic biomedical research in this area remains an important objective for developing new, successful biotechnology.

Table 33.1 Licensed Biotechnology-Derived Products

Product	Year Licensed	Company (Trade Name)	Clinical Indications
Hematopeietic Growth Factors			
Epotin alpha	1989	Amgen (EPOGEN®) Ortho Biotech Products (Procrit®)	Anemia associated with renal failure
Sargramostlm engraftment	1991	Betlex (Leukine®)	Enhanced myeloid-simulating leukocytes; neutropenia
Oprelvekin	1997	Genetics Institute (Neumega®)	Thrombocytopenia
Coagulation factor IX	1997	Genetics Institute (BeneFIX®)	Hemophilia B; clotting disorders
Coagulation factor VIIA	1999	Novo Nordisk (NovoSeven®)	Hemorrhagic episodes in hemophilia A and B
Antihemophilic factor	2000	Pharmacia (ReFacto®)	Uncontrolled bleeding
	1998	Baxter Healthcare (Advate®)	Hemophilia A
	1998	Genetics Institute (Recombinate®)	—
	2000	Bayer (Kogenate®, Kogenate® FS)	—
Lepirudin	1998	Berlex (REFLUDAN®)	Anticoagulation for thrombocytopenia, thromboembolic disease
Bivalirudin	2000	BenVenue Labs (Angiomax®)	Ischemic complications in angina
Eptifibatide	1998	COR Therapeutics (Integrilin®)	Acute coronary syndrome
Darbepoetin alpha	2001	Amgen (Aranesp®)	Anemia with chronic renal failure
Pegfilgrastim	2002	Amgen (Neulasta®)	Infections in cancer chemotherapy
Interferons			
Interferon alfacon-1	1997	Amgen (Infergen®)	Chronic hepatitis C virus (HCV) infection
Interferon alpha-2a	1998	Roche Laboratories (Roferon-A®)	Chronic HCV, hairy-cell leukemia, AIDS-related Kaposi's sarcoma, chronic myelogenous leukemia
Interferon alpha-2b	1997	Schering–Plough (Intron® A)	Hairy-cell leukemia, malignant melanoma, follicular non-Hodgkin's lymphoma, Kaposi's sarcoma, HCV, skin disorder
Interferon beta-1a	1996	Biogen (Avonex®)	Multiple sclerosis
Interferon beta-1b	1993	Chiron (BETASERON®)	Multiple sclerosis
Aldesleukin	1992	Chiron (PROLEUKIN®)	Metastatic renal cell carcinoma and melanoma
Denileukin diftitox	1999	Seragen (Ontak®)	Cutaneous T-cell lymphoma
Anakinra	2001	Amgen (Kineret®)	Rheumatoid arthritis
Peginterferon alpha-2b	2001	Schering–Plough (PEG-Intron®)	Chronic hepatitis C
Interferon beta-1a	2002	Serono (Rebif®)	Multiple sclerosis
Hormones			
Human insulin (recombinant)	1982	Eli Lilly (Humulin®)	Diabetes mellitus
	1996	Novo Nordisk (Novolin®)	
	1999	Novo Nordisk (Velosulin® BR)	
Insulin lispro	2000	Eli Lilly (Humalog®)	Diabetes mellitus
Insulin glargine	2000	Aventis (Lantus®)	Diabetes mellitus
Insulin aspart	2000	Novo Nordisk (NovoLog®)	Diabetes mellitus
Glucagon	1998	Novo Nordisk (GlucaGen®) Eli Lilly (Glucagon®)	Hypoglycemia
Somatrem	1985	Genentech (Protropin®)	Growth hormone deficiency
Follitropin alpha	2000	Serono (Gonal-F®)	Induction of ovulation and pregnancy
Follitropin beta	1998	Organon (Follistim®)	Induction of ovulation and pregnancy

Table 33.1 Licensed Biotechnology-Derived Products (cont.)

Product	Year Licensed	Company (Trade Name)	Clinical Indications
Somatropin (recombinant)	1997 2000	Eli Lilly (Humatrope®) Serono (Saizen®, Serostim®) Pharmacia (Genotropin®) Novo Nordisk (Norditropin®) Genentech (Nutropin®)	Growth hormone deficiency
Nafarelin	1999	Searle (Synarel®)	Endometriosis, central precocious puberty
Goserelin	1998	Zeneca (Zoladex®)	Carcinoma of prostate, endometriosis
Ganirelix	1999	Vetter Pharma-Fertigung (Antagon™)	Inhibition of premature leutenizing hormone surges
Oxytocin	1997	King Pharmaceuticals (Pitocin®) Wyeth Ayerst, Eon Labs, Fujisawa (Oxytocin®)	Induction and augmentation of labor; postpartum bleeding
Octreotide	1998	Sandoz Pharmaceuticals (Sandostatin®)	Reduction of blood growth hormone and IGF-I in acromegaly; metastatic tumors

Enzymes

Alglucerase	1991	Genzyme (Ceredase®)	Type 1 Gaucher's disease
Imiglucerase	1999	Genzyme (Cerezyme®)	—
Pegademase	1990	Enzon (Adagen®)	Adenosine deaminase deficiency
Bovine dornase alpha	1993	Genentech (Pulmozyme®)	Cystic fibrosis
Pegaspargase	1994	Enzon (Oncaspar®)	Acute lymphoblastic leukemia
Reteplase	1996	Centocor (Retavase®)	Acute myocardial infarction
Tenecteplase	2000	Genentech (TNKase®)	Acute myocardial infarction
Drotrecogin alpha	2001	Eli Lilly (Xigris®)	Severe sepsis

Monoclonal Antibodies

Muromonab-CD3	1986	Ortho Biotech (Orthoclone® OKT3)	Acute allograft rejection
Daclizumab	1997	Roche Pharmaceuticals (Zenapax®)	Prophylaxis of acute organ rejection
Basiliximab	1998	Novartis (Simulect®)	Prophylaxis of acute organ rejection
Etanercept	1998	Amgen (Enbrel®)	Polyarticular-course juvenile rheumatoid arthritis
Infliximab	1998	Centocor (Remicade®)	Crohn's disease
Gemtuzumab ozogamicin	2000	Wyeth Ayerst (Mylotarg®)	CD33 positive acute myeloid leukemia
Rituximab	1997	Genentech (Rituxan®)	B-cell non-Hodgkin's lymphoma
Trastuzumab	1998	Genentech (Herceptin®)	Metastatic breast cancer
Palivizumab	1998	MedImmune (Synagis®)	Prophylaxis of respiratory syncytial virus infection
Abciximab	1998	Centocor (ReoPro®)	Prevention of cardiac ischemic complications
Ibritumomab tiuxetan	2002	IDEC Pharmaceuticals (Zevalin®)	B-cell non-Hodgkin's lymphoma

Other Products

Becaplermin	1997	OMJ Pharmaceuticals (Regranex® Gel)	Diabetic neuropathic ulcers
Fomivirsen	1998	Abbott (Vitravene®)	Cytomegalovirus retinitis
Alpha$_1$-proteinase	1987	Bayer (Prolastin®)	Congenital alpha-1 antitrypsin deficiency

During a period of explosive growth in the number of human gene transfer studies, a patient died in the course of a gene transfer in 1999, apparently as a direct consequence of the use of an adenovirus gene transfer reagent. The regulatory agency and many other research groups have now recognized the need for greater attention and awareness of human subject protection issues. As a result, changes to the procedures for clinical trial protocol review have been designed to promote interagency collaboration. The FDA continues to review gene transfer protocols and issues INDs for carrying out clinical trials. In addition, as of October 2000, every human clinical gene transfer protocol requires evaluation by the Recombinant DNA Advisory Committee (RAC) of the National Institutes of Health (NIH). Any protocol involving gene therapy investigation is submitted for RAC review before final approval can be granted by the institutional biosafety committee (IBC) and institutional review board (IRB). Furthermore, changes to the reporting of serious adverse events (SAEs) have been proposed to simplify and harmonize the NIH and FDA reporting systems.[30] With the proposed coordination of the SAE reporting procedures, investigators and sponsors may file an SAE report simultaneously to the two agencies.

The changes proposed by the RAC also include the establishment of a gene transfer safety assessment board (GTSAB) and a publicly accessible SAE database. The GTSAB would consist of clinical experts, biostatisticians, FDA reviewers, and members of the RAC. The GTSAB would review and assess the SAE reports. The incidence and type of SAE data would then be entered into the public database to enhance the usefulness of the information, maximally protecting patient and subject safety while enhancing and protecting the commercial and intellectual property interests of study sponsors.[31]

33.3.2 DNA Vaccines

A DNA vaccine consists of a foreign gene for the desired antigen; the gene is cloned into a bacterial plasmid. Plasmid DNA, a small ring of double-stranded DNA derived from bacteria but unable to produce an infection, is engineered for expression in eukaryotic cells. The plasmid also frequently contains a bacterial antibiotic resistance gene, such as ampicillin or kanamycin resistance gene, and a promoter from cytomegalovirus (CMV) or simian virus 40, for example, for optimal expression in mammalian cells. The vaccine is usually immunized intramuscularly by a gene gun, which can deliver plasmids into skin cells or mucous membranes. After entering the cells, some of the recombinant plasmids make their way to the nucleus and instruct the cell to synthesize the encoded antigenic proteins. These proteins leave the cell and are taken up by antigen-presenting cells (APCs), such as macrophages or dendritic cells. Protein molecules are broken into fragments to interact with major histocompatibility class (MHC) I or II molecules. After such processing, the complexes are displayed on the cell surface and bind to Th cells. The activation of Th cells helps to elicit humoral (antibody-type) and cellular (killer-type) immunity.

In 1996, the FDA issued a guidance document to assist manufacturers developing DNA vaccines. Entitled *Points To Consider on Plasmid DNA Vaccines for Preventive Infectious Disease Indications*,[32] this document presents manufacturing, preclinical, and clinical issues related to the development of DNA vaccines and describes potential safety concerns that manufacturers should address before initiating clinical trials. Later, the World Health Organization (WHO) issued a document entitled "WHO Guidelines for Assuring the Quality of DNA Vaccines" to advise vaccine developers regarding methods for production, control of DNA plasmids, and regulatory issues.[33] In addition, a guidance document is also available from European Union regulatory agencies that addresses manufacturing, preclinical, and clinical issues related to DNA vaccine development.[34]

REFERENCES

1. Vadham-Raj, S., Clinical experience with recombinant human thrombopoeitin in chemotherapy-induced thrombocytopenia, *Semin. Hematol.*, 37, 28–34, 2000.

2. Sandhu, J., Engineered human vaccines, *CRC Crit. Rev. Biotechnol.*, 14, 1–27, 1994.

3. Walsh, G., *Biopharmaceuticals: Biochemistry and Biotechnology*, Wiley, Chichester, 1999.

4. Masci, P., Bukowski, R.M., Patten, P.A. et al., New and modified interferon alfas: preclinical and clinical data, *Curr. Oncol. Rep.*, 5, 108–113, 2003.

5. Ergie, J.C. and Goa, K.L., Development and the characterization of novel erythropoiesis stimulating protein (NESP), *Br. J. Cancer*, 84(Suppl. 1), 3–10, 2001.

6. Bonig, H., Silbermann, S., Weller, S. et al., Glycosylated vs. non-glycosylated granulocyte colony-stimulating factor (G-CSF): results of a prospective randomised monocentre study, *Bone Marrow Transplant.*, 28, 259–264, 2001.

7. King, D.J. and Adair, J.R., Recombinant antibodies for diagnosis and therapy of human disease, *Curr. Opin. Drug Discov. Dev.*, 2, 110–117, 1999.

8. Cater, P., and Merchant, A., Engineering antibodies for imaging and therapy, *Curr. Opin. Biotechnol.*, 8, 449–454, 1997.

9. Hudson, P.J. and Souriau, C., Engineered antibodies, *Nat. Med.*, 9, 129–134, 2003.

10. Pluckthun, A. and Pack, P., New protein engineering approaches to multivalent and bispecific antibody fragments, *Immunotechnology*, 3, 83–105, 1997.

11. Adair, J.R., Antibody engineering and expression, in *Biotechnology*. Vol. 5a. *Recombinant Proteins, Monoclonal Antibodies and Therapeutic Genes*, Rehm, H.J. and Reed, G., Eds., Wiley, Weinheim, 1999, pp. 219–244.

12. Hudson, P.J., Recombinant antibody fragments, *Curr. Opin. Biotechnol.*, 9, 395–402, 1998.

13. Sandhu, J., Engineered human vaccines, *CRC Crit. Rev. Biotechnol.*, 14, 1–27, 1994.

14. Russo, S., Turin, L., Zanella, A. et al., What's going on in vaccine technology?, *Med. Res. Rev.*, 17, 277–301, 1997.

15. Jackson, D.C., Purcell, A.W., Fitzmaurice, C.J. et al., The central role played by peptides in the immune response and the design of peptide-based vaccines against infectious diseases and cancer, *Curr. Drug Targets*, 3, 175–196, 2002.

16. Lee, C.J., Lee, L.H., and Frasch, C.E., protective immunity of pneumococcal glycoconjugates, *CRC Crit. Rev. Microbiol.*, 29(4), 333–349, 2003.

17. Kang, S.M. and Compans, R.W., Enhancement of mucosal immunization with virus-like particles of simian immunodeficiency virus, *J. Virol.*, 77, 3615–3623, 2003.

18. Mason, H.A., Warzecha, H., Mor, T. et al., Edible plant vaccines: applications for prophylactic and therapeutic molecular medicine, *Trends Mol. Med.*, 8, 324–329, 2002.

19. Donnelly, J., DNA vaccines, *Annu. Rev. Immunol.*, 15, 617–648, 1997.

20. Crystal, R., The gene as a drug, *Nat. Med.*, 1, 15–17, 1995.

21. Tirapu, I., Rodriguez-Calvillo, M., Qian, C. et al., Cytokine gene transfer into dendritic cells for cancer treatment, *Curr. Gene Ther.*, 2, 79–89, 2002.

22. Chiou, H.C., Lucas, M.A., Coffin, C.C. et al., Gene therapy strategies for the treatment of chronic viral hepatitis, *Expert Opin. Biol. Ther.*, 1, 629–639, 2001.

23. Trucco, M., Robbins, P.D., Thomson, A.W. et al., Gene therapy strategies to prevent autoimmune disorder, *Curr. Gene Ther.*, 2, 341–354, 2002.

24. Smith, A.E., Viral vectors in gene therapy, *Annu. Rev. Microbiol.*, 49, 807–838, 1995.

25. Lai, C.M., Lai, Y.K., and Rakoczy, P.E., Adenovirus and adeno-associated virus vectors, *DNA Cell Biol.*, 21, 895–913, 2002.

26. Darji, A., Guzman, C.A., Gerstel, B. et al., Oral somatic transgene vaccination using attenuated *S. typhimurium*, *Cell*, 91, 765–775, 1997.

27. Friedmann, T., Overcoming the obstacles to gene therapy, *Sci. Am.*, June, 80–85, 1997.

28. Anderson, W.F., Human gene therapy, *Science*, 256, 808, 1992.

29. Kasid, A., Morecki, S., Aebersold, P. et al., Human gene transfer: characterization of human tumor-infiltrating lymphocytes as vehicles for retroviral-mediated gene transfer in man, *Proc. Natl. Acad. Sci. USA*, 87, 473, 1990

30. U.S. Food and Drug Administration, Proposed rule on public disclosure, *Fed. Reg.*, January 18, 2001 (66FR 4688).

31. Friedmann, T., Noguchi, P., and Mickelson, C., The evolution of public review and oversight mechanisms in human gene transfer research: joint roles of the FDA and NIH, *Curr. Opin. Biotechnol.*, 12, 299–303, 2001.

32. FDA, *Points To Consider on Plasmid DNA Vaccines for Preventive Infectious Disease Indications*, Docket No. 96-N-0400, Office of Vaccine Research and Review, Center for Biologics Evaluation and Research, U.S. Food and Drug Administration, Washington, D.C., 1996.

33. World Health Organization, WHO guidelines for assuring the quality of DNA vaccines, *Biologicals*, 26(3), 205–212, 1998.

34. Robertson, J.S. and Cichutek, K., Development and clinical progress of DNA vaccines: European Union guidance on the quality, safety and efficacy of DNA vaccines and regulatory requirements, *Dev. Biol.*, 104, 53–56, 2000.

PART XIV

Future Perspectives

CHAPTER **34**

Future Perspectives in Drug Development

Christopher L. Wu, Benjamin R. Lee, and Mei-Ling Chen

CONTENTS

34.1 INTRODUCTION

At the heart of the National Institutes of Health campus in Bethesda, MD, stands the NIH Clinical Center, a research hospital combined with laboratories to conduct clinical studies for development of drugs and biopharmaceuticals. Patients come from all over the nation — and, in some cases, from all corners of the world — to participate in clinical trials. Other hospitals do research, but one half of the beds in the NIH Clinical Center are reserved for research studies. It serves as an international model of collaborative excellence and innovation in clinical research. It provides an ideal environment for elucidating the knowledge that will help prevent, diagnose, and treat disease and disability and for developing new drugs and biologics to cure the rarest genetic disorders, cancers, and cardiovascular disease.

Clinical trials of novel drugs account for approximately half the protocols in the NIH Clinical Center. Most of the clinical trials conducted there have been phase I or II trials with the objective of evaluating safety and preliminary efficacy. These trials mark the first time these agents have been tested in humans. After these early studies, the drugs move into phase III trials, which are usually conducted off campus in large populations by extramural researchers. The intramural researchers at the NIH Clinical Center turn their attention to other challenges requiring innovative or original research that cannot be easily performed elsewhere.

The other half of the protocols involving the NIH Clinical Center are designed to study the natural process of rare diseases to elucidate their pathogenesis and possible targets of drug action and to develop new medical therapies for diagnosis, prevention, and treatment. It is the final common pathway for translating scientific endeavor in the laboratory to practical clinical applications in humans.

The NIH Clinical Center supports about 1000 active clinical research protocols. In 2003, it had 6723 hospital admissions plus an additional 98,172 outpatient visits. Investigators examined 9175 new patients in 2003, bringing the total number of active patients to more than 80,000, representing the largest population of patients with rare diseases anywhere. Critical to the success of the biomedical research is the proximity of research laboratories to the patients. The NIH Clinical Center allows investigators to work in both the laboratory and the clinic. The idea is to bring both basic and clinical science to the patient's bedside; moreover, it encourages informal interactions in the corridors between clinicians and scientists. It provides a critical mass of intellectually curious scientists and medical experts and the world's best supply of patients with rare and research-worthy medical conditions.[1]

The dawn of a new age in biomedical and pharmaceutical sciences is on the horizon. New technologies contribute to the production of better and safer drugs. Major changes are taking place in the development and evaluation of chemical compounds for their therapeutic application and the elucidation of their pharmacologic mechanisms at the molecular level. This exciting age has arisen from advances in our understanding of the molecular basis of changes in body functions during various stages of disease. Biotechnology and computer science are making significant contributions to the field of new drug discovery. Further, progress in our understanding of how quantitative structure–activity relationships can be used to modify, design, and synthesize chemical compounds has led to the development of many effective pharmaceutical products and further understanding of the interactions of drugs with their biologic target molecules.

Many diseases are targeted by conventional small-molecule drugs. A revolutionary technology in small-molecule drug discovery is combinatorial chemistry combined with high-throughput screening, which aids in the evaluation of many new and unique potential drug compounds. Another new technique is computer-assisted drug design for systematic exploration of the physicochemical properties of a candidate drug molecule and its possible modes of interaction with a target receptor. This procedure, known as structure-based drug design, works best when the target has been identified and isolated and its three-dimensional structure elucidated.

Modern drug development is still a slow and expensive process. The time from discovery of a drug to its availability on the market is quite long, ranging from 8 to 20 years. The cost to bring a conventional, small-molecule drug to market has been estimated to be between $800 and $880 million. The marketing success rate for drug development was found to be 5% for 140 leading drug candidates; all 140 drugs made it through preclinical animal testing, 65 made it through phase I trials, 27 made it through phase II trials, 9 made it through phase III trials, and 7 were approved for marketing.[2] Phase I of these trials can be up to 1 year; phase II, up to 2 years; and phase III, 1 to 4 years, with an additional FDA review time of 2 months to 7 years.

Pharmaceutical scientists have taken advantage of every opportunity or technology available to facilitate the long, costly drug development process to change the way drug research is conducted and optimize conditions necessary for identifying novel chemical leads. The process of modern drug development involves three critical elements: (1) identification of new targets by genomics and related technology; (2) rapid, sensitive bioassays utilizing high-throughput screening methods; and (3) rapid synthesis of new molecules by combinatorial chemistry. The critical elements are carried out with the assistance of bioinformatics.

Traditionally, drug discovery relied mainly upon random screening followed by analog synthesis and lead optimization through structure–activity relationship studies. The search for new, effective, and safe drugs is an increasing costly and complex process. Thus, any technology allowing for a reduction in time and expense is extremely important. Advances in biomedical and pharmaceutical sciences have contributed to a greater understanding of the causes and process of disease and have identified new therapeutic targets that serve as the bases for novel drug screens. These advances have facilitated the discovery of new drugs with novel mechanisms of action for diseases that were previously difficult or impossible to treat. In an effort to facilitate identifying useful, effective drug leads against a disease target, investigators have implemented high-throughput screening (HTS) and efficient synthesis methods.

34.2 HIGH-THROUGHPUT SCREENING AND COMBINATORIAL CHEMISTRY

Recombinant DNA technology has provided the capability to clone, express, and isolate receptor enzymes, membrane bound proteins, in large quantities. Instead of using receptors present in animal tissues or enzymes for screening or *in vitro* bioassay, it is now possible to utilize human protein targets. Biotechnology has been applied to isolate and purify various receptor molecules for *in vitro* screening: (1) cloned membrane-bound receptors expressed in cell lines; (2) immobilized receptors, antibodies, and other ligand-binding proteins; and (3) soluble enzymes and extracellular protein receptors. Screening synthetic compounds and natural products can be performed directly based on structural information about the receptor or natural ligand. Newly developed sensitive radioligand binding assays and automated robotic techniques have facilitated the screening process.

High-throughput screening (HTS) provides the bioassay for thousands of compounds in multiple assays at the same time.[3,4] The process is automated and utilizes multiple-well microtiter plates. While 96-well microtiter plates are standard in HTS, the development of 1536- and 3456-well nanoplate formats and enhanced robotics have brought small size and rapid speed to cell-based and biochemical assays. At present, investigators can perform 100,000 bioassays each day. In addition, modern drug discovery and lead optimization with DNA microarrays allow scientists to monitor hundreds to thousands of genes. Enzyme inhibition and radioligand binding assays are the most common biochemical analyses conducted. In most cases, biotechnology contributes directly to the understanding and identification of the drug target being screened.

The genomic age has changed the early discovery paradigm and introduced an abundance of uncharacterized genes as targets. New technologies are being applied to detect and characterize cell systems. In addition, novel amplification strategies for receptor readout have been developed, allowing the identification of receptor agonists and antagonists. Chip-based technology will be integrated into the overall screening process. These chips may provide the ability to evaluate millions of compounds in a short time at reduced cost. The validation of targets by using gene chips, cell-based assays, proteomics, and other validation approaches will lead to the integration of all available technology into an effective high-throughput drug development.

The trials for most drugs developed prior to the biotechnology age were conducted based on a combination of luck and intuition with regard to drug function and optimization, coupled with systematic chemical synthesis. Drugs discovered in the past originated from the screening of natural products, followed by isolation, chemical synthesis, and elimination of side effects. This procedure required the time-consuming sequential synthesis of each identifiable candidate (lead) molecule and modifying different functional groups to improve potency.

One of the most effective methods to optimize drug discovery is automated high-throughput synthesis. When conducted in a combinatorial approach, such synthesis provides for simultaneous preparation of hundreds or thousands of related drug candidates.[5,6] The molecular libraries generated are screened in high-throughput screening assays for the desired activity, and the most active molecules are identified and isolated for further development.

The advantage of combinatorial chemistry over conventional synthetic chemistry is that it can lead to compounds that might not be synthesized using the traditional methods. For example, the benzodiazapenes possess a range of biological activities and interact with a broad range of biological receptors in addition to the diazapene receptor, which is responsible for the antianxiety effects of the inhibitor valium. A combinatorial synthesis has allowed libraries of related compounds to be prepared, such as the prostaglandin family or the α- and β-blockers. In the solid-phase synthesis of benzodiazapene, a 2-aminobenzophone derivative is linked to a solid support and then reacted with a fluoroenyl methoxycarbonyl (FMOC)-protected amino acid. A cyclization step followed by cleavage from the support with an alkylating agent releases a 1,4-benzodiazapene derivative that can be isolated and screened against the desired target.[7] Biologically active molecules isolated in this way include inhibitors to the opioid receptor and the human immunodeficiency virus (HIV) Tat protein.

The parallel procedures of combinatorial chemistry apply automation to the synthetic process. These procedures can be conducted on solid-phase supports or in solution. Applying the automatic synthesizing equipment results in the rapid production of large collections, as many as 10,000 compounds of diverse molecules. When coupled with high-throughput screening, thousands of compounds can be generated, screened, and evaluated in a period of weeks.

34.3 CANCER AND CHRONIC DISEASES IN AN AGING SOCIETY

Since the beginning of the 20th century, the size of the elderly population in the United States has been steadily increasing. At present, people 65 years of age and older are expected to live an average of an additional 16 years. Cancer and chronic diseases are becoming a serious health problem, and the medicines used as treatments have limitations. In the United States, cancer is the second leading cause of mortality and is expected to become the leading cause in the near future. The medical treatment of cancer still has many shortcomings. The main approach of cancer treatment, surgery, and radiation is usually only effective if the cancer is found at an early and localized stage. When the disease has progressed to an advanced metastatic stage, these therapies are less successful. In many cases, the chemotherapies are effective only for a short period.

The development of new drugs and biologics for cancer therapy involves several critical issues. Ideal therapies would include targeted and lasting antitumor activity, low toxicities, and avoidance of drug resistance caused by the genome instability of tumors. Biomedical research discoveries based on disease mechanisms often lead to the most direct pharmaceutical approaches to counter the disease. The past 20 years have witnessed a basic change in the way target identification in cancer is approached. Advances in molecular genetics now allow scientists to identify genes that become deranged in cancer. At first, just a few cancer genes were identified (e.g., *src*, *abl*, *ras*). Today, many genes are known to affect tumorigenesis and tumor growth. Various areas of signal transduction, cell-cycle regulation, apoptosis, telomere biology, and angiogenesis are being studied extensively to select potential therapeutic molecular targets against tumor cells. These molecular targets include epidermal growth factor (EGF) receptor, estrogen receptor (ER), farnesyltransferase (Ftase), and protein kinase C (PKC). The choice of target is often based on the underlying gene mutation. Overexpression of specific gene products, such as HER-2, epidermal growth factor, and insulin-like growth factor receptor, has been considered a causative factor in cancers.

In addition, a normal gene product may be correlated with cancer progression. Elevated telomerase activity is observed in all human cancers, and increased serum vascular endothelial growth factor (VEGF) has been found to correlate with decreased survival rates in patients with breast, ovarian, lung, gastric, and colon cancer. These findings indicate that the telomerase enzyme and the receptor of VEGF are good targets for cancer drug development. Some of the most exciting results have been reported for agents directed against tyrosine kinase, either as therapeutic antibodies or as small-molecule kinase inhibitors. Many molecular mechanisms have been examined as new targets for drug development in the hope that they have more effective antitumor activity.[8]

A hard medical reality is that prostate cancer kills. This disease is the second leading cause of cancer death in men in the United States and results in more than 32,000 deaths each year. It is especially prevalent in men older than 65 years of age. The goal of surgery for the prostate is threefold: (1) to remove cancer within the prostate, (2) to preserve urinary control following surgery, and (3) to preserve erectile function. Recent advances in surgical techniques can further extend survival time and improve the quality of life for many prostate cancer patients. Prior to the advent of laparoscopic surgery, for example, the typical incision for open radical prostatectomy would be 8 inches. Now, with a groundbreaking new technique known as laparoscopic prostatectomy, improved surgical outcome and a better quality of life are possible. This revolutionary approach uses a videocamera to magnify the operative field 12-fold. Better operative precision leads to greater preservation of vital anatomic structures. Careful attention is paid to avoiding delicate nerves adjacent to the cancer. The best news of all is that this technique offers the advantage of smaller scars, less pain medication, less blood loss, and quicker return to normal life.

Because many human diseases are caused by heredity and central nervous system disorders, it is exciting to see how biomedical research has contributed to the early detection, prevention, and treatment of geriatric conditions such as Alzheimer's disease, depression, and Parkinson's disease. The dramatic rise in life expectancy has enabled many of us to reach the age at which degenerative chronic disorders, such as Alzheimer's disease and stroke, become common. Approximately 15% of people who live to the age of 65 will develop some form of dementia; by age 85, the proportion increases to at least 35%. Of all the dementias, Alzheimer's disease is the most common. Understanding why an accumulation of β-amyloid protein plaques occurs in the brain can provide significant clues about disease mechanisms. Deposits of amyloid protein gather in the spaces between nerve cells. Amyloid plaques are usually accompanied by reactive inflammatory cells referred to as microglia, which are part of the brain's immune system trying to degrade and remove damaged neurons. Such plaques are present in most elderly people. Their extensive presence in the hippocampus and cerebral cortex, however, is specific to Alzheimer's patients. The amyloid protein is a small fragment, made up of either 40 or 42 amino acids. Identification of the β-amyloid peptide was made possible by sequencing the 695-amino acid protein referred to as the β-amyloid precursor protein

The βAPP gene is located on chromosome 21. People with Down's syndrome have three rather than two copies of chromosome 21 and invariably display some features of Alzheimer's by the age of 40. These findings suggest that the amyloid protein is involved in the onset of Alzheimer's disease, and the βAPP gene may be the site of mutations. In the course of Alzheimer's disease, βAPP is processed in one of two ways. The protein is first cleaved by the alpha-secretase and gamma-secretase enzyme. The resulting product is the harmless peptide fragment p3. The second way in which βAPP is cleaved involves another two-step process. First, the protein is cleaved by a beta-secretase to form a C99-βAPP fragment. This fragment is then cleaved by gamma-secretase to form the β-amyloid peptide. The peptide may act in several ways. First, it disrupts calcium regulation, which can lead to cell death. Second, it damages the mitochondria, causing the release of free oxygen radicals, which then damage proteins, lipids, and DNA. Third, it causes neuronal injury and release of cellular compounds. An inflammatory response may occur that creates a cycle of escalating damage.

New treatments for Alzheimer's disease focus on blocking the ability of either the beta- or gamma-secretase enzyme to cleave APP, thus preventing β-amyloid peptide formation. Other alternative approaches include antioxidants, such as glycoaminoglycans, which can break down β-amyloid aggregates. Attempts have also been made to develop a therapeutic vaccine to neutralize the activity of β-amyloid peptide.[9] Whatever the future holds, it is increasingly likely that, in the years to come, more effective products and treatments will be generated.

REFERENCES

1. McNee, P., *50 Years of Clinical Research at the NIH Clinical Center*, National Institutes of Health, U.S. Department of Health and Human Services, Bethesda, MD, 2003, pp. 21–33.
2. Shapiro, B., The Impact of Biotechnology on Drug Discovery, paper presented at the 9th International Congress of Immunology, San Francisco, CA, 1955.
3. Kenny, B.A., Bushfield, M., Parry-Smith, D.J. et al., The application of high-throughput screening to novel lead discovery, *Prog. Drug. Res.*, 51, 245–269, 1998.
4. Oldenburg, K.R., Current and future trends in high-throughput screening for discovery, *Ann. Rep. Med. Chem.*, 33, 301–311, 1988.
5. Fenniri, H., *Combinatorial Chemistry: A Practical Approach*, Oxford University Press, Oxford, 2000.
6. Sucholeiki, I., *High-Throughput Synthesis: Principles and Practices*, Marcel Dekker, New York, 2001.

7. Bunin, B.A., Plunkett, M.J., and Ellman, J.A., The combinatorial synthesis and chemical and biological evaluation of a 1,4-benzodiazepene library, *Proc. Natl. Acad. Sci.*, 91(11), 4708–4712, 1994.
8. Gibbs, J.B., Mechanism-based target identification and drug discovery in cancer research, *Science*, 287, 1969–1973, 2000.
9. George-Hyslop, P.H., Piecing together Alzheimer's disease, *Sci. Am.*, December, 76–83, 2000.

CHAPTER 35

Future Perspectives in Biopharmaceutical Development

Chi-Jen Lee, Lucia H. Lee, Christopher L. Wu, and Benjamin R. Lee

CONTENTS

35.1 INTRODUCTION

The medical and pharmaceutical sciences have progressed greatly over the past several decades due to advances in biotechnology such as recombinant DNA techniques, monoclonal antibody production, and new chemical analysis techniques. An extensive, expanding understanding of molecular biology and clinical medicine has been achieved. We have begun to understand the basic mechanisms of the natural process of disease and the pharmacological actions of drugs and biologics. Together with the new biotechnologies, these fundamental insights have opened up a window of opportunity for biopharmaceutical development. Biotechnology has revolutionized research in biomedicine and created an entirely new field of pharmaceutical industry. Today, many proteins are produced through rDNA technology and used for the treatment and prevention of diseases such as cancer, autoimmune and neurologic diseases, infections, heart attacks, and genetic abnormalities. Furthermore, biotechnology has been used to improve the efficacy and safety of therapeutic biologics.[1]

The analogs of natural polypeptides can be produced by the *in vitro* recombination of hybrid genes. Using DNA polymerase to prepare mutant synthetic oligonucleotide primers, site-specific mutagenesis can be induced in cloned genes prior to insertion into a vector. Insertion or deletion of a few nucleotides can be achieved using restriction enzymes. With the polymerase chain reaction (PCR), it is feasible to carry out site-specific, directed mutagenesis of single nucleotides within a cloned gene; thus, restriction enzyme digestion in conjugation with the PCR technique can produce truncated or fusion hybrid proteins. This new technology allows the determination of amino acid sequences of bioregulatory peptides and the design of their pharmacologic antagonists.

In the 1980s, advances in DNA cloning and expression facilitated the discovery and development of novel biopharmaceuticals. These achievements expanded the ability to develop the therapeutic molecules. These techniques, however, were complicated and only provided a modest increase in the number of targets available before the 1980s. The total number of targets available for drug screening was limited to about 500 between 1940 and 1990.[2] Today, however, the number of drug targets has increased greatly, which can be attributed to the accomplishments of the Human Genome Project. The human genome sequencing effort has provided access to many unique genes with assigned protein products. About 1700 genes within the human genome sequences have been identified as producing functional proteins suitable for serving as drug targets.

35.2 STRATEGIES FOR PROTEIN DISCOVERY IN A POST-GENOMIC AGE

The Human Genome Project (HGP) has had a major impact on the biomedical research and pharmaceutical industries due to its translation of the genomic sequence and the functional genomics information gained that will prove useful to the discovery of new therapeutics and diagnostic devices. In the genomic age, efforts were directed toward the sequencing of genes and identification of pharmaceutical targets, as well as therapeutic proteins and genes. In the post-genomic age, the focus will shift to the broader use of biological and molecular information within a new paradigm of drug development and health care. The emphasis in the laboratory is on the possible association of genes with disease and the identification of targets for drug screening. The pharmaceutical industry must deal with the challenges of how to manage biotechnology effectively to produce more effective and safe drugs and biologics.

Several strategies and technologies have been applied to discovering and analyzing human genes, including: (1) homology in protein or gene families, (2) gene expression and regulation, (3) identification by function, and (4) genetic linkage and cloning. Homology is a powerful technique for identifying new genes of certain classes and classifying many proteins into families. Sequence homology may translate into functional similarity.[3] Approaches for cloning homologs include degenerate polymerase chain reaction (PCR) and low-stringency hybridization. Homology sequencing has been applied to developing broad patent positions and selecting the most useful growth factors from a gene family. Regulation of gene expression at the messenger RNA (mRNA) and protein level has become an important approach for the discovery and characterization of genes. DNA microarrays have been used for measurement of changes in gene expression. A gene can be identified by its function. Expression cloning, or the screening of complementary DNA (cDNA) libraries for the expression of specific activities in transfected cells, has been used to identify growth and differentiation factors, interleukins, and receptors of various classes.

The development of dense genome linkage maps in 1990s made the identification and cloning of genes by genetic linkage feasible. For example, positional cloning in humans was used to identify the BRCA1 gene, a major predisposing factor in breast cancer.[4] A more recent example in inbred mice is the cloning of the mahogany gene, a gene involved in obesity and weight control.[5,6] In addition, the development of high-resolution, single-nucleotide polymorphism (SNP) maps will contribute to the power of genetic linkage as a tool for gene identification.

DNA sequence analysis has helped to create protein product libraries and related databases to facilitate the drug discovery process. Proteomic data are mainly derived from large-scale sequencing of full-length cDNA, which is reverse transcribed from mRNA transcripts. The mRNA sequences are translated into unique proteins that exhibit specific functions, such as enzymes or hormones. In the past, protein structure and function were characterized one protein at a time. While a DNA sequence allows one to predict the amino acid sequence of a protein, it can neither ensure expression nor provide information about protein function. Proteins can be glycosylated, phosphorylated, acylated, or sulfated, but these processes cannot be predicted by DNA sequence analysis. In addition, a single gene can encode multiple proteins through several mechanisms, including alternative splicing of mRNA and varying start as well as stop protein translation sites. Protein synthesis and stability may also be regulated by changing cellular processes and extracellular signals. These processes can lead to changes in protein localization and interactions, the generation of protein fragments, and alterations in protein function and metabolism.

The continuous accumulation of genomic data and innovations in proteomics have had a significant impact on drug discovery. Because the Human Genome Sequence project is essentially completed, we must now identify the functions of proteins that the newly discovered genes encode. Many of these newly identified targets still lack information on how and when they act in cells and whole living system. Progress in genomics and proteomics along with integration of the sciences involved in drug development will allow the removal of drug candidates with poor efficacy and unacceptable safety profiles early in the research and development stages. The successful integration of discovery and development with the help of genomics and proteomics is likely to reduce costs and increase the number of novel drugs produced by the pharmaceutical industry.

35.3 MANAGING BIOINFORMATICS FOR INDIVIDUALIZED DRUG THERAPY

Patients on drug therapy display different responses to the same medication. A drug may have poor therapeutic effects in some patients and elicit adverse reactions at low doses in others. Individual variation in drug effectiveness and safety has resulted in failed efficacy trials and the withdrawal of products from the market. Variation in drug response affects the treatment of diseases and increases healthcare costs.[7] Matching the patient with the appropriate drug and tailoring the dosage to that individual's therapeutic need could overcome this problem. Advances in molecular genetics and determining the genetic basis of variation in drug disposition and pharmacologic activity can help predict individual variability. These advances have also led to the development of drugs designed to address specific disease processes and to be therapeutic in only certain defined patients. Genetic information on genotyping and phenotyping can account for differences in drug response among patients and identify individuals with disease-causing mutations. Analysis of genetic information with regard to genotyping is an effective and better approach to apply to the individualization of drug therapy.

The study of the association between genetics and response to drug therapy is known as pharmacogenetics. It refers to gene identification and selecting the appropriate medicine for each patient. An important application of pharmacogenetics is to predict drug response. CYP2D6, a cytochrome P-450 drug-metabolizing enzyme, is involved in the metabolism of at least 30 drugs. A least 48 nucleotide variations that create 53 CYP2D6 alleles have been identified in the CYP2D6 gene. Some of these variations lead to multiple copies of the enzyme, while others lead to the absence of the enzyme; consequently, a drug dose that produces the optimum response in the average person can be therapeutically ineffective in some people or unsafe in others.[9,10]

Genetic polymorphism in drug metabolism is one reason for differences in patients' responses to drugs. Another factor is mutations in genes coding for receptors or proteins that control drug response. The genes for more than a dozen inherited traits or polymorphisms (e.g., cystic fibrosis, insulin receptor resistance, HIV resistance) have been identified. In these conditions, pharmacogenetics may serve as a guide to the development and application of drug therapy. For example, in thrombophilia, variation in the structure of a blood-clotting protein predicts susceptibility to thrombosis. Genetic studies have shown that the susceptible phenotype is associated with a single change in factor V that substitutes a glutamine for an arginine in the structure. Not all patients who carry the variant protein suffer thrombosis, but these carriers become lifelong candidates for drug therapy with anticoagulation and require close monitoring to maintain an effective dose and avoid serious bleeding.

By applying pharmacogenetics to determine a patient's genotype, physicians will be able to make better prescribing decisions. Candidate genes can be examined to establish a genetic basis for individual drug responses. Examining a patient's genotype prior to prescribing a medication may improve the quality of health care by increasing the proportion of patients for whom the drug is beneficial or decreasing the risk of adverse reactions.

A genome-wide map of thousands of single nucleotide polymorphisms will be useful for pharmacogenetic discovery. SNPs are the locations along chromosomes where a single base varies among different people. Where some have a thymine in a given string of nucleotide, for example, others might have a guanine. It has been suggested that common diseases such as cancer might be caused by common mutations, and the most common mutations in the genome are SNPs, which occur about every 1000 bases.

Cytochrome P-450 (CYP) enzymes catalyze the final step in the incorporation of oxygen into organic molecules. These enzymes usually convert foreign chemicals and drugs into less toxic metabolites. Humans have more than 50 P-450 genes. The most highly expressed subfamily is CYP3A, which includes the isoforms CYP3A4, CYP3A5, CYP3A7, and CYP3A43. These isoforms account for as much as 30% of total P-450 content in liver and play an important role in the oxidative metabolism of more than 50% of all drugs. The most abundant CYP isoform expressed in liver and the gastrointestinal tract is CYP3A4.

The level of CYP3A4 expression may determine which patients best respond to certain drugs and which patients experience side reactions or toxicity when the same dosage is given; however, hepatic expression of CYP3A4 is observed to vary more than 50-fold among individuals, and its function in drug clearance varies by more than 20-fold. Genetic factors cause 60 to 90% of patient variability in CYP3A4 function to drug metabolism. The variability in CYP3A4 expression may be regulated at the transcriptional level, either through polymorphisms in regulatory elements or in the genes encoding the transcription factors. For example, rifampin, an antiinfectious agent to tuberculosis that induces CYP3A4 transcription, activates a member of the nuclear receptor super-family PXR. Rifampin is a ligand of PXR, bound at regulatory regions of CYP3A4 gene, allowing it to activate transcription.

A map of human genome sequence variation, reported to contain 1.42 million SNPs, will permit a comprehensive search for genetic loci that are likely to regulate expression of CYP3A4 enzymes. Polymorphism in the CYP3A4 or other genetic loci controlling the expression and function of CYP3A4 would explain the individual variations observed in the intensity and duration of drug action, as well as the extent of adverse effects. A better understanding of the genetic basis of differences in CYP3A function will assist in determining the optimum drug dosages for individual patients and achieving a more effective therapeutic response with fewer adverse effects.[10]

It is now recognized that all patients do not react in the same way to chemotherapy, but in some cases treatment response can be predicted. Pharmacogenetics provides a way to tailor drug therapy and reduce uncertainty in its effectiveness. The SNP screening approach has been used to examine drug disposition in patients with advanced breast cancer. The results showed that 22 unique SNPs in 12 genes were involved in drug metabolism, as well as a statistically significant association of 3 genes with drug metabolism rates, tumor response, and patient survival following chemotherapy with cyclophosphamide, cisplatin, and carmustine. Approximately one quarter of patients with decreased metabolism of cyclophosphamide correlated with shorter survival. Decreased cyclophosphamide metabolism was linked to a SNP in the promoter region of CYP3A4 or CYP3A5. These observations could lead to a pretreatment genotype analysis to determine what dose of drug would be most effective for each patient. Oncologists who correlate genetic data with phenotypic data could use this information to forecast a patient's response to drug treatment and potential adverse events.

Alteration of a single nucleotide in a gene can determine whether the gene will predispose an individual to developing cancer. At the same time, these SNPs can alter gene function in ways that affect response to drug treatment. For example, SRD5A2 encodes for steroid type 2,5-alpha reductase, an enzyme that catalyzes the conversion of testosterone to dihydrotestosterone (DHT).

Higher levels of this enzyme result in higher levels of DHT and increase the possibility for developing benign prostate hypertrophy (BHP) and prostate cancer. It was observed that a particular variant of SRD5A2 was associated with a sevenfold increased risk of prostate cancer in African–American men, a fourfold risk in Hispanic men, and a threefold risk in Caucasian men.

The observed ten SNP variants of SRD5A2 differ in their biologic effects, not only in affecting the levels of DHT but also in their response to finasteride, a competitive inhibitor of 2,5-alpha reductase. Finasteride (Proscar®) is used for the treatment of BHP and the prevention of prostate cancer. A 200-fold range in activity of the enzymes encoded by these gene variants has been observed, and as much as a 60-fold difference in the ability of finasteride to inhibit the activity of the enzyme has been found. It is necessary to investigate further whether certain genotypes are linked to a particular response to finasteride.[11]

In addition, women who exhibit mutations in BRCA1, a gene implicated in hereditary breast cancer, respond differently to chemotherapy than those lacking such mutations. The BRCA1 gene normally functions as a tumor suppressor and transcriptional regulator. Moreover, it encodes a protein involved in the cellular response to DNA damage. BRCA1 mutations increase the susceptibility to breast, ovarian, and prostate cancer. The frequency of BRCA1 mutations in the general population is 1 in 833; in Jewish women, 1 in 107. Women with BRCA1 mutations face a 50 to 80% lifetime risk of developing breast cancer and develop it in earlier age than those without such mutations.

Human breast cancer cell lines with BRCA1 mutations have shown a two- to fourfold increase in apoptosis after treatment with radiation, cisplatin, or dexorubicin, compared with cells free of mutations. In addition, BRCA1 tumor cell lines are resistant to other agents, such as paclitaxel (Taxol®) and docetaxel (Taxotere®), both treatments commonly used in ovarian and advanced breast cancers. Differences in drug sensitivity are also related to the levels of another protein, Bcl2, which is also implicated in apoptosis. Loss of Bcl2 results in higher levels of apoptosis after DNA damage. BRCA1 regulates the expression of Bcl2. In contrast, breast tumors expressing BRCA1 mutations lack the Bcl2 protein and are resistant to chemotherapy with taxanes, which induce cell death through a Bcl2 pathway. Women with BRCA1 mutations who develop breast or ovarian cancer are not good candidates for treatment with certain types of chemotherapy agents such as Taxol®. Doxorubicin, cisplatin, or other newly approved agents will be a better choice. In the future, genetic analysis will undoubtedly improve the treatment of cancer.

A recently approved monoclonal antibody for the treatment of breast cancer — trastuzumob (Herceptin®) — is indicated only for those tumors measurably expressing the protein expressed by the gene erbB-2. This observation is based on the finding that the oncogene product of erbB-2 is produced in fewer than 30% of breast cancer patients and patients with no erbB-2 protein (HER2) in metastatic cancer cells exhibit no benefit from treatment with Herceptin®. HER2 antigen testing was an important process in the development of this product, and the Herceptin® label indicates that its use should be based on diagnostic testing using the available reagent, HER2/neu. Thus, identifying the appropriate breast cancer patient for Herceptin therapy became the first example of individualized drug therapy. A therapy requiring prescreening of a patient's genetic makeup is a significant step toward a new clinical practice pattern.

Pharmacogenetic testing has been applied in renal disease patients who lack thiopurine methyltransferase and are receiving low doses of azathioprine therapy to reduce the risk of drug toxicity. Individuals who lack glucose-6-phosphate dehydrogenase show increased sensitivity toward dapsone-related hemolytic anemia. Physicians routinely screen for this case before prescribing dapsone to treat Pneumocystis carinii pneumonia in patients with AIDS. In these cases, pharmacogenetic testing has been beneficial to predict the drug efficacy and safety outcomes.

The pharmaceutical industry strives to develop drugs and biologics that are effective in as large a population as possible to obtain maximum profits. Genetic analysis can be a time-consuming task that can limit the potential market for the product; however, manufacturers tend to develop targeted drugs such as Herceptin® when they realize that, although the user population is limited, these drugs are likely to be profitable in the long term. It is anticipated that a day will come when patients will carry gene chip identification cards, similar to electronic IDs, that contain their complete genetic information for use in therapeutic decision making. New drugs will be targeted to only some patients — those who display a specific genetic marker that is critically involved in the efficacy and safety of the drug.

35.4 GENE TECHNOLOGY, DNA VACCINE, AND STEM CELLS FOR THERAPEUTICS

As we enter the 21st century, we are approaching a historic transition in medicine and the pharmaceutical sciences. A few years ago, only little pieces of the genetic information of life, the genomes, were understood in detail. After dramatic advances in molecular genetics and biotechnology, the complete sequence of the human genome has become available. Information processing on computers and biomedical science are crucial to this process and the epic transition. The potential impact on biomedicine, health care, and quality of life is expected to be enormous. In 1955, two lambs were born from a surrogate mother that received genetic material from cultured embryonic cells. The successful cloning proved that, even though the cultured cells are partially differentiated, they can be genetically reprogrammed to function like those in an early embryo. Later, the cultured cells taken from a 26-day-old fetus and from a mature ewe were cloned to animals. In February 1997, the ewe's cells produced Dolly, the first mammal to be cloned from an adult. The possibility to create clones from tissue culture cells brought forth alternative ways to develop beneficial medical therapeutic drugs, practical benefits in animal husbandry, and a more in-depth understanding of the mechanisms contributing to cell development.

Cloning is based on nuclear transfer that involves the use of two cells. The recipient cell is an unfertilized egg taken from an animal soon after ovulation. The donor cell is the one to be copied. During the cloning process, chromosomes from the recipient egg are gently removed by a micropipette. Then, the donor cell with an intact nucleus is fused with the recipient egg. When implanted into a surrogate mother, the fused cells continue to develop similarly to a normal embryo. The cloning of Dolly from the mammary-derived culture and the cloning of other lambs from the cultured fibroblasts showed that the cloned offspring looked like the sheep that donated the nucleus rather than like their surrogate mother. Genetic tests prove that Dolly is indeed a clone of an adult.[12]

Investigators then inserted the gene for human factor IX, a blood-clotting protein used to treat hemophilia, into sheep. Also, an antibiotic-resistance gene was transferred to the donor cells along with the factor IX gene, so a high dose of the antibiotic neomycin added to cultured cells selected only those contained the transferred gene. In 1997, the first transgenic sheep was produced by this method. The transgenic animals secreted the human protein in their milk.[13]

Cloning has many other practical applications. One is the supply of genetically modified animal organs that are suitable for human transplantation. At present, thousands of patients die before a replacement of heart, liver, or kidney becomes available. A normal animal organ would be rapidly destroyed by the human body's immune system, a reaction that is triggered by an alpha-galactosyl transferase enzyme, if it were transplanted into a human. Thus, animal organs have been genetically altered so that they no longer contain this enzyme and are better tolerated in the host. Cloning technology provides a means to quickly produce large animal models that mimic human diseases, such as cystic fibrosis. These techniques are also useful in evaluating cell-based therapies for genetic disorders such as muscular dystrophy, diabetes, and Parkinson's disease for which no fully effective treatment currently exists.

DNA immunization provides several advantages over current vaccines:

- DNA vaccines mimic the effects of live attenuated vaccines in their ability to induce cell-mediated immune response.
- DNA vaccines are relatively inexpensive to manufacture and are easy to produce in large quantities.

- They are stable and can be stored at room temperature, eliminating the need for a cold chain.
- They can be engineered to carry genes from different strains of a pathogen to provide immunity against several strains at once.

DNA vaccine consists of a foreign gene for the desired antigen; the gene is cloned into a bacterial plasmid and engineered for expression in mammalian cells. The vaccine is injected intramuscularly or administered by a gene gun, which can deliver plasmids into skin cells or mucous membrane. After entering the cells, the recombinant plasmids make their way to the nucleus and instruct the cell to synthesize the encoded protein antigens. These protein antigens are processed to activate helper T-cells to elicit cellular and humoral immune responses. DNA vaccines have initiated a new era of biomedical research by providing a powerful means to develop novel vaccines and immunotherapies. Several investigational DNA vaccines for the prevention of malaria, tuberculosis, and HIV infections are currently being evaluated in clinical trials. Further studies are necessary to overcome the issues of safety concerns as well as technical challenges of improving delivery system and efficacy so low-dose DNA vaccines can effectively prevent infectious disease.[14-17]

One of the most important biomedical research initiatives involves the production of universal donor cells. A difficult challenge is to create cells for transplantation that are not regarded as foreign by the recipient immune system. Scientists are investigating the possibility of using undifferentiated embryonic stem cells to repair or replace tissue damaged by disease. Stem cells matched to a patient can be made by using nuclear transfer cloning techniques, in which one of the patient's cells serves as the donor and a human egg serves as the recipient. The resulting embryo develops until it is possible to separate and culture stem cells from it. When stem cells divide, some of the progeny differentiate and mature into cells of specific types. Other progeny remain as stem cells. Thus, intestinal stem cells continually regenerate the lining of the intestine, and hematopoietic stem cells produce the cells found in blood. The stem cells allow our bodies to repair disease tissues and perhaps can be used to treat AIDS, muscular dystrophy, and Parkinson's disease.

Stem cells can be manipulated to differentiate into specific cells and tissues. Investigators have shown that treating mouse embryonic stem cells with a vitamin A derivative, retinoic acid, stimulates them to produce neurons. Specific growth factors stimulate cells derived from embryonic stem cells to produce the complete range of cells found in blood. Embryonic stem cells could even generate useful tissues without special treatment. Spontaneous differentiation of stem cells was observed to form cardiomyocyte of greater than 99% purity.

This century will be very exciting and challenging and will witness an explosion of new drugs and biologics that, until recently, were only the dreams of investigators in research laboratories. In this century, effective AIDS and cancer vaccines are anticipated, as well as safer blood supply and tissue products. We will have new and more effective treatments for Alzheimer's and other chronic diseases. Advances in proteomics and genomics research will produce individualized medicines that have practical therapeutic benefits and fewer adverse reactions. We welcome the new era of pharmaceutical sciences and look forward to continuing progress to fulfill the dreams of better health and quality of life.

REFERENCES

1. Hentschel, C., Recombinant DNA proteins and drug discovery, in *Genetically Engineered Human Therapeutic Drugs*, Copsey, D.N. and Delantte, S.Y.J., Eds., Macmillan, New York, 1988, p. 3.
2. Goodfellow, P.N., The impact of genomics on drug discovery, *Novartis Found. Symp.*, 229, 131–135, 2000.
3. Tatusoy, R.L., Koonin, E.V., and Lipman, D.J., A genomic perspective on protein families, *Science*, 278(5338), 631–637, 1997.
4. Miki, Y., Swensen, J., Shatluck-Eidens, D. et al., A strong candidate for 17q linked breast and ovarian cancer susceptibility gene BRCA1, *Science*, 266, 66–71, 1994.

5. Gunn, T.M., Miller, K.A., Le, L. et al., The mouse mahogany locus encodes a transmembrane form of human attactin, *Nature*, 398(6723), 152–156, 1999.

6. Nagle, D.L., McGrail, S.H., Vitale, J. et al., The mahogany protein is a receptor involved in suppression of obesity, *Nature*, 398(6723), 148–152, 1999.

7. Dormann, H., Muth-Sellbach, U., Kreb, S. et al., Incidence and costs of adverse drug reactions during hospitalization: computerized monitoring versus stimulated spontaneous reporting, *Drug Saf.*, 22(2), 161–168, 2000.

8. Mahgoub, A., Idle, J.R., Dring, R. et al., Polymorphic hydroxylation of debrisoquine in man, *Lancet*, 2(8038), 584–586, 1977.

9. Scarlett, L.A., Madani, S., Shen, D.D. et al., Development and characterization of a rapid and comprehensive genotyping assay to detect the most common variants in cytochrome P450 2D6, *Pharm. Res.*, 17(2), 242–246, 2000.

10. Eichelbaum, M. and Burk, O., CYP3A genetics in drug metabolism, *Nat. Med.*, 7(3), 285–287, 2001.

11. Stephenson, J., As genes differ, so should interventions for cancer, *JAMA*, 285(14), 1829–1830, 2001.

12. Campbell, K.H.S., McWhir, J., Ritchie, W.A. et al., Sheep cloned by nuclear transfer from a cultured cell line, *Nature*, 385, 810–813, 1997.

13. Schnieke, E. et al., Human factor IX transgenic sheep produced by transfer of nuclei from transfected fetal fibroblasts, *Science*, 278, 2130–2133, 1997.

14. Gurunathan, S., Klinman, D.M., and Seder, R.A., DNA vaccines: immunology, application, and optimization, *Annu. Rev. Immunol.*, 18, 927–974, 2000.

15. Weiner, D.B. and Kennedy, R.C., Genetic vaccines, *Sci. Am.*, July, 50–57, 1999.

16. Tuteja, R., DNA vaccines: a ray of hope, *CRC Crit. Rev. Biochem. Mol. Biol.*, 34(1), 1–24, 1999.

17. Seder, R.A. and Gurunathan, S., DNA vaccines: designer vaccines for the 21st century, *N. Engl. J. Med.*, 341, 277–278, 1999.

Index

Index